Workbook and Competency Evaluation Review

MOSBY'S TEXTBOOK FOR NURSING ASSISTANTS

Tenth Edition

Candice K. Kumagai, RN, MSN
Formerly, Instructor in Clinical Nursing
School of Nursing
University of Texas at Austin
Austin, Texas

ELSEVIER

Elsevier
3251 Riverport Lane
St. Louis, Missouri 63043

WORKBOOK AND COMPETENCY EVALUATION REVIEW   ISBN: 978-0-323-67288-7
MOSBY'S TEXTBOOK FOR NURSING ASSISTANTS, TENTH EDITION

Notices

Practitioners and researchers must always rely on their own experience and knowledge in evaluating and using any information, methods, compounds or experiments described herein. Because of rapid advances in the medical sciences, in particular, independent verification of diagnoses and drug dosages should be made. To the fullest extent of the law, no responsibility is assumed by Elsevier, authors, editors or contributors for any injury and/or damage to persons or property as a matter of products liability, negligence or otherwise, or from any use or operation of any methods, products, instructions, or ideas contained in the material herein.

Previous editions copyrighted 2017, 2012, 2008, 2004.

Senior Content Strategist: Nancy O'Brien
Senior Content Development Manager: Luke Held
Senior Content Development Specialist: Kelly Skelton
Publishing Services Manager: Deepthi Unni
Project Manager: Srividhya Vidhyashankar

Working together
to grow libraries in
developing countries

www.elsevier.com • www.bookaid.org

Printed in the United States of America

Last digit is the print number: 9 8 7 6 5 4 3 2

PREFACE

This workbook is written to be used with Sorrentino and Remmert's *Mosby's Textbook for Nursing Assistants,* Tenth Edition. You will not need other resources to complete the exercises in this workbook.

This workbook is designed to help you apply what you have learned in each chapter of the textbook. You are encouraged to use this book as a study guide. Each chapter is thoroughly covered in the multiple-choice questions, which will help prepare you to take the NATCEP test. In addition, other exercises such as fill-in-the-blank, matching, labeling, and crossword puzzles are used in many chapters. The section titled Optional Learning Activities may be used as an alternative exercise to give you more practice in studying the materials. The FOCUS ON PRIDE critical thinking and discussion questions offer opportunities to reflect on and improve clinical practice. The Evolve Student Learning Resources also include Independent Learning Activities for each chapter that can be used to apply the information you will learn in a practical setting.

In addition, Procedure Checklists that correspond with the procedures in the textbook are provided. These checklists are designed to help you become skilled at performing procedures that affect quality of care. In addition to NATCEP skills being identified for you, icons indicate skills that are (1) in Mosby's Nursing Assistant Video Skills 4.0 and (2) on the Evolve Student Learning Resources website (video clips).

The Competency Evaluation Review includes a general review section and two practice exams with answers to help you prepare for the written certification exam. It also features a skills evaluation review to help you practice procedures required for certification.

Assistive personnel are important members of the health team. Completing the exercises in this workbook will increase your knowledge and skills. The goal is to prepare you to provide the best possible care and to encourage pride in a job well done.

Candice K. Kumagai

CONTENTS

1 Health Care Agencies

Fill in the Blank: Key Terms

Acute illness
Assisted living residence
 (ALR)
Case management
Chronic illness

Functional nursing
Health team
Hospice
Licensed practical nurse
 (LPN)

Licensed vocational nurse
 (LVN)
Nursing assistant
Nursing team
Patient-focused care

Primary nursing
Registered nurse (RN)
Survey
Team nursing
Terminal illness

1. _____ is a nursing care pattern where the RN is responsible for the person's total care.

2. A person who performs delegated nursing tasks under the supervision of an RN or LPN/LVN is a _____.

3. An illness or injury from which the person will not likely recover is a _____.

4. A nurse who has completed a practical nursing program and has passed a licensing test is a _____.

5. The _____ are those who provide nursing care—RNs, LPNs/LVNs, and nursing assistants.

6. An illness from which the person is expected to recover is an _____.

7. _____ is a nursing care pattern that focuses on tasks and jobs, and each nursing team member is assigned certain tasks and jobs.

8. An _____ provides housing, personal care, support services, health care, and social activities in a home-like setting to persons needing help with daily activities.

9. _____ is an illness or injury that is ongoing, slow or gradual in onset, and has no known cure.

10. _____ is a health care agency or program that promotes comfort and quality of life for the dying person and the family.

11. _____ have training and licensing that is similar to the LPNs.

12. _____ is a nursing care pattern in which services for the person's care are obtained and monitored from admission through discharge to the home or long-term care setting.

13. A _____ is a nurse who has completed a 2-, 3-, or 4-year nursing program and has passed a licensing test.

14. The _____ includes many health care workers whose skills and knowledge focus on the person's total care.

15. _____ is a nursing care pattern in which an RN leads a team of nursing staff and the RN decides the amount and kind of care each person needs.

16. When services are moved from departments to the bedside, this is a nursing care pattern called _____.

17. A _____ is the formal review of an agency through the collection of facts and observations.

Circle the Best Answer

18. Which person is most likely to need the type of care that is provided in a memory care unit?
    A. Has chronic cardiac and respiratory problems
    B. Has Alzheimer disease with wandering behaviors
    C. Needs some assistance with activities of daily living
    D. Has cancer and death is expected within 6 months

19. Which nursing assistant action contributes to health promotion?
    A. Assists doctor with the person's physical examination
    B. Obtains stool and urine specimens as ordered
    C. Encourages person to do daily recommended exercises
    D. Holds infant while RN administers an immunization

20. Which nursing assistant action contributes to detection and treatment of disease?
    A. Transports person to the radiology department
    B. Assists elderly person to a standing position
    C. Shows respect and maintains person's privacy
    D. Assists vision-impaired person to read a lunch menu

21. Which nursing assistant action helps the person to meet the goal of rehabilitation and restorative care?
    A. Reassures person that all needs will be meet in a timely fashion
    B. Encourages person to independently do as much self-care as possible
    C. Takes and reports vital signs according to facility protocol
    D. Helps to organize and pack person's belongings for discharge

22. Which health care agency offers care and treatment for an acute illness?
    A. A hospital
    B. A long-term care center
    C. An assisted living facility
    D. A rehabilitation agency

23. Which person needs sub-acute care?
    A. Had minor surgery for a skin condition
    B. Discharged from hospital but needs complex wound care
    C. Needs help with toileting, bathing and meal preparation
    D. Has terminal illness and death is imminent

24. Which elderly person needs the care that is provided in a long-term care center?
    A. Developed pneumonia and now has trouble breathing
    B. Sustained a hip fracture and needs physical therapy
    C. Has chronic heart and respiratory problems
    D. Has depression and thoughts about suicide

25. The primary difference between long-term care centers and skilled nursing facilities is the
    A. Length of stay.   C. Funding sources.
    B. Complexity of care.   D. Certification of staff.

26. A person may have an apartment and receive help with personal care when living in
    A. A long-term care center
    B. An assisted living facility
    C. A rehabilitation care agency
    D. A skilled nursing facility

27. Persons who have thoughts of harm to self or others may be treated in a
    A. Mental health center   C. Skilled care facility
    B. Long-term care center   D. Hospice

28. To work for a home care agency you must be comfortable with
    A. Performing more complex care
    B. Calling the doctor if the person is very ill
    C. Providing care with offsite supervision
    D. Helping families to resolve interpersonal problems

29. Which action would you perform to fulfill your role in hospice care?
    A. Do everything for person until he/she recovers
    B. Ensure that person is clean and comfortable
    C. Encourage person to eat and exercise to regain strength
    D. Provide care only to meet person's physical needs

30. The primary goal of a health care system that includes several clinics, a hospital, a pharmacy, a skilled nursing facility and a home health agency is to
    A. Decrease the overall cost of comprehensive health care.
    B. Share resources and cross-train members of the health team
    C. Make medical records readily accessible across the system
    D. Meet all health care needs for persons and their families

31. Which member of the health care team can recommend treatments for a person who is having trouble swallowing?
    A. Speech therapist   B. Occupational therapist
    C. Podiatrist   D. Physician

32. Who would you notify if a family member has a complaint about the nursing care?
    A. Person's primary care doctor
    B. RN team leader
    C. Director of nursing
    D. All health care team members

33. In which circumstance are you most likely to seek assistance from the nursing education staff?
    A. You need tutoring to pass the NATCEP competency evaluation
    B. You are unsure how to use a new automatic blood pressure machine
    C. You know that an elderly person has questions about his medications
    D. You suspect that an LPN is doing tasks that should be done by an RN

34. Which health care team member will you notify if a resident tells you he has pain in his foot?
    A. Podiatrist   C. Physical therapist
    B. Physician's assistant   D. RN

35. An RN
    A. is responsible for all of your actions and performance
    B. is expected to give you clear and specific instructions
    C. will complete your tasks if you cannot finish them
    D. has authority to fire you for using assertive communication

36. Which action is the LPN/LVN most likely to perform?
    A. Assists the nursing assistants to complete tasks
    B. Assists the RN in caring for an acutely ill person
    C. Assumes RN responsibilities if no RN is available
    D. Claims limited authority in supervising nursing assistants

37. What is the best description of your role in the nursing care pattern of team nursing?
    A. You do whatever the team leader tells you to do
    B. You help all persons who need assistance with bathing
    C. Your skills and abilities are matched to persons' needs
    D. You assist the RNs and LPNs when they need help

38. In the nursing care pattern of functional nursing, you would
    A. Take vital signs on all patients and report data to the licensed nurse
    B. Talk to the other nursing assistants and decide how to divide duties
    C. Assist the RNs and LPNs after you receive specific instructions
    D. Perform total care for all patients that are assigned to you

39. In patient-focused care,
    A. You would transport the patient to the diagnostic testing center
    B. The patient directs the focus and type of the care and treatment
    C. The RN would draw blood sample at the patient's bedside
    D. The patient is invited to actively participate in care conferences

40. Which action would you perform to contain health care costs for a person who has Medicare coverage?
    A. Complete care and duties as quickly and efficiently as possible
    B. Assist the person to be discharged to home as soon as possible
    C. Limit the amount and use of supplies that are charged to the person
    D. Follow the RN's instructions for the prevention of pressure injuries

41. Which action should you perform to help your health care agency to meet the standards of licensure, certification, or accreditation?
    A. Close the door when assisting a patient or resident to bathe
    B. Describe the NATCEP testing process to the surveyor
    C. Memorize all policies and procedures related to your job
    D. Assist patients or residents whenever they ask for your help

42. A confused elderly resident tells you he doesn't have any money to pay you for your help or to pay the bill for the long-term care center. What should you do?
    A. Reassure him that you will care for him no matter how much money he has
    B. Tell him not to worry about it and change the subject
    C. Find out who is paying the bills for the resident
    D. Tell the charge nurse about the resident's concerns

43. Which rationale would support your choice to work for an accredited health care agency?
    A. All health care team members are licensed and experienced
    B. Any person needing care is accepted regardless of income level
    C. Voluntary review shows that a high quality of care is provided
    D. Facility is likely to offer promotions, a good salary and benefits

44. Which action should you take if a deficiency is found during a survey of a health care agency where you work?
    A. Seek a new job with a different agency within 60 days
    B. Ask if your responses to surveyor's questions created a problem
    C. Give honest information about the deficiency to patients/residents
    D. Follow instructions from the team leader to correct the deficiency

45. If you do not understand a question that is posed by a surveyor, what should you do?
    A. Explain that you are not allowed to answer any questions
    B. Answer the question to the best of your ability
    C. Tell the surveyor that you do not know the answer
    D. Ask the surveyor to restate or rephrase the question

Matching

Match the type of health care agency with the service provided.

A. hospital
B. rehabilitation agency
C. long-term care center
D. mental health center
E. home care agency
F. hospice
G. skilled nursing facility
H. assisted living residence

46. _____ Promotes comfort and quality of life for dying persons and the families

47. _____ Provides complex care for persons with severe health problems who needs time to recover or rehabilitation

48. _____ Provides services to persons who do not need hospital care but cannot care for themselves at home

49. _____ Serves people of all ages for acute, chronic, or terminal illnesses

50. _____ Treats people who may have difficulty dealing with events in life

51. _____ Provides housing, personal care, and other services in a home-like setting

52. _____ Serves people who do not need hospital care but need complex equipment and care measures

53. _____ Provides care to persons at home

Fill in the Blank

54. Write out the abbreviations.
    A. DON _____
    B. LPN _____
    C. LVN _____
    D. RN _____
    E. SNF _____
    F. PPS _____

Write the name of the health team member described.

55. _____ Supervises LPNs/LVNs and assistive personnel

56. _____ Diagnoses and prescribes treatment for diseases and injuries

57. _____ Collects samples and performs tests on blood, urine, and other body fluids and secretions

58. _____ Takes x-rays and processes film for viewing

59. _____ Gives respiratory treatments and therapies

60. _____ Assesses and plans for nutritional needs

61. _____ Assists persons with movement, prevention of disability, and rehabilitation

62. _____ Assists persons to learn or retain skills needed to perform activities of daily living

63. _____ Treats persons with communication, and swallowing disorders

64. _____ Assists persons with their spiritual needs

65. _____ Helps patients and families with social, emotional, and environmental issues affecting illness and recovery

66. _____ Treats hearing, balance and ear problems

Labeling

67. Fill in members of nursing service on the organizational chart (A–F).

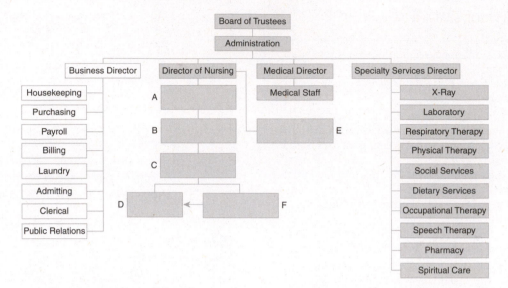

68. The nursing assistant reports to 2 groups of nursing service. They are

    A. _____

    B. _____

Optional Learning Exercises

Name the member of the health team who provides the service described.

69. Mr. Williams needs assistance to regain skills to dress, shave, and feed himself (ADLs). He is assisted by the _____.

70. Mrs. Young needs the corns on her feet treated. The nurse notifies the _____.

71. Ms. Stewart has the responsibility of doing physical examinations, health assessments, and health education in the center where she works. She is a _____.

72. Mr. Gomez keeps turning up the volume of his TV. His hearing is tested by the _____.

73. The _____ meets with a new resident and his family to discuss his nutritional needs.

74. Mr. Fox had a stroke and has weakness on his left side. The _____ assists him by developing a plan that focuses on restoring function and preventing disability from his illness.

75. The doctor orders x-rays after Mr. Jackson falls. The x-rays are done by the _____.

76. Mr. Ling has chronic lung disease and needs respiratory treatments. These are given by the _____.

77. Ms. Walker plans the recreational needs of a nursing center. She is an _____.

78. After a stroke, Mr. Stubbs has difficulty swallowing. He is evaluated by the _____.

79. When the doctor orders blood tests, the samples are collected by the _____.

Name the nursing care pattern described in the following examples.

80. Ms. Hines works with Dr. Hogan. When his patient, Harry Forbes, is admitted to the hospital, Ms. Hines coordinates his care from admission to discharge. She also communicates with the insurance company and community agencies involved in Mr. Forbes' care. This is an example of _____.

81. When Mr. Holcomb reports for work as a nursing assistant, he is assigned to make all beds on the unit. The RN gives all drugs and the LPN gives all treatments. This nursing care pattern is _____.

82. Ms. Conroy works on the same nursing unit each day. She has a group of patients and she gives total care to each of them. She teaches and counsels the person and family and plans for home care or long-term care when needed. This is an example of _____.

83. Ms. Ryan is a nursing assistant. She gives care that is delegated by an RN. The RN leads a team of nursing staff members and she decides the amount and kind of care each person needs. This is called _____.

84. Mrs. Young receives her care and physical therapy on the nursing unit. She does not have to go to different departments to receive treatments and care. This care is provided by the nursing team instead of by other health team members. This is called _____.

Use the FOCUS ON PRIDE section to complete these statements and then use the critical thinking and discussion questions to develop your ideas.

85. The word PRIDE used in the chapter stands for:

P _____

R _____

I _____

D _____

E _____

Critical Thinking and Discussion Questions

86. List three or four personal behaviors that will help you achieve your goals in the nursing assistant program; then share, compare and discuss your list with your classmates.

87. Identify three or four professional behaviors that you believe are necessary to be an excellent nursing assistant. Discuss your rationale for identifying those professional behaviors with your classmates.

Fill in the Blank: Key Terms

Involuntary seclusion   Ombudsman   Representative   Treatment

1. A _____ is any person who has the legal right to act on the resident's behalf when he or she cannot do so for himself or herself.

2. Separating a person from others against his or her will, keeping the person in a certain area, or keeping the person away from his or her room without consent is _____.

3. The care provided to maintain or restore health, improve function, or relieve symptoms is

_____.

4. An _____ is someone who supports or promotes the needs and interests of another person.

Circle the Best Answer

5. Which of these ideas is a part of the Patient Care Partnership?
   A. The person must follow all recommended treatments or plans of care.
   B. The doctor makes the treatment decisions if the person is unable to do so.
   C. The person should know when students or other trainees are involved in his or her care.
   D. Hospital charges are not given to the person, only to the insurance companies.

6. Which action violates a resident's rights?
   A. The resident is asked to share a room with another resident
   B. You help the resident to arrange personal items and clothing
   C. You decline to discuss a resident's care with another resident
   D. The resident is not told that his health status has changed

7. For which circumstance must the resident's representative be consulted?
   A. The resident refuses to brush his teeth or comb his hair.
   B. A resident with dementia needs a medical procedure.
   C. The resident has out of town visitors including children.
   D. A resident would like to see a physical therapist.

8. If a resident refuses treatment, what should you do?
   A. Avoid giving care and move on to other duties.
   B. Report the refusal to the nurse.
   C. Tell the resident the treatment is necessary.
   D. Tell the resident's family.

9. Which action is correct if a student wants to observe a treatment, but the resident does not want any observers?
   A. The student cannot watch as this violates the resident's right to privacy.
   B. The student may observe from the doorway where the resident cannot see her.
   C. The staff nurse tells the resident he must allow the student to watch.
   D. The nurse calls the resident's wife to get her permission.

10. Which consideration is the most important when a resident is making a personal choice?
    A. Safety   C. Doctor's orders
    B. Personal rights   D. Personal pride

11. Which resident is exercising his right to voice a dispute or grievance?
    A. Resident A tells Resident B that he talks too much.
    B. Resident C tells the doctor that he is not getting his pain medication.
    C. Resident D requests that you bring extra sugar packets for his coffee.
    D. Resident E refuses to allow you to take his blood pressure.

12. A resident volunteers to take care of houseplants at the center. Which action violates the resident's rights?
    A. The resident's desire to work is reflected in the care plan.
    B. The resident tends the plants in exchange for care items.
    C. The resident incorporates the plant care into his schedule.
    D. The resident's rehabilitation goals include volunteering.

13. Which action violates the residents' right to participate in resident and family groups?
    A. Residents are encouraged to meet and discuss concerns about the care center.
    B. Several families gather to celebrate birthdays and holidays.
    C. Resident is invited to attend a church service, but invitation is declined.
    D. Residents with dementia are not invited to attend a musical performance.

14. Which action denies the resident her rights to keep and use personal items?
    A. You store resident's belongings when he leaves for emergency surgery.
    B. You take soiled items to the laundry and hang clean clothes in the closet.
    C. You throw away her old holiday decorations without her permission.
    D. You wipe off the surface of her nightstand and dust her picture frames.

15. Which action infringes on the resident's right of freedom from abuse, mistreatment, and neglect?
    A. A staff member tells a resident he cannot leave his room because he talks too much.
    B. A nurse explains the problems that can result when a resident refuses a medication.
    C. You coach a resident to perform certain portions of self-care as identified by the RN
    D. A nurse accompanies a resident to a private room to discuss an upsetting incident.

16. When a resident is given certain drugs that affect his mood, behavior, or mental function, it may deny his right to
    A. Freedom from abuse, mistreatment, and neglect
    B. Personal choice
    C. Privacy
    D. Freedom from restraint

17. Which of these actions will promote courteous and dignified care?
    A. Using terms of endearment such as "Honey," or "Sweetheart" to address the residents
    B. Assisting with dressing the resident in clothing appropriate to the time of day
    C. Using frequent touch, hugs, and handshakes with all residents and staff
    D. Leaving the bathroom door open so you can see the resident

18. Which question is a surveyor most likely to ask to determine if you are promoting the residents' rights?
    A. What can the resident expect from the treatment plans?
    B. How much time does it take you to help a resident to bathe?
    C. What tasks must you complete when a resident is discharged?
    D. How do you prevent unnecessary exposure of the resident's body?

19. Which information must you give to a co-worker when you need help to assist residents to and from activities?
    A. Which residents require a wheelchair, cane, or walker
    B. How to politely address the residents using proper name and title
    C. Which residents take offense to scolding or hurried actions.
    D. How to provide privacy and draping during transport

20. You provide privacy and self-determination for a resident when you
    A. Knock on the door before entering and wait to be asked in
    B. Allow her to smoke in designated areas
    C. Listen with interest to what the person is saying
    D. Groom his beard as he wishes

21. You allow the resident to maintain personal choice and independence when you
    A. Obtain her attention before interacting with her
    B. Provide extra clothing for warmth such as a sweater or lap robe
    C. Assist him to take part in activities according to his interests
    D. Use curtains or screens during personal care and procedures

22. What is the best action to encourage social interaction among residents?
    A. Tell residents about activities and offer help to and from activities.
    B. Place wheelchair residents in a close circle after mealtimes.
    C. Talk to individual residents whenever you have extra time.
    D. Encourage residents to sit by different people during meals.

23. You are giving a report about a resident's care to the oncoming staff. Which people should be present during your report?
    A. All oncoming staff including nursing students
    B. Resident's family and legal representative
    C. Any licensed health care professional
    D. Any staff directly involved in the resident's care

24. Which response is best to give a family member who asks you about a resident's weight?
    A. "I weigh him every morning and his weight is about the same as it has been."
    B. "I told the nurse about your question and she will speak to you soon."
    C. "It will take me a couple of minutes, but I can go and look at the records."
    D. "I am sorry, but I am not allowed to give you any information."

25. Which of these activities would be carried out by an ombudsman?
    A. Organize activities for a group of residents
    B. Accompany residents to a religious service at a house of worship
    C. Investigate and resolve complaints made by a resident
    D. Assist the resident to choose friends

Fill in the Blank

26. CMS _____

27. OBRA _____

28. According to the Patient Care Partnership, list 6 things that the patient needs to understand in to make informed decisions about treatment choices.
    A. _____
    B. _____
    C. _____
    D. _____
    E. _____
    F. _____

29. What should the health care staff do if a person refuses treatment?
    A. _____
    B. _____
    C. _____
    D. _____

30. List three circumstances that would be considered involuntary seclusion.

    A. _____

    B. _____

    C. _____

Optional Learning Activities

OBRA-Required Actions to Promote Dignity and Privacy (Box 2-3) p 17

Match the action to promote dignity and privacy with the example.

A. Courteous and dignified interaction
B. Courteous and dignified care
C. Privacy and self-determination
D. Maintain personal choice and independence

31. _____ File fingernails and apply polish as the resident requests.

32. _____ Cover the resident with a blanket during a bath.

33. _____ Gain the person's attention before giving care.

34. _____ Show interest when a resident tells stories about his past.

35. _____ Open containers and arrange food at meal times to assist the resident.

36. _____ Close the door when the person asks for privacy.

37. _____ Allow a resident to smoke in a designated area.

38. _____ Make sure the resident is wearing his dentures when he goes to the dining room.

39. _____ Take the resident to her weekly card game.

Use the FOCUS ON PRIDE section and the critical thinking and discussion questions to develop your ideas.

Critical Thinking and Discussion Questions

40. Discuss how leaving the familiar setting of home and community to move into a nursing care facility would influence a person's independence.

41. Identify ways to help residents maintain their independence.

3 The Nursing Assistant

Fill in the Blank: Key Terms

Certification   Equivalency   Misappropriation   Reciprocity
Endorsement   Job description   Nursing task

1. A _____ is nursing care or a nursing procedure, activity, or work that can be delegated to nursing assistants when it does not require a nurse's professional knowledge or judgment.

2. When a state recognizes the certificate, license, or registration issued by another state it is

_____.

3. A _____ is a document that describes what the agency expects you to do.

4. Another name for equivalency or endorsement is

_____.

5. Official recognition by a state that standards or requirements have been met is _____.

6. _____ is also called endorsement or reciprocity.

7. _____ is the dishonest use of property.

Circle the Best Answer

8. How do nursing assistants contribute to the efforts to reduce health care costs?
   A. Nursing assistants can perform nurse duties during the nurse shortages.
   B. Staff mixing reduces costs by including RNs, LPN/LVNs and nursing assistants.
   C. Nursing assistants have the lowest salaries; therefore, the hospitals save money.
   D. Many nursing assistants use their experience and eventually become nurses.

9. What should you do if you believe that a nurse is performing an action that violates the state's nurse practice act?
   A. There is nothing you can do, because the nurse has more authority than you do.
   B. Watch to see if the nurse's actions are causing harm to anyone.
   C. Call the Board of Nursing and make an anonymous report.
   D. Go up the chain of command and give the facts to the nurse's supervisor.

10. Which nurse is performing an action that violates the nurse practice act?
    A. Nurse A recently graduated and seems unsure about the facility policies.
    B. Nurse B makes many unreasonable demands on the nursing assistants.
    C. Nurse C comes to work and is under the influence of alcohol and drugs.
    D. Nurse D is tired after working dayshift, but agrees to stay and cover night shift

11. How are the state's nurse practice acts relevant to nursing assistants?
    A. RNs and LPNs/LVNs are affected; nursing assistants are not affected.
    B. Nurse practice acts bestow protection from liability for nursing assistants.
    C. Roles, tasks, actions, and education of nursing assistants can be affected.
    D. Nurse practice acts are less relevant for nursing assistants than facility policies.

12. If you do something beyond the legal limits of your role, you could be
    A. Protected by the nurse practice act
    B. Practicing nursing without a license
    C. Protected by the nurse who supervises your work
    D. Accused of a criminal act

13. Nursing assistants can face disciplinary charges and possible loss of certification for
    A. Being absent from work frequently
    B. Failing to maintain confidentiality of information
    C. Refusing to care for a certain patient
    D. Having frequent arguments with co-workers

14. How many hours of instruction are required by OBRA for nursing assistant training and competency evaluation programs?
    A. 16   C. 120
    B. 75   D. 200

15. In a training program for nursing assistants, which skill would you be expected to master?
    A. Interpreting vital signs
    B. Positioning people in bed
    C. Transcribing the doctor's orders
    D. Drawing blood for laboratory testing

16. What should you say first when you meet a patient in your student clinical experience?
    A. "Hello. Please state your name and may I see your identification band."
    B. "Hello. Are you Mr. Smith? I will be caring for you today."
    C. "Hello. My name is Ms. Jones. I am a student nursing assistant."
    D. "Hello. Would you like me to call you Mr. Smith or use your first name?"

17. According to the nursing assistant registry, if you had an incident of misappropriation. What rights do you have?
    A. Right to include a statement disputing the findings
    B. Right to have record expunged for good behavior
    C. Right to sue the nursing assistant registry
    D. Right to have incident withheld from employers

18. How does the nursing assistant registry benefit you as an individual?
    A. Records dates and times of your excellent work ethic
    B. Is a permanent record of your interactions with patients
    C. Allows you the freedom to move from state to state for work
    D. Shows that you successfully completed the state's approved NATCEP

19. OBRA requires that re-training and a new competency evaluation test must be taken if you have not worked as a certified nursing assistant for
    A. 24 months
    B. 5 years
    C. 1 year
    D. 6 months

20. Which action is best if a mandatory in-service training is scheduled during the middle of your shift?
    A. Tell the nurse that you can't go because of your patient care duties
    B. Ask the in-service trainer to provide you copies of the handouts
    C. Explain to the patients that you must go and to call the nurse as needed
    D. Plan with co-workers; some do patient care while others attend the training

21. Which action could result in a discipline with a possible loss of certification?
    A. You go to a patient's home after he is discharged and provide care without the supervision of a nurse.
    B. You inform the nurse that you recorded the vital signs on the wrong person's medical records.
    C. There is family emergency in the middle of your shift and you tell the nurse you have to leave.
    D. A confused resident rubs your breasts while you are helping him to complete morning hygiene.

22. Which circumstance is most important for you to report to the supervising nurse?
    A. A new nursing assistant is unable to complete her duties and is frequently asking for your help.
    B. The off-going nursing assistant frequently fails to leave the work areas tidy and asks you to do the cleaning.
    C. You overhear another nursing assistant asking a resident to lend her money for her child's school fees.
    D. An experienced nursing assistant, gives you tips about how to interact with confused residents.

23. As a nursing assistant, you never give medications unless
    A. The nurse is busy and asks you to give the medications
    B. The person is in the shower and the nurse leaves the medications at the bedside
    C. You have completed a state-approved medication assistant training program
    D. You are feeding the person and the nurse asks you to mix the medications with the food.

24. You are alone in the nurses' station and you answer the phone. Dr. Smith begins to give you verbal orders. You should
    A. Tell the doctor that you are not allowed to take phone orders.
    B. Politely give your name and title and then promptly get the nurse.
    C. Quickly write down the orders and promptly give them to the nurse.
    D. Politely tell her to call back later when the nurse is there.

25. The nurse asks you to assist him as he changes sterile dressings. You should
    A. Assist him as needed
    B. Tell him you cannot assist
    C. Offer to change the dressings
    D. Report him to the director of nursing.

26. Which member of the health care staff can tell the person or family a diagnosis or prescribe treatments?
    A. Director of nursing
    B. RN
    C. Physician
    D. Experienced nursing assistant

27. The nurse asks you carry out a task that you do not know how to do. You should
    A. Ignore the order because it would not be safe for you to carry out the task
    B. Promptly explain to the nurse why you cannot carry out the task
    C. Look up information about the task and then do your best to do the task
    D. Ask another nursing assistant to show you how to carry out the task.

28. The nurse knows you are an EMT in addition to being a CNA. She is very busy and asks if you will start an IV on a patient. You should
    A. Politely tell her that you cannot start an IV as a CNA
    B. Start the IV since you start IVs routinely as an EMT
    C. Ask her to spend a few minutes supervising you as you start the IV
    D. Report her to the director of nursing services.

29. If you are giving care in a home, you may be expected to
    A. Give medications and physical therapy treatments
    B. Provide personal care and prepare meals
    C. Do any household chores that the person is unable to do
    D. Drive the person's car so the person can shop or run errands.

30. Which action should you take if an elderly home care patient offers you extra money if you will help his wife to paint the house?
    A. Make private arrangements to do the work on your days off.
    B. Consult the supervising nurse about what to do and say.
    C. Help him to locate a reliable handyman to help the wife.
    D. Tell him that it would be illegal for you to accept any money.

31. Which information must be immediately reported to the nurse?
    A. Resident is upset because he didn't get any coffee with breakfast.
    B. Resident wants to take a tub bath, but his doctor has ordered showering.
    C. Resident's blood pressure and pulse are higher than usual.
    D. Resident's daily weight was recorded on the flowsheet.

32. When you read a job description, you should not take a job if it requires you to
    A. Carry out duties you do not like to do
    B. Function beyond your training limits
    C. Maintain required certification
    D. Attend in-service training.

Fill in the Blank

33. Write out the abbreviations.
    A. CNA _____
    B. LNA _____
    C. LPN _____
    D. LVN _____
    E. OBRA _____
    F. NATCEP _____
    G. BON _____
    H. RN _____
    I. RNA _____
    J. SRNA _____
    K. STNA _____

34. When hospitals seek to reduce costs with a staffing mix, nursing care is given by a mix of
    A. _____
    B. _____
    C. _____

35. Identify at least 7 areas of study that are included in a nursing assistant training program.
    A. _____
    B. _____
    C. _____
    D. _____
    E. _____
    F. _____
    G. _____

36. What information does the nursing assistant registry have about each nursing assistant?
    A. _____
    B. _____
    C. _____
    D. _____

37. Why does OBRA require 12 hours of educational programs and performance reviews each year for every nursing assistant? _____
    _____

38. List at least four observations that a surveyor could make to assess your competence to perform your job.
    A. _____
    B. _____
    C. _____
    D. _____

39. If you wanted to work in another state, what would you do first? _____
    _____

40. List 7 "nevers" that are role limits for nursing assistants
    A. _____
    B. _____
    C. _____
    D. _____
    E. _____
    F. _____
    G. _____

41. List three reasons for declining a job offer; based on your understanding of a written job description.
    A. _____
    B. _____
    C. _____

42. Identify at least 7 of the Nursing Assistant Standards in Box 3-4 (p 27) that are particularly meaningful to you.
    A. _____
    B. _____
    C. _____
    D. _____
    E. _____
    F. _____
    G. _____

43. List 4 roles and responsibilities for nursing assistants who provide home care.
    A. _____
    B. _____
    C. _____
    D. _____

Optional Learning Exercises

OBRA requirements related to the nursing assistant.

44. OBRA requires many areas of study. Write the area of study where you learn the skill used in each example.
    A. _____ You make a bed.
    B. _____ You close Mr. Smith's door to give him privacy.
    C. _____ You tell Mrs. Forbes the time of day and the day of the week frequently because she is mildly confused.
    D. _____ You apply lotion to a resident's skin.
    E. _____ You assist a person to put on his shirt.

F. _____ When assigned to a new unit, you check the location of the fire alarm.

G. _____ You practice hand hygiene before and after giving care.

H. _____ You get help to move a person from his bed to the chair.

I. _____ When speaking to Mr. Jackson, you maintain good eye contact.

J. _____ The nurse tells you to exercise a person's extremities (limbs).

K. _____ You position a urinal for a resident in bed.

L. _____ You assist Mrs. Young to walk in the hall.

M. _____ You notice that Mrs. Peck has an elevated temperature and her skin is warm.

N. _____ You cut up the meat on Mr. Sanyo's plate before helping him to eat.

Use the FOCUS ON PRIDE section to complete these statements and then use the critical thinking and discussion questions to develop your ideas.

45. If a patient refuses to have a student care for him, you should kindly _____ the person's rights to choose who is involved in his care.

46. Practicing skills in the classroom or laboratory will make you feel more _____.

47. When the nurse asks you to do a task, the nurse is _____ the task to you.

Critical Thinking and Discussion Questions

Recall the areas of knowledge and skills that will be included in your training program: (1) communication, (2) infection control, (3) safety and emergency procedures, (4) resident's rights, (5) basic nursing skills and personal care skills, (6) feeding methods, (7) elimination methods, (8) skin care, (9) transferring, positioning and turning methods, (10) dressing, (11) helping the person to walk, (12) range of motion exercises, (13) signs and symptoms of common diseases, and (14) care for cognitively impaired persons.

48. After considering the list, identify 3 or 4 areas that seem the most difficult or challenging for you. Discuss your selections and your concerns with your classmates or instructors.

49. Discuss how you plan to take personal and professional responsibility for achieving excellence and mastery in the areas that seem to be the most difficult for you.

4 Delegation

Fill in the Blank: Key Terms

Accountable   Delegated nursing   Delegation   Routine nursing task
Delegate   responsibility   Nursing task

1. Being responsible for one's actions and the actions of others who perform delegated tasks is being _____.

2. To _____ means to authorize another person to perform a nursing task in a certain situation.

3. A _____ is nursing care or a nursing procedure, activity, or work that can be delegated to nursing assistants when it does not require an RN's professional knowledge or judgment.

4. A _____ is a nursing task that a nurse transfers to a nursing assistant when it does not require a nurse's professional knowledge or judgment.

5. _____ is the process a nurse uses to direct a nursing assistant to perform a nursing task; allowing a nursing assistant to perform a nursing responsibility that is beyond the nursing assistant's usual role and not routinely done by the nursing assistant.

6. A _____ is a nursing task that is part of a nursing assistant's routine job description and commonly assigned to the nursing assistant; a nursing task that was learned in a Nursing Assistant Training and Competency Evaluation Program (NATCEP).

Circle the Best Answer

7. Which health care team member is exceeding his/her authority to delegate?
   A. An APRN delegates a task to a nursing assistant.
   B. An RN delegates a task to a nursing assistant.
   C. An LPN/LVN delegates a task to a nursing assistant.
   D. A nursing assistant delegates a task to another nursing assistant.

8. When a nurse decides how to delegate tasks, the decision depends on
   A. What is best for the person at the time
   B. How many staff members are available to assist
   C. Priorities of care for persons needing care
   D. Whether the person likes the nursing assistant.

9. You have been caring for a person for several weeks. The nurse tells you that she will give his care today. Her delegation decision is based on
   A. How well you gave his care in the past
   B. Changes in the person's condition today
   C. Your need to spend time caring for other people
   D. How much supervision you need.

10. At which step of the delegation process would you tell the nurse that you have never performed a task before?
    A. Assess and plan
    B. Communication
    C. Supervision
    D. Evaluation and feedback

11. Which nurse is performing supervision of the nursing assistant's performance?
    A. Nurse A tells the nursing assistant how to perform and complete the task.
    B. Nurse B determines the skills that are needed to safely perform the nursing task.
    C. Nurse C observes as the nursing assistant performs the nursing task.
    D. Nurse D gives the nursing assistant feedback about task performance.

12. Which nursing assistant has the greatest need for a good communication plan with the supervising nurse?
    A. Nursing assistant A has been asked to do a task that she has never done before.
    B. Nursing assistant B does home care for an elderly person with many health problems.
    C. Nursing assistant C is assisting in the orientation of a newly hired assistant.
    D. Nursing assistant D is assigned extra patients because someone called in sick.

13. Which of these tasks cannot be delegated to a nursing assistant?
    A. Give perineal care
    B. Supervise others
    C. Assist with coughing and deep-breathing exercises
    D. Collect specimens

14. You have the right to refuse a task if
    A. You have never cared for the person before
    B. The task is too time-consuming
    C. The task is not in your job description
    D. It's the end of your shift

15. Which task would generally be considered one of your routine nursing tasks?
    A. Measuring the height and weight
    B. Inserting a urinary catheter
    C. Administering an enema
    D. Helping a person to swallow medication

16. A newly graduated nurse asks you to go and check on a patient, see if he is breathing okay and put oxygen on if he needs it. What should you do?
    A. Tell the charge nurse about the new nurse's inappropriate delegation.
    B. Count his respiratory rate, put the oxygen on him and report back to the nurse.
    C. Check on the patient and ask him if he is okay and if he needs oxygen.
    D. Tell the nurse that you are not sure how to assess his breathing or need for oxygen.

Fill in the Blank

17. Write out the abbreviations.
    A. LPN _____
    B. LVN _____
    C. NATCEP _____
    D. RN _____
    E. APRN _____

18. List 10 reasons that support your right to refuse to do a task.
    A. _____
    B. _____
    C. _____
    D. _____
    E. _____
    F. _____
    G. _____
    H. _____
    I. _____
    J. _____

19. What directions must be given when the nurse communicates with the nursing assistant about a delegated task?
    A. _____
    B. _____
    C. _____
    D. _____
    E. _____
    F. _____

20. What are the five rights of delegation?
    A. _____
    B. _____
    C. _____
    D. _____
    E. _____

Optional Learning Experiences

21. What are the 4 steps in the delegation process? (See Figure 4-2 p 34 of textbook)
    A. Step 1 _____
    B. Step 2 _____
    C. Step 3 _____
    D. Step 4 _____

22. Read the following statements and for each indicate which of the four steps of the delegation process it describes.
    A. The nurse makes sure that you complete the task correctly. _____
    B. How will delegating the task help the person? What are the risks to the person?
       _____
    C. The nurse tells you when to report observations.
       _____
    D. Was the desired result achieved?
       _____

23. Look at the Five Rights of Delegation for Nursing Assistants in Box 4-1 (p 36). For each question, list the Right that is fulfilled.
    A. Did you review the task with the nurse?
       _____
    B. Were you trained to do the task? _____
    C. Do you have concerns about performing the task?
       _____
    D. Is the nurse available if the person's condition changes or if problems occur?
       _____
    E. Do you have the equipment and supplies to safely complete the task? _____

Use the FOCUS ON PRIDE section to complete these statements and then use the critical thinking and discussion questions to develop your ideas.

24. You show responsibility when you refuse a task to protect _____.

25. List 5 behaviors that indicate that you are respectful and willing to receive corrective feedback from the supervising nurse that will help to improve your performance.
    A. _____
    B. _____
    C. _____
    D. _____
    E. _____

26. List four things that the staff can do to facilitate positive interactions during delegation experiences
    A. _____
    B. _____
    C. _____
    D. _____

Critical Thinking and Discussion Questions

27. You are providing care for an elderly resident who lives in a long-term care center. What should you do if the nurse delegates the nursing task (measuring blood glucose) that is beyond your routine nursing assistant role?

28. You are caring for a resident who falls in the bathroom. You tell the nurse at once. The nurse says: "Take him to the dining room. I'll check him after lunch." You are aware that the agency policy states that a nurse must immediately assess the resident after a fall. What should you do?

Fill in the Blank: Key Terms

Abuse
Assault
Battery
Boundary crossing
Boundary sign
Boundary violation
Child abuse and neglect
Civil law
Code of ethics

Crime
Criminal law
Defamation
Elder abuse
Ethics
False imprisonment
Fraud
Informed consent
Intimate partner violence

Invasion of privacy
Law
Libel
Malpractice
Neglect
Negligence
Professional boundary
Professional sexual
  misconduct

Protected health
  information
Self-neglect
Slander
Standard of care
Tort
Vulnerable adult
Will

1. Physical, sexual, or psychological abuse by a current of former partner or spouse is _____.

2. Any knowing, intentional, or negligent act by a caregiver or any other person to an older adult is _____.

3. A rule of conduct made by a government body is a _____.

4. _____ is injuring a person's name and reputation by making false statements to a third person.

5. An act, behavior, or comment that is sexual in nature is _____.

6. Touching a person's body without his or her consent is _____.

7. _____ are laws concerned with offenses against the public and society in general.

8. _____ is the failure by caregiver or other person to protect a vulnerable person or failure to provide food, water, clothing shelter, health care or other activities of daily living.

9. _____ are rules, or standards of conduct, for group members to follow.

10. An act, behavior, or thought that warns of a boundary crossing or violation is a _____.

11. _____ is the skills, care, and judgments required by a health team member under similar conditions.

12. A _____ is a legal document of how a person wants property distributed after his or her death.

13. _____ is saying or doing something to trick, fool, or deceive a person.

14. The intentional mistreatment or harm of another person is _____.

15. An unintentional wrong in which a person did not act in a reasonable and careful manner and causes harm to a person or to the person's property is _____.

16. _____ is a person's behaviors and way of living that threaten his or her health, safety, and well-being.

17. A wrong committed against a person or the person's property is a _____.

18. _____ is a brief act or behavior outside of the helpful zone.

19. Making false statements in print, writing, or through pictures or drawings is _____.

20. A _____ is an act that violates a criminal law.

21. _____ is knowledge of what is right and wrong conduct.

22. Violating a person's right not to have his or her name, photo, or private affairs exposed or made public without giving consent is an _____.

23. Identifying information and information about the person's health care is _____.

24. A _____ is a person 18 years old or older who has a disability or condition that makes him or her at risk to be wounded, attacked, or damaged.

25. A _____ is an act or behavior that meets your needs, not the person's.

26. Negligence by a professional person is _____.

27. Making false statements orally or by using sign language _____.

28. _____ are laws concerned with relationships between people.

29. _____ is that which separates helpful actions and behaviors from those that are not helpful.

30. Unlawful restraint or restriction of a person's freedom of movement is _____.

31. _____ is intentionally attempting or threatening to touch a person's body without the person's consent.

32. The intentional harm or mistreatment of a child under 18 years old is _____.

33. _____ is the process by which a person receives and understands information about a treatment or procedure and is able to decide if he or she will receive it.

Circle the Best Answer

34. Which situation is unethical behavior for a nursing assistant?
    A. The nursing assistant believes that children should care for their elderly parents.
    B. The nursing assistant asks to be assigned to care for people of the same race.
    C. The nursing assistant reports that an elderly patient says her son sometimes hits her.
    D. The nursing assistant disagrees with a man's decision to refuse life-saving measures.

35. What should you do if you saw a co-worker drinking alcohol at work?
    A. Report the facts and details of the event to the nurse.
    B. Tell the co-worker that his actions are endangering patients.
    C. Give the co-worker information about a program for alcoholics.
    D. Ignore the behavior to be loyal to the co-worker.

36. You schedule your lunch to finish giving personal care to a person. According to the code of conduct for nursing assistants, which principle are you following?
    A. Perform no act that will cause the person harm.
    B. Know the limits of your role and knowledge.
    C. Consider the person's needs to be more important than your own.
    D. Respect each person as an individual.

37. Which action constitutes boundary crossing?
    A. Telling the patient the steps of a procedure
    B. Inviting the patient to your house for Thanksgiving dinner
    C. Avoiding a patient because he has made sexual advances
    D. Showing interest when the patient is talking

38. You may be accused of negligence when giving care if you
    A. Tell the nurse that you know the person you are assigned to care for.
    B. Assist a person to the bathroom and the toilet paper dispenser is empty.
    C. Give the wrong care to the wrong person because they both have the same name.
    D. Report to the nurse that the person is complaining of chest pain.

39. You tell another nursing assistant that you think the housekeeper is stealing money from the staff. This is an example of
    A. Defamation   C. Invasion of privacy
    B. Boundary crossing   D. Libel

40. In the cafeteria, you overhear two nursing assistants talking about a person they are caring for. This is an example of
    A. Defamation   C. Boundary crossing
    B. Libel   D. Invasion of privacy

41. If you begin to give care to a person without asking permission, you may be guilty of
    A. Battery   C. Invasion of privacy
    B. Assault   D. Slander

42. Which person can give informed consent for treatment?
    A. He or she is under the legal age (usually 18 years)
    B. He or she is the responsible party
    C. He or she is sedated
    D. He or she has dementia

43. If you are asked to witness the signing of a consent, you
    A. Must know the agency policy on whether you may do this
    B. Should always refuse as it is not legal to do this
    C. Cannot ethically or legally witness a will
    D. Cannot refuse as it is part of your responsibility.

44. If you are convicted of abuse, neglect, or mistreatment, this information:
    A. Will be in your nursing assistant registry information
    B. Should not be disclosed during a job application or interview
    C. Is available only in the court records and attorney's notes
    D. Is deleted if you make amends to the abused person.

45. You notice a home care patient has no food in the house and the water has been turned off. This could be a sign of
    A. Self-neglect   C. Involuntary seclusion
    B. Physical abuse   D. Emotional abuse

46. If you suspect an elderly person is being abused, you should
    A. Ask the person to tell you who is abusing him or her.
    B. Discuss your suspicions with the caregiver.
    C. Call the police or social services.
    D. Discuss your observations with the nurse.

47. A child asks you for food or money for food because, "mom's not home and there's nothing to eat." What do you suspect?
    A. Physical abuse   C. Sexual abuse
    B. Neglect   D. Emotional abuse

48. If you suspect a child is being abused
    A. Ask the child whether he or she is being abused.
    B. Share your concerns with the nurse.
    C. Call the local child welfare agency.
    D. Talk to the parents.

49. Which health care team member is committing wrongful use of electronic communications?
    A. Physical therapist uses a cell phone to make an appointment for a home visit.
    B. Nurse uses computer to enter assessment data and treatment outcomes.
    C. Physician obtains informed consent to photography a wound on a patient's foot.
    D. Nursing assistant student takes photos of residents and posts them on Facebook.

50. Which action should you take to avoid being accused of assault and battery when you assist a person to take a shower?
    A. Ask the nurse to give you specific instructions related to the procedure.
    B. Keep the person covered and warm before and after showering.
    C. Explain what you are going to do and get verbal or implied consent.
    D. Validate with the nurse that general consent was obtained which covers your duties.

51. Which nursing assistant could be accused of abandonment?
    A. Nursing assistant is doing home care an elderly person but leaves before giving report to a nurse who will assume responsibility.
    B. Nursing assistant spends extra time with the resident and often trades assignments in order to care for that resident.
    C. Nursing assistant does not like to answer questions about the care given or the relationship with the resident.
    D. Nursing assistant sends text messages about patient's health condition to family members and the patient's friends.

52. You are giving care in a home and you notice the person is not taking the prescribed medications. What do you suspect?
    A. Substance abuse
    B. Self-neglect
    C. Physical abuse
    D. Financial misappropriation

53. Which action would you take when you notice another nursing assistant forcing food into a 90-year-old person's mouth. She says, "He needs to eat and this is the only way I can get done with my assignments."
    A. Offer to feed the person, so that the other assistant can finish her assignments.
    B. Tell her that force feeding is considered a form of physical abuse.
    C. Show her how to feed the person and share tips for time management.
    D. Discuss your observations and the assistant's remarks with the nurse.

54. Which rationale defines your negligence when a person sustains a hot water burn while showering because you forgot to test the water temperature?
    A. You did not act in a reasonable and careful manner.
    B. You were acting outside your scope of practice.
    C. You did not ask for clarification and supervision.
    D. You were focusing on the task, not the person.

55. In which circumstance would the nursing assistant be liable?
    A. The nurse tells the nursing assistant to see if a pain pill relieved the patient's pain.
    B. The nurse tells the nursing assistant that hygiene is deferred because of patient's condition.
    C. The nursing assistant is correctly assisting a resident to eat, but he chokes and coughs.
    D. The nursing assistant records the vital signs and weight on the wrong chart.

Matching

Match the statements to the correct term.

A. Rules for maintaining professional boundaries
B. Boundary signs
C. Boundary crossing
D. Boundary violation

56. _____ You keep the person's information confidential.

57. _____ You borrow money from a patient's family.

58. _____ You do not go out on a date with a current patient or resident or family members of a current patient or resident.

59. _____ You believe you are the only person who understands the person and his or her needs.

60. _____ You hug a person because he or she is crying.

61. _____ You tell a person about your personal relationships or problems.

62. _____ You select what you report and record. You do not give complete information.

63. _____ You trade assignments with other nursing assistants so you can provide the person's care.

Fill in the Blank

64. Write out the meaning of the abbreviations.
    A. CDC _____
    B. HIPAA _____
    C. IPV _____
    D. OBRA _____

65. If a nursing assistant causes unintentional harm to a person, it is called _____. If a nurse or other professional person causes unintentional harm, it is called _____.

66. When giving care, you must follow standards of care. Standards of care come from:
    A. _____
    B. _____
    C. _____
    D. _____
    E. _____
    F. _____
    G. _____

67. Define the two forms of defamation.
    A. Libel _____
    B. Slander _____

68. What problems would cause a person to be considered a vulnerable adult?
    A. _____
    B. _____
    C. _____

69. Name the type of child abuse described in these examples.
    A. The child is injured mentally.

    _____

    B. The child was left in circumstances where the child suffers serious harm.

    _____

    C. The child has been kicked, burned, or bitten.

    _____

    D. The child has engaged in sexual activity with a family member.

    _____

    E. Drug activity has taken place when the child is present.

    _____

    F. Parents withhold praise and affection.

    _____

70. What kinds of violence are considered intimate partner violence?
    A. _____
    B. _____
    C. _____
    D. _____

71. List three actions that would be considered false imprisonment.
    A. _____
    B. _____
    C. _____

Optional Learning Exercises

Which principle in the Code of Conduct for Nursing Assistants applies to the situations?

72. A nursing assistant has back pain and takes her mother's medication to treat it. _____

    _____

73. A nursing assistant is caring for a person her sister knows. The sister asks for information about the person. _____

74. A nursing assistant changes her lunch time because her assigned patient needs unexpected care.

    _____

75. The nursing assistant tells the nurse that he recorded information on the wrong patient. _____

    _____

76. The nursing assistant knows that she is not allowed to care for very ill patients by herself. _____

    _____

77. The nursing assistant declines to start an IV when the nurse delegates that task. _____

    _____

78. The nursing assistant carefully cleans and store the resident's dentures.

    _____

Use the FOCUS ON PRIDE section to complete these statements and then use the critical thinking and discussion questions to develop your ideas.

79. Persons who must report abuse and neglect are called

    _____.

80. If you suspect a person is being abused, tell

    _____

81. Accepting a task beyond the legal limits of your role can lead to _____.

Critical Thinking and Discussion Questions

You notice that the door to a resident's room is shut, when you enter the room, you see that the call bell has been removed. This resident frequently calls out, demands help and never seems to be satisfied with the care that any of the staff provides. The resident has been rude towards staff.

82. Discuss the ethical and legal implications of the staff's reaction and behaviors towards this resident.

83. What can the staff do to improve the situation?

6 Student and Work Ethics

Fill in the Blank: Key Terms

Bullying   Conflict   Harassment   Stress

Burnout   Courtesy   Priority   Teamwork

Confidentiality   Gossip   Professionalism   Work ethics

1. A clash between opposing interests or ideas is _____.

2. _____ is job stress resulting in being physically or mentally exhausted.

3. Following laws, being ethical, having good work ethics, and having the skills to do your work is _____.

4. The most important thing at the time is the _____.

5. Trusting others with personal and private information is _____.

6. _____ is behavior in the workplace.

7. _____ is to spread rumors or talk about the private matters of others.

8. The response or change in the body caused by any emotional, physical, social, or economic factor is _____.

9. _____ is a polite, considerate, or helpful comment or act.

10. _____ means to trouble, torment, offend, or worry a person by one's behavior or comments.

11. When staff members work together as a group it is called _____.

12. Repeated attacks or threats of fear, distress, or harm by a bully toward a target is _____.

Circle the Best Answer

13. Which nursing assistant is demonstrating good work ethics?
    A. Nursing Assistant A does his or her duties quickly and avoids interaction.
    B. Nursing Assistant B incorporates his or her religious beliefs at work.
    C. Nursing Assistant C respects others and works well with others.
    D. Nursing Assistant D has similar cultural beliefs as his or her residents.

14. Which nursing assistant action involves the use of good body mechanics?
    A. Turning a patient during a bed bath
    B. Opening a milk carton for a patient
    C. Recording a patient's vital signs
    D. Buttoning a patient's shirt

15. Which action will best help you to maintain your weight?
    A. You limit intake of salty and sweet foods.
    B. You eat fewer calories on your days off.
    C. You avoid consumption of fat and oils.
    D. You balance calorie intake and energy needs.

16. Adults need about _____ hours of sleep daily.
    A. 7 to 8   C. Less than 6
    B. 10 to 11   D. 12

17. You recognize that you need to exercise, but you have spent the past several months sitting and studying. Which form of exercise is the best to start with?
    A. Hiking   C. Cycling
    B. Running   D. Walking

18. Which statement about smoking odors is true?
    A. The odors disappear quickly when the person finishes smoking.
    B. Smoke odors can be covered up by using mouthwash or gum.
    C. The smoker is the only one who can actual smell residual odor.
    D. Odors stay on a person's breath, hands, clothing, and hair.

19. Which rationale is the best explanation for health care workers to avoid using drugs or alcohol while on the job?
    A. Usage affects the safety of self and others.
    B. Intoxication creates personal disorganization.
    C. Drug usage is an unlawful criminal offense.
    D. Alcohol or drug use can result in termination.

20. Tattoos should be covered when working because they
    A. May offend persons you care for, their families, and co-workers
    B. Can become infected while caring for persons who have infections
    C. May cause persons with dementia to hallucinate or become fearful
    D. Increase the risk of skin injuries because the skin has been pierced.

21. When working, the nursing assistant may wear
    A. Any type of clothing if it is clean and neat
    B. Wrist watch with second hand
    C. Decorative pins that relate to health care
    D. Professionally applied nail polish

22. Which nursing assistant needs to be counseled to change and correct his professional presentation?
    A. Nursing Assistant A has a beard and mustache that is clean and trimmed.
    B. Nursing Assistant B has long hair that he wears pulled back in a pony tail.
    C. Nursing Assistant C uses a fragrant smelling cologne and after-shave.
    D. Nursing Assistant D wears a large black wristwatch with a second hand.

23. When in school or working, the most important reason to plan good childcare and transportation in advance is it
    A. Makes your instructor or employer like you
    B. Shows you are a responsible student or employee
    C. Prevents undue stress for you and your children
    D. Shows that you are a conscientious parent

24. What is a common reason for losing a job?
    A. Lacking knowledge about a task
    B. Being absent or tardy
    C. Being disorganized or slow
    D. Lacking self-confidence

25. You are scheduled to begin work at 3 PM, which plan do you make?
    A. To arrive by 2:30 PM and clock in just before 3 PM
    B. To arrive at exactly 3 PM and ready to work at 3:05PM
    C. To arrive a few minutes early and be ready to work at 3 PM
    D. To arrive within a few minutes before or after 3 PM

26. Which of these statements would signal you have a good attitude?
    A. "I will do that right away."
    B. "My turn is tomorrow."
    C. "That's not my patient."
    D. "It's not my fault."

27. You can avoid being part of gossip by
    A. Remaining quiet when you are in a group where gossip is occurring
    B. Talking about persons and family members only to co-workers
    C. Advising people that gossiping is unethical and grounds for dismissal
    D. Removing yourself from a situation where gossip is occurring

28. The person's information can be shared
    A. With the person's immediate family
    B. With staff members involved in the care
    C. With co-workers who know the person
    D. With health care facility administrators

29. Slang or swearing should not be used at work because
    A. This language can be offensive to others.
    B. Older people may not understand you.
    C. Communication should be clear and precise.
    D. Usage violates the professional code of ethics.

30. Which nursing assistant is displaying a courtesy act?
    A. Nursing Assistant A completes his or her work in a timely fashion.
    B. Nursing Assistant B arrives for work at the scheduled time.
    C. Nursing Assistant C understands his or her job description.
    D. Nursing Assistant D greets a family member who is visiting.

31. It is acceptable at work if you
    A. Borrow a pen or notepad to use at home
    B. Sell cookies for your child's school project
    C. Use a cell phone on your break to call your child
    D. Use the copier to copy a textbook page

32. What is the best rationale for telling the nurse when you leave and return to the unit for breaks or lunch?
    A. Nurse expects you to behave professionally.
    B. Nurse will do your tasks while you are gone.
    C. Nurse knows when you are available.
    D. Nurse knows why your tasks are not done.

33. Which action will help you to maintain safety practices?
    A. Allow family members to enter the elevator first.
    B. Follow the agency's rules, policies and procedures.
    C. Be mindful of the cost and usage of supplies.
    D. Be cheerful, friendly and have a good attitude.

34. Which nursing assistant is not displaying a good safety practice?
    A. Nursing Assistant A checks the stability of the person's walker.
    B. Nursing Assistant B asks the nurse to clarify instructions for a task.
    C. Nursing Assistant C forgets to take vital signs and doesn't tell anyone.
    D. Nursing Assistant D requests training to use a new piece of equipment.

35. When setting priorities they are planned around
    A. Your break and lunch time
    B. The person's needs
    C. The time of day
    D. The time scheduled by the nurse

36. Which circumstance would be considered a pleasant stressor?
    A. You and a co-worker are competing for the same promotion.
    B. You plan a celebration for your grandmother's 85th birthday.
    C. You feel like you need to lose weight; so, you go on a diet.
    D. You experience stress out every minute of every day because of work.

37. What physical effects of stress can be life-threatening?
    A. High blood pressure, heart attack, strokes, ulcers
    B. Increased heart rate, faster and deeper breathing
    C. Anxiety, fear, anger, depression
    D. Headaches, insomnia, muscle tension

38. When you are dealing with a conflict, the first step to resolve the problem is to
    A. Talk to the supervisor.
    B. Collect the information.
    C. Define the problem.
    D. Identify possible solutions.

39. Burnout
    A. Occurs because caring for people is stressful
    B. Is a signal to quit your job or change occupations
    C. Can lead to physical and mental health problems
    D. Will improve if you just ignore the symptoms

40. Which of these actions is harassment?
    A. Offending others with gestures or remarks
    B. Gossiping about a patient or his family
    C. Voicing doubts about the nurse's instructions
    D. Ignoring a conflict among staff members

41. If you resign from a job, it is good practice to give
    A. One week's notice
    B. Two weeks' notice
    C. Four weeks' notice
    D. Three months

42. Which nursing assistant is displaying a courtesy?
    A. While working with Mr. Smith, Nursing Assistant A tries to understand and feel what it must be like to be paralyzed on one side.
    B. Nursing Assistant B realizes that he or she is good at giving basic care, but he or she knows that he or she needs to improve his or her communication skills.
    C. Nursing Assistant C works with attention to detail and performs delegated tasks quickly and efficiently.
    D. Nursing Assistant D thanks co-workers when they help him or her and remembers to wish residents happy birthday as appropriate.

43. Which nursing assistant is performing an action that contributes to patient safety?
    A. When Mrs. Gibson is upset and angry, Nursing Assistant A remembers to respect her feelings and to be kind.
    B. Nursing Assistant B reports the blood pressure and temperature readings promptly and accurately to the nurse.
    C. Nursing Assistant C realizes that giving care to residents is important and she is excited about her work.
    D. Even though Mr. Acevado has different cultural and religious views, Nursing Assistant D values his feelings and beliefs.

44. Which nursing assistant is managing his or her personal matters in a professional way?
    A. Nursing Assistant A had an argument with his or her child; when he or she got to work, he or she made every effort to put that aside and be pleasant and happy.
    B. The nurse discusses a resident problem and Nursing Assistant B knows to keep the information confidential.
    C. Nursing Assistant C is assigned to give care to a resident, he or she makes sure that the care is done thoroughly and exactly as instructed.
    D. Nursing Assistant D adjusts the schedule when the patient has a visitor and care cannot be given when planned.

45. Which nursing assistant is demonstrating the best example of good teamwork?
    A. Nursing Assistant A knows that patients, residents, families, visitors, and co-workers depend on him or her to give safe and effective care.
    B. Nursing Assistant B cheerfully offers to help when a co-worker needs help to turn and bathe a resident.
    C. Nursing Assistant C tries to do small things to make elder residents happy or to find ways to ease their pain.
    D. Nursing Assistant D plans for his or her child's care in advance and makes sure that the car has enough gas.

46. Which situation would be considered a legitimate reason to be absent from class or clinical?
    A. You are unable to get a baby sitter.
    B. You can't afford to get your car fixed.
    C. You have a high fever and a cough.
    D. You haven't finished your assignment.

47. If a nursing assistant leaves before the care of a home health patient is completed, this would be considered
    A. Conflict that can be fixed with the problem-solving process
    B. Abandonment if no other health care staff arrives to assume care
    C. Discourteous to the patient, but not a serious legal error
    D. Acceptable if the patient can independently finish the care

48. A new nursing assistant is hired to work at a long-term care center, but the other nursing assistants won't talk to him or her and he or she feels shunned. Which type of bullying is occurring?
    A. Verbal bullying
    B. Cyber-bullying
    C. Emotional bullying
    D. Prejudicial bullying

Fill in the Blank

49. NATCEP means _____.
50. Work ethics involves
    A. _____
    B. _____
    C. _____
    D. _____

Matching

Match the related health, hygiene, or appearance factor with the examples.

A. Smoking
B. Alcohol
C. Diet
D. Drugs
E. Exercise
F. Eyes
G. Body Mechanics
H. Sleep and Rest

51. _____ Hand-washing and good personal hygiene are needed to remove odors on your breath, hands, clothing, and hair.
52. _____ If you have fatigue, lack of energy, and irritability, it may mean you need more of this.
53. _____ You will feel better physically and mentally if you walk, run, swim, or bike regularly.
54. _____ Some of these affect thinking, feeling, behavior, and function. This may affect the person's safety.
55. _____ Avoid foods from the fats, oils, and sweets group. Also avoid salty foods and crash diets.
56. _____ You may not be able to read instructions and take measurements accurately if you do not have these checked.

57. _____ Practice this when you bend, carry heavy objects, and lift, move, and turn persons.

58. _____ This substance depresses the brain and affects thinking, balance, coordination, and mental alertness.

59. List three things that should you do if you will be late or cannot attend school or go to work.
    A. _____
    B. _____
    C. _____

60. How can you promote teamwork and manage your time when someone is late or does not show up for work?
    A. _____
    B. _____
    C. _____

61. You hear a co-worker say, "It's not my turn. I did it yesterday." This is an example of having a

    _____

62. If you make or repeat any comment that you do not know to be true, or a comment that can hurt a person or family member, you are _____.

63. You are caring for a friend of your mother and your mother asks for information about her friend's illness and care. If you repeat this information to your mother, you will violate the person's _____ and _____.

64. If your friends or family need to visit with you when you are working, they must meet you

    _____.

65. Setting priorities involves deciding
    A. _____
    B. _____
    C. _____
    D. _____
    E. _____
    F. _____
    G. _____

66. What physical symptoms may occur when a person has stress?
    A. _____
    B. _____
    C. _____
    D. _____
    E. _____

67. When you have a conflict with another person, what are steps (in correct order) to take when resolving the conflict?
    A. Step 1 _____
    B. Step 2 _____
    C. Step 3 _____
    D. Step 4 _____
    E. Step 5 _____
    F. Step 6 _____

68. What are the causes of burnout?
    A. _____
    B. _____
    C. _____
    D. _____
    E. _____
    F. _____
    G. _____
    H. _____

69. When you resign from a job, you tell the employer by doing one of the following:
    A. _____
    B. _____
    C. _____

Optional Learning Exercises

70. Use Box 6-1 (p 59), Professional Appearance, in the text to answer these questions.
    A. It is best to wear your name badge

       _____

    B. Why should undergarments be the correct color for your skin tone?

       _____

    C. You should follow the dress code for jewelry and not wear necklaces or dangling earrings because

       _____.

    D. Chipped nail polish may provide a

       _____

    E. Perfume, cologne, or after-shave lotion scents may

       _____

Use the FOCUS ON PRIDE section to complete these statements and then use the critical thinking and discussion question to develop your ideas.

71. When you greet patients and residents and politely introduce yourself, you are displaying good social

    _____.

72. When you offer to help others, ask the nurse if you can help others, and return from breaks on time, you are displaying actions that help build a strong

Critical Thinking and Discussion Questions

73. Think back to the first time you entered the nursing school or the first time you walked into a new clinical unit. Discuss: How were you greeted? Who made you feel welcome? Were people friendly? How did they act towards you and each other? Did anyone offer to help? Why is it important to smile and greet people as they enter a new environment?

74. Two nursing assistants are having a conflict. Nursing Assistant A who works the dayshift says that Nursing Assistant B who works the nightshift leaves patient care tasks undone. Nursing Assistant B says that the comments are unfounded and unsubstantiated. Discuss how this conflict can be resolved.

7 Communicating With the Person

Fill in the Blank: Key Terms

Bariatrics
Body language
Comatose
Communication
Culture
Disability

Esteem
Geriatrics
Holism
Morbid obesity
Need
Nonverbal communication

Obesity
Obstetrics
Optimal level of
    functioning
Paraphrasing
Pediatrics

Psychiatry
Religion
Self-actualization
Self-esteem
Verbal communication

1. _____ is defined as weight that is 20% or more above what is considered normal for that person's height and age.

2. _____ is the characteristics of a group of people—language, values, beliefs, habits, likes, dislikes, customs—passed from one generation to the next.

3. Communication that uses spoken words is _____.

4. _____ is re-stating the person's message in your own words.

5. The branch of medicine concerned with the problems and diseases of old age and older persons is _____.

6. Messages sent through facial expressions, gestures, posture, hand and body movements, gait, eye contact, and appearance is _____.

7. The field of medicine focused on the treatment and control of obesity is _____.

8. The worth, value, or opinion one has of a person is _____.

9. _____ is communication that does not use words.

10. The branch of medicine concerned with mental health disorders is _____.

11. Thinking well of oneself and seeing oneself as useful and having value is _____.

12. _____ is a concept that considers the whole person; physical, social, psychological, and spiritual parts are woven together and cannot be separated.

13. A lost, absent, or impaired physical or mental function is a _____.

14. The branch of medicine concerned with the care of women during pregnancy, labor, and childbirth and for 6 to 8 weeks after birth is _____.

15. _____ is experiencing one's potential.

16. _____ is the branch of medicine concerned with the growth, development, and care of children who range in age from newborn to teenagers.

17. A _____ is something necessary or desired for maintaining life and well-being.

18. _____ is spiritual beliefs, needs, and practices.

19. A person who is unable to respond to stimuli is _____.

20. _____ is a person's highest potential for mental and physical performance.

21. The person has _____ when he or she weighs 100 pounds or more over his or her normal weight.

22. _____ is the exchange of information—a message sent is received and correctly interpreted by the intended person

Circle the Best Answer

23. Who is the most important person in the health care agency?
    A. The patient or resident
    B. The doctor
    C. The director of nursing
    D. The administrator

24. When you are caring for a person, you should
    A. Focus only on the person's priority physical problems or needs.
    B. Treat the physical, social, psychological, and spiritual parts separately.
    C. Minimize the person's experiences, life-style, culture, joys, and sorrows.
    D. Consider the whole person—physical, social, psychological, and spiritual.

25. Which of these statements, show that you see the person as a whole person?
    A. "I need to give a bath to the gallbladder."
    B. "The gentleman in 220 needs pain medication."
    C. "Mrs. Jones reports having pain in her leg."
    D. "Room 235 needs to speak to the charge nurse."

26. Which basic needs have the lowest priority?
    A. Physical needs
    B. Safety and security needs
    C. Love and belonging needs
    D. Self-esteem needs

27. Oxygen, food, water, elimination, rest, and shelter needs
    A. Relate to feeling safe from harm, and danger
    B. Relate to the needs to live and survive
    C. Relate to love, closeness, and affection
    D. Relate to feelings of self- worth, and value

28. It is important to tell a person why a procedure is needed because it
    A. Helps the person feel more secure
    B. Makes the person feel important
    C. Fulfills the person's legal rights
    D. Helps the person to self-actualize

29. You may need to repeat information many times to a person who is newly admitted to a long-term care nursing center because the person
    A. May have hearing or visual loss
    B. Is senile and cannot remember anything
    C. Is in a strange place with strange routines
    D. Is not able to understand what you are saying

30. Who can meet love and belonging needs?
    A. The spouse or relationship partner
    B. Family, friends and the health care team
    C. The mother and the father
    D. Best friends if family is unavailable

31. A need that is rarely, if ever, totally met is
    A. Safety and security
    B. Love and belonging
    C. Self-actualization
    D. Self-esteem

32. When you are caring for a person from a different culture or religion than your own, you must
    A. Judge the person's behavior according to the community norms.
    B. Assume that standard health practices override cultural beliefs.
    C. Give needed care and not worry about culture or religious beliefs.
    D. Respect and accept the person's culture and religion.

33. A culture that believes hot and cold imbalances cause disease is
    A. Mexico
    B. England
    C. The United States
    D. Russia

34. When a person does not follow all beliefs and practices of his or her religion, you
    A. Assume the person is not religious or that the beliefs are not important.
    B. Should know and accept that each person is unique in beliefs and practices
    C. Can call a spiritual leader to help the person follow the religious beliefs
    D. Should not be concerned about the person's religious beliefs when giving care

35. When people are ill, they
    A. Will feel better if you keep talking to them all the time
    B. May fear death, disability, chronic illness, and loss of function
    C. Want to be left alone, so avoid entering their room
    D. Want someone to be around and do everything for them

36. A person who is having the appendix removed is
    A. An adult with medical problems
    B. A person having surgery
    C. A child with a mental health disorder
    D. A person needing sub-acute care

37. Which of these persons would need to see a pediatrician?
    A. A woman who has breast cancer
    B. An older person with disorders of old age
    C. A 7-year-old child with pneumonia
    D. A person receiving kidney dialysis

38. A person who weighs 600 pounds would need
    A. Sub-acute care
    B. Bariatric care
    C. Psychiatric care
    D. Geriatric care

39. Which of these persons is not a candidate for a long-term care center?
    A. A man who is recovering from minor surgery and needs antibiotics
    B. An alert person with a chronic illness who needs help with personal care
    C. A 63-year-old who is unable to care for himself due to dementia
    D. A person with a terminal illness who needs assistance with care

40. Which nursing assistant is not using effective communication?
    A. Nursing Assistant A uses words that the person understands.
    B. Nursing Assistant B communicates in a logical and orderly manner.
    C. Nursing Assistant C gives specific facts and information to the person.
    D. Nursing Assistant D uses medical terminology when talking to the person.

41. When using verbal communication, a rule to follow is
    A. Ask one question at a time, then wait for an answer.
    B. Speak in a loud voice so the person can hear you.
    C. Ask several questions at a time, then wait for answers.
    D. Use slang words to make the person comfortable.

42. Mrs. Stevens cannot speak. What is the best way to replace verbal communication?
    A. She may use touch, as a non-verbal method.
    B. Her body language sends messages.
    C. She can use gestures to communicate.
    D. She may write messages on a pad of paper.

43. When you use touch to communicate, it is important to
    A. Be aware of the person's culture and practices about touch.
    B. Write a note to the person to ask if touch is permitted.
    C. Check the doctor's order to see if touch is ordered.
    D. Touch the person before you speak or begin care.

44. Which of these would be a sign that Mrs. Green is not happy or is not feeling well?
    A. Her hair is well groomed.
    B. She has a slumped posture.
    C. She smiles when you come into the room.
    D. She has applied her make-up.

45. Which action shows that you are effectively listening?
    A. You focus on what is said and observe nonverbals.
    B. You lean back, relax, smile, and cross your arms.
    C. You frequently interrupt to offer suggestions.
    D. You change the subject to a more interesting topic.

46. Mrs. Smith says, "I am used to farm life. I am not sure what I am supposed to do.Which of these is paraphrasing?
    A. "The routine is different than what you are used to."
    B. "That's okay. We are here to help you with things."
    C. "Tell me about living on a farm and your daily life."
    D. "Can you explain what you mean? I don't understand."

47. When you say, "Mr. Davis, have you taken a shower this morning?" you are
    A. Paraphrasing his thoughts
    B. Asking a direct question
    C. Focusing his thoughts
    D. Asking an open-ended question

48. Responses to open-ended questions generally
    A. Invite the person to share thoughts, feelings, or ideas
    B. Are "yes" or "no" answers
    C. Ensure that you understand the message
    D. Focus on dealing with a certain topic

49. Which communication technique would you use if you do not understand the person's message?
    A. Ask an open-ended question.
    B. Clarify what he is saying.
    C. Use nonverbal communication.
    D. Use silence and wait.

50. Mr. Parker often rambles and his thoughts wander while he tells long stories. You need to know if he had a bowel movement today, so you will
    A. Make a clarifying statement.
    B. Ask an open-ended question.
    C. Ask a focusing question.
    D. Paraphrase his thoughts.

51. What is the best action to use if the person takes long pauses between statements?
    A. Just being there shows that you care.
    B. Try to cheer the person up by talking.
    C. Leave the room and come back later.
    D. Find another resident to talk with him.

52. Which nursing assistant is using a barrier to communication?
    A. Nursing Assistant A asks, "Are you saying that you want to go home?"
    B. Nursing Assistant B says, "I think you should follow your doctor's advice."
    C. Nursing Assistant C asks, "Would you like me to help you take a shower?"
    D. Nursing Assistant D says, "I understand that this is upsetting for you."

53. When you care for a person who is comatose, you
    A. Explain to the person what you are going to do.
    B. Remain silent so you do not disturb the person.
    C. Enter the room quietly so you do not startle the person.
    D. Speak in a loud voice so the person can hear you.

54. Mrs. Duke has visitors and you need to give care. What would you do?
    A. Tell the nurse that you can't give the care because of the visitors.
    B. Politely ask the visitors to leave the room until you are finished.
    C. Ask the visitors if they would like to participate in the care.
    D. Tell the visitors that they must leave the nursing center.

55. When you are caring for a person who becomes angry, you should
    A. Avoid the person until he or she calms down.
    B. Stay calm. Listen to his or her concerns.
    C. Explain to the person why being angry is hurtful.
    D. Tell the person that you have rights too.

56. If a person hits, pinches, or bites you when you are giving care, what is the first action you should take?
    A. Protect the person, others, and yourself from harm.
    B. Write a report and explain the incident to the nurse.
    C. Firmly tell the person to stop being so aggressive.
    D. Ask for help when you are assigned to care for the person.

57. What is the meaning of touch to some people from the Philippines?
    A. Some would feel embarrassed.
    B. The person would feel comforted.
    C. It would be considered a friendly gesture.
    D. Some would think it is rude behavior.

58. If you are meeting a male family member of a resident from India, what might you notice about his practice of greeting people?
    A. He will not shake your hand if you are a woman.
    B. He will put his palms together and bow his head.
    C. He will nod and bow slightly when meeting you.
    D. He will give you a very firm handshake.

59. You are caring for a person who cannot speak or hear. What should you do first?
    A. Find someone on the staff who knows sign language to help you.
    B. Ask the nurse or check the care plan for the communication method.
    C. Get a pad of paper and a felt pen and write messages in large block letters.
    D. Get a picture board and point at the figures that convey your message.

60. A nursing assistant is not listening to people as she provides care. Which outcome is the most serious?
    A. Person feels unnoticed and disrespected and this decreases his self-esteem.
    B. Person feels that the nursing assistant doesn't like him, so he stops talking.
    C. Person's requests are ignored, and he makes an official complaint.
    D. Person has pain and other symptoms that do not get reported to the nurse.

Fill in the Blank

61. What are the parts of the person you consider when you use the concept of holism?

    A. _____

    B. _____

    C. _____

    D. _____

62. List the basic needs according to Maslow's theory.

    A. _____

    B. _____

    C. _____

    D. _____

    E. _____

63. Name the culture that may follow the listed belief or custom.

    A. _____ or _____ Food and medicine is given to restore the hot–cold balance

    B. _____ Folk healers called *yerbero* may use herbs and spices to prevent or cure disease.

    C. In Vietnam or _____, men shake hands with other men but do not touch women they do not know.

    D. _____ Eyes are rolled upward to express disapproval.

    E. _____ Facial expressions may mean the opposite of what the person is feeling. Negative emotions may be concealed with a smile.

    F. In _____ and Asian cultures, eye contact is impolite and an invasion of privacy.

    G. In some _____ cultures, silence is a sign of respect, particularly toward an older person.

    H. In _____, family members are involved in the person's care.

64. If a person can hear but cannot speak or read, ask questions that have _____.

65. Nonverbal communication messages reflect a person's _____ more accurately than words do.

66. Body language is nonverbal communication that is shown with

    A. _____

    B. _____

    C. _____

    D. _____

    E. _____

    F. _____

    G. _____

67. When you listen, you follow these guidelines.

    A. _____

    B. _____

    C. _____

    D. _____

    E. _____

68. List nine communication barriers

    A. _____

    B. _____

    C. _____

    D. _____

    E. _____

    F. _____

    G. _____

    H. _____

    I. _____

Crossword

Fill in the crossword by answering the clues below with the words from this list:

Clarifying   Esteem   Nonverbal   Touch
Comatose   Focusing   Paraphrasing   Verbal
Culture   Holism   Silence
Direct   Need

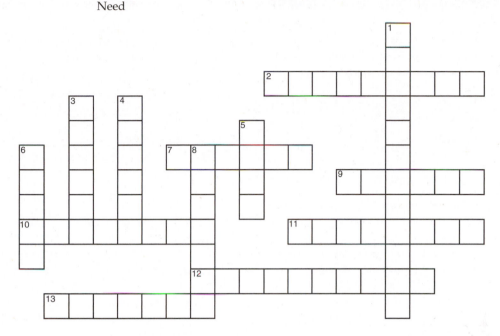

Across

2. Communication expressed with gestures, facial expressions, posture, body movements, touch, and smell

7. The worth, value, or opinion one has of a person

9. Communication in which the words are spoken

10. An unconscious person who cannot respond to others

11. A communication method that is useful when a person rambles or wanders in thought

12. A communication method in which you can ask the person to repeat the message, say you do not understand, or restate the message

13. The characteristics of a group of people—language, values, beliefs, habits, likes, dislikes, customs—passed from one generation to another

Down

1. Restating the person's message in your own words

3. A concept that considers the whole person—physical, social, psychological, and spiritual parts

4. A question that focuses on certain information and may require a "yes" or "no" answer or more information

5. Something necessary or desired for maintaining life and mental well-being

6. Nonverbal communication that conveys comfort, caring, loving, affection, interest, concern, and reassurance

8. Communicating by not saying anything

Optional Learning Exercises

Basic Needs

Physical Needs

69. What are the six physical needs required for survival?

   A. _____

   B. _____

   C. _____

   D. _____

   E. _____

   F. _____

70. Give one example of how a serious problem with urinary elimination could cause death.

_____

Safety and Security

71. Safety and security needs relate to protection from

   A. _____

   B. _____

   C. _____

72. You can help meet safety and security needs when you explain the following for every task.

   A. _____

   B. _____

   C. _____

   D. _____

Love and Belonging

73. The need for love and belonging relates to

   A. _____

   B. _____

   C. _____

Self-Esteem

74. Self-esteem means to

   A. Think _____

   B. See _____

   C. See oneself as having _____

75. Why is it important to encourage residents to do as much as possible for themselves? _____

_____

Self-Actualization

76. What does self-actualization involve?

   A. _____

   B. _____

   C. _____

Culture and Religion Practices

Religion

77. How can you help a resident observe religious practices if services are held in the nursing center?

_____

78. If the resident wants a spiritual leader or advisor to visit in the room, you should tell the nurse and

   A. _____

   B. _____

   C. _____

Cultural Health Care Beliefs

79. List three examples of "hot" conditions according health beliefs for people from Mexico.

   A. _____

   B. _____

   C. _____

Cultural Sick Practices

80. How are Vietnamese folk practices used to treat these illnesses?

   A. Common cold _____

   B. Headache and sore throat _____

81. Which illnesses are treated by using these Russian folk practices?

   A. _____ An ointment placed behind the ears and temples and also on the back of the neck

   B. _____ Placing a dough made of dark rye flour and honey on the spinal column

Cultural Touch Practices

82. Residents from which country may not like to be touched, especially by those they do not know?

_____

83. If the family is from Mexico, why would you touch the infant if you are complimenting the child? _____

_____

Eye Contact Practices

84. If a resident from Vietnam blinks when you explain a procedure, it probably means that the message

_____.

85. Eye contact in American culture signals

_____.

Family Roles in Sick Care

86. You are caring for a resident from China. You might expect the family members to provide _____, _____, and _____ to the person.

Using Communication Methods

You have completed your duties for the morning and have some free time. Mr. Harry Donal is a resident of the nursing center. He rarely has visitors and you try to spend time with him when you can. Answer the following questions about communication techniques you use when you visit with Mr. Donal.

87. You sit in a chair next to Mr. Donal so you can see each other. This position will help you to have better

_____.

88. You should lean _____ Mr. Donal to show interest.

89. Mr. Donal says, "I know this is the best place for me but I miss my flower garden at home." You respond, "You miss your home." This is an example of

    _____.

90. You ask Mr. Donal, "You told me you did not sleep well last night. Can you tell me what was happening?" He replies, "There was a lot of noise in the hall." This is an example of a _____ question.

91. You say to Mr. Donal, "Tell me about your flower garden at home." This is an _____ question.

92. When you say, "Can you explain what that means?" you are asking a person to _____.

93. Mr. Donal says he "hurts all over" and then begins to talk about the weather. You say, "Tell me more about where you hurt. You said you hurt all over." This statement helps in _____ the topic.

94. Mr. Donal begins to cry when he talks about his flower garden. How can you show caring and respect for his situation and feelings? _____

    _____.

95. When Mr. Donal begins to cry, you quickly begin to talk about the activities planned this morning. Changing the subject is a _____

    _____.

Use the FOCUS ON PRIDE section to complete these statements and then use the critical thinking and discussion questions to develop your ideas.

96. To promote a sense of identity, worth, and belonging when communicating, you should

    A. _____

    B. _____

    C. _____

    D. _____

    E. _____

    F. _____

    G. _____

    H. _____

Critical Thinking and Discussion Questions

Think back to a conversation that you recently had with someone who needed you to listen, for example, your child was trying to explain a school project, or a friend just ended a serious romantic relationship. Cite examples of good (attentive listening, making good eye contact, asking questions, using open-ended questions or paraphrasing) and poor (changing the subject, giving opinions, talking too much, failure to listen or pat answers) communication that you used during the conversation with your child or friend.

97. What can you do to improve?

    You are assigned to take care of a resident who has recently moved into the long-term care facility. During the shift, the resident calls you repeatedly and orders you around using a commanding tone. Whatever you do, doesn't seem to please the resident and she asks you to do things over and over. At the end of the day, you feel exhausted and frustrated. The next day you are assigned to the same resident and her behavior is the same.

98. A. Discuss some of the reasons that may be causing the resident to be so demanding.

    B. What can you do to improve the care experience for the resident and yourself?

8 Health Team Communications

Fill in the Blank: Key Terms

Assessment
Chart
Clinical record
Electronic health record
Electronic medical record
End-of-shift report

Evaluation
Implementation
Medical record
Nursing care plan
Nursing diagnosis
Nursing intervention

Nursing process
Objective data
Observation
Planning
Progress note
Recording

Reporting
Signs
Subjective data
Symptoms

1. An electronic version of a person's medical record is the _____; also called electronic medical record.

2. Another term for medical record is _____.

3. The medical record is also called the _____.

4. The legal account of a person's condition and response to treatment and care is the _____ _____; also referred to as the chart or clinical record.

5. _____ are things a person tells you about that you cannot observe through your senses; symptoms.

6. The method RNs use to plan and deliver nursing care is the _____.

7. _____ is to perform or carry out measures in the care plan; a step in the nursing process.

8. Another name for subjective data is _____.

9. A written guide about the person's nursing care is the _____.

10. _____ is collecting information about the person; a step in the nursing process.

11. Another name for objective data is _____.

12. The _____ describes a health problem that can be treated by nursing measures; a step in the nursing process.

13. Information that is seen, heard, felt, or smelled is _____ data.

14. A step in the nursing process that is used to measure if goals in the planning step were met is called _____.

15. _____ is setting priorities and goals; a step in the nursing process.

16. A _____ is an action or measure taken by the nursing team to help the person reach a goal.

17. Using the senses of sight, hearing, touch, and smell to collect information is _____.

18. The oral account of care and observations is _____.

19. A report that the nurse gives at the end of the shift to the on-coming staff is _____.

20. _____ is the written account of care and observations.

21. Another name for an electronic health record is _____.

22. _____ describes the care given and the person's response and progress.

Circle the Best Answer

23. Which member of the health care team needs a reminder about inappropriate sharing of patient information?
    A. Nurse relates a personal story about the patient and his family.
    B. Nursing assistant reports that the patient's vital signs are recorded.
    C. Nursing assistant informs the nurse that patient is reporting pain.
    D. Doctor informs the team that the patient is not responding to therapy.

24. A nursing assistant tells the nurse that Mr. Jones ate a small amount of his lunch. The nurse
    A. Knows this means Mr. Jones ate one half of his meal
    B. Thinks Mr. Jones ate two or three bites of food
    C. Thinks Mr. Jones ate between 0% to 25% of his meal
    D. Is unsure about exactly how much food Mr. Jones ate

25. When giving information to another health team member
    A. Be brief and concise and include important details.
    B. Be professional by using unfamiliar medical terminology.
    C. Give a lot of details, so that nothing is overlooked.
    D. Use general phases, such as, "He's doing great."

26. The medical record or chart is
    A. A temporary tool for staff
    B. Discarded when the person dies
    C. A permanent legal document
    D. Given to the person upon discharge

27. Which information can be found in the person's chart?
    A. Person's selections from the daily menu
    B. Person's current and previous x-ray reports
    C. Outstanding debt that the person owes the agency
    D. History of person bring lawsuits against staff

28. A nursing assistant
    A. May read the charts in all health care agencies
    B. Is never allowed to read the person's chart
    C. Must know the agency policy before reading the chart
    D. Can tell the person what is in the chart if he gives consent

29. If a person asks to see his or her record, the nursing assistant
    A. Advises that the nurse will be notified about the request
    B. Checks agency policy about letting a person see the chart
    C. Gives the chart to the person's legal representative
    D. Makes a photocopy of the chart for the person

30. The admission record contains
    A. Doctor's orders for medications and treatments
    B. The name, birth date, age, and gender of the person
    C. Test results, such as laboratory and radiology
    D. Special diet information related to religion or culture

31. The health history is completed
    A. When the person is discharged
    B. When the person is admitted
    C. By the doctor or his assistant
    D. By the nursing assistant

32. In which section of the chart would you find the person's reason for seeking health care?
    A. Health history
    B. Graphic sheet
    C. Progress notes
    D. Kardex

33. In which area of the chart, would you record the vital signs taken during the shift?
    A. Health history
    B. Nurses notes
    C. Flow sheet
    D. Progress notes

34. In long-term care, what is your role to make sure that the medical record reflects the requirements of the Centers for Medicare and Medicaid?
    A. On the monthly summary, you record actions for each shift.
    B. You summarize your actions to the nurse every 3 months.
    C. You contribute to the written summary every 3 months.
    D. On the weekly record, you record on the day care is given.

35. In which setting, are you are more likely to document on a weekly care record?
    A. Home care
    B. Hospital
    C. Long-term care
    D. Special care unit

36. The Kardex is
    A. Used to record visits by health team members
    B. A sheet used to record vital signs taken every 15 minutes
    C. A record of the person's family history
    D. A quick, easy source of information about the person

37. What is the primary purpose of the nursing process?
    A. The doctor communicates orders for diagnosis and treatment.
    B. Care is planned and delivered according to the person's needs.
    C. Care tasks are described in detail with step-by-step instructions.
    D. Process describes tasks that can delegated to nursing assistants.

38. The nursing process
    A. Is fixed from admission to discharge
    B. Is used in all health care settings
    C. Cannot be used in home care
    D. Can be used only for adults

39. What is your role in nursing process?
    A. You report your observations to the nurse.
    B. You plan care and develop the care plan.
    C. You assess symptoms as instructed by the nurse.
    D. You choose tasks according to the care plan.

40. Which observation displays the sense of hearing?
    A. You notice that the person's ankle is swollen.
    B. You use a stethoscope to take a blood pressure.
    C. You smell a strong odor on the person's breath.
    D. You touch a person's wrist to take a pulse.

41. You notice that the person feels hot to the touch. In which area are you assisting the nurse?
    A. Assessment of the person
    B. Planning how to reduce fever
    C. Ensuring that the person is comfortable
    D. Evaluating the person's response to touch

42. Which of these is an example of objective data you can collect?
    A. Mrs. Hewitt complains of pain and nausea.
    B. Mr. Stewart tells you he has a dull ache in his stomach.
    C. While taking Mrs. Jensen's pulse, you notice that she is very pale.
    D. Mrs. Murano tells you she is tired because she could not sleep last night.

43. Mr. Young's blood pressure is 50 points higher than when you took it in the morning. You
    A. Chart the results on the flow sheet
    B. Report the difference at the end of the shift
    C. Tell the nurse immediately
    D. Ask Mr. Young if he feels okay

44. A Minimum Data Set (MDS) is used
    A. For nursing center residents
    B. In all health care settings
    C. In acute care settings
    D. In home care

45. What is an important role for the nursing assistants related to the MDS?
    A. Be courtesy and polite and respond to the nurses' requests.
    B. Report changes in the level of assistance required for ADLs.
    C. Attend and actively contribute at the care conferences.
    D. Record and report vital signs promptly and accurately.

46. On the care plan you see the nursing diagnosis: Bathing self-care deficit-inability to independently complete cleansing activities. Which question would you ask the nurse to clarify your duties?
    A. "When should I help the person with hygiene?"
    B. "What type of deficits does the person have?"
    C. "Are the supplies in the person's room?"
    D. "Should I do everything for the person?"

47. You report that the person is having problems moving from a prone to a supine position. Your observations and report help the nurse to make which nursing diagnosis?
    A. Bathing self-care deficit
    B. Impaired bed mobility
    C. Impaired walking
    D. Urinary retention

48. Which nursing assistant is contributing to the planning step of the nursing process?
    A. Nursing Assistant A tells the nurse that the person prefers to shower in the evening.
    B. Nursing Assistant B assists the person to ambulate in the hallway after lunch.
    C. Nursing Assistant C tells the nurse that the person ate 75% of her breakfast.
    D. Nursing Assistant D reports that the person is following the toilet schedule.

49. What is the most important reason for nursing assistants to attend care conferences?
    A. Conferences are educational because the nurses teach new skills.
    B. Attendance demonstrates interest and commitment to the job and agency.
    C. Nursing assistants spend time caring for people and make many observations.
    D. Conferences are required for funding from Medicare and Medicaid.

50. CMS requires a comprehensive care plan, which is a
    A. Conference held to update the care plan
    B. Written guide about the person's care
    C. Conference about one problem that affects the care
    D. Conference held regularly to review care plans

51. What part of the nursing process is being carried out when you give personal care to a person?
    A. Assessing
    B. Planning
    C. Implementation
    D. Evaluation

52. A goal for a person is to achieve independence to do morning hygiene. When you report to the nurse that the person continues to need help with brushing his teeth, which step of the nursing process are you contributing to?
    A. Assessing
    B. Planning
    C. Implementation
    D. Evaluation

53. The nursing assistant reports information about the person
    A. Only at the end of the shift
    B. When a change in condition occurs
    C. Each time care is given
    D. Only in writing

54. The oncoming staff is listening to the end-of-shift report, who should answer the call lights?
    A. The oncoming staff will answer when the report is finished.
    B. The staff going off duty will answer so the report can continue.
    C. The lights are answered by the first person who is available.
    D. The nurse will assign one nursing assistant to answer all lights.

55. Below is a section of the assignment sheet. When would you obtain Ms. Jone's weight?

Room # 202   Name: Mary Jones   ID Number: S1514491530
Date of birth: 11/04/1934 VS: Daily at 0700 T _____
P _____ R _____ BP _____
Wt: Weekly (Monday at 0700) Intake _____
Output _____ BM _____ Bath: Shower

    A. Every day at 0700
    B. Every Monday at 0700
    C. After the shower
    D. At Ms. Jones' request

56. If you are recording using the 24-hour clock, which of these is correct?
    A. 8 AM
    B. 0100 PM
    C. 1300
    D. 5:30 PM

57. When you are given a computer password, you
    A. Must never change or alter it in anyway
    B. Can share it with your nursing supervisor
    C. Should never tell anyone your password
    D. Can use a friend's password with their permission

58. Which staff member has made an error in using the agency computer?
    A. Laboratory technician sends the blood work results to the nursing unit.
    B. Physician prints outs an x-ray report, reads it and then shreds it.
    C. Nurse updates the family on the patient's condition via e-mail.
    D. Nursing Assistant enters vital sign data for assigned patients.

59. Which staff member has created a potential lack of privacy?
    A. Nurse A responds to a call light and leaves the computer screen on.
    B. Social worker changes his or her password every three to four months.
    C. Nursing assistant puts his or her assignment worksheets through the shredder.
    D. Nursing assistant logs off an soon as he or she is done using the computer.

60. When you answer the telephone, do not put the caller on hold if
    A. The person has an emergency
    B. The caller is a physician
    C. The call needs to be transferred
    D. You are too busy to find the nurse

61. When you answer a phone when giving home care, you should
    A. Give your name, title, and location.
    B. Simply answer with "Hello".
    C. Explain that you are giving homecare.
    D. Hand the receiver to the person in the home.

Fill in the Blank

62. Write out the meaning of the abbreviations.
    A. ADL _____
    B. BMs _____
    C. CAA _____
    D. CMS _____
    E. EHR _____
    F. EMR _____
    G. EPHI; ePHI _____
    H. IDCP _____
    I. MDS _____
    J. OASIS _____
    K. PHI _____

63. On the figure below, write in the five steps of the nursing process in correct order.

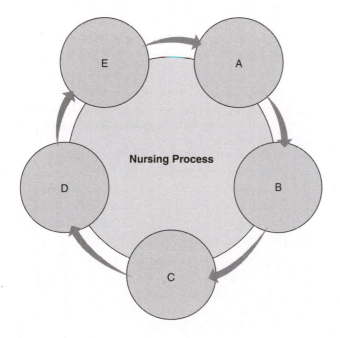

64. When you make observations while you give care, what senses are used?
    A. _____
    B. _____
    C. _____
    D. _____

65. Name the body system or other area you are observing in each of these examples (from Box 8-3, p 92 Basic Observations).
    A. Is the abdomen firm or soft?

    _____
    B. Is the person sensitive to bright lights?

    _____
    C. Are sores or reddened areas present?

    _____
    D. What is the frequency of the person's cough?

    _____
    E. Can the person bathe without help?

    _____
    F. Is the person eating and drinking?

    _____
    G. What is the position of comfort?

    _____
    H. Does the person answer questions correctly?

    _____
    I. Does the person complain of stiff or painful joints?

    _____

66. When planning care, needs that are required for life and survival must be met before _____.

67. List at least 6 observations that you need to immediately report to the nurse.
    A. _____
    B. _____
    C. _____
    D. _____
    E. _____
    F. _____

68. The assignment sheet tells you about
    A. _____
    B. _____
    C. _____

69. You have a key role in the nursing process. How do your actions assist the nurse?
    A. The nurse uses your observations for
    _____ and _____.
    B. You may help develop the _____.
    C. In the _____ step, you perform nursing actions and measures.
    D. Your observations are used for the
    _____ step.

70. Next to each time, write the military time using the 24-hour clock. Use the figure as a guide.

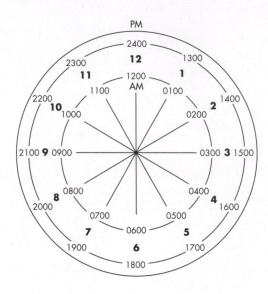

A. _____ 11:00 AM   G. _____ 3:00 AM
B. _____ 8:00 AM   H. _____ 4:50 AM
C. _____ 4:00 PM   I. _____ 5:30 PM
D. _____ 7:30 AM   J. _____ 10:45 PM
E. _____ 6:45 PM   K. _____ 11:55 PM
F. _____ 12 Noon   L. _____ 9:15 PM

71. Convert the times from military time to standard time
    A. 0200 = _____ AM/PM
    B. 2030 = _____ AM/PM
    C. 0500 = _____ AM/PM
    D. 0930 = _____ AM/PM
    E. 1545 = _____ AM/PM
    F. 2345 = _____ AM/PM
    G. 0600 = _____ AM/PM
    H. 1145 = _____ AM/PM
    F. 1800 = _____ AM/PM
    G. 2200 = _____ AM/PM

72. The Nursing Diagnosis is Feeding Self Care Deficit related to weakness in right arm. Briefly describe how you might help this person.
    _____
    _____

73. Nursing Diagnosis: Hygiene Self Care Deficit related to forgetfulness. In your own words, briefly describe what this means.
    _____
    _____

Optional Learning Exercises

Case Study

Mr. Larsen was admitted to a sub-acute care center after his abdominal surgery 1 week ago. This morning, the nursing assistant gave Mr. Larsen a shower and assisted him to sit in a comfortable chair. The nursing assistant noticed that he sat there very still and held his arms across his abdomen. He asked for a pillow and held it tightly against his abdomen.

74. Imagine you are the patient and answer these questions.
    A. What would you like the nursing assistant to ask you?
    _____
    _____
    _____

    B. How would you communicate your feelings to the nursing assistant?
    _____
    _____
    _____

    C. How could you let the nursing assistant know that you had pain without telling her?
    _____
    _____
    _____

75. Imagine you are the nursing assistant and answer these questions.
    A. As the nursing assistant, what observations would be important to make about Mr. Larsen?
    _____
    _____
    _____

    B. What questions could you ask Mr. Larsen?
    _____
    _____
    _____

    C. What nonverbal communication would give you information about Mr. Larsen?
    _____
    _____
    _____

Case Study

Mrs. Miller was admitted to the health care center since you last worked 3 days ago. You have just started your shift and have been assigned to Mrs. Miller.

76. What information would you need to know before giving care?

   _____

   _____

   _____

Use the FOCUS ON PRIDE section to complete the statements.

77. The person has the right to take part in the care

   _____.

78. _____ action can be taken against persons who record false information.

Review the assignment sheet and use the principles of communication and teamwork to answer the questions.

79. It is 0650 on Tuesday morning. You are assigned to care for Ms. Lopez. Review the assignment sheet and answer the following questions
   A. What will you do first?

   _____

   _____

   _____

   B. What (if anything) do you need to clarify with the nurse?

   _____

   _____

   _____

   C. What do you need help with?

   _____

   _____

   _____

Room # 501A   Name: Mrs. Ann Lopez
ID Number: S1514491530   Date of birth: 11/04/1934
VS: Daily at 0700 T _____ P _____ R _____ BP _____
Wt: Weekly (Monday at 0700)   Intake _____
Output _____ BM _____ Bath: Portable tub
Functional status/care measures and procedures
Total assist with ADL
Stand-pivot transfers
Uses w/c
Incontinent of bowel and bladder – uses briefs
Passive ROM exercises to extremities twice daily
Turn and re-position q2h when in bed
Wears eyeglasses and dentures
Diet: High fiber (total assist)

9 Medical Terminology

Fill in the Blank: Key Terms

Abbreviation   Lateral   Proximal   Ventral

Anterior   Medial   Root   Word element

Distal   Posterior   Suffix

Dorsal   Prefix

1. _____ is at or near the middle or mid-line of the body or body part.

2. Another word for dorsal is _____.

3. At or toward the front of the body or body part is ventral or _____.

4. A _____ is a word element placed after a root; it changes the meaning of the word.

5. At the side of the body or body part is _____.

6. An _____ is a shortened form of a word or phrase.

7. A part of a word is a _____.

8. A word element containing the basic meaning of the word is the _____.

9. A word element placed before a root is the _____. It changes the meaning of the word.

10. The part nearest to the center or the point of origin is _____.

11. _____ is the part farthest from the center or from the point of attachment.

12. Another term for anterior is _____.

13. _____ is at or toward the back of the body or body part; posterior.

Circle the Best Answer

14. If a person points to the left side of his body below the umbilicus and tells you he has pain, you will tell the nurse he has pain in the
    A. Right upper quadrant   C. Left upper quadrant
    B. Left lower quadrant   D. Right lower quadrant

15. When describing the position of body parts, the hands and fingers are
    A. Medial   C. Proximal
    B. Distal   D. Posterior

16. For a person who has paraplegia, which type of assistance would you be prepared to offer?
    A. Opening a milk carton
    B. Reminding to use the hearing aid
    C. Assisting in moving the legs
    D. Fastening the shirt and pants

17. The nurse tells you that the patient has occasional episodes of cyanosis that need to be reported. What do you watch for?
    A. Bluish hue to the skin   C. Difficulty swallowing
    B. Tremors in the hands   D. Blood in the urine

18. In caring for a person who has fecal incontinence, which equipment will you obtain?
    A. Disposable pads for the bed
    B. Blood pressure cuff
    C. Measurement cylinder
    D. Thermometer

19. Which type of pain and discomfort is the person likely to report if he or she has a gastrointestinal disorder?
    A. Headache   C. Abdominal pain
    B. Joint stiffness   D. Backache

20. Which vital sign data indicates that the person is having tachycardia?
    A. 130/80 mmHg   C. 40 breaths/min
    B. 103°F (39.4°C)   D. 130 beats/min

21. The nurse tells you to immediately report hematemesis. What do you watch for?
    A. Blood in the person's vomit
    B. Redness and warmth of the skin
    C. Bleeding at a wound site
    D. Red or pinkish urine

22. Which patient is mostly likely to need a glucometer measurement?
    A. Patient has a tracheostomy
    B. Patient has a urinary tract infection
    C. Patient had a stroke last year
    D. Patient has diabetes mellitus

23. Which type of equipment will you use to protect yourself in caring for a person who has dermatitis?
    A. Radiation badge   C. Gloves
    B. Eyeshield   D. Mask

24. A person has rhinorrhea. Which type of equipment will you obtain?
    A. Stethoscope   C. Extra laundry bags
    B. Box of tissues   D. Otoscope

25. The nurse tells you that the person has risk for polyuria. Which question do you ask to clarify your duties?
    A. Should I apply the gait belt for ambulation?
    B. How often should I measure the urine output?
    C. How often should I perform range-of-motion?
    D. Should I cut up the food in smaller bites?

26. If you are caring for a person who has dysphagia, you would
    A. Allow extra time for communication
    B. Ask the nurse for feeding instructions
    C. Assist the person to the bathroom
    D. Watch for vaginal bleeding

27. Which condition is the most serious and needs to be immediately reported?
    A. Dyspnea
    B. Polyphagia
    C. Dermatitis
    D. Otitis

28. Which person is most likely to have dysmenorrhea?
    A. 3-year old female
    B. 23-year old female
    C. 84-year old male
    D. 55-year old male

29. Anemia is a condition of the
    A. Heart
    B. Lungs
    C. Blood
    D. Bones

30. If a person has pharyngitis, which question would you ask to clarify your duties?
    A. What types of food and fluids should I offer?
    B. How often should I offer to help with toileting?
    C. How often should I take the vital signs?
    D. Is the person on fall precautions?

In questions 31 to 38, choose the correct spelling of the medical term.

31. Slow heart rate
    A. Bradecardia
    B. Bradycardia
    C. Bradacordia
    D. Bradicardia

32. Difficulty urinating
    A. Dysuria
    B. Dysurya
    C. Dysuira
    D. Disuria

33. Blue color or condition
    A. Cyonosis
    B. Cyinosis
    C. Cyanosis
    D. Cianosys

34. Rapid breathing
    A. Tachepnea
    B. Tachypinea
    C. Tachypnea
    D. Tachypnia

35. Opening into the trachea
    A. Tracheastomy
    B. Trachiostomy
    C. Tracheostome
    D. Tracheostomy

36. Inflammation of the kidneys
    A. Nephytisis
    B. Nephretis
    C. Nefritis
    D. Nephritis

37. Removal of the breast
    A. Mastectomy
    B. Massectomy
    C. Masectomy
    D. Mastecomy

38. Record of the electrical activity in the heart
    A. Electrocartiogram
    B. Electrocardiogram
    C. Eletrocardeogram
    D. Elegtocardeeogram

Matching

Match the word with the correct definition.

A. arthroscopy
B. bronchoscope
C. cholecystectomy
D. colostomy
E. cyanotic
F. dermatology
G. dysuria
H. enteritis
I. gastrostomy
J. gastritis
K. glossitis
L. nephritis
M. neuralgia
N. oophorectomy
O. proctoscopy

39. _____ Difficulty urinating
40. _____ Inflammation of kidneys
41. _____ Pertaining to blue coloration
42. _____ Joint examination with a scope
43. _____ Study of the skin
44. _____ Creating an opening into the large intestine
45. _____ Instrument used to examine bronchi
46. _____ Inflammation of the tongue
47. _____ Nerve pain
48. _____ Examination of rectum with instrument
49. _____ Excision of gallbladder
50. _____ Excision of ovary
51. _____ Creating an opening into stomach
52. _____ Inflammation of stomach
53. _____ Inflammation of intestine

Fill in the Blank

54. Write out the meaning of these abbreviations.
    A. ADL _____
    B. BP _____
    C. TPR _____
    D. NPO _____
    E. ROM _____
    F. I&O _____

Write the definition of each prefix.

55. anti- _____
56. auto- _____
57. brady- _____
58. dys- _____
59. ecto- _____
60. leuk- _____
61. macro- _____
62. neo- _____
63. supra- _____
64. uni- _____

Write the definition of each root word.

65. adeno _____
66. angio _____
67. broncho _____
68. cranio _____
69. duodeno _____
70. entero _____
71. gyneco _____

72. masto _____
73. pyo _____

Write the definition of each suffix.

74. -asis _____
75. -genic _____
76. -oma _____
77. -phasia _____
78. -ptosis _____
79. -plegia _____
80. -megaly _____
81. -scopy _____
82. -stasis _____

Write the correct abbreviations.

83. Weight _____
84. Fahrenheit _____
85. Bowel movement _____
86. Intake and output _____
87. Lower left quadrant _____
88. Vital signs _____
89. Urinary tract infection _____
90. Milliliter _____
91. Centigrade; Celsius _____

Labeling

92. Label the 4 abdominal regions. Use RUQ, LUQ, RLQ, LLQ to label.

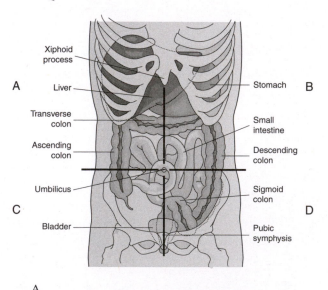

A. _____
B. _____
C. _____
D. _____

Optional Learning Exercises

Use the FOCUS ON PRIDE section to complete the statement and then take pride in learning and conduct the class experiment.

93. Only use abbreviations allowed by your

_____.

Class Experiment

94. It is often difficult to describe fluids in a clear and precise manner. Set up the following examples that imitate situations where you need to describe intake, output, or drainage. Describe as accurately as possible what you see in terms of amounts, colors, and textures. Compare your notes with classmates to see if you are using words that all have the same meaning. What words were used that were easy to understand? What words were used that had more than one meaning?
   1. Bloody drainage: Mix a teaspoon of ketchup and a teaspoon of water. Pour onto the center of a paper napkin.
   2. Urine: Pour a tablespoon of tea into the center of a paper towel.
   3. Bleeding: Smear a teaspoon of red jelly in the center of a paper towel.
   4. Broth: Pour 4 ounces of tea into a bowl.

Class Experiment	
Substance	**Observations**
Bloody drainage	
Urine	
Bleeding	
Broth	

10 Body Structure and Function

Fill in the Blank: Key Terms

Artery   Hemoglobin   Metabolism   System
Capillary   Hormone   Organ   Tissue
Cell   Immunity   Peristalsis   Vein
Digestion   Menstruation   Respiration

1. The substance in red blood cells that carries oxygen and gives blood its color is _____.

2. _____ is protection against a disease or condition.

3. The process of supplying the cells with oxygen and removing carbon dioxide from them is

_____

4. The process of physically and chemically breaking down food so that it can be absorbed for use by the cells is _____.

5. _____ is the burning of food for heat and energy by the cells.

6. A blood vessel that carries blood away from the heart is an _____.

7. _____ is the involuntary muscle contractions in the digestive system that move food through the alimentary canal.

8. Organs that work together to perform special functions form a _____.

9. The basic unit of body structure is a _____.

10. Groups of tissues with the same function form an

_____.

11. A _____ is a tiny blood vessel.

12. A group of cells with similar function is

_____.

13. _____ is the process in which the lining of the uterus breaks up and is discharged from the body through the vagina.

14. A chemical substance secreted by the glands into the bloodstream is a _____.

15. A _____ is a blood vessel that carries blood back to the heart.

Circle the Best Answer

16. A cell
    A. Has no independent purpose
    B. Is the basic unit of body structure
    C. Has the same function as an organ
    D. Is a group of tissues

17. The control center of a cell is the
    A. Membrane   C. Cytoplasm
    B. Protoplasm   D. Nucleus

18. Genes control a person's
    A. Level of physical activity
    B. Dietary practices
    C. Skin and eye color
    D. Hygiene and odor

19. What is an example of connective tissue?
    A. Stomach   C. Femur
    B. Brain   D. Heart

20. How would the person be affected if the epidermis is damaged?
    A. There is loss of sensation to touch and pain.
    B. Hair growth could cease because of root damage.
    C. There is an increased risk for infection.
    D. Sensitivity to temperature would decrease.

21. Sweat glands help
    A. The body regulate temperature
    B. Keep the hair soft and shiny
    C. Protect the nose from dust
    D. The skin to interpret sensations

22. Long bones
    A. Allow skill and ease in movement
    B. Bear the weight of the body
    C. Protects the vital organs
    D. Allow degrees of flexion

23. Blood cells are manufactured in
    A. The heart   C. Blood vessels
    B. The liver   D. Bone marrow

24. Joints move smoothly because of
    A. Cartilage   C. Muscle
    B. Synovial fluid   D. Ligaments

25. What is an example of a hinge joint?
    A. Elbow   C. Shoulder
    B. Hip   D. Spine

26. Voluntary muscles are
    A. Found in the stomach   C. Found in the heart
    B. Attached to bones   D. Attached to sphincters

27. Muscles produce heat by
    A. Contracting   C. Maintaining posture
    B. Relaxing   D. Working automatically

28. The central nervous system consists of
    A. A myelin sheath
    B. Nerves throughout the body
    C. The brain and spinal column
    D. Cranial nerves

29. How would the person be affected if the medulla was damaged?
    A. Muscle control would stop.
    B. Breathing could cease.
    C. Memory loss would occur.
    D. Vision would be blurry.

30. Which safety precaution would you use if a person has a disorder that affects the cerebellum?
    A. Watch for and immediately report problems with swallowing.
    B. Remind to test water temperature before getting in the shower.
    C. Use a gait belt when assisting person to stand or ambulate.
    D. Help the person to clean and don corrective eyewear.

31. If the person has a disorder that affects the cerebral cortex, which behavior are you most likely to observe?
    A. He can't recall the name of his eldest grandchild.
    B. His movements are jerky and he has muscle weakness.
    C. He has a hard time coughing up secretions.
    D. He seems a little unsteady when he first gets up.

32. Cerebrospinal fluid
    A. Cushions the brain and spinal cord
    B. Controls voluntary muscles
    C. Lubricates movement
    D. Controls involuntary muscles

33. Cranial nerves conduct impulses between the
    A. Brain and the head, neck, chest, and abdomen
    B. Brain and the skin and extremities
    C. Brain and internal body structures
    D. Spinal cord and lower extremities

34. Which part of the nervous system is stimulated when a person gets frightened?
    A. Sympathetic   C. Central
    B. Parasympathetic   D. Cranial

35. Receptors for vision and nerve fibers of the optic nerve are found in the
    A. Sclera   C. Retina
    B. Choroids   D. Cornea

36. What happens to a person if the semi-circular canals of the ear are not functioning properly?
    A. Ability to interpret sounds is lost
    B. Person will have inner ear pain
    C. Ability to hear low tones will occur
    D. Person will have trouble with balance

37. Which important function does hemoglobin perform?
    A. Carries oxygen   C. Fights infection
    B. Helps blood to clot D. Contains water

38. If the nurse tells you to gently handle the person, because he bruises and bleeds very easily, which component of the blood is likely to be contributing to the problem?
    A. There are too few red blood cells.
    B. There are too few white blood cells.
    C. The number of platelets is insufficient.
    D. The amount of plasma is decreased.

39. White blood cells or leukocytes
    A. Protect the body against infection
    B. Are necessary for blood clotting
    C. Carry food, hormones, and waste products
    D. Pick up carbon dioxide

40. The left atrium of the heart
    A. Receives blood from the lungs
    B. Receives blood from the body tissues
    C. Pumps blood to the lungs
    D. Pumps blood to all parts of the body

41. Arteries
    A. Return blood to the heart
    B. Pass food, oxygen, and other substances into the cells
    C. Pick up waste products, including carbon dioxide, from the cells
    D. Carry blood away from the heart

42. If the spleen is seriously damaged in an accident, which problem would occur first?
    A. Old red blood cells would remain in the bloodstream.
    B. Bacteria and other substances would not be filtered.
    C. There would be significant blood loss; at least 500 milliliters.
    D. The recovered and stored iron would not be available for use.

43. In the lungs, oxygen and carbon dioxide are exchanged
    A. In the epiglottis
    B. Between the right bronchus and the left bronchus
    C. By the bronchioles
    D. Between the aveoli and capillaries

44. The lungs are protected by
    A. The diaphragm and other muscles
    B. The fluid-filled pleural space
    C. The ribs, sternum, and vertebrae
    D. The division between the lobes

45. Food is moved through the alimentary canal (GI tract) by
    A. Chyme   C. Swallowing
    B. Peristalsis   D. Bile

46. Water is absorbed from chyme in the
    A. Small intestine   C. Esophagus
    B. Stomach   D. Large intestine

47. Digested food is absorbed through tiny projections called
    A. Jejunum   C. Villi
    B. Ileum   D. Colon

48. A function of the urinary system is to
    A. Remove waste products from the blood
    B. Rid the body of solid waste
    C. Remove oxygen from the blood
    D. Burn food for energy

49. A person feels the need to urinate when the bladder contains about
    A. 1000 mL of urine   C. 250 mL of urine
    B. 500 mL of urine   D. 125 mL of urine

50. Which observation would you report to the nurse because sodium (one type of electrolyte) and water loss are being lost?
    A. Headache   C. Nausea
    B. Vomiting   D. Constipation

51. Testosterone is needed for
    A. Male secondary sex characteristics
    B. Female secondary sex characteristics
    C. Prostate gland function
    D. Ova to be produced

52. The prostate gland lies
    A. In the scrotum   C. Just below the bladder
    B. Under the testes   D. In the penis

53. The ovaries secrete progesterone and
    A. Estrogen   C. Ova
    B. Testosterone   D. Semen

54. When an ovum is released from an ovary, it travels first through the
    A. Uterus   C. Endometrium
    B. Fallopian tubes   D. Vagina

55. Menstruation occurs when
    A. The hymen is ruptured
    B. The ovary releases an ovum
    C. The endometrium breaks up
    D. Fertilization occurs

56. A fertilized cell implants in the
    A. Ovary   C. Endometrium
    B. Fallopian tubes   D. Vagina

57. The master gland is the
    A. Thyroid gland   C. Adrenal gland
    B. Parathyroid gland   D. Pituitary gland

58. If a person has insufficient thyroid hormone, what would you expect to observe?
    A. Nervous behavior   C. Muscle spasms
    B. Slowed movements   D. Weight loss

59. If too little insulin is produced by the pancreas, the person has
    A. Decrease urine output   C. Diabetes mellitus
    B. Irregular menstruation D. High blood pressure

60. When antigens enter the body, they are attacked and destroyed by
    A. Antibodies   C. B cells
    B. Lymphocytes   D. T cells

Fill in the Blank

61. Write out these abbreviations.
    A. CNS _____
    B. CO_2 _____
    C. GI _____
    D. mL _____
    E. O_2 _____
    F. RBC _____
    G. WBC _____

Matching

Match the terms with the descriptions.
Musculo-Skeletal System
    A. Periosteum   E. Striated muscle
    B. Joint   F. Smooth muscle
    C. Cartilage   G. Cardiac muscle
    D. Synovial fluid   H. Tendons

62. _____ Connective tissue at end of long bones

63. _____ Skeletal muscle

64. _____ Membrane that covers bone

65. _____ Connects muscle to bone

66. _____ Point at which two or more bones meet

67. _____ Heart muscle

68. _____ Involuntary muscle

69. _____ Acts as a lubricant so the joint can move smoothly

Sensory System
    A. Sclera   D. Cerumen
    B. Cornea   E. Middle ear
    C. Retina   F. Inner ear

70. _____ Contains eustachian tubes and ossicles

71. _____ White of the eye

72. _____ Inner layer of eye; receptors for vision are contained here

73. _____ Light enters eye through this structure

74. _____ Waxy substance secreted in auditory canal

75. _____ Contains semicircular canal and cochlea

Nervous System
    A. Autonomic nervous system
    B. Cerebral cortex
    C. Brainstem
    D. Peripheral nervous system

76. _____ Has 12 pairs of cranial nerves and 31 pairs of spinal nerves

77. _____ Outside of cerebrum; controls highest function of brain

78. _____ Contain midbrain, pons, and medulla

79. _____ Controls involuntary muscles, heart beat, blood pressure, and other functions

Circulatory System
    A. Plasma   G. Myocardium
    B. Erythrocytes   H. Endocardium
    C. Hemoglobin   I. Arteries
    D. Leukocytes   J. Veins
    E. Thrombocytes   K. Capillaries
    F. Pericardium

80. _____ Liquid part of blood

81. _____ Thin sac covering the heart

82. _____ Very tiny blood vessels

83. _____ Substance in blood that picks up oxygen

84. _____ Carry blood away from heart

85. _____ White blood cells

86. _____ Carry blood toward heart

87. _____ Red blood cells

88. _____ Thick muscular portion of heart

89. _____ Platelets; necessary for clotting

90. _____ Membrane lining inner surface of heart

Lymphatic System
A. Lymph nodes
B. Tonsils
C. Spleen

91. _____ Stores blood and saves iron

92. _____ Bean shaped and found in the neck, underarm, groin, chest, abdomen, and pelvis

93. _____ Traps microorganisms in the mouth to prevent infection

Respiratory System
A. Epiglottis   E. Aveoli
B. Larynx   F. Diaphragm
C. Bronchiole   G. Pleura
D. Trachea

94. _____ Air passes from larynx into this structure

95. _____ A two-layered sac that covers the lungs

96. _____ Piece of cartilage that acts like a lid over larynx

97. _____ Separates lungs from the abdominal cavity

98. _____ The voice box

99. _____ Several small branches that divide from the bronchus

100. _____ Tiny one-celled air sacs

Digestive System
A. Liver   E. Anus
B. Chyme   F. Saliva
C. Colon   G. Pancreas
D. Rectum   H. Gallbladder

101. _____ Feces passes out of the body

102. _____ Semi-liquid food mixture formed in stomach

103. _____ Receives feces passed from colon

104. _____ Stores bile

105. _____ Portion of GI tract that absorbs water

106. _____ Produces bile

107. _____ Moistens food particles in the mouth

108. _____ Produces digestive juices

Urinary System
A. Bladder   E. Nephrons
B. Urethra   F. Ureter
C. Kidney   G. Tubule
D. Meatus

109. _____ Basic working unit of the kidney

110. _____ Fluid and waste products form urine in this structure

111 _____ Bean-shaped structure that produces urine

112. _____ Opening at the end of the urethra

113. _____ Structure that allows urine to pass from the bladder

114. _____ A tube attached to the renal pelvis of the kidney

115. _____ Hollow muscular sac that stores urine

Reproductive System
A. Scrotum   E. Vagina
B. Testes   G. Labia
C. Urethra   H. Vulva
D. Gonads   F. Endometrium

116. _____ Male or female sex organs

117. _____ Two folds of tissue on each side of the vagina

118. _____ Sac between thighs that contains testes

119. _____ External genitalia of female

120. _____ Testicles; sperm produced here

121. _____ Muscular canal that receives the penis during intercourse

122. _____ Outlet for urine and semen

123. _____ Tissue lining the uterus

Endocrine System
A. Epinephrine   D. Parathormone
B. Estrogen   E. Testosterone
C. Insulin   F. Thyroxine

124. _____ Regulates sugar in blood; allows sugar to enter the cells

125. _____ Sex hormone secreted by testes

126. _____ Sex hormone secreted by ovaries

127. _____ Regulates metabolism

128. _____ Regulates calcium levels in the body

129. _____ Stimulates the body to produce energy during emergencies

Immune System
A. Antibodies   D. Lymphocytes
B. Antigens   E. B cells
C. Phagocytes   F. T cells

130. _____ Normal body substances that recognize abnormal or unwanted substances

131. _____ Type of cell that destroys invading cells

132. _____ Type of white blood cell that digests and destroys microorganisms

133. _____ Type of cell that causes production of antibodies

134. _____ Substances that cause an immune response

135. _____ Type of white blood cell that produces antibodies

Labeling

136. Identify the subcutaneous fatty tissue, dermis, and epidermis in the skin.

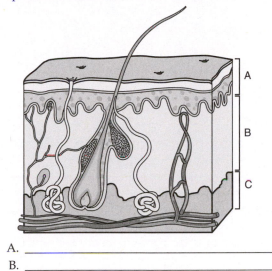

A. _____

B. _____

C. _____

137. Name each type of joint in the figures.

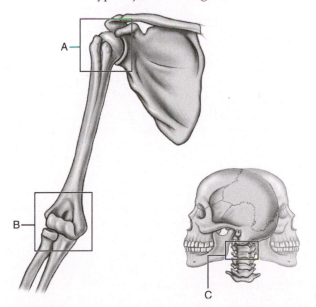

Modified from Herlihy B: The human body in health and illness, ed 6, St Louis, 2018, Elsevier.

A. _____

B. _____

C. _____

138. Identify the structures in the chest cavity

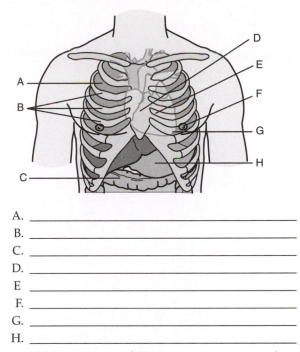

A. _____

B. _____

C. _____

D. _____

E. _____

F. _____

G. _____

H. _____

139. Name the structures of the respiratory system in the figure.

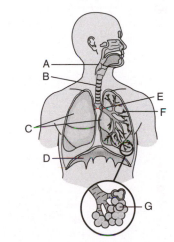

A. _____

B. _____

C. _____

D. _____

E. _____

F. _____

G. _____

140. Name the structures of the digestive system in the figure.

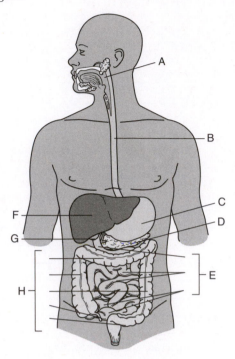

A. _____
B. _____
C. _____
D. _____
E. _____
F. _____
G. _____
H. _____

141. Name the structures of the urinary system in the figure.

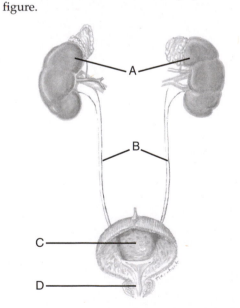

A. _____
B. _____
C. _____
D. _____

142. Name the structures of the male reproductive system in the figure.

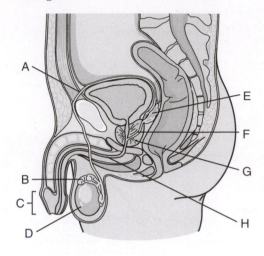

A. _____
B. _____
C. _____
D. _____
E. _____
F. _____
G. _____
H. _____

143. Name the external female genitalia in the figure.

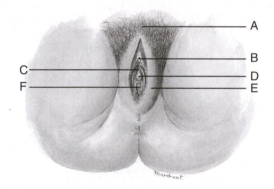

A. _____
B. _____
C. _____
D. _____
E. _____
F. _____

Optional Learning Exercises

144. List what structures are contained in the two skin layers.
    A. Epidermis _____
    B. Dermis _____

145. Explain the function of the types of bone.
    A. Long bones _____
    B. Short bones _____
    C. Flat bones _____
    D. Irregular bones _____

146. Describe how each type of joint moves and give an example of each type.
     A. Ball and socket _____
        Ex. _____
     B. Hinge _____
        Ex. _____
     C. Pivot _____
        Ex. _____

147. Explain what happens when muscles contract.
     _____

148. Explain how the sympathetic and parasympathetic nervous systems balance each other.
     _____
     _____

149. What happens to the pupil of the eye in bright light?
     _____

150. What is the function of the acoustic nerve?
     _____

151. When an infection occurs, what do white blood cells do?
     _____
     _____
     _____

152. Explain the function of the four atria of the heart.
     A. Right atrium _____
     B. Left atrium _____
     C. Right ventricle _____
     D. Left ventricle _____

153. Explain what happens in the aveoli.
     _____
     _____

154. After food is swallowed, explain what happens in each of these parts of the digestive tract.
     A. Stomach _____
     B. Duodenum _____
     C. Jejunum and ileum _____
     D. Colon _____
     E. Rectum _____
     F. Anus _____

155. What is the function of the endometrium?
     _____
     _____

156. Menstruation occurs about every _____ days. Ovulation usually occurs on or about day _____ of the cycle.

157. What is the function of each of these pituitary hormones?
     A. Growth hormone _____
     B. Antidiuretic hormone _____
     C. Oxytocin _____

158. What is the function of insulin? _____
     _____

159. What happens if too little insulin is produced?
     _____

160. What happens when the body senses an antigen?
     _____
     _____

161. What is a reflex?
     _____
     _____

Optional Learning Exercises

Use the FOCUS ON PRIDE section to complete the statement and then use the critical thinking and discussion question to develop your ideas.

162. If the person's decision about his own body may cause _____, tell the nurse at once.

Critical Thinking and Discussion Question

163. You are caring for a person who can walk independently, but he moves very slowly. He also has pain in his finger joints, and this causes problems with tasks, such as buttoning his shirt. He is otherwise healthy and other body systems function properly.
     A. Discuss how these changes in the musculoskeletal system could affect his toileting abilities.
     B. What could you do to help this person?

164. You are caring for a person with a low red blood cell count.
     A. Based on your knowledge of the function of red blood cells, what would you expect to observe?
     B. What could you do to assist him?

11 Growth and Development

Fill in the Blank: Key Terms

Adolescence
Development
Developmental task
Ejaculation

Growth
Infancy
Menarche
Menopause

Milestone
Peer
Primary caregiver
Puberty

Reflex
Sexual orientation
Stage
Teen dating violence

1. The first menstruation and the start of menstrual cycles is _____.

2. _____ is the time between puberty and adulthood; a time of rapid growth and physical and social maturity.

3. The release of semen is _____.

4. The period when reproductive organs begin to function and secondary sex characteristics appear is _____.

5. _____ is the first year of life.

6. Changes in mental, emotional, and social function is _____.

7. An involuntary movement is a _____.

8. _____ is the physical changes that can be measured and that occur in a steady, orderly manner.

9. The person mainly responsible for providing or assisting with the child's basic needs is the _____.

10. A skill that must be completed during a stage of development is a _____.

11. _____ is the time when menstruation stops and menstrual cycles end.

12. A person of the same age-group and background is a _____.

13. _____ refers to sexual arousal or romantic attraction to persons of the other gender, the same gender, or both genders.

14. _____ is the physical, sexual, psychological, or emotional violence within a dating relationship as well as stalking.

15. _____ is a behavior or skill that occurs in a stage of development

16. _____ is a period of time (age range) in which a person learns certain skills.

Circle the Best Answer

17. Growth and development begin
    A. At fertilization
    B. At birth
    C. When the baby sits up
    D. When children have growth spurts

18. Growth and development occur from the center of the body outward. Based on this principle, what would you expect to observe about a baby's movements?
    A. Baby would move legs and arms, but movements would be uncontrolled.
    B. Baby would control shoulder movements before controlling hand movements.
    C. Baby would control the hand movements before controlling the legs.
    D. Baby would move the legs before moving the arms or hands

19. You observe that a neonate is not cooing or babbling. What would you do?
    A. Immediately report your observation to the nurse.
    B. Ask the mother if she has heard the baby making any sounds.
    C. Verify with nurse that this is normal behavior for the neonate.
    D. Talk to and play with the neonate to stimulate a social response.

20. Which newborn is within the range of average birth weight?
    A. Newborn A weighs 12 pounds
    B. Newborn B weighs 10 pounds
    C. Newborn C weighs 8 pounds
    D. Newborn D weighs 5 pounds

21. Which reflex would be useful for a newborn and a mother who are attempting to master breast feeding?
    A. Moro reflex   C. Palmar grasp reflex
    B. Rooting reflex   D. Step reflex

22. The nurse is teaching the mother of a newborn to gently touch the cheek near the mouth. Which result would you expect to observe?
    A. Newborn opens mouth and turns head towards the nipple.
    B. Newborn opens eyes and looks at the mother's face.
    C. Newborn begins to coo and socialize with the mother.
    D. Newborn closes his fingers around the mother's finger.

23. Infants can play peek-a-boo by
    A. 2 to 3 months   C. 8 to 9 months
    B. 4 to 5 months   D. The first birthday

24. Which child is most likely to have a temper tantrum and say "no"?
    A. You are changing the diaper of a 9-month old child.
    B. You are helping an 18-month old child to get undressed.
    C. You are bathing and dressing a 4-month old child.
    D. You are reading a bedtime story to a 4-year old child.

25. A task that will begin in toddlerhood is
    A. Learning to stand and walk
    B. Learning to feed themselves
    C. Learning to share toys with others
    D. Learning to control bowel and bladder function
26. Toddlers learn to feel secure when
    A. Primary caregivers are consistently present when needed
    B. Long periods of separation from primary caregivers are planned
    C. Primary caregivers teach that needs cannot be met quickly
    D. They are alone for long periods of time with primary caregivers
27. The nurse asks you to watch a three-year-old while the mother has a laboratory test. Which activity would you use to engage the child?
    A. Have the child name and number objects in the waiting room.
    B. Ask the child to draw mommy and self going to the hospital.
    C. Ask the child to start counting numbers until mommy is done.
    D. Have the child play make believe hospital with dolls and animals.
28. During the pre-school years, children grow
    A. Much more rapidly than during infancy
    B. 2 to 3 inches per year and gain about 5 pounds per year
    C. Very slowly, if at all, especially if parents are short
    D. 6 to 7 inches per year and gain about 10 pounds per year
29. Baby teeth are lost and permanent teeth erupt at about
    A. 2 years of age
    B. 12 months of age
    C. 6 years of age
    D. 9 or 10 years of age
30. Reading, writing, grammar, and math skills develop during
    A. Toddlerhood
    B. Pre-school years
    C. School-age years
    D. Late childhood
31. Which girl is most likely to be taller and heavier than the boys in her age group?
    A. 3-year old
    B. 8-year old
    C. 12-year old
    D. 17-year old
32. Which child is most likely to be interested in "helping" you to take his vital signs to get praise and a token reward?
    A. 7-year old
    B. 2- year old
    C. 18-year old
    D. 12-year old
33. Girls reach puberty
    A. When menarche occurs
    B. When hips widen, and breast buds appear
    C. When they stop growing in height
    D. When they begin to show interest in sex
34. You are volunteering at your child's school and the school nurse asks you to watch for signs of bullying on the playground. Which behavior would you report to the nurse?
    A. Children are running, and one child can't keep up.
    B. Children are playing, and one child falls on the grass.
    C. Children are teasing and pointing at one child.
    D. Children are sitting together and trading snack items.
35. Which adolescent behavior indicates that there is a need for guidance and discipline?
    A. Adolescent asks his or her parents for spending money.
    B. Adolescent drinks some beer because a friend does.
    C. Adolescent thinks he or she should be allowed to date.
    D. Adolescent asks a teacher for clarification of homework.
36. Teens usually do not understand why parents worry about sexual activities, pregnancy, and sexually transmitted diseases because
    A. They are emotionally unstable and mood swings take over.
    B. Independence from adults is the overriding task for this age group.
    C. They don't always consider the consequences of sexual activity.
    D. They do not have a sense of right and wrong, or good and bad.
37. Which teen has the greatest risk for dating violence?
    A. 15-year old has never dated before
    B. 16-year old frequently disagrees with parents
    C. 14-year old engages in early sexual activity
    D. 16-year old has a 17-year old male partner
38. Development ends
    A. When puberty occurs
    B. When physical growth is complete
    C. At young adulthood
    D. At death
39. Which behavior is expected for a young adult?
    A. Adjusting to physical changes
    B. Adjusting to aging parents
    C. Developing a satisfactory sex life
    D. Accepting changes in appearance
40. A 45-year old adult is likely to tell you about
    A. Plans for traveling during retirement
    B. Embarking on a chosen career path
    C. Death of a partner or spouse
    D. A daughter's upcoming wedding

Fill in the Blank

41. Write out the meaning of the abbreviations
    A. CDC _____
    B. CNS _____
    C. IPV _____

Matching

Match the description with the correct reflex of a newborn.

A. Moro (startle) reflex   D. Grasp (palmar) reflex
B. Rooting reflex   E. Step reflex
C. Sucking reflex

42. _____ Legs extend and then flex

43. _____ Occurs when baby is held upright and the feet touch a surface

44. _____ Guides baby's mouth to the nipple

45. _____ Occurs when lips are touched

46. _____ Fingers close firmly around the object

Match the milestone/task with the correct age-group.

A. Infancy (birth–1 year)
B. Toddler (1–3 years)
C. Preschooler (3–6 years)
D. School Age (6–9 or 10 years)
E. Late Childhood (9 or 10–12 years)
F. Adolescence (12–18 years)
G. Young Adulthood (18–40 years)
H. Middle Adulthood (40–65 years)
I. Late Adulthood (65 years and older)

47. _____ Accepting changes in body and appearance

48. _____ Developing leisure-time activities

49. _____ Gaining control of bowel and bladder functions

50. _____ Becoming independent from parents and adults

51. _____ Learning to eat solid foods

52. _____ Adjusting to decreased strength and loss of health

53. _____ Learning how to study

54. _____ Learning how to get along with persons of the same age group and background

55. _____ Increasing ability to communicate and understand others

56. _____ Tolerating separation from primary caregiver

57. _____ Learning to live with a partner

58. _____ Developing moral or ethical behavior

59. _____ Learning basic reading, writing, and arithmetic skills

60. _____ Developing stable sleep and feeding patterns

61. _____ Performing self-care

62. _____ Using words to communicate with others

63. _____ Adjusting to aging parents

64. _____ Develop appropriate relationships with others and begin to attract partners

65. _____ Cope with a partner's death

66. _____ Choosing education and a career

Optional Learning Exercises

Infancy

67. List six tasks of growth and development that occur during the stage of infancy.

    A. _____

    B. _____

    C. _____

    D. _____

    E. _____

    F. _____

68. What are three language and communication behaviors that a 2-month old should display?

    A. _____

    B. _____

    C. _____

Toddlerhood

69. What are four developmental tasks of toddlerhood?

    A. _____

    B. _____

    C. _____

    D. _____

Preschool

70. What personal skills can be performed by 3-year-olds?

    A. Put on _____

71. What are five communication skills that 5-year-olds should be using?

    A. _____.

    B. _____.

    C. _____.

    D. _____.

    E. _____.

School-Age

72. Play activities in school-age children have a _____.

    A. They like household tasks such as _____

    _____.

    B. Rewards are important, such as _____

    _____.

Late Childhood

73. What are six developmental tasks of late childhood?

    A. _____

    B. _____

    C. _____

    D. _____

    E. _____

    F. _____

Adolescence

74. What are six developmental tasks of adolescence?
   A. _____
   B. _____
   C. _____
   D. _____
   E. _____
   F. _____

75. During adolescence, girls and boys need about _____ hours of sleep at night because of _____.

76. Girls usually complete development by age _____. Boys usually stop growing between _____ years.

77. What is the definition of teen dating violence?
   _____

Young Adulthood

78. What are seven factors that affect the selection of a partner during young adulthood?
   A. _____
   B. _____
   C. _____
   D. _____
   E. _____
   F. _____
   G. _____

Middle Adulthood

79. During middle adulthood, weight control becomes a problem because _____.

80. What are four developmental tasks of middle adulthood?
   A. _____
   B. _____
   C. _____
   D. _____

Late Adulthood

81. What are five developmental tasks of late adulthood?
   A. _____
   B. _____
   C. _____
   D. _____
   E. _____

Use the FOCUS ON PRIDE section to complete the statements and then use the critical thinking and discussion questions to develop your ideas.

82. For children, the _____ is an important part of the health team.

83. When interacting with caregivers you should
   A. _____
   B. _____
   C. _____
   D. _____
   E. _____

Critical Thinking and Discussion Questions

84. You are making a home visit to assist an adult who had surgery and who needs some temporary assistance to bath and ambulate. During the visit, you notice that there is a 4-month old infant who has been crying continuously for the past hour.
   A. What could be causing the infant to cry?
   B. If the crying continues and you and the caregiver cannot calm and comfort the infant, what would you do?
   C. Discuss how you feel about advocating or intervening for someone (such as this infant) who is not your responsibility or the person who is assigned to your care.

Crossword

Fill in the crossword by answering the clues below with the words from this list:

Development	Menopause	Pre-adolescence	Step
Grasp	Moro	Puberty	Sucking
Growth	Neonatal	Rooting	

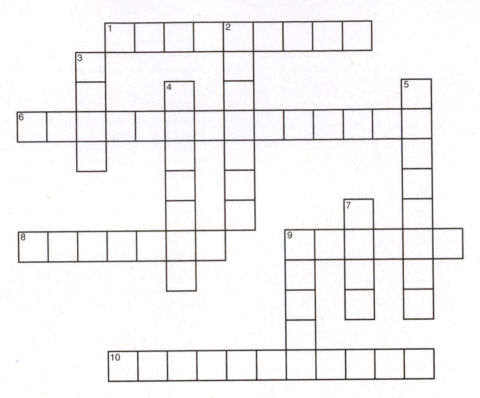

Across

1. Event that occurs to women between ages 45 and 55
6. Time between childhood and adolescence (late childhood)
8. Reflex that occurs when the lips are touched
9. Physical changes that can be measured and that occur in a steady, orderly manner
10. Changes in mental, emotional, and social function

Down

2. Period between ages 9 and 16 years that girls reach; period between ages 13 and 15 years that boys reach
3. Reflex in which the feet move up and down as in stepping motions
4. Reflex that occurs when the cheek is touched near the mouth
5. Period of infancy from birth to 1 month of age
7. Reflex that occurs when a loud noise, a sudden movement, or the head falling back startles the baby
9. Reflex that occurs when the palm is stroked

12   The Older Person

Fill in the Blank: Key Terms

Geriatrics   Menopause

Gerontology

1. _____ is the care of aging people.
2. _____ occurs when menstrual cycles stop and there is at least one year with no menstrual period.
3. The study of the aging process is _____.

Circle the Best Answer

4. In caring for an elderly person who had hip surgery, which every day activity is most likely to be included in your assigned tasks?
   A. Helping her to manage her money
   B. Administering her prescribed medications
   C. Assisting her with toileting and hygiene
   D. Doing her shopping and housework

5. You are assigned to care for an 86-year old man, who retains physical mobility but needs help with every day activity because of dementia. Which action are you most likely to use?
   A. Supervise him while he prepares meals.
   B. Coach him step-by-step to put on his shirt.
   C. Spoon feed him and hold his drink cup.
   D. Escort him around the shopping center.

6. Which nursing assistant has provided a care measure that is insufficient to meet the needs of an elderly person who has limited mobility?
   A. Nursing Assistant A assists the person into a wheelchair and pushes her to the dining area.
   B. Nursing Assistant B helps the person to sit up and to wash her hands before eating.
   C. Nursing Assistant C places the unwrapped food tray on a table in the person's room.
   D. Nursing Assistant D cuts up the meat and puts the food within the person's reach.

7. A myth about aging is
   A. Many older people enjoy a fulfilling sex life
   B. Most older people have memory loss and dementia
   C. Many older persons have jobs or do volunteer work
   D. Most older persons frequently interact with family

8. Based on the social changes that occur with aging, which topic is the oldest of the old most likely to talk about?
   A. Changes in physical appearance
   B. Attending a family reunion in the summer
   C. Death of a friend or family member
   D. Investments and savings for retirement

9. Which basic need, as described by Maslow, is met when a retired older person decides to do volunteer work?
   A. Self-actualization   C. Love and belonging
   B. Physical   D. Safety and security

10. You are providing care in the home setting, which observation should be reported to the nurse, because the elderly person is probably experiencing a reduced income?
    A. Elderly person is living with an adult child.
    B. Elderly person rarely goes out to eat dinner.
    C. Elderly person often talks about trips he used to take.
    D. Elderly person has stopped taking prescribed medication.

11. You notice that a foreign-born person rarely interacts with other the other residents in the nursing center. Which action would you take?
    A. Ask the nurse to invite the family to visit more frequently.
    B. Ask native-born residents to accept foreign-born persons.
    C. Identify residents or staff who can speak the person's language.
    D. Be pleasant and cheerful, but recognize nothing can be done.

12. Which older person may be having trouble adjusting to changes in social relationships?
    A. Person stays at home alone to save money.
    B. Person attends church and community activities.
    C. Person takes up a new hobby to meet new people.
    D. Person maintains regular contact with family.

13. What is a source of disagreement when an older person moves in with an adult child?
    A. The older person tries to maintain dignity.
    B. The older person expresses a feeling of security.
    C. Family members experience a lack of privacy.
    D. Older person spends time with the grandchildren.

14. You are caring for an older couple in the home setting and the wife dies after a long illness. Which observation would you report to the nurse?
    A. The husband seems to accept his wife's death as a part of life.
    B. The husband develops headaches, and insomnia and seems sad.
    C. The husband starts socializing and forming new friendships.
    D. The husband has prepared for this change and he seems at peace.

15. What changes in the integumentary system would you expect to observe in an older person?
    A. Skin is fragile and is easily bruised.
    B. Skin is moist and the fatty layer increases.
    C. Skin appears pale or a may be slightly bluish.
    D. Skin appears puffy and indents with pressure.

16. Which observation needs to be immediately reported to the nurse?
    A. Person gets up slowly from bed or chair.
    B. There is a small skin tear on the buttocks.
    C. Person refuses to wear his hearing-aid.
    D. There is a thin layer of earwax in the ear.

17. Hot water bottles and heating pads are not used with older persons because
    A. Older people don't understand how to adjust the temperature for safety.
    B. You could be liable if the equipment fails and the person is injured.
    C. Fragile skin and changes in sensation create an increased risk for burns.
    D. Heat causes the blood vessels to dilate and this causes changes in circulation.

18. Older persons can prevent bone loss and loss of muscle strength by
    A. Activity, exercise, and diet
    B. Taking hormones
    C. Resting with feet elevated
    D. Taking vitamins

19. In an elderly person, bones may break easily; therefore, which care measure would you use?
    A. Ask the nurse for permission to leave the person in bed.
    B. Put the person into a wheelchair; never let him walk.
    C. Remind the person that the bones are weak.
    D. Turn and move the person gently and carefully.

20. For an older person who is experiencing dizziness, which care measure would you use?
    A. Encourage the person to take naps in the daytime.
    B. Remind the person to get up slowly from bed or chair.
    C. Have the person eat a snack before exercise or activity.
    D. Use memory aids and prompts according to the care plan.

21. Which older person is displaying expected behavior related to aging of the nervous system?
    A. Person A talks happily and continuously but most of it is nonsense.
    B. Person B talks about events that happened when he or she was a teenager.
    C. Person C is usually calm and cooperative, but today he or she is angry and hostile.
    D. Person D has periods of confusion that seem to be related to his or her medication.

22. You recognize that an older person has a reduced sensitivity to touch, pressure or pain; therefore, you will immediately report which of the following?
    A. Person asks for an icepack because his or her ankle is swollen and deformed.
    B. Person asks you to give him or her a soothing back rub with warmed lotion.
    C. Person wants the air-conditioning turned down, even though it is hot weather.
    D. Person wants to take a deep warm bath to relieve muscle aches and stiffness.

23. An older people is complaining about the taste of the food. Which care measure would you use?
    A. Provide or encourage oral hygiene.
    B. Offer the person salt and pepper.
    C. Tell the person to drink extra fluids.
    D. Suggest raw fruits and vegetables.

24. An older person reports decreased vision in dark rooms and at night. Which care measure would you use?
    A. Tell the person to wear his glasses all the time.
    B. Open curtains in the day and turn on a night light.
    C. Ask the nurse if the person needs eyedrops.
    D. Advise the person not to walk around at night.

25. Which sound is an older person most likely to have difficulty in hearing?
    A. Loud music on television
    B. High-pitched alarm on cell phone
    C. Pastor giving a sermon in church
    D. German shepherd dog barking outside

26. When severe circulatory changes occur, the person
    A. May be encouraged to walk long distances
    B. May need to rest during the day
    C. Should not do any kind of exercise
    D. Should exercise only once a week

27. When a person has difficulty breathing, it is easier to breathe when
    A. Lying flat in bed
    B. Covered with heavy bed linens
    C. Allowed to be on bedrest
    D. Resting in the semi-Fowler's position

28. For an older person, which type of food is generally avoided?
    A. Fried food   C. Puddings
    B. Whole grain foods   D. Fruit juices

29. To prevent constipation, you would encourage which type of foods?
    A. Foods with fewer calories
    B. High fiber foods
    C. Foods that supply calcium
    D. Low-protein foods

30. You are assigned to care for four people. Which person is likely to need the most assistance throughout the day?
    A. Person has flatulence
    B. Person has genitalia atrophy
    C. Person has urinary incontinence
    D. Person has earwax impaction

31. An older woman may find intercourse uncomfortable or painful because
    A. Partner has a delayed erection
    B. There is vaginal dryness
    C. Arousal takes longer
    D. Orgasm is less intense

32. You notice that an older person living in a nursing center seems lonely. Which care measure would you use?
    A. Visit with the person a few times during your shift.
    B. Take the person to your own home during the holidays.
    C. Call the family and tell them that the person is lonely.
    D. Tell the person that he must attend social activities.

33. Adult day-care centers
    A. Provide meals, supervision, and activities for older persons
    B. Accept only self-care persons and those who can walk without help
    C. Provide complete care for physical, social and emotional needs
    D. Provide sleeping facilities for older persons who have no family

34. When an older person rents an apartment, it allows the person to
    A. Remain independent and keep personal items
    B. Share common meals with other older persons
    C. Enjoy gardening and yard work opportunities
    D. Repair appliances and maintain the property

35. Elder Cottage Housing Opportunity or accessory dwelling units allow the person to
    A. Have meals with other people
    B. Have supervision and activities
    C. Live independently but near family
    D. Receive medical care in the home

36. Senior citizen housing is available to
    A. Only those who can afford the rent
    B. Those who have no disabilities
    C. Older and disabled persons
    D. Families who live with an older person

37. Home-sharing is a way to avoid
    A. Living alone
    B. Paying rent
    C. Doing housework
    D. Dealing with disabilities

38. Assisted living facilities are for persons who
    A. Need daily nursing care
    B. Need help getting in and out of bed
    C. Need help with daily living
    D. Are dependent on others for all care

39. Continuing care retirement communities (CCRCs)
    A. Only have independent living units
    B. Only have 24-hour nursing care
    C. Add services as the person's needs change
    D. Require the person to leave if care needs increase

40. Nursing centers are housing options for older persons who
    A. Need companionship only
    B. Cannot care for themselves
    C. Need care during the day-time
    D. Are developmentally disabled

41. A quality nursing center must meet OBRA and CMS requirements to
    A. Be approved by the medical society
    B. Receive Medicare and Medicaid funds
    C. Give care to people over 65 years of age
    D. Be licensed by the local health department

42. Which environmental observation needs to be reported?
    A. Ventilation is adequate to control odors
    B. Temperature levels are comfortable and safe
    C. Bed and bath linens are clean and in good condition
    D. Call light system is functional only in the bathrooms

43. A feature of a quality nursing center is
    A. Hand rails are provided in hallways.
    B. Each resident has a private bathroom.
    C. Residents provide furniture for their rooms.
    D. Tablecloths and cloth napkins are used for dining.

Matching

Match physical changes during the aging process with the body system affected.

A. Integumentary   E. Respiratory
B. Musculo-skeletal   F. Digestive
C. Nervous   G. Urinary
D. Cardiovascular

44. _____ Reduced blood flow to kidneys
45. _____ Arteries narrow and become stiffer
46. _____ Forgetfulness
47. _____ Gradual loss of height
48. _____ Decreased strength for coughing
49. _____ Decreased secretion of oil and sweat glands
50. _____ Difficulty digesting fried and fatty foods
51. _____ Heart pumps with less force
52. _____ Bladder muscles weaken
53. _____ Difficulty seeing green and blue colors
54. _____ Difficulty swallowing
55. _____ Lung tissue less elastic
56. _____ Bone mass decreases
57. _____ Facial hair in some women

Fill in the Blank

58. Write out the meaning of the abbreviations.
    A. ADU _____
    B. CCRC _____
    C. CMS _____
    D. ECHO _____

59. List eleven everyday activities that can be affected by disabilities, illness, or changes related to aging.
    A. _____
    B. _____
    C. _____
    D. _____
    E. _____
    F. _____
    G. _____
    H. _____
    I. _____
    J. _____
    K. _____

60. What changes can be made in the bathroom to make it safer for a person with poor eyesight?
    A. _____ flooring
    B. Grab bars by _____
    C. _____ surfaces in showers and tubs
    D. Rugs with _____
    E. _____ devices on faucets and shower-heads
    F. Toilet with raised _____ or toilet _____
    G. _____ lighting

61. Name the housing options described in each of the following:
    A. A small portable home that can be placed in the yard of a single-family home _____
    B. Provides meals, supervision, activities, and sometimes rehabilitation to elderly during day-time _____
    C. The elderly person lives with older brothers, sisters, or cousins for companionship or to share living expenses _____
    D. The elderly person pays rent and utility bills but does not need to do maintenance, yard work, or snow removal _____
    E. The elderly person who needs help with activities of daily living but does not need nursing care may live in a _____.
    F. A _____ meets the changing needs of older persons. Services change as the person's needs change.

62. List five myths about aging.
    A. _____
    B. _____
    C. _____
    D. _____
    E. _____

Optional Learning Exercises

63. When bathing an older person, what kind of soap should be used? _____
    Often, no soap is used on the _____.

64. Because bone mass decreases, why is it important to turn an older person carefully?
    _____

65. Why does an older person often have a gradual loss of height? _____
    _____

66. What types of exercise help prevent bone loss and loss of muscle strength? _____
    _____

67. What problems can occur because of the physiologic changes related to aging?
    A. Nerve conduction and reflexes are slower.
    _____
    B. Blood flow to brain is reduced.
    _____
    C. Touch and sensitivity to pain and pressure are reduced.
    _____

68. When you are eating with an older person, you notice she puts salt on vegetables that taste fine to you. What may be a reason she does this?
    _____

69. What exercises will help a person with circulation changes who must stay in bed?
    _____

70. What can the nursing assistant do to prevent respiratory complications from bedrest?
    _____

71. The stomach and colon empty slower and flatulence and constipation are common in the older person. What causes these problems?
    _____

72. How will good oral hygiene and denture care improve food intake?
    _____

73. How can a nursing assistant help prevent urinary tract infections in an older person?
    _____

74. Why should you plan to give most fluids to the older person before 1700 (5:00 PM)?
    _____

Use the FOCUS ON PRIDE section to complete these statements then use the critical thinking and discussion question to develop your ideas.

75. You can promote social interaction when caring for an older person when you
    A. Encourage _____
    B. Ask _____
    C. Use _____
    D. Take _____

Critical Thinking and Discussion Question

76. Discuss some beliefs or ideas that you have about older people. After studying and caring for older people in the clinical setting have your ideas changed? If so, give examples.

13 Safety

Fill in the Blank: Key Terms

Coma
Dementia
Disaster
Electrical shock
Elopement

Ground
Hazard
Hazardous chemical
Hemiplegia
Incident

Paralysis
Paraplegia
Poison
Quadraplegia
Suffocation

Tetraplegia
Workplace violence

1. When a patient or resident leaves the agency without staff knowledge it is _____.

2. The loss of cognitive and social function caused by changes in the brain is _____.

3. _____ are violent acts (including assault or threat of assault) directed toward persons at work or while on duty.

4. Paralysis from the neck down is _____.

5. _____ is any chemical that is a physical hazard or a health hazard.

6. A _____ is a sudden catastrophic event in which many people are injured and killed and property is destroyed.

7. _____ occurs when breathing stops from the lack of oxygen.

8. Paralysis on one side of the body is _____.

9. A _____ is a state of being unaware of one's surroundings and being unable to react or respond to people, places, or things.

10. That which carries leaking electricity to the earth and away from an electrical appliance is a _____.

11. _____ is paralysis from the waist down.

12. _____ occurs when electrical current passes through the body.

13. Any event that has harmed or could harm a patient, resident, visitor, or staff member is an _____.

14. _____ means loss of muscle function, loss of sensation, or loss of both muscle function and sensation.

15. _____ is any substance harmful to the body when ingested, inhaled, injected, or absorbed through the skin.

16. Another term for quadraplegia is _____.

17. A _____ is anything in the person's setting that could cause injury or illness.

Circle the Best Answer

18. Safety measures needed by a person can be found
    A. In the doctor's orders
    B. In the person's care plan
    C. By talking to the family
    D. By asking the person

19. When checking for safety issues, a survey team will observe
    A. How well you give care
    B. For actual or potential hazards
    C. How quickly you answer questions
    D. Identity of persons at risk for harm

20. For a person who takes a drug that causes loss of balance as a side effect, which safety issue is the biggest concern?
    A. Potential for suffocation
    B. Risk for injuries due to falls
    C. Burning self with hot water
    D. Unintentional poisoning

21. Young children are at risk of injury because they
    A. Have not learned the difference between safety and danger
    B. Have limited control over their environment
    C. Have poor motor control and no self-discipline
    D. Have not learned how to read and interpret information

22. When a person has dementia, there is a risk for injury because
    A. There is an inability to smell and interpret hazardous odors.
    B. Judgment and ability to discriminate danger are lacking.
    C. Physical immobility prevents moving to a safe place.
    D. Dementia increases sensitive to hazardous materials.

23. What is the most important reason for you to correctly identify persons who are under your care?
    A. Life and health are threatened if the wrong care is given.
    B. Visitors or doctors may ask for your help to find someone.
    C. It is polite and professional to call a person by the right name.
    D. You must care for two people if you go to the wrong person first.

24. Which nursing assistant is not using a reliable way to identify the person?
    A. Nursing Assistant A checks the person's identification bracelet.
    B. Nursing Assistant B uses the person's picture and compares it to the person.
    C. Nursing Assistant C follows the center's policy to identify the person.
    D. Nursing Assistant D recognizes the person and greets him by name.

25. A leading cause of death, especially among children and older persons, is
    A. Falls   C. Poisoning
    B. Burns   D. Suffocation

26. When children are in the kitchen
    A. Use the burners at the back of the stove.
    B. Turn pot and pan handles so they point outward.
    C. Supervise children to help you cook at the stove.
    D. Leave cooking utensils in pots and pans.

27. Burns can be avoided if oven mitts and pot-holders are kept dry because
    A. Dry material provides a thicker layer.
    B. Water conducts heat and can cause burns.
    C. Moisture allows bacteria to penetrate the cloth.
    D. Mitts and pot-holders are not waterproof.

28. Accidental poisoning of children can occur when
    A. Harmful products are kept in their original containers.
    B. Harmful substances are labeled and stored in locked areas.
    C. Drugs are carried in purses, backpacks, and briefcases.
    D. Safety latches are used on cabinets and storage spaces.

29. Which item needs a "Mr. Yuk" sticker?
    A. A sealed box of dog biscuits
    B. An unopened bottle of red wine
    C. An opened jar of mayonnaise
    D. A spray bottle of bathroom cleaner

30. Which child has the greatest risk for lead poisoning?
    A. 6-month old infant is being switched from breast feeding to bottle feeding.
    B. 8-month old infant is crawling and likes to put objects in his or her mouth.
    C. 10-year old frequently plays with his or her friends in a nearby forested area.
    D. 15-year old is learning to shoot guns and some bullets are made of lead.

31. What should you do if water is contaminated with lead from inside the home?
    A. Use only bottled water until the plumbing is complete renovated.
    B. Run the water until it is hot before drinking or using it for baby formula.
    C. Boil all water for at least 20 minutes, cool and then use in cooking.
    D. Let cold water run 1 to 2 minutes before using it for cooking or coffee.

32. Which gas is associated with accidental poisoning in the household?
    A. Oxygen   C. Carbon monoxide
    B. Carbon dioxide   D. Nitrogen

33. Which of these is a source of carbon monoxide?
    A. Computer   C. Furnace
    B. Vacuum cleaner   D. Electric heater

34. A choking hazard for older persons can be
    A. Loose dentures that fit poorly
    B. Sitting up in a wheelchair to eat
    C. Using supplemental oxygen
    D. Eating a snack after dinner time

35. Which toy would be the best to prevent accidental choking?
    A. Mobile hanging over the crib
    B. Stuffed toy with no removable parts
    C. Small plastic action figure
    D. Toy car with interchangeable parts

36. The universal sign of choking is when the
    A. Person begins to cough forcefully
    B. Conscious person clutches at the throat
    C. Person tells you he is choking
    D. Person becomes unconscious

37. Abdominal thrusts given for choking can be used on
    A. Pregnant women
    B. Obese people
    C. Neonates and infants
    D. Adults or children aged over 1 year

38. When giving abdominal thrusts, the correct procedure is to
    A. Make a fist, place the thumb side on the abdomen, and quickly thrust upward.
    B. Press your fist against the abdomen and slowly push straight down.
    C. Gently thrust upward on the abdomen with the palmar surface of the hand.
    D. Lay the hands on top of each other over the abdomen and push down.

39. If you see a foreign object in the mouth of a conscious person, you should
    A. Turn the head to one side and pat the person's back.
    B. Leave the object in place and do abdominal thrusts.
    C. Grasp and remove the object if it is within reach.
    D. Ask the person to forcefully cough out the object.

40. If an infant is choking, you should
    A. Call 911 or take the infant to the nearest emergency room.
    B. Give five abdominal thrusts using the same hand position and motions as for adults.
    C. Hold the infant face down; give fiveforceful back slaps between the shoulder blades.
    D. Reach in the mouth and try to retrieve the object or use finger sweeping motions.

41. If a choking person becomes unresponsive you should
    A. Make sure EMS or RRT was called.
    B. Begin abdominal thrusts.
    C. Give 2 rescue breaths.
    D. Finger sweep mouth for foreign objects.

42. Which occurrence suggests that there is a fault in the electrical item?
    A. You hear a sizzling or buzzing sound when the toaster oven is on.
    B. The lamp on the person's bedside table was left on overnight.
    C. You notice that a vacuum cleaner is not picking up dirt and dust.
    D. The light in the back of the refrigerator doesn't come on.

43. What is the primary purpose of the three-pronged plug?
    A. It acts as ground to carry leaking electricity away from the appliance.
    B. It stabilizes the contact with outlet so that the connection is more secure.
    C. It protects the function of the appliance if there is a power surge.
    D. It prevents fires by distributing the current if usage is prolonged.

44. An electrical shock is especially dangerous to which body system?
    A. Urinary system
    B. Circulatory system
    C. Lymphatic system
    D. Reproductive system

45. If you are shocked by electrical equipment, you should
    A. Report the shock at once.
    B. Label the equipment as damaged.
    C. Make sure it has a ground prong.
    D. Test the equipment in a different outlet.

46. Which entity requires that health care employees understand the risks of hazardous substances and how to handle them safely.
    A. Omnibus Budget Reconciliation of 1987 (OBRA)
    B. Occupational Safety and Health Administration (OSHA)
    C. Centers for Medicare and Medicaid Services (CMS)
    D. Safety data sheet (SDS)

47. Which information is not included on the SDS of a hazardous chemical?
    A. Physical hazards and health hazards
    B. What protective equipment to wear
    C. Contact information for local resources
    D. Storage and disposal information

48. For which situation would you refer to the safety data sheets (SDSs) for hazardous materials?
    A. You are trying to safely store the product.
    B. You need to order additional product.
    C. You need to replace the warning label.
    D. You want to know if you are allergic to it.

49. For which circumstance are you most likely to don gloves for personal protection?
    A. A person is choking, you perform abdominal thrusts.
    B. An electrical fan is sparking and you need to unplug it.
    C. You are using a cleaning solution to disinfect a bedpan.
    D. The nurse asks you to help during an elopement situation.

50. When a person is receiving oxygen, which of these is allowed in the room?
    A. Visitors may smoke if they use caution.
    B. Wool or synthetic blankets in good condition
    C. Electrical items that are in good working order
    D. Alcohol-based after shave in a glass container

51. If a fire occurs, what should you do first?
    A. Rescue people in immediate danger.
    B. Sound the nearest fire alarm.
    C. Close doors and windows to confine the fire.
    D. Use a fire extinguisher on a small fire

52. If evacuation is necessary, persons who are
    A. Closest to the outside door are rescued first
    B. Able to walk are rescued last
    C. Closest to the fire are evacuated first
    D. Helpless are rescued last

53. If a space heater is used in a home, a safety practice is to
    A. Place the heater in doorways or in hallways, away from the bed.
    B. Keep the heater 3 feet away from curtains, drapes, and furniture.
    C. Use an extension cord and place the heater in a distant corner.
    D. Keep the heater on the lowest temperature throughout the night.

54. If there is a disaster, you
    A. Are expected to go to your agency immediately.
    B. May be called into work if you are off duty.
    C. Should stay away or leave to get out of the way.
    D. May go home to check on your family.

55. According to OSHA, which nursing assistant the greatest risk for workplace violence?
    A. Nursing Assistant A cares for elderly residents at a nursing center located in a farming community.
    B. Nursing Assistant B works in an urban clinic that serves persons with a history of violence and drug abuse.
    C. Nursing Assistant C has attended several training sessions for management of hostile and assaultive behaviors.
    D. Nursing Assistant D is paired with a co-worker, and they work together when transporting patients and residents.

56. You are caring for a person who becomes angry and aggressive. What is the immediate action to use to prevent and control workplace violence?
    A. Stand far enough away from the person to avoid being hit or kicked.
    B. Identify and remove any objects that can be used as weapons.
    C. Sit quietly with the person in his room and hold his hand.
    D. Assume an authoritative posture, hands on hips and chest thrust forward.

57. Which nursing assistant is dressed to prevent workplace violence?
    A. Nursing Assistant A has long hair up and off the collar.
    B. Nursing Assistant B wears white shoes with leather soles.
    C. Nursing Assistant C wears a long necklace and drop earrings.
    D. Nursing Assistant D has a uniform that is loose and large.

58. If you are threatened in a home setting, you should
    A. Call the agency for help, call the police or leave the setting.
    B. Refuse to go back and resolve the matter over the phone.
    C. Confront the person who is making the threats.
    D. Ignore the situation and continue to give care.

59. A yellow color-coded wristband may indicate that the person
    A. Has allergies
    B. Is "Do Not Resuscitate"
    C. Has a restricted diet
    D. Is at risk for falling

Matching

Match each safety measure to the risk it prevents.

A. Burns   D. Equipment accident
B. Poisoning   E. Hazardous substances
C. Suffocation   F. Fire

60. _____ Do not allow person to sleep with a heating pad.

61. _____ Apply sunscreen to children before they go outside.

62. _____ Keep child-resistant caps on all harmful products.

63. _____ Wear PPE to clean spills and leaks.

64. _____ Report loose teeth or dentures to the nurse.

65. _____ Turn off an electrical appliance when you are done using it.

66. _____ Attend to food cooking on the stove.

67. _____ Have water heaters set at 120°F or less.

68. _____ Never call drugs or vitamins "candy."

69. _____ Store flammable liquids outside in their original containers.

Fill in the Blank

70. Write out the meaning of the abbreviations.
    A. AED _____
    B. CMS _____
    C. CDC _____
    D. CO _____
    E. CPR _____
    F. EMS _____
    G. F _____
    H. HCS _____

    I. NFPA _____
    J. OSHA _____
    K. PASS _____
    L. RACE _____
    M. RRS _____
    N. SDS _____
    O. MRN _____
    P. MSDS _____

71. As part of the team, you can help provide a safe setting by correcting something that is unsafe. What could you do if
    A. You see a water spill _____
    B. You see a person sliding out of a wheelchair

       _____
    C. A person is having problems holding a cup of coffee _____
    D. Food is left unattended in a microwave

       _____
    E. A grab bar is loose in the bathroom

       _____

72. A person who is agitated or aggressive may be at risk for injuries. What can cause these behaviors?
    A. _____
    B. _____
    C. _____
    D. _____

73. What health hazards can be caused by hazardous chemicals?
    A. _____
    B. _____
    C. _____
    D. _____

74. You have permission from the nurse and patient to discard outdated medication in the household trash. List four steps that you would take.
    A. _____
    B. _____
    C. _____
    D. _____

75. The word PASS is used to remember how to use a

    _____.
    What action is taken for each of these steps?
    A. P _____
    B. A _____
    C. S _____
    D. S _____

76. If a disaster occurs, the agency usually has an emergency preparedness plan that generally provides for
    A. _____
    B. _____
    C. _____
    D. _____
    E. _____

77. When giving _____, the rescuer is trying to dislodge a foreign body to relieve choking.

Short Answer

78. Identify the steps of RACE as depicted in the figure.

A. _____
B. _____
C. _____
D. _____

What should you do in these situations related to hazardous chemicals? (Box 13-8) p 177

79. When cleaning up a hazardous chemical, how do you know what equipment to wear?
_____

80. When a spill occurs, what is the correct way to wipe it up? _____
_____

81. The nurse tells you that the person is having an x-ray done in her room.
_____

What measures to prevent or control workplace violence are being used or should be used in these examples? (Box 13-10) p 184

82. What types of jewelry can serve as a weapon?
_____
_____

83. Why is long hair worn up? _____
_____

84. Why are pictures, vases, and other items removed from certain areas?
_____

85. What clothing items should be worn by staff in order to safely manage aggressive persons?
_____

List personal safety practices that apply in these situations (Box 13-11) p 185.

86. What safety practices should be used when parking your car in a parking garage?
_____
_____

87. What items should you keep in the car for safety?
_____
_____

88. Why is a "dry run" important?
_____
_____

89. If you think someone is following you, what should you do? _____
_____

Optional Learning Exercises

90. Identify at least five symptoms that you might observe in a child who has lead poisoning.
A. _____
B. _____
C. _____
D. _____
E. _____

91. Identify at least five symptoms that accompany carbon monoxide poisoning.
A. _____
B. _____
C. _____
D. _____
E. _____

Use the FOCUS ON PRIDE section to complete these statements then use the critical thinking and discussion question to develop your ideas.

92. What can you do ensure the safety of self and other staff when arriving and leaving the agency?
A. _____
B. _____
C. _____
D. _____
E. _____

Critical Thinking and Discussion Question

93. You are caring for an older person who has dementia and occasionally, he or she is combative during morning hygiene. Today, he or she suddenly strikes out at you and bumps his or her arm on a siderail and sustains a laceration.
A. Discuss how you would feel.
B. Explain why it would be important to complete an incident report.

Fill in the Blank: Key Terms

Bed rail   Position change alarm
Gait belt   Transfer belt

1. A device used to support a person who is unsteady or disabled is a _____.

2. A _____ is a device that serves as a guard or barrier along the side of the bed.

3. Another name for a transfer belt is a _____.

4. A physical or electronic device that monitors a person's movement and alerts staff of movement is a _____.

Circle the Best Answer

5. In nursing centers the most common causes of falling are
   A. Confusion and dementia
   B. Weakness and walking problems
   C. Throw rugs and clutter on the floor
   D. Loose or missing hand rails and grab bars

6. Which of these measures would the staff use to prevent falls?
   A. Answer call lights promptly.
   B. Restrain people who have risk factors.
   C. Always keep side rails up.
   D. Wait for position change alarms to sound.

7. A safety measure that can help prevent falls would be to
   A. Have the person wear reading glasses when walking.
   B. Assist the person with bedpan, urinal, commode or bathroom.
   C. Re-arrange the furniture and personal belongings.
   D. Dim lights or limit use of night-lights at night.

8. A position change alarm
   A. Prevents the person from getting out of bed or the chair
   B. Can be turned off and on by the person
   C. Warns when the person is getting up unassisted
   D. Is a substitute for restraints

9. Bed rails
   A. Are used for all older persons
   B. Must be in the person's best interest
   C. Prevent falls and reduce risk for injury
   D. Are never used when giving care

10. Information about when to use the bed rails for a person can be found in the
    A. Safety data sheet
    B. Doctor's orders
    C. Manufacturers' instructions
    D. Care plan

11. Which nursing assistant has correctly used the wheel locks?
    A. Nursing Assistant A transfers the person to the bed and then locks wheels.
    B. Nursing Assistant B locks the wheelchair wheels before transferring the person.
    C. Nursing Assistant C unlocks the wheels on the bed before giving care.
    D. Nursing Assistant D unlocks the stretcher wheels and then transfers the person.

12. What is your primary responsibility in preventing falls during shift change?
    A. Quickly give and get shift report.
    B. Know your role during shift change.
    C. Ask the nurse to provide supervision.
    D. Stay with your assigned patients/residents.

13. Check with the nurse before using a transfer belt when a person
    A. Is unsteady when moving from a chair to the bed
    B. Has diabetes or a heart problem
    C. Has an abdominal wound or incision
    D. Needs help to stand up and walk

14. An elderly person is agitated and upset. Which measure might help to calm him/her?
    A. Bright lights and cheerful music
    B. Warm drink and a back massage
    C. Card game or a jigsaw puzzle
    D. Walk the person up and down the hallways

15. If a bariatric person starts to fall, you should
    A. Grasp the gait belt and pull him close.
    B. Ease the person to the floor.
    C. Quickly move items that could cause injury.
    D. Call for help and hold the person up.

Fill in the Blank

16. Tubs and showers may be made safer if they have _____ surfaces.

17. You raise the bed to give care. If the person uses bed rails and you are working alone, what do you do with the side rails?
    A. _____
    B. _____

18. After you are done giving care, how is the bed positioned? _____ _____.

19. When using position change alarms safely, you should
    A. _____
    B. _____
    C. _____

20. Hand rails in hallways and stairways give support to persons who are _____.

21. Bed wheels are locked when
    A. _____
    B. _____

22. When a transfer belt is applied, you should be able to slide _____ under the belt.

23. Check with the nurse before using a transfer belt if the person has
    A. _____
    B. _____
    C. _____
    D. _____
    E. _____
    F. _____
    G. _____

24. When a person starts to fall, you can protect the person's _____ as you ease the person to the floor.

Optional Learning Exercises

25. What kinds of equipment and safety measures help to make bathrooms and showers safer?
    A. _____
    B. _____
    C. _____
    D. _____
    E. _____

26. Why should floor coverings be one color in areas where older persons are living? _____
    _____

27. What kind of footwear and clothing will help to prevent falls?
    A. Footwear

    _____

    _____

    B. Clothing

    _____

    _____

28. Why is it important to answer call lights promptly?
    _____
    _____

29. If a person does not use bed rails and you are giving care, how do you protect him or her from falling?
    _____

30. Wheels are locked at all times except when
    _____.

31. If a bariatric person starts to fall, you should
    A. _____
    B. _____
    C. _____
    D. _____
    E. _____

32. What is depicted in the figure?
    _____

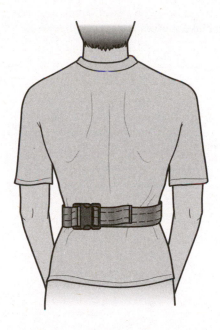

33. According to the documentation below, what safety measures were preformed on 6/16 at 1415?

DATE: 06/16	TIME: 1415
ACTIVITY AND POSITIONING	
☐ Ambulate	☐ Chair
☐ Self	☒ Bed
☒ Assist of 1	☒ Right side
☐ Assist of 2	☐ Left side
☐ Mechanical lift	☐ Back

Turned Mr. Adams from his back to his right side. Placed pillows under his head, against his back, and under his left leg. He stated he was comfortable with needed items in reach (water mug, phone, tissues, urinal, call light). I told him that I will check on him every 15 minutes and to use the call light if he needs anything.

DATE: 06/16	TIME: 1415
SAFETY	
☐ Gait belt	☒ Belongings in reach
☐ Slip-resistant shoes	☒ Bed rails raised
☒ Call light in reach	☐ Bed rails lowered
☒ Bed in low position	☐ Bed/chair alarm

A. _____
B. _____
C. _____
D. _____

Use the FOCUS ON PRIDE section to complete these statements and then use the critical thinking and discussion question to develop your ideas.

34. To show personal and professional responsibility, you do not take short cuts and take time to

    A. _____

    B. _____

    C. _____

    D. _____

    E. _____

35. When assisting a co-worker with a transfer, what information do you need?

    A. _____

    B. _____

    C. _____

    D. _____

    E. _____

    F. _____

Critical Thinking and Discussion Question

36. An elderly resident has frequent episodes of falling, despite everyone's best efforts to follow the care plan. There is no medical reason that warrants the use of restraints. The family is worried and upset. The charge nurse has called a care conference to elicit everyone's ideas about how to decrease falls for this resident. What suggestions could you offer?

15 Restraint Alternatives and Restraints

Fill in the Blank: Key Terms

Chemical restraint   Discipline   Freedom of movement   Physical restraint
Convenience   Enabler   Medical symptom   Remove easily

1. Any action taken to control or manage a person's behavior that requires less effort by the staff is a

   _____.

2. Any manual method or physical or mechanical device, material, or equipment attached to or near the person's body that he or she cannot remove easily is a

   _____.

3. _____ is a term used when a manual method device, material, or equipment can be removed intentionally by the person in the same way that it was applied by the staff.

4. A device that limits freedom of movement but is used to promote independence is an

   _____.

5. Any change in place or position of the body that the person is physically able to control is called

   _____.

6. An indication or characteristic of a physical or psychological condition is a

   _____.

7. A _____ is any drug used for discipline or convenience that is not required to treat medical symptoms.

8. Any action taken by the agency to punish or penalize a patient or resident is _____.

Circle the Best Answer

9. Restraints are used
   A. To control aggression
   B. To treat a medical symptom
   C. To prevent falls
   D. To stop wandering

10. Which person is under chemical restraint?
    A. Person A is given his or her daily blood pressure medication
    B. Person B is wearing a mitt restraint to prevent self-scratching
    C. Person C is given a sleeping medication to prevent wandering
    D. Person D is sitting in a chair that has a position change alarm.

11. Which potential cause for harmful behaviors is the most serious and needs to be reported immediately to the nurse?
    A. Person is scratching at his or her skin and you can see blood.
    B. Person is breathing fast and you can hear wheezing.
    C. Person walks toward the bathroom while struggling to get his or her pants off.
    D. Person seems afraid and is anxiously looking around the room.

12. To meet a person's love and belonging needs, which restraint alternative could the health care staff use?
    A. Encourage family, friends and volunteers to visit
    B. Pad the walls and corners of furniture
    C. Place knob guards on doors that go outside
    D. Make sure that sleep is not interrupted

13. Which person is displaying a physical need that could be relieved with a restraint alternative measure?
    A. Person A likes to talk about memories of his or her friends and family.
    B. Person B is not sure who you are, what time it is or where he or she is at.
    C. Person C often talks to her dead husband and tries to touch him.
    D. Person D is always going to the bathroom to prevent incontinence.

14. Which of these is a type of restraint?
    A. A soft chair with a footstool to elevate the feet
    B. A bed that is in the lowest position
    C. A chair with a tray that prevents the person from rising
    D. A drug that helps a person function at his or her highest level

15. Which risks from restraints are the most common?
    A. Cuts, bruises, and fractures
    B. Death from strangulation
    C. Constipation or incontinence
    D. Depression, anger, and agitation

16. You are assigned to care for a person who is in restraints. You do not know the reason. What should you do?
    A. Refuse to participate in possible false imprisonment.
    B. Politely ask the nurse why the person is restrained.
    C. Ask the person if he gave informed consent.
    D. Follow the care plan for frequency of care.

17. Which method would be considered the least restrictive?
    A. Vest restraint
    B. Elbow splint
    C. Wedge cushion
    D. Jacket restraint

18. In which circumstance might the doctor order use of leather restraints?
    A. Obese person cannot fit into belt restraint.
    B. Strong person is agitated and combative.
    C. Small person has risk for strangulation with vest restraint.
    D. Confused person has fallen out of bed several times.

19. If you do not know how to apply a restraint, you should
    A. Ask the nurse to show you the correct way to apply it.
    B. Tell the nurse that you are unable to apply the restraint.
    C. Watch another nursing assistant apply it to a person.
    D. Apply it to the person by using general safety principles.

20. Which of these is a physical restraint?
    A. Vest
    B. Position change alarm
    C. Gait belt
    D. A sleeping pill

21. When restraining a combative and agitated person, it should be done
    A. Slowly by only one person in a private area
    B. Only after explaining to the person what will be done
    C. With enough staff to complete the task safely and quickly
    D. In a public area so there are witnesses to the person's rights

22. The person who is restrained must be observed every
    A. 5 minutes
    B. 15 minutes
    C. Hour
    D. 2 hours

23. When a person is restrained, at least every 2 hours you should
    A. Look in on the person and make sure he is breathing.
    B. Remove restraints, re-position the person, and meet basic needs.
    C. Make sure the restraints are secure and person cannot get loose.
    D. Change the restraints to a different type or a different position.

24. Wrist restraints are used when a person
    A. Tries to get out of bed without calling for help
    B. Moves the wheelchair without permission
    C. Pulls at tubes used in medical treatments
    D. Slides down or out of a chair easily

25. A roll guard
    A. Is more restrictive than other restraints
    B. Allows the person to turn from side to side
    C. Must be released by the staff
    D. Can be used only in a chair

26. What is the best rationale for using a quick release tie when securing restraints?
    A. Tie can be immediately released if there is an emergency.
    B. Person who is restrained cannot release the tie by themselves.
    C. Ensures that the restraint is snug but not restricting the person
    D. Is quick to tie if the person is struggling while being restrained

27. Elbow restraints are used
    A. To remind adults not to pull on tubes
    B. To prevent children from touching incisions
    C. To limit use of the dominant hand
    D. To prevent injury to the staff by a confused person

28. When applying wrist restraints
    A. Tie the straps to the bed rail.
    B. Tie firm knots in the straps.
    C. Place the restraints over clothing.
    D. Place the soft or foam part toward the skin.

29. If you are using padded mitt restraints, you should
    A. Give the person a hand roll to hold
    B. Pad the mitt with soft material
    C. Make sure the person's hands are clean and dry
    D. Insert the hand into the restraint, palm upward

30. What would you check after applying a belt restraint?
    A. Person's understanding of informed consent
    B. Quick release tie secured to the bedrail
    C. Comfort and good body alignment
    D. Pulses and skin temperature

31. When using a vest restraint in bed
    A. The ties are secured to the bed frame out of the person's reach.
    B. The ties are secured to the bed rail within the person's reach.
    C. The vest crosses in the back and "V" is in the back.
    D. The person can turn over or roll side to side.

32. When you check a person in vest, jacket, or belt restraint, report at once if
    A. The skin is slightly reddened under the restraint
    B. The person needs to urinate or have a bowel movement
    C. The person is not breathing or is having difficulty breathing
    D. You need to re-position the person

Matching

Match the laws and safety guidelines with the correct example.

A. Restraints must protect the person.
B. Restraints require a written doctor's order.
C. The least restrictive method of restraint is used
D. Restraints are used only after other methods fail to protect the person.
E. Unnecessary restraint is false imprisonment.
F. Informed consent is required for restraint use.
G. The manufacturer's instructions are followed.
H. Restraints are applied with enough help to protect the person and staff from injury.
I. Restraints can increase a person's confusion and agitation.
J. Quality of life must be protected.
K. The person is observed at least every 15 minutes or more often as required by the care plan.
L. The restraint is removed, the person repositioned, and basic needs are met at least every 2 hours.

33. _____ Injuries and deaths have occurred from improper restraint and poor observation.

34. _____ A restraint is used only when it is the best safety precaution for the person.

35. _____ You are provided the manufacturer's instructions for applying and securing restraints.

36. _____ Restrained persons need repeated explanations and reassurance.

37. _____ The doctor gives the reason for the restraint, what to use, and how long to use the restraint.

38. _____ Persons in immediate danger of harming themselves or others are restrained quickly.

39. _____ Wedge cushions are used whenever possible, instead of vest or jacket restraints.

40. _____ Restraints are used only for a brief time.

41. _____ If told to apply a restraint, you must clearly understand the need for restraints and the risks.

42. _____ Restraint is removed. Person is ambulated or range-of-motion exercises are performed.

43. _____ The care plan must include measures to protect the person and to prevent the person from harming others.

44. _____ The person must understand the reason for the restraints.

Fill in the Blank

45. Write out the abbreviations.
    A. CMS _____
    B. FDA _____
    C. ID _____
    D. ROM _____
    E. TJC _____

46. When using restraints, what information is reported and recorded?
    A. _____
    B. _____
    C. _____
    D. _____
    E. _____
    F. _____
    G. _____
    H. _____
    I. _____
    J. _____
    K. _____
    L. Complaints to report at once:
       i. _____
       ii. _____
       iii. _____
       iv. _____

47. When you check a mitt, wrist, or ankle restraint every 15 minutes, tell the nurse at once if you observe these signs or symptoms.
    A. _____
    B. _____
    C. _____
    D. _____

48. When you remove the restraints every 2 hours, what are the basic needs that should be met?
    A. _____
    B. _____
    C. _____
    D. _____
    E. _____
    F. _____
    G. _____

49. Persons restrained in a supine position must be monitored constantly because they are at great risk for _____.

50. You should carry scissors with you because in an emergency _____ _____.

51. When you are delegated to apply restraints, what information do you need from the nurse and the care plan?

A. _____

B. _____

C. _____

D. _____

E. _____

F. _____

G. _____

H. _____

I. _____

J. _____

K. _____

L. _____

M. _____

N. _____

Optional Learning Exercises

52. Drugs or drug dosages are restraints if they

A. _____

B. _____

53. How can a geriatric chair be an enabler instead of a restraint?

_____

_____

54. What life-long habits and routines could be included in the nursing care plan as alternatives to restraints?

_____

_____

55. Why would a person in restraints be at risk for dehydration?

_____

56. What is the purpose of padded hip protectors and floor cushions?

_____

_____

Use the FOCUS ON PRIDE section to complete these statements and then use the critical thinking and discussion question to develop your ideas.

57. When a person has restraints in place, your professional responsibilities mean you must

A. _____

B. _____

C. _____

D. _____

E. _____

Critical Thinking and Discussion Question

58. You are assigned to take over the care of a person who has been in restraints for the past 8 hours. As you are checking the person, you find that the person has urinated and defecated in the bed, the skin underneath the restraints is red and a small sore is noted in one area. The person immediately begs you for water and food. What will you do?

16 Preventing Infection

Fill in the Blank: Key Terms

Antibiotic
Antisepsis
Asepsis
Carrier
Clean technique
Contamination
Cross-contamination
Disinfectant

Disinfection
Healthcare-associated
   infection (HAI)
Immunity
Infection
Infection control
Medical asepsis
Microbe

Microorganism
Non-pathogen
Normal flora
Pathogen
Spore
Sterile
Sterile field
Sterile technique

Sterilization
Surgical asepsis
Vaccination
Vaccine
Vector
Vehicle

1. _____ is passing microbes from person to person by contaminated hands, equipment, or supplies.

2. A carrier (animal, insect) that transmits disease is a _____.

3. A _____ is a small living plant or animal seen only with a microscope; a microbe.

4. A human or animal that is a reservoir for microbes but does not have signs and symptoms of infection is a _____.

5. Protection against a certain disease is _____.

6. A preparation containing dead or weakened microbes is a _____.

7. A work area free of all pathogens and non-pathogens is a _____.

8. Practices and procedures that prevent the spread of disease are _____.

9. _____ are the practices used to remove or reduce pathogens and to prevent their spread from one person or place to another person or place; clean technique.

10. An _____ is a drug that kills microbes that cause infections.

11. An _____ is a disease state resulting from the invasion and growth of microorganisms in the body.

12. _____ is the practices that keep equipment and supplies free of all microbes; sterile technique.

13. Any substance that transmits microbes is a _____.

14. The process of destroying pathogens is _____.

15. The processes, procedures, and chemical treatments that kill microbes or prevent them from causing an infection are _____.

16. A _____ is an infection that develops in a person cared for in any setting where health care is given.

17. _____ is being free of disease-producing microbes.

18. Another name for a microorganism is a _____.

19. A _____ is a liquid chemical that can kill many or all pathogens except spores.

20. Medical asepsis is also called _____.

21. The process of becoming unclean is _____.

22. The absence of all microbes is _____.

23. Surgical asepsis is also called _____ _____.

24. A bacterium protected by a hard shell is a _____.

25. _____ are microbes that usually live and grow in a certain area.

26. A microbe that does not usually cause an infection is a _____.

27. _____ is the process of destroying all microbes.

28. A microbe that is harmful and can cause an infection is a _____.

29. The administration of a vaccine to produce immunity against an infectious disease is _____.

Circle the Best Answer

30. Which type of microbe can cause an infection in any body system?
   A. Protozoa   C. Viruses
   B. Fungi   D. Bacteria

31. Rickettsiae are transmitted to humans by
   A. Plants   C. Insect bites
   B. Other humans   D. One-celled animals

32. In order to live and grow, all microbes require
   A. Oxygen   C. A hot environment
   B. A reservoir   D. Plenty of light

33. *Escherichia coli (E. coli)* is considered normal flora in the colon but is a pathogen if it enters the urinary system. How does this knowledge impact the nursing assistant's duties?
    A. Do not sit on the person's bed.
    B. Raw fruits and vegetables are washed.
    C. Attention is given to perineal care.
    D. Hand hygiene is performed.

34. Why are multidrug-resistant organisms (MDROs) a concern?
    A. The medications for MDROs have side effects.
    B. Infections caused by MDROs are hard to treat.
    C. MDROs are easily spread by coughing or sneezing.
    D. Health care staff are more susceptible to MDROs.

35. Which of these is a sign or symptom of infection?
    A. Weight gain
    B. Constipation
    C. Confusion
    D. Increased appetite

36. An older person is at higher risk for infection because of changes in
    A. Diet preferences
    B. The immune system
    C. Activities
    D. Independence

37. Which care measure breaks the chain of infection at the portal of entry?
    A. Giving a person a tissue to cover the mouth while coughing
    B. Asking a visitor with a cold to defer a visit to a vulnerable person
    C. Washing your hands between caring for different people
    D. Helping a vulnerable person preform good oral hygiene

38. Which care measure breaks the chain of infection at the portal of exit?
    A. Putting a mask on a patient who has a cough
    B. Putting a susceptible host in a private room
    C. Helping a person wash his hands before eating
    D. Checking a child, who played outside for ticks

39. Healthcare-associated infections often occur when
    A. Insects are present.
    B. Hand-washing is poor.
    C. Items are left on the floor.
    D. A person is in isolation.

40. Which situation requires surgical asepsis?
    A. Person vomited and you are helping her clean up.
    B. You are assisting the nurse with a sterile dressing change.
    C. You are caring for person who has a MDRO infection.
    D. Person has a urine infection and needs help to the bathroom.

41. To prevent the spread of microbes
    A. Sterilize all equipment.
    B. Use only disposable equipment.
    C. Keep all residents in private rooms.
    D. Wash your hands.

42. When washing hands, you should
    A. Use hot water.
    B. Keep hands lower than the elbows.
    C. Turn off faucets after lathering.
    D. Use a disinfectant.

43. Clean under the fingernails by rubbing your fingers against your palms
    A. Each time you wash your hands
    B. If you have long nails
    C. Only for the first hand-washing of the day
    D. For at least 10 seconds

44. To avoid contaminating your hands, turn off the faucets
    A. After soap is applied
    B. Before drying hands
    C. With clean paper towels
    D. With your elbows

45. In which situation could you use an alcohol-based hand sanitizer to decontaminate your hands?
    A. Your gloves are covered with blood after changing a person's peri-pad.
    B. You finished your lunch and used the restroom before going back to work.
    C. You took a person's blood pressure and the person's skin was intact.
    D. You are preparing a person's meal tray and will assist her to eat.

46. Which common aseptic practice prevents the spread of microbes in long-term care settings?
    A. Clean the tub or shower if the person has a cold.
    B. Use a disinfectant to clean surfaces in the bathroom.
    C. Wash bath and hand towels if they look soiled.
    D. Keep the bathroom door closed to reduce odors.

47. For older persons with dementia, what would you do to protect them from infection?
    A. Gently explain the need for aseptic practices.
    B. Repeatedly tell them to wash their hands.
    C. Frequently check and clean their hands and nails.
    D. Ask the nurse what to do about their hygiene practices.

48. When cleaning contaminated equipment
    A. Wear personal protective equipment (PPE).
    B. Rinse it in hot water first.
    C. Use the clean utility room.
    D. Remove organic materials with a paper towel.

49. Organic material is removed from re-usable items with
    A. Soap and hot water
    B. An autoclave
    C. Cold water rinse
    D. A disinfectant

50. A good, cheap disinfectant to use in the home is
    A. Chlorine bleach
    B. Ammonia
    C. White vinegar solution
    D. Soap and water

51. To sterilize items in the home, boil the items for 10 minutes. Add 1 minute for each 1000 feet of elevation. If the home is at 2000 feet above sea level, how long should you boil the items?
    A. 1 minute
    B. 10 minutes
    C. 12 minutes
    D. 20 minutes

52. What viruses are bloodborne pathogens?
    A. Influenza and pneumococcus
    B. Measles and chicken pox
    C. Human immunodeficiency virus (HIV) and hepatitis B virus (HBV)
    D. Staphylococcus and streptococcus

53. Which item has the greatest risk for transmitting bloodborne pathogens?
    A. Blood pressure cuff
    B. Computer keyboard
    C. Needle used to draw body fluid
    D. Shirt with perspiration stains

54. Staff who are at risk for exposure to bloodborne pathogens receive free training. Which information is included?
    A. Which tasks or circumstances might cause exposure
    B. Which patients/residents have pathogens
    C. How to respond to patients/residents with pathogens
    D. How to differentiate pathogens from non-pathogens

55. The hepatitis B virus (HBV) vaccine
    A. Requires only 1 vaccination
    B. Must be given every year
    C. Involves 3 injections
    D. Is required by law

56. Which nursing assistant is using a work practice control to reduce exposure risks?
    A. Nursing Assistant A discards a broken glass in the bedside trash can.
    B. Nursing Assistant B puts her lunch in the unit's specimen refrigerator.
    C. Nursing Assistant C breaks a contaminated needle and puts it in the sharps box.
    D. Nursing Assistant D wash her hands after removing her gloves.

57. Which situation would prompt you to obtain personal protective equipment?
    A. Person is elderly, and the nurse tells you that a urinary tract infection is suspected.
    B. Person has a health care associated infection and needs help getting out of bed.
    C. Person had an organ transplant last month and needs to be transported to x-ray.
    D. Person has diarrhea and the nurse tells you *Clostridium difficile*— is suspected.

58. Broken glass is cleaned up by
    A. Picking it up carefully with gloved hands
    B. Using a brush and dustpan or tongs
    C. A person trained to remove biohazardous materials
    D. Wiping it up with wet paper towels

59. Which waste would need to be treated and disposed of as regulated waste, in containers that are closable, puncture-resistant, leak-proof and labeled with the BIOHAZARD symbol?
    A. Paper towels used for hand washing
    B. Tissues used for sneezing or coughing
    C. Leftover food and fluids
    D. Contaminated sharps or needles

60. If you are working in a home and need to dispose of sharps, you may need to
    A. Place needles and other sharp items into hard plastic containers.
    B. Rinse off organic materials and flush them down the toilet.
    C. Place them in a plastic bag labeled with the BIOHAZARD symbol.
    D. Discard them with the regular trash each day.

61. You accidentally get stuck in the finger with a used needle. What should you do first?
    A. Report it at once to the supervising nurse.
    B. Wash your hands thoroughly with soap and water.
    C. Save the needle in a puncture proof container for testing.
    D. Observe yourself for any symptoms of the disease.

62. If a sterile item touches a clean item, the sterile item
    A. Is still sterile if there is no visible contamination
    B. Is contaminated and should not be used
    C. Should be handled with sterile gloves
    D. May still be used, but it depends on the purpose

63. When working with a sterile field, you should
    A. Always wear a mask and sterile gloves.
    B. Keep items within your vision and above your waist.
    C. Keep the door open or use a fan for good ventilation.
    D. Wash your hands before and after donning clean gloves.

64. What would you do when arranging the inner package of sterile gloves?
    A. Arrange the gloves so they are in the middle of the package.
    B. Have the fingers pointing toward you.
    C. Have the right glove on the right and the left glove on the left.
    D. Straighten the gloves to remove the cuff.

65. When picking up the first sterile glove
    A. Pick it by the cuff and touch only the inside.
    B. Reach under the cuff with your fingers.
    C. Grasp the edge of the glove with your hand.
    D. Unfold the cuff carefully before picking up the glove.

Fill in the Blank

66. Write out the meaning of the abbreviations.

A. EPA _____

B. GI _____

C. HAI _____

D. HBV _____

E. HIV _____

F. MDRO _____

G. MRSA _____

H. OPIM _____

I. OSHA _____

J. PPE _____

K. VRE _____

L. AIDS _____

M. *C. diff* _____

N. cm _____

Matching

Match the kind of asepsis being used with each example.

A. Medical asepsis (clean technique)

B. Surgical asepsis (sterile technique)

67. _____ An item is placed in an autoclave.

68. _____ Each person has his or her own toothbrush, towel, washcloth, and other personal care items.

69. _____ Hands are washed before preparing food.

70. _____ Contaminated items are boiled in water for at least 10 minutes.

71. _____ Disposable supplies and equipment reduce the spread of infection.

72. _____ Liquid or gas chemicals are used to destroy microbes.

73. _____ Hands are washed every time you use the bathroom.

Match the aseptic measures used to control the related chain of infection with the step in the chain.

A. Reservoir (host)   D. Portal of entry

B. Portal of exit   E. Susceptible host

C. Transmission

74. _____ Provide the person with tissues to use when coughing or sneezing.

75. _____ Make sure linens are dry and wrinkle-free to protect the skin.

76. _____ Use leak-proof plastic bags for soiled tissues, linens, and other materials.

77. _____ Do not take equipment from one person to use on another person

78. _____ Hold equipment and linens away from your uniform.

79. _____ Assist with cleaning or clean the genital area after elimination.

80. _____ Clean from cleanest area to the dirtiest.

81. _____ Label bottles with the person's name and the date it was opened.

82. _____ Follow the care plan to meet the person's nutritional and fluid needs.

83. _____ Make sure drainage tubes are properly connected.

84. _____ Do not use items that are on the floor.

85. _____ Assist the person with cough and deep-breathing exercises as directed.

86. _____ Do not sit on a person's bed. You will pick up microorganisms and transfer them.

Match the practices with the correct principles for surgical asepsis.

A. A sterile item can only touch another sterile item.

B. Sterile items or a sterile field is always kept within your vision and above your waist.

C. Airborne microbes can contaminate sterile items or a sterile field.

D. Fluid flows down, in the direction of gravity.

E. The sterile field is kept dry, unless the area below it is sterile.

F. The edges of a sterile field are contaminated.

G. Honesty is essential to sterile technique.

87. _____ Consider any item as contaminated if it touches a clean item.

88. _____ Wear a mask if you need to talk during the procedure.

89. _____ Place all sterile items inside the 1-inch margin of the sterile field.

90. _____ Do not turn your back on a sterile field.

91. _____ Prevent drafts by closing the door and avoiding extra movements.

92. _____ Avoid spilling and splashing when pouring sterile fluids into sterile containers.

93. _____ If you cannot see an item, then it is contaminated.

94. _____ You report to the nurse that you contaminated an item or a field.

95. _____ Point sterile forceps downward if holding a wet item.

Optional Learning Exercises

96. Compare medical asepsis to surgical asepsis.

A. Medical asepsis is _____

_____

B. Surgical asepsis is

_____

_____

_____

97. Why are hands and forearms kept lower than elbows in hand-washing?

_____

_____

98. Why is lotion applied after hand-washing?

_____

99. When you wear gloves, you protect yourself and the person.
   A. They protect you from _____

   _____.

   B. They protect the person from _____

   _____.

100. What information is included in training about bloodborne pathogens?
   A. _____
   B. _____
   C. _____
   D. _____
   E. _____
   F. _____
   G. _____

101. What are measures for safely handling and using personal protective equipment?
   A. _____
   B. _____
   C. _____
   D. _____
   E. _____
   F. _____
   G. _____
   H. _____

102. If you are asked to assist with a sterile procedure, what information do you need before beginning?
   A. _____
   B. _____
   C. _____
   D. _____
   E. _____
   F. _____

Use the FOCUS ON PRIDE section to complete these statements and then use the critical thinking and discussion question to develop your ideas.

103. You show personal and professional responsibility when you prevent infections by
   A. Practicing good hand hygiene _____ and _____ giving care

104. If delegated care of a person at increased risk for infection, you must
   A. _____
   B. _____
   C. _____
   D. _____
   E. _____
   F. _____
   G. _____
   H. _____
   I. _____

Critical Thinking and Discussion Question

105. You observe another nursing assistant delivering meal trays to bedridden patients. The assistant is kind and prepares the trays by opening containers and cutting up food. However, you notice that the assistant is not offering to assist patients with hand hygiene before they start eating. What could you do or say to improve the quality of care?

Crossword

Fill in the crossword by answering the clues below with the words from this list:

Asepsis   HBV   Parenteral   Sharps
Autoclave   HIV   PPE   Sterilize
Bacteria   Isolation   Protozoa   Viruses
Fungi   OPIM   Rickettsiae

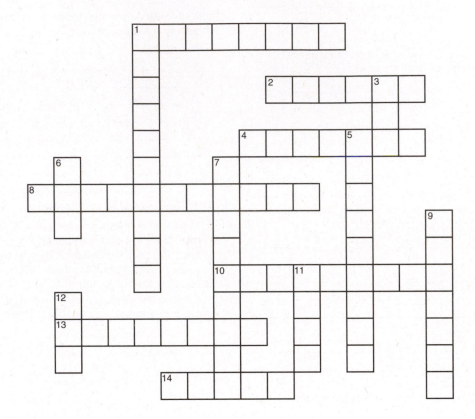

Across

1. One-celled animals; can infect the blood, brain, intestines, and other body areas
2. Any object, such as needles, scalpels, broken glass, and broken capillary tubes, that can penetrate the skin
4. Grows in living cells; causes many diseases such as the common cold, herpes, and hepatitis
8. Found in fleas, lice, ticks, and other insects; spread to humans by insect bites
10. A pressure-steam sterilizer
13. One celled organisms that multiply rapidly; can cause infection in any body system
14. Plant-like organisms that live on other plants or animals; can infect the mouth, vagina, skin, feet, and other body areas

Down

1. Piercing mucous membranes or the skin barrier through such events as needle-sticks, human bites, cuts, and abrasions
3. Clothing or equipment worn by an employee for protection against a hazard
5. The use of physical or chemical procedure designed to destroy all microbial life, including highly resistant bacterial spores
6. Human immunodeficiency virus
7. When a person has a skin infection with drainage, he could be placed in an _____ room.
9. Being free of disease-producing microbes
11. Other potentially infectious materials; human body fluids, any tissue or organ from a human, HIV-containing cell or tissue cultures
12. Hepatitis B virus

Fill in the Blank: Key Terms

Biohazardous waste   Communicable disease   Contagious disease   Personal protective equipment (PPE)

1. A communicable disease is also called a
   _____

2. A _____ is a disease caused by pathogens that spread easily; contagious disease.

3. _____ are items contaminated with blood, body fluids, secretions, and excretions that may be harmful to others.

4. The clothing or equipment worn by the staff for protection against a hazard is _____
   _____

Circle the Best Answer

5. Isolation precautions are used
   A. To reduce infection for all patients
   B. To guide care for surgical patients
   C. To protect older persons from self-harm
   D. To prevent the spread of communicable diseases

6. Standard Precautions are used
   A. For a person with a respiratory infection
   B. For a person with a wound infection
   C. For a person with tuberculosis
   D. For any person whenever care is given

7. Gloves worn in Standard Precautions
   A. Are worn for all tasks for the same person
   B. Can be worn until they tear or are punctured
   C. Are changed before caring for another person
   D. Are worn only if the person has an infection

8. When you are working in a room with isolation precautions, you use clean and dry paper towels to
   A. Handle clean items.
   B. Turn faucets on and off.
   C. Give personal care.
   D. Wipe up spills on the floor.

9. Wash your hands
   A. After removing gloves
   B. After donning a gown
   C. If PPE is not available
   D. As a substitute for gloving

10. If you are allergic to latex gloves, you should
    A. Wash your hands after removing the gloves.
    B. Wear gloves only for heavy contamination.
    C. Wear latex-free gloves.
    D. Never wear any gloves.

11. Which principle do you need to remember about use of gloves when giving care?
    A. The inside of the gloves is always considered contaminated.
    B. Changing gloves is not necessary if caring for the same person.
    C. You may need more than one pair of gloves for a task.
    D. Gloves are easier to put on when your hands are slightly damp.

12. When removing gloves
    A. Make sure that glove touches only glove.
    B. Pull the gloves off by the fingers.
    C. Reach inside the glove with the gloved hand to pull it off.
    D. Hold the discarded gloves tightly in your ungloved hand.

13. When you wear a gown for isolation precautions, the contaminated areas are
    A. The ties at the neck and waist
    B. The gown front and sleeves
    C. The gown back and sleeves
    D. Only the areas that touch the patient

14. When you remove gown and gloves worn for isolation precautions, what step is done first?
    A. Untie the neck and waist strings.
    B. Remove and discard your gloves.
    C. Turn the gown inside out as it is removed.
    D. Pull the gown down from each shoulder toward the same hand.

15. For which circumstance would it be most important to make sure that a box of tissues is within the person's reach?
    A. Person has a wound infection and is on contact precautions.
    B. Person has respiratory symptoms and is on droplet precautions.
    C. Person had knee surgery and is on standard precautions.
    D. Person has measles and is on airborne precautions.

16. When removing a mask, only the ties or elastic bands are touched because
    A. The front of the mask is contaminated.
    B. The front of the mask is sterile.
    C. Your gloves are contaminated.
    D. Your hands are contaminated.

17. When donning a gown, which of these is done first?
    A. Tie the strings at the back of the neck.
    B. Tie the waist strings at the back.
    C. Put on the gloves.
    D. Overlap the back of the gown.

18. When removing personal protective equipment, which of these is done *first*?
    A. Remove the face mask.
    B. Remove and discard the gloves.
    C. Remove the gown.
    D. Untie the waist strings of the gown.

19. For which circumstance would you anticipate the need to wear an eye shield?
    A. You are assisting a doctor to irrigate a contaminated wound.
    B. You are helping a person in contact precautions to walk around the room.
    C. You are coaching a person with mild dementia to put on his clothes.
    D. You are taking the vital signs of a person who needs standard precautions.

20. When contaminated items are sent to the laundry or trash collection, bags are
    A. Transparent so materials are visible.
    B. Labeled as "contaminated."
    C. Always double-bagged.
    D. Labeled with the BIOHAZARD symbol.

21. Which nursing assistant has correctly collected a specimen from a person who is on transmission-based precautions?
    A. Nursing assistant A avoids contaminating the outside of the specimen container and the biohazard specimen bag.
    B. Nursing assistant B uses a paper towel to place the specimen inside the container, seals container and puts it outside the room.
    C. Nursing assistant C puts the specimen inside the biohazard specimen bag and puts the bag in the specimen container.
    D. Nursing assistant D double bags the specimen and applies the warning labels according to agency policy.

22. You are asked to transport a person to the x-ray department; the person is currently in Transmission-Based Precautions. Which question is the most important to ask the nurse?
    A. How long does the person have to stay in x-ray?
    B. What kind of infection does the person have?
    C. What type of PPE does the person need to wear?
    D. Does the stretcher need to be disinfected before use?

23. When a person is in isolation, you can help to meet love, belonging, and self-esteem needs when you
    A. Talk a lot while you are giving care.
    B. Open the door so the person can see others.
    C. Stop by often and say "hello" from the doorway.
    D. Explain why people are avoiding the room.

24. When a child is in isolation, it may be helpful if
    A. Favorite toys or blankets are brought from home.
    B. PPE is put on before entering the room.
    C. The child can hold and touch PPE (e.g. mask, eyewear).
    D. You avoid using PPE so the child is not scared.

25. You can help a person with poor vision, confusion, or dementia to tolerate isolation by
    A. Letting the person touch your face and hold your gloved hand
    B. Keeping the door open so they can see people in the hall
    C. Letting the person see your face before putting on PPE
    D. Not wearing a mask or face shield when in the room

26. A person with measles, chicken pox, or tuberculosis would be isolated with
    A. Contact precautions
    B. Bloodborne Pathogen Standard
    C. Droplet precautions
    D. Airborne precautions

27. When the person has airborne precautions, you do not need to wear a mask when
    A. The person no longer has skin lesions.
    B. You are transporting the person.
    C. The person is not sneezing or coughing.
    D. The skin lesions are covered.

28. For contact precautions, gloves are worn
    A. Upon entering the room or care setting
    B. Only if the skin has open lesions
    C. If you must touch the person
    D. When the person has symptoms

29. Which transmission-based precaution is specific to caring for a person who has tuberculosis?
    A. Placing reusable dishes and drinking vessels in a leak proof bag
    B. Removing the approved respirator after leaving the room
    C. Washing hands after removing all PPE and before leaving the room
    D. Wearing gloves to touch the person's intact skin or items near the person

Fill in the Blank

30. Standard Precautions are used to prevent the spread of infection from:
    A. _____
       _____
    B. _____
       _____
    C. _____
       _____
    D. _____
       _____

31. What is commonly needed in the set up for an isolation room?

    A. _____

    _____

    B. _____

    _____

    C. _____

    _____

    D. _____

    _____

32. According to the CDC, what is the correct order for donning PPE?

    A. _____

    _____

    B. _____

    _____

    C. _____

    _____

    D. _____

    _____

Labeling

33. The figure shows how to remove gloves. List the steps of the procedure shown in each drawing.

    A. _____
    B. _____
    C. _____
    D. _____

Optional Learning Exercises

34. When are the following worn for Standard Precautions?

    A. Gloves _____

    _____

    B. Masks, eye protection, and face shield _____

    _____

35. If a person has measles and you are susceptible, what should you do? _____

36. If a person in airborne precautions must leave the room, the person must wear a _____

    _____

37. Why is a gown turned inside out as you remove it?

    _____

38. Why is a moist mask or gown changed?

    _____

39. What basic needs may not be met when a person is in isolation? _____

Use the FOCUS ON PRIDE section to complete these statements and then use the critical thinking and discussion questions to develop your ideas.

40. What can you do to help the person on Transmission-Based Precautions from feeling lonely and isolated?

    A. _____
    B. _____
    C. _____
    D. _____
    E. _____
    F. _____
    G. _____
    H. _____

Critical Thinking and Discussion Question

41. Caring for people who need Transmission-Based Precautions is very time consuming. Consider the needs and circumstances of the four people and then discuss the following questions.

    Person A needs contact precautions and is likely to require frequent linen changes and help with perineal hygiene during the shift for infectious diarrhea

    Person B needs standard precautions and requires assistance to ambulate in the hallway several times during the shift

    Person C needs airborne precautions and is self-care, but is unable to leave the room for meals, socialization or any other activities.

    Person D needs standard precautions and must be transported in the early am for a procedure that will take approximately 6 hours.

    A. Which person is going to require the most time to complete care?

    B. Which person is going to require the least amount of your time?

    C. Discuss how you would organize and accomplish care for these four people.

Fill in the Blank: Key Terms

Base of support
Body alignment
Body mechanics
Dorsal recumbent position

Ergonomics
Fowler's position
Lateral position
Posture

Prone position
Semi-prone side position
Side-lying position
Sims' position

Supine position
Musculo-skeletal disorders

1. Another name for the lateral position is

   _____.

2. The way in which the head, trunk, arms, and legs align with one another is _____ or posture.

3. The _____ is also called the side-lying position.

4. The _____ is the same as the back-lying or supine position.

5. The area on which an object rests is the

   _____.

6. _____ are injuries and disorders of the muscles, tendons, ligaments, joints, and cartilage.

7. _____ is a left side-lying position in which the upper leg is sharply flexed so that it is not on the lower leg and the lower arm is behind the person.

8. A semi-sitting position with the head of the bed elevated 45 to 60 degrees is _____.

9. Lying on the abdomen with the head turned to one side is _____.

10. _____ is using the body in an efficient and careful way.

11. The back-lying or dorsal recumbent position is also called the _____.

12. _____ or body alignment is the way in which body parts are aligned with one another.

13. _____ is the science of designing the job to fit the worker.

14. Another name for the Sims' position is

    _____.

Circle the Best Answer

15. What is the best rationale for using good body mechanics?
    A. Complies with facility policies
    B. Strengthens the back muscles
    C. Reduces the risk of injury
    D. Reduces muscle fatigue

16. For a wider base of support and balance
    A. Keep your knees slightly bent.
    B. Align head, trunk, arms, and legs.
    C. Stand with your feet apart.
    D. Maintain your physical condition.

17. When you bend your knees and squat to lift a heavy object, you are
    A. Using good body alignment
    B. Using good ergonomics
    C. Using your back muscles
    D. Using good body mechanics

18. Which nursing assistant is using the rules of good body mechanics to move a heavy object?
    A. Nursing Assistant A pushes, slides, or pulls the object.
    B. Nursing Assistant B reaches upwards to grab the object.
    C. Nursing Assistant bends forward to lift the object.
    D. Nursing Assistant D works alone to control the object.

19. Which factor creates the biggest risk for musculo-skeletal disorders (MSDs)?
    A. Worker does not exercise regularly or eat healthy foods.
    B. Worker is small-framed and lacks upper body strength.
    C. Worker uses force or repetitive action when moving objects.
    D. Worker has not memorized the rules of good body mechanics.

20. If you have pain when standing or rising from a seated position, you
    A. May have a back injury
    B. Are using poor body mechanics
    C. Have worked too many hours
    D. Should exercise more

21. According to the Occupational Safety and Health Administration (OSHA), which of these is a factor that can lead to MSDs?
    A. Resting between repetitive tasks
    B. Getting help to lift a heavy object
    C. Anticipating sudden movements
    D. Lifting with forceful movement

22. Which of these activities will help to prevent back injury?
    A. Reach across the bed to give care.
    B. Bend at the waist to pick up an object.
    C. Lift an object above your shoulder.
    D. Carry objects close to your body.

23. Regular position changes and good alignment
    A. Can substitute for exercise
    B. Promote comfort and well-being
    C. Interrupt rest and sleep
    D. Limit full range of motion

24. A resident who depends on the nursing team for position changes needs to be positioned
    A. At least every 2 hours   C. Every 15 minutes
    B. Once an hour   D. Once a shift

25. Linens need to be clean, dry, and wrinkle-free to help prevent
    A. Pressure injuries
    B. Contractures
    C. Breathing problems
    D. Frequent repositioning

26. Persons with heart and respiratory disorders usually can breathe more easily in the
    A. Fowler's position
    B. Semi-Fowler's position
    C. Supine position
    D. Prone position

27. Most older persons have limited range of motion in their necks and so do not tolerate the
    A. Lateral position
    B. Semi-Fowler's position
    C. Fowler's position
    D. Prone position

28. When positioning a person in the supine position, the nurse may ask you to place a pillow under the person's lower legs to
    A. Improve the circulation to feet.
    B. Assist the person to breathe easier.
    C. Prevent heels from rubbing on sheets.
    D. Prevent swelling of the legs and feet.

29. A small pillow is positioned against the person's back in the
    A. Lateral position   C. Supine position
    B. Prone position   D. Semi-Fowler's position

30. When a person cannot keep his or her upper body erect in a chair
    A. A vest restraint may be used.
    B. Postural supports help maintain alignment.
    C. A geriatric chair with a tray provides support.
    D. A belt restraint can be applied.

31. In the chair position, a pillow is not used
    A. To position paralyzed arms
    B. To support the feet
    C. Under the upper arms or hands
    D. Behind the back if restraints are used

Fill in the Blank

32. Write out the abbreviations.
    A. MSD _____
    B. OSHA _____

33. What are the four sets of strong, large muscles that are used to lift and move heavy objects?
    A. _____
    B. _____
    C. _____
    D. _____

34. Identify four friction-reducing devices that you could use to move a person in bed.
    A. _____
    B. _____
    C. _____
    D. _____

35. Describe these risk factors for musculo-skeletal disorders (MSDs) in nursing centers.
    A. Force _____
    B. Repeating action _____
    C. Awkward postures _____
    D. Heavy lifting _____

36. Early signs and symptoms of MSDs are
    _____.

37. Name 17 nursing tasks that are known to be high risk for MSDs.
    A. _____
    B. _____
    C. _____
    D. _____
    E. _____
    F. _____
    G. _____
    H. _____
    I. _____
    J. _____
    K. _____
    L. _____
    M. _____
    N. _____
    O. _____
    P. _____
    Q. _____

38. Instructions to re-position a person are received from the _____ and the _____.

39. If you are delegated the task of positioning the person, which 11 items of information do you need?
    A. _____
    B. _____
    C. _____
    D. _____
    E. _____
    F. _____
    G. _____
    H. _____
    I. _____
    J. _____
    K. _____

In the following questions, list the measures needed for good alignment in each position.

40. What measures are needed for good alignment when the person is in Fowler's position?

A. _____

B. _____

C. _____

41. For supine position?

A. _____

B. _____

C. _____

42. For prone position?

A. _____

B. _____

C. _____

43. For lateral position?

A. _____

B. _____

C. _____

D. _____

E. _____

F. _____

44. For Sims' position?

A. _____

B. _____

C. _____

D. _____

45. For chair position?

A. _____

B. _____

C. _____

Labeling

46. Label the positions in each of the drawings.

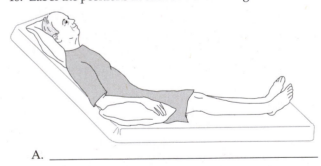

A. _____

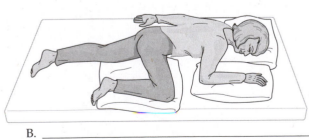

B. _____

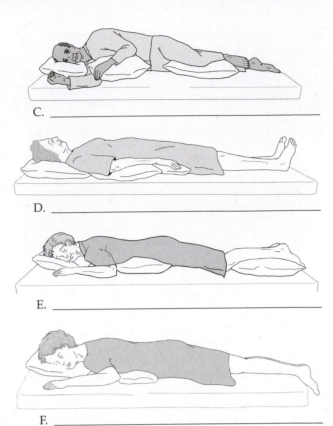

C. _____

D. _____

E. _____

F. _____

Optional Learning Exercises

47. According to OSHA, there are four risk factors (Force, Repeating action, Awkward postures, Heavy lifting) that contribute to MSD. Read the examples and identify the risk factor that could cause MSD in each scenario.

A. The nursing assistant does not raise the level of the bed when changing linens.

_____

B. While you are walking with Mr. Smith, he slips and starts to fall. _____

C. Mrs. Tippett often slides down in bed and always looks uncomfortable. _____

D. You assist Mrs. Miller, who is a large and heavy woman, to use the toilet in her small bathroom.

_____

E. Mr. Thomas is confused and incontinent and you frequently clean and reposition him.

_____

F. You lean across the bed to hold the person while the nurse washes his back.

_____

48. Regular position changes and good alignment promote

A. _____

B. _____

C. _____

D. _____

and position changes and alignment prevent

E. _____

F. _____

49. When you properly position and re-position a person, you help prevent a lack of joint or mobility or

_____.

Use the FOCUS ON PRIDE section to complete these statements then use the critical thinking and discussion question to develop your ideas.

50. You take responsibility for protecting yourself from harm when moving patients. What decisions do you make about protecting yourself?

A. _____

B. _____

C. _____

D. _____

E. _____

51. How can you promote comfort, independence, and social interaction for a person you are caring for?

A. _____

B. _____

Critical Thinking and Discussion Question

52. Are you a strong young male? A slender petite female? Are you older with a history of back problems? Are you stronger than you appear? Consider your own stature, strength and physical condition and discuss how you will protect yourself and your co-workers from sustaining MSDs.

19 Moving the Person

Fill in the Blank: Key Terms

Bed mobility   Logrolling
Friction   Shearing

1. Turning the person as a unit, in alignment, with one motion is _____.

2. _____ occurs when skin sticks to a surface and muscles slide in the direction the body is moving.

3. How a person moves to and from a lying position, turns from side to side, and re-positions in bed or other furniture is _____.

4. The rubbing of one surface against another is

_____.

Circle the Best Answer

5. An elderly person with dementia is grabbing and hitting while you and a co-worker are trying to turn him. What could you do to distract him?
   A. You firmly hold his hands and arms, while the co-worker turns him.
   B. You talk very cheerfully and ask him questions about his family.
   C. You give him something soft to hold, such as a washcloth or stuffed animal.
   D. You turn up the volume on the television and instruct him to watch the program.

6. **To prevent injuries when moving older persons**
   A. Do not move the person unless it is necessary.
   B. Grasp a body part where there is no pain or injury.
   C. Allow the person to move himself or herself.
   D. Provide for comfort and avoid causing pain.

7. When moving a person up in bed, prevent hitting the head on the head-board by
   A. Placing the person's hand against the head-board
   B. Placing the pillow upright against the head-board
   C. Placing your hand on the person's head
   D. Asking the person to bend his or her neck forward

8. When moving residents, it is best if you move the person
   A. Only if he/she is very small
   B. With at least 2 staff members
   C. Using a mechanical lift
   D. Only if they totally dependent

9. To prevent work-related injuries, OSHA recommends that
   A. Manual lifting be minimized or eliminated when possible
   B. Manual lifting be used at all times with 3 staff members
   C. You never lift any person or object alone
   D. You always use mechanical lifts for any lifting

10. Which term describes the level of help that is needed if a person requires help to turn, re-position, sit up, and move in bed?
    A. Total dependence
    B. Extensive assistance
    C. Limited assistance
    D. Supervision

11. Why is the bed raised before moving the person?
    A. It prevents the person from falling out of bed.
    B. It reduces friction and shearing.
    C. It prevents pulling on drainage tubes.
    D. It reduces bending and reaching for staff members.

12. How can you reduce friction and shearing?
    A. Raise the head of the bed before moving the person.
    B. Roll the person or use a lift sheet.
    C. Grasp the person under the arms and pull him up.
    D. Massage the skin before and after moving.

13. If a person with dementia resists being moved, you should
    A. Move the person by yourself very slowly.
    B. Proceed slowly and use a calm voice.
    C. Let the person alone and do not re-position.
    D. Firmly tell the person that moving is necessary.

14. When you are delegated to move a person in bed, what do you need to know?
    A. The person's level of knowledge about assist devices
    B. Previous work-related injuries of other staff members
    C. The person's medical history and diagnosis
    D. Limits in the person's ability to move or be repositioned

15. When raising an older person's head and shoulders
    A. It is best to have help to prevent pain and injury.
    B. A mechanical lift should be used.
    C. You first try to accomplish this yourself.
    D. A transfer belt will be needed.

16. To correctly raise the head and shoulders
    A. Both of your hands are placed under the person's back as you move forward.
    B. The person puts his/her near arm behind your near arm and your shoulder.
    C. Use a lift sheet to raise or drag the person upwards towards the head of the bed.
    D. Your free arm rests on the edge of the bed, as you brace and pull up.

17. You may move a person up in bed by yourself if the
    A. Person can assist using a trapeze.
    B. Rest of the staff is busy and cannot help.
    C. Nurse tells you to use a lift sheet or slide sheet.
    D. Nurse tells you to move the person alone.

18. What is the position of the bed when you are moving a person up in bed?
    A. Fowler's if the person is having a hard time breathing
    B. Flat, even if the person can only tolerate it temporarily
    C. As flat as possible for the person's condition
    D. Semi-Fowler's if the person can help by pushing with feet

19. The person is generally moved
    A. On the "count of 3"
    B. On the "count of 2"
    C. When the person says "go"
    D. When the workers are in position

20. An assist device such as a lift sheet can be used for
    A. A person who can use the trapeze to help
    B. Any person regardless of size
    C. A person who is totally dependent
    D. Moving a person when you are working alone

21. How is the lift (or turning) sheet positioned?
    A. Under the head and shoulders
    B. Under the hips and buttocks
    C. From the head to above the knees or lower
    D. From the hips to below the knees

22. When using a lift sheet as an assist device, how do the workers hold the device?
    A. Hold the sheet near the shoulders and hips.
    B. Grasp the sheet at the four corners.
    C. Hold and pull one side of the sheet at a time.
    D. Grasp the sheet only at the top edge.

23. A person is moved to the side of the bed before turning because
    A. Otherwise, after turning, the person lies on the side of the bed.
    B. It makes it easier to turn the person if he/she is closer to you.
    C. It prevents injury and reduces the need for siderails.
    D. It prevents friction and reduces shearing.

24. When using a drawsheet to move a person to the side of the bed, support the person's
    A. Back
    B. Knees
    C. Head
    D. Hips

25. After the person is turned
    A. Put up all the siderails.
    B. Position him or her in good body alignment.
    C. Elevate the head of the bed.
    D. Raise the bed to its highest position.

26. When delegated to turn a person, which information do you need from the nurse and the care plan?
    A. Whether the person has given informed consent
    B. Which staff helped when the person was last turned
    C. Whether the doctor has ordered turning
    D. What supportive devices are needed for positioning

27. When a person is turned, musculo-skeletal injuries, skin breakdown, and pressure injuries could occur if a person is not in
    A. A special bed
    B. Good body alignment
    C. A supine position
    D. The middle of the bed

28. How do you decide whether to turn the person toward you or away from you?
    A. Check the doctor's order.
    B. It depends on the person's condition and the situation.
    C. Use the method that helps you to maintain your balance.
    D. Ask the person which way is best.

29. Why do you need 2 or 3 staff members to logroll a person?
    A. A person who is being logrolled is usually in pain.
    B. It is important to keep the spine straight and in alignment.
    C. The person is probably totally dependent and needs extra help.
    D. No assist devices are used when the logroll method is used.

30. When preparing to logroll a person, place a pillow
    A. At the head of the bed
    B. Between the knees
    C. Under the head
    D. Under the shoulders

31. What information do you need before dangling a person?
    A. The person's medical diagnosis
    B. When the person ate last
    C. The person's areas of weakness
    D. What kind of medication the person takes

32. What should you do if a person becomes faint or dizzy while dangling?
    A. Lay the person down and tell the nurse.
    B. Report this at the end of the shift.
    C. Tell the person to take deep breaths.
    D. Have the person move the legs around in circles.

33. When preparing to dangle a person, the head of the bed should be
    A. Flat
    B. Slightly raised
    C. In a sitting position
    D. Comfortable for the person

34. Which person needs to be re-positioned while sitting in a wheelchair?
    A. The person is in good alignment, but is motioning for you.
    B. The person's back and buttocks are against the back of the chair.
    C. The person has slid downwards and cannot move himself.
    D. The person is bored after sitting in the same position all day.

Fill in the Blank

35. To prevent injuries in older persons with fragile bones and joints, what safety measures would be used?
    A. _____
    B. _____
    C. _____
    D. _____
    E. _____
    F. _____

36. To promote mental comfort when handling, moving, or transferring the person, you should
    A. _____
    B. _____

37. To prevent work-related injuries when moving a person, what should be done?
    A. _____
    B. _____
    C. _____
    D. _____

38. Explain how a person is moved for each level of assistance.
    A. Independent

    _____

    B. Supervision

    _____

    C. Limited Assistance

    _____

    D. Extensive Assistance

    _____

    E. Total Dependence

    _____

39. When you move a person in bed, report and record the following:
    A. _____
    B. _____
    C. _____
    D. _____
    E. _____

40. When you move a person, you move the body in segments. List the three steps in the correct order.
    A. _____
    B. _____
    C. _____

41. Friction and shearing can be reduced when moving a person in bed by
    A. _____
    B. _____

42. When moving a person up in bed and the person can assist, ask the person to
    A. Grasp the _____
    B. Flex _____
    C. Move on the count of _____

43. Identify five assist devices, other than mechanical lifts, that are used to move persons to the side of the bed.
    A. _____
    B. _____
    C. _____
    D. _____
    E. _____

44. Before turning and re-positioning a person, what information do you need from the nurse and care plan?
    A. _____
    B. _____
    C. _____
    D. _____
    E. _____
    F. _____
    G. _____
    H. _____

45. What should you report and record after you turn or move a person?
    A. _____
    B. _____
    C. _____
    D. _____
    E. _____

46. After turning and re-positioning a person, it is common to place a small pillow under the
    _____.

47. When a person is logrolled, the spine is
    _____.

48. Logrolling is used to turn these persons.
    A. _____
    B. _____
    C. _____
    D. _____

49. When a person is dangling, the circulation can be stimulated by having the person move
    _____.

50. What observations should be reported and recorded after dangling a person?
    A. _____
    B. _____
    C. _____
    D. _____
    E. _____
    F. _____
    G. _____

51. While you are helping a person to dangling, she becomes pale and reports dizziness and chest pain. What should you do?

_____

52. When re-positioning a person in a chair or wheelchair, you *do not* _____.

Optional Learning Exercises

53. When planning to move a person, why is it important to know the person's height and weight, physical abilities, and cognitive function?

_____

54. If you need to move a person with dementia, he or she may resist because he or she may not _____ _____. What care measures will help you give safe care?
    A. _____
    B. _____
    C. _____

55. It is safe to move a person up in bed alone only if
    A. _____
    B. _____
    C. _____
    D. _____
    E. _____
    F. _____
    G. _____

56. What three features must an under-pad or draw sheet have to accomplish a safe lift?
    A. _____
    B. _____
    C. _____

57. How does moving a person to the side of the bed avoid work-related injuries for you? _____

58. When you are delegated to turn a person, how will you know whether to turn them alone, with help, or by using logrolling?

_____

59. When you turn a person and re-position them, what must be done to the bed level before you leave the room? _____

60. When two staff members are logrolling a person without a turning sheet, where does each person place the hands? (See Figure 19-11, p 281)
    A. Staff at head _____
    B. Staff at legs _____

61. Why should a person dangle for 1 to 5 minutes before walking or transferring? _____

62. What simple hygiene measures can be performed while the person is dangling? _____ _____ In addition to refreshing the person, what is another benefit this activity will provide? _____

63. Refer to the charting sample below and answer the following questions:

DATE: 09/10	TIME: 1530
ACTIVITY AND POSITIONING	

☒ Dangle	☐ Chair
☐ Self	☒ Bed
☒ Assist of 1	☒ Right side
☐ Assist of 2	☐ Left side
☐ Mechanical lift	☐ Back

Assisted to sit on the side of the bed. Active leg exercises performed. Tolerated procedure without complaints of pain or discomfort. Denied dizziness. Assisted to lie down on right side after 5 minutes.

FLOWSHEET

Date / Time	09/10 1530	09/15
Temperature	98.4	
Pulse	72	
Respiration	18	
Blood Pressure	118/76	
ACTIVITY:	DANGLE	CH
POSITIONING:	R SIDE	
SAFETY:	BED	C
	CALL	

DATE: 09/10	TIME: 1530
SAFETY	

☐ Gait belt	☒ Belongings in reach
☐ Slip-resistant shoes	☒ Bed rails raised
☒ Call light in reach	☐ Bed rails lowered
☒ Bed in low position	☐ Bed/chair alarm

A. What activity and positioning were performed on 9/10 at 1530?

B. How did the person tolerate the activity?

_____

C. How long did the activity last?

_____

Use the FOCUS ON PRIDE section to complete these statements and then use the critical thinking and discussion question to develop your ideas.

64. When moving a person, you promote pride and independence when you

   A. _____

   B. _____

   C. _____

   D. _____

Critical Thinking and Discussion Question

65. You are newly hired at a long-term care center. You notice that the other nursing assistants are always pairing up to help each other when moving and turning people. You can get help if you ask around, but no one seems overly eager to offer you help, and you feel a little awkward and left out. What could you do?

Fill in the Blank: Key Terms

Lateral transfer   Transfer
Pivot

1. _____ is how a person moves to and from a surface.

2. When a person moves between 2 horizontal surfaces, it is a _____.

3. To turn one's body from a set standing position is to _____.

Circle the Best Answer

4. If an agency has a lift team, they will
   A. Perform all lifts in the agency.
   B. Only do manual lifts.
   C. Carry out scheduled lifts.
   D. Only assist when you ask.

5. When preparing to transfer a person, you should
   A. Arrange the furniture for a safe transfer.
   B. Keep furniture in the position the resident likes.
   C. Remove all furniture from the room.
   D. Shift all furniture away from the door.

6. The person being transferred should wear slip-resistant footwear to
   A. Protect the person from falls
   B. Comply with agency policy
   C. Promote the person's dignity
   D. Keep the feet warm

7. Lock the bed, wheelchair, or assist device wheels when transferring to
   A. Prevent the staff from moving the bed or the device.
   B. Prevent damage to the bed or other equipment.
   C. Prevent the bed and the device from moving.
   D. Prevent the person from moving the equipment.

8. When a person is transferring to a chair or wheelchair, help the person out of bed on
   A. The right side of the bed
   B. His or her strong side
   C. His or her weak side
   D. The side closest to the door

9. If not using a mechanical lift, which of these is the preferred method for chair or wheelchair transfers?
   A. Use a gait/transfer belt.
   B. Ask the person to grasp your neck.
   C. Perform a two-person manual lift.
   D. Have the person use a trapeze.

10. When a person is seated in a wheelchair, you can increase the person's comfort by
    A. Placing pillows around the person
    B. Making sure nothing covers the vinyl seat and back
    C. Covering the back and seat with a folded bath blanket
    D. Removing any cushions or positioning devices

11. When you transfer a person, the nurse may ask you to report the _____ before and after the transfer.
    A. Blood pressure, pulse and respirations
    B. Height and weight
    C. Muscular strength and balance
    D. Level of confusion and ability to cooperate

12. When using a transfer belt, you can prevent the person from sliding or falling by
    A. Bracing your knees against the person's knees
    B. Holding the person close to your body
    C. Having another staff member hold the person's feet in place
    D. Grasping the belt in the back to give you better balance

13. A transfer belt must be used for a transfer unless
    A. The doctor has written an order that states no belt is needed.
    B. You are directed by the nurse and care plan to transfer without a belt.
    C. The person asks you not to use the belt.
    D. You feel safer moving the person without the belt.

14. When you are transferring a person back to bed from a chair or wheelchair, the person should be positioned
    A. With the weak side near the bed
    B. With the strong side near the bed
    C. In the same position as getting out of bed
    D. At the foot of the bed, facing the head of the bed

15. When moving a person from a bed to a stretcher, it is most important that you prevent
    A. The person from becoming chilled
    B. Friction and shearing injuries
    C. The person from assisting with the move
    D. Leaving wrinkles in the linens

16. When moving a person to a stretcher, you should
    A. Position the stretcher to an equal level of the assist device
    B. Position the stretcher so it is 2 inches lower than the bed
    C. Position the stretcher so it is ½ inch lower than the bed
    D. Position the stretcher so it is 1 inch higher than the bed

17. A mechanical lift is used
    A. For all persons regardless of physical abilities
    B. For persons who are too heavy for the staff to move
    C. When staff members prefer mechanical to manual lifting
    D. Only when ordered by the doctor

18. You have been delegated to transfer a person using the mechanical sling lift. Which question would you ask that is specific to the use this equipment?
    A. "Is person strong enough to stand and pivot?"
    B. "Which type of sling should I use for this person?"
    C. "How many staff members are needed to use the lift?"
    D. "Which type of friction reducing device should I use?"

19. As a person is lifted in the sling of the mechanical lift, the person
    A. Holds the swivel bar
    B. Holds the straps or chains
    C. Crosses the arms across the chest
    D. Holds your hand

20. When transferring a person from a wheelchair to the toilet
    A. The toilet should have a raised seat.
    B. The toilet seat should be removed.
    C. The wheelchair should be removed.
    D. The wheelchair should be unlocked.

21. A slide board may be used to transfer a person from a wheelchair to a toilet if
    A. The person can stand and pivot.
    B. There is room to position the wheelchair next to the toilet.
    C. The wheelchair can be positioned in front of the toilet.
    D. The person has lower body strength.

22. When moving a person who weighs more than 200 pounds to a stretcher
    A. Use a lateral sliding aid and 2 staff members.
    B. Use a mechanical ceiling lift and 3 staff members.
    C. Use a friction-reducing device and 1 staff member.
    D. Use a drawsheet or a turning pad and 2 staff members.

Fill in the Blank

23. A person can transfer from the bed to the chair with a stand and pivot transfer if
    A. _____
    B. _____
    C. _____

24. During a chair or wheelchair transfer, the person must not put his or her arms around your neck because
    _____ .

25. Locked wheelchairs may be considered restraints if the person _____ .

26. When using a transfer belt to transfer a person to a chair or wheelchair, grasp the belt at _____ and from _____ .

27. If you transfer a person to a chair without a transfer belt, place your hands _____ and around the person's _____ .

28. What is the purpose of each type of sling?
    A. Standard full sling _____
    B. Bathing sling _____
    C. Toileting sling _____
    D. Amputee sling _____
    E. Bariatric sling _____

29. What information do you need when you are delegated to use a mechanical lift?
    A. _____
    B. _____
    C. _____
    D. _____
    E. _____
    F. _____
    G. _____

30. To promote mental comfort when using a mechanical lift, you should explain _____ and show the person _____ .

Optional Learning Exercises

31. When transferring a person to and from the toilet, why should the person have a raised toilet seat?
    _____

32. What safety measures are important when transferring a bariatric person to and from the toilet?
    A. _____
    B. _____
    C. _____

33. When moving a person to a stretcher, you know that for a safe transfer
    A. A _____ device is used
    B. At least _____ staff are needed
    C. If the person weighs less than 200 pounds, a _____ device or _____ is used

34. When moving a person to a stretcher, if a person weighs more than 200 pounds, what are 2 devices that may be used?
    A. _____
    B. _____

35. What should you do after using a shared device, such as a mechanical lift, to be considerate of other staff members?
    A. _____
    B. _____

36. Stand-assist lifts are used for persons who can
    A. _____
    B. _____
    C. _____
    D. _____

37. Why should you know the person's weight before using a mechanical lift? _____
_____

38. What should you do if the mechanical lift available is different than one you have used before?
_____

Use the FOCUS ON PRIDE section to complete these statements and then use the critical thinking and discussion questions to develop your ideas.

39. When transferring a person, you respect the person's privacy when you
A. _____
B. _____

40. When giving directions about transferring, what should you do to encourage independence and social interaction?
A. _____
B. _____
C. _____
D. _____
E. _____
F. _____
G. _____

Critical Thinking and Discussion Questions

41. The nurse tells you that an elderly resident, who is newly admitted, is at the "supervision" level for transfers and that the long-term goal is independence in mobility. However, when you give the resident the cues to transfer to the chair, she says, "You have to lift me up, my daughter says so."
A. What would you do first?
B. If the resident is newly admitted and you are unfamiliar with the resident's usual behavior, how would this effect your approach?

Fill in the Blank: Key Terms

Entrapment   High-Fowler's position   Reverse Trendelenburg's   Trendelenburg's position
Fowler's position   Hospital bed system   position
Full visual privacy   Person's unit   Semi-Fowler's position

1. The space, furniture, and equipment used by the person in the agency is the

   _____.

2. In _____,
   the head of the bed is raised 30 degrees and the knee portion is raised 15 degrees; or the head of the bed is raised 30 degrees.

3. _____ is a semi-sitting position; the head of the bed is raised 45 to 60 degrees.

4. The head of the bed is raised and the foot of the bed is lowered in _____.

5. Getting caught, trapped, or entangled in spaces created by the bed rails, the mattress, the bed frame, the head-board, or the foot-board is _____.

6. In _____, the head of the bed is lowered and the foot of the bed is raised.

7. The person has the means to be completely free from public view while in bed when they have

   _____.

8. _____ is a semi-sitting position with the head of the bed raised 60 to 90 degrees.

9. The _____ is the bed frame and its parts: the mattress, bed rails, head- and foot-boards, and bed attachments.

Circle the Best Answer

10. Which resident's behavior should be reported to the nurse?
    A. A resident asks you to keep the door of her room closed.
    B. A resident is using her roommate's shampoo and lotion.
    C. A resident has placed family pictures on her bedside table.
    D. A resident asks to borrow a roommate's romance novel.

11. CMS require that nursing centers maintain a temperature range of
    A. 68°F to 74°F
    B. 61°F to 71°F
    C. 71°F to 81°F
    D. 78°F to 85°F

12. Older persons or those who are ill may
    A. Need cooler room temperatures
    B. Need higher room temperatures
    C. Be insensitive to room temperature changes
    D. Need a warmer room at night

13. Which factor that affects comfort can the nursing staff control?
    A. Illness   C. Noise
    B. Age   D. Facility design

14. What is the best way to protect a person who is sensitive to drafts?
    A. Putting the person to bed
    B. Giving the person a hot shower
    C. Offering a lap cover
    D. Turning off the air conditioning

15. Older persons are sensitive to cold because they
    A. Have poor circulation and a loss of fatty tissue.
    B. Get confused about the season and time of day.
    C. Have poor nutrition and are underweight.
    D. Are unable to select warm clothes and dress themselves.

16. Which action would the nursing assistant use to reduce unpleasant odors?
    A. Use spray deodorizers before cleaning up feces or urine.
    B. Report poor personal hygiene to the charge nurse.
    C. Place soiled linens and clothing in the far corner of the room.
    D. Empty and clean bedpans, commodes, and urinals promptly.

17. A surveyor is observing for comfortable sound levels at your health care agency. Which circumstance is the surveyor most likely to query?
    A. Noise levels in the evening are decreased as the residents get ready to retire to bed.
    B. During a social activity, the residents converse with each other in conversational tones.
    C. At mealtime, a nursing assistant calls across the dining room to ask what people want to drink.
    D. The nurse answers the intercom and the volume is low enough to prevent others from overhearing.

18. Which measure helps to reduce noises in a health care agency?
    A. Control the volume and tone of your voice.
    B. Use metal equipment, such as meal trays.
    C. Step outside to answer your cell phone.
    D. Move residents outside when housekeepers are cleaning.

19. For which person and circumstance is bright lighting the best choice?
    A. A person with poor vision is trying to read a medication label.
    B. The nursing assistant is helping a person to put on a shirt.
    C. A person who is hard of hearing wants to watch television.
    D. The person had a busy day and wants to rest and relax.

20. A low bed position
    A. Is the safest position to give care, such as a bed bath
    B. Allows the person get out of bed with ease
    C. Facilitates the transfer of the person to a stretcher
    D. Helps the person to maintain good body alignment

21. Cranks on manual beds are kept down when not in use to
    A. Prevent persons from operating the bed
    B. Prevent anyone walking past the crank from bumping into it
    C. Keep the bed in the correct position
    D. Make sure they are ready to use at all times

22. How can the staff prevent a person from adjusting an electric bed to unsafe positions?
    A. Lock the bed into a position.
    B. Unplug the bed.
    C. Put the person in a bed that cannot be re-positioned.
    D. Keep reminding the person not to change the position.

23. Which bed position raises the head of the bed and the knee portion?
    A. Fowler's
    B. Semi-Fowler's
    C. Trendelenburg's
    D. Reverse Trendelenburg's

24. The bed wheels are locked
    A. Only when giving care
    B. When the person is not using bed rails
    C. At all times except when moving the bed
    D. When indicated in the care plan

25. Hospital bed entrapment is more likely to occur for persons who are
    A. Alert and oriented
    B. Able to move easily in bed independently
    C. Older, frail, and confused
    D. Large in size

26. A person who weighs 600 pounds will need
    A. An electric bed
    B. A manual bed
    C. A bariatric bed
    D. Bed rails

27. Hospital bed entrapment zone 4 is between
    A. The top of the compressed mattress and the bottom of the bed rail and at the end of the bed rail
    B. The split bed rails
    C. The top of the compressed mattress and the bottom of the bed rail and between the rail supports
    D. The bed rail and the mattress

28. A child can become entrapped in a crib if the
    A. Mattress is larger than the crib
    B. Mattress is smaller than the crib
    C. Mattress is too soft
    D. Bumper pad does not fit correctly

29. Which items are never placed on the over-bed table?
    A. Meals, snacks and drinks
    B. Personal care items
    C. Writing and reading materials
    D. Bedpans, urinals, and soiled linens

30. Where are the bedpan and urinal stored?
    A. Wherever the person wants them kept
    B. On the top shelf of the person's closet
    C. On the lower shelf or drawer of the bedside stand
    D. In the top drawer of the person's chest of drawers

31. Privacy curtains
    A. Are always closed if there is more than one person in the room
    B. Are pulled completely around the bed before giving care
    C. Can block sounds and conversations
    D. Are only closed if the person requests privacy

32. Which action achieves full visual privacy as required CMS?
    A. Covering the person with a bath blanket
    B. Placing a movable screen around the person
    C. Assisting the person to don a full-length robe
    D. Asking other persons in the room to look away

33. Personal care items
    A. May be supplied by the agency
    B. Must be supplied by the person
    C. Are supplied when ordered by the doctor
    D. Must be purchased from the agency by the person

34. When the person is weak on the left side, the call light is
    A. Placed on the left side
    B. Replaced by a phone
    C. Placed on the right side
    D. Replaced by an intercom

35. If a confused person cannot use a call light
    A. Use simple language to explain how to use the call light.
    B. Instruct the person to call out loudly for assistance.
    C. Advise the family to find a solution.
    D. Check the person often to make sure needs are met.

36. When a person turns on a call light, who should answer it?
    A. Only the person assigned to give care to the person.
    B. Any available nursing team member should answer and assist the person.
    C. The charge nurse will decide and delegate the task to someone.
    D. Another team member may answer but is not expected to give any care.

37. Elevated toilet seats
    A. Help persons with joint problems
    B. Make wheelchair transfers more difficult
    C. Help when using a mechanical lift
    D. Are used if the person is very tall

38. When a person uses a bathroom call light
    A. It flashes red above the room door and at the nurses' station.
    B. It makes the same sound as the room call light.
    C. It activates the intercom, so the person can speak.
    D. It flashes the same color as the room call light.

39. Closet and drawer space
    A. Is shared by persons in a room with more than 1 person
    B. Can be cleaned out as needed by a staff member
    C. Can be searched without the person's permission
    D. Must be freely accessible by the person

40. Which nursing assistant has exceeded his/her responsibilities in maintaining the person's unit?
    A. Nursing Assistant A throws away papers and knickknacks that are cluttering the room.
    B. Nursing Assistant B arranges personal items after discussing the person's preferences.
    C. Nursing Assistant C empties the wastebasket and linen receptacle at least once a day.
    D. Nursing Assistant D explains that the unusual noises are related to building repairs.

Fill in the Blank

41. Write out the abbreviations.
    A. CMS _____
    B. IV _____
    C. F _____

42. If you smoke, list three things you should do before giving care.
    A. _____
    B. _____
    C. _____

43. According to the CMS, list three criteria of a "comfortable" sound level.
    A. _____
    B. _____
    C. _____

44. List three functions that are served by safe and comfortable lighting.
    A. _____
    B. _____
    C. _____

45. Describe each hospital bed system entrapment zone
    A. Zone 1 _____
    B. Zone 2 _____
    C. Zone 3 _____
    D. Zone 4 _____
    E. Zone 5 _____
    F. Zone 6 _____
    G. Zone 7 _____

Labeling

46. In this figure

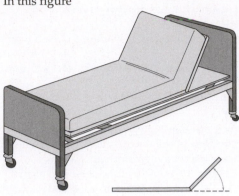

    A. What is the bed position called?

    _____

    B. What is the angle of the head of the bed?

    _____

47. In this figure

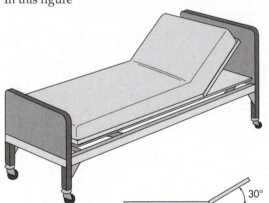

    A. What is the bed position called?

    _____

    B. What is the angle of the head of the bed?

    _____

48. In this figure

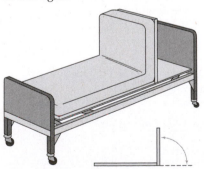

    A. What is the bed position called?

    _____

    B. What is the angle of the head of the bed?

    _____

49. In this figure

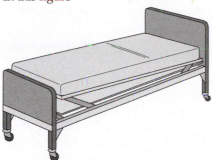

   A. What is the bed position called?

   _____

   B. What is the position of the head of the bed and the foot of the bed?

   _____

   C. Who decides this position is to be used?

   _____

50. In this figure

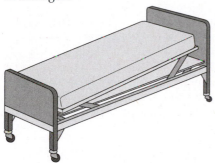

   A. What is the bed position called?

   _____

   B. What is the position of the head of the bed and the foot of the bed?

   _____

   C. Who decides this position is to be used?

   _____

Optional Learning Exercises

51. List five questions/statements that you could ask to determine if the person feels comfortable.

   A. _____
   B. _____
   C. _____
   D. _____
   E. _____

52. List five factors that you can control that affect the person's comfort.

   A. _____
   B. _____
   C. _____
   D. _____
   E. _____

53. In these situations, how would you protect a person from drafts?
   A. The person is dressing for the day.

   _____

   B. The person is sitting in a wheelchair.

   _____

   C. You are assisting a person who is going to bed for the night.

   _____

   D. You are giving personal care to the person.

   _____

54. How can you help to eliminate odors in these situations?
   A. You are caring for a person who is frequently incontinent. _____

   B. The person is vomiting and has wound drainage.

   _____

   C. The person changes his own ostomy drainage bag in his bathroom. _____
   D. The person keeps a urinal at his bedside and uses it himself during the day. _____

   _____

55. When the staff talks loudly and laughs in hallways, some persons may think that

   _____.

56. List four measures that the staff can use to reduce noises and increase the person's comfort.
   A. Control _____
   B. Handle _____
   C. Keep _____
   D. Answer _____

57. For a person with poor vision, how does good lighting contribute to safety?
   A. _____

58. What does CMS require for the furniture and equipment listed?
   A. Closet space _____
   B. Bed and bath linens _____
   C. Chair _____
   D. Temperature _____
   E. Toilet seat _____
   F. Number of persons in a room _____
   G. Windows _____
   H. Call system _____
   I. Lighting _____
   J. Hand rais _____

59. List three circumstance where the bed is in flat position.
    A. _____
    B. _____
    C. _____

60. Semi-Fowler's has 2 different definitions. They are
    A. _____
    B. _____

61. Which 2 methods are used to raise the foot of the bed with Trendelenburg's position?
    A. _____
    B. _____

62. How can you place a person in Fowler's or semi-Fowler's position if the person has a regular bed?

    _____
    _____

63. When the nursing team uses the over-bed table as a work area, which items can be placed on it?

    _____

64. What are your responsibilities in these situations regarding the call light?
    A. The person is sitting in a chair next to the bed.

    _____
    _____

    B. The person is weak on the right side.

    _____
    _____

    C. The person calls out instead of using the call light.

    _____
    _____

    D. The person is embarrassed because she soiled the bed after calling for assistance.

    _____
    _____

    E. The call light in a bathroom rings while you are busy in another room.

    _____
    _____

Use the FOCUS ON PRIDE section to complete these statements and then use the critical thinking and discussion question to develop your ideas

65. You help to protect the rights of the person and respect the person when you allow personal choice when arranging items. Make sure the person's choices
    A. _____
    B. _____
    C. _____

66. The location of items in the person's unit can prevent injuries when you help the person to
    A. _____
    B. _____
    C. _____

Critical Thinking and Discussion Question

67. You know that Resident B's family brought a special box of candy for her yesterday. When you enter the room, Resident A says, "Look, my family brought this candy for me." Resident A proceeds to eat the candy and then stores the box with her personal items. Resident B looks tearful but says nothing and looks away. Later, you see Resident A walk up to Resident B and grab B's lap cover. Resident B says, nothing and acts like nothing has happened. The next day, you notice that Resident B's furniture and other personal items have been pushed into a far corner and Resident A has taken over much of the space in the room. When you ask Resident B about the furniture, she quietly says, "It's okay. I don't want any trouble." You suspect that Resident A is intimidating her roommate Resident B. What would you do?

22 Bedmaking

Fill in the Blank: Key Terms

Cotton drawsheet   Padded waterproof drawsheet
Drawsheet

1. A drawsheet made of an absorbent top and waterproof bottom used to protect the mattress and bottom linens from dampness and soiling is a

   _____.

2. A _____ is a small sheet placed over the middle of the bottom sheet.

3. A drawsheet made of cotton that helps keep the mattress and bottom linens clean is a

   _____.

Circle the Best Answer

4. In nursing centers, a complete linen change is usually done
   A. When the person is out visiting family
   B. Every day
   C. On the person's bath or shower day
   D. Every other day

5. What is the primary purpose of keeping beds clean, dry and wrinkle-free?
   A. To promote good posture and body alignment
   B. To meet the expectations of surveyors and visitors
   C. To promote comfort and prevent skin breakdown
   D. To provide a home-like atmosphere for residents

6. A closed bed is
   A. Not in use
   B. Made with the top linens fan-folded
   C. Made with the person in it
   D. For a person to transfer from a stretcher to the bed

7. An open bed is
   A. Made when the person cannot easily get in and out of bed
   B. In use; the top linens are folded back so that the person can get into bed
   C. Not in use until bedtime; the bed linens are tightly tucked
   D. Made when a person needs to transfer from a stretcher to the bed

8. When making a bed, medical asepsis is practiced by
   A. Putting used or heavily soiled linens on the floor
   B. Shaking the linens as you place them on the bed
   C. Raising the bed to prevent bending and reaching
   D. Holding the linens away from your uniform

9. If extra clean linens are brought to a person's room, you should
   A. Return the un-used linens to the linen room.
   B. Use the linens for the person's roommate.
   C. Put the un-used linens in the laundry.
   D. Use the linens for a person in the next room.

10. Which of these linens will be collected first when making a bed?
    A. Bath towel
    B. Bath blanket
    C. Mattress pad (if needed)
    D. Top sheet

11. When you remove used linens, which of these actions is correct?
    A. Gather all used linens in 1 large roll and double bag them.
    B. Wear gloves and roll each piece of soiled linen towards your body.
    C. Top sheet, and drawsheets may be re-used if not visibly soiled.
    D. The blanket and bedspread may be re-used for the same person.

12. You allow the person the right of personal choice when you
    A. Allow the person to choose the time when you make the bed.
    B. Decide which linens will look best in the room.
    C. Tell the person you will make the bed at 9 AM.
    D. Choose the pillows and blanket the person needs for comfort.

13. When caring for a person in the home, the linens are usually changed
    A. Once a day
    B. Twice a week
    C. Only if the person gives you permission
    D. Weekly or more often at the person's request

14. A padded waterproof drawsheet
    A. Protects against skin breakdown and pressure injuries
    B. Protects the blankets and bedspread from moisture and soil
    C. Protects the mattress and bottom linens from dampness and soiling
    D. Protects the person from getting wet or soiled

15. You are caring for a person at home, for which observation would you need to speak to the caregiver or the supervising nurse?
    A. A flat sheet is folded in half and is being used as a drawsheet.
    B. A plastic trash bag is placed between the mattress and linens.
    C. A cotton drawsheet is directly underneath the person.
    D. A plastic mattress protector is between the mattress and linens.

16. When you are delegated to make a bed, why do you need to know the person's schedule for treatments, therapies, and activities?
    A. You need to make sure the bed is flat and that bedrails and frame are clean.
    B. It is best to change linens after the treatment or when the person is out of the room.
    C. You need to lock beds that may have been unlocked after being moved.
    D. You will know what type of bed to make and what type of linen to obtain.

17. When making a bed in the home, you should
    A. Always follow the person's wishes.
    B. Make the bed only as stated in the care plan.
    C. Follow the person's wishes unless the request is unsafe.
    D. Use the most convenient method to make the bed.

18. When making a bed, you are using good body mechanics when you
    A. Bend from the waist to remove and replace linens.
    B. Stretch across the bed to smooth linens.
    C. Raise the bed to a comfortable height to work.
    D. Lock the wheels and raise the head of the bed.

19. When a person is discharged, what is done in addition to changing the bed?
    A. New pillows are placed on the bed.
    B. The bed system is cleaned and disinfected.
    C. The bed system and all linens are sterilized.
    D. The bedspread and blanket may be re-used.

20. When making a bed, position the bottom flat sheet with
    A. The lower edge even with the top of the mattress
    B. The hem stitching facing away from the person
    C. The large hem at the bottom and the small hem at the top
    D. The crease cross-wise on the bed.

21. When the top sheet, blanket, and bedspread are in place on the bed
    A. Each one is tucked under the mattress separately.
    B. The sheet and blanket are tucked together and the bedspread is allowed to hang loose over them.
    C. All top linens are tucked together under the foot of the bed and the corners are mitered.
    D. All three are allowed to hang loose over the foot of the bed.

22. The pillow is placed on the bed
    A. With the open end away from the door
    B. With the seam of the pillowcase toward the foot of the bed
    C. Leaning against the head of the bed
    D. With the open end toward the window

23. An open bed is made
    A. With the linens fan-folded to one side
    B. With the top linens fan-folded to the foot of the bed
    C. With the person in the bed
    D. When the room is unoccupied

24. When you change the linens for a comatose person, it is important to
    A. Keep the bed in the lowest position.
    B. Have several co-workers assist you.
    C. Keep the bedrails up at all times.
    D. Explain each step before it is done.

25. When making an occupied bed, a bath blanket is used to
    A. Protect the person while he is being bathed.
    B. Cover the person for warmth and privacy.
    C. Protect the bed linens.
    D. Protect the person from used linens.

26. When making an occupied bed for a person who does not use bed rails, you should.
    A. Have a co-worker work on the other side of the bed
    B. Push the bed against the wall.
    C. Always keep a hand on the person while you are making the bed.
    D. Change linens only when the person is out of the bed for tests or therapies.

27. When making an occupied bed
    A. Remove all used linens from the bed first.
    B. Have the person roll from side to side for each piece of the bottom linens.
    C. Tuck the used bottom linens and the clean bottom linens under the person.
    D. Ask the person to raise his or her hips so you can push the linens under the buttocks.

28. Which nursing assistant needs a reminder about how to make a surgical bed?
    A. Nursing Assistant A tucks the sides and bottom of top linens under the mattress.
    B. Nursing Assistant B removes and discards soiled linens in a used laundry receptacle.
    C. Nursing Assistant C positions a clean mattress pad on the mattress.
    D. Nursing Assistant D smooths the wrinkles from the bottom flat sheet.

Fill in the Blank

29. Number this list from 1 to 13 in the order you would collect the linens to make a bed.

    _____ Pillowcase(s)

    _____ Top sheet

    _____ Gown

    _____ Bottom sheet (flat or fitted)

    _____ Mattress pad (if needed)

    _____ Bedspread

    _____ Waterproof under-pad (if needed)

    _____ Bath blanket

    _____ Hand towel

    _____ Cotton or padded waterproof drawsheet (if needed)

    _____ Bath towel(s)

    _____ Blanket

    _____ Washcloth

30. Beds are made every day to
    A. Promote _____
    B. Prevent _____
    C. Prevent _____

31. When doing home care, list three guidelines that you should follow for doing the laundry.
    A. _____
    B. _____
    C. _____
    D. _____

32. How will you be able to tell the difference between a closed bed and an open bed?

    _____

    _____

33. When you make a surgical bed, fan-fold linens

    _____

    _____.

Optional Learning Exercises

34. Compare how often linen changes are made in a hospital and nursing center.
    A. How often is a complete linen change made in a nursing center? _____

    _____

    B. How often are linens changed in a hospital?

    _____

35. Even when a complete linen change is not scheduled, you should do the following to keep beds neat and clean.
    A. _____
    B. _____
    C. _____
    D. _____
    E. _____

36. The mattress pad, waterproof drawsheet, blanket, and bedspread are re-used when making a bed unless they are _____.

37. If you were making a bed in a home, how would you use a twin sheet for a drawsheet? _____

    _____

38. When giving care in a home, what should you tell a family member who suggests using a plastic trash bag to protect the linens and mattress?
    A. _____
    B. _____
    C. _____

Use the FOCUS ON PRIDE section to complete these statements and then use the critical thinking and discussion question to develop your ideas.

39. When handling used linens, it is important as a team member that you
    A. Do not _____
    B. Linens must not _____
       If you see a full cart, _____

       _____

    C. Remember to wear _____
       when you are handling used linen
    D. Place used linens _____

       _____

    E. Follow agency policy for _____

       _____

Critical Thinking and Discussion Question

40. You are caring for a woman in a nursing center who has been bedridden for several years. She is alert and conversant but is very frail and has limited mobility. Discuss how a clean and tidy bed could contribute to the woman's quality of life and her physical health.

23 Oral Hygiene

Fill in the Blank: Key Terms

Aspiration   Hygiene   Oral hygiene   Tartar
Denture   Mouth care   Plaque

1. _____ is the set of practices that promote healthy tissues and structures of the mouth.

2. Hardened plaque on teeth is _____

3. _____ occurs when breathing fluid, food, vomitus, or an object into the lungs.

4. _____ is a thin film that sticks to the teeth. It contains saliva, microbes, and other substances.

5. _____ are a removable replacement for missing teeth.

6. _____ is the cleanliness practices that promote health and prevent disease.

7. _____ is another name for oral hygiene.

Circle the Best Answer

8. If good oral hygiene is not performed regularly, the person may develop tartar, which will lead to
   A. A dry mouth
   B. Periodontal disease
   C. A bad taste in the mouth
   D. Plaque

9. Which activity is most likely to cause a dry mouth?
   A. Walking
   B. Sleeping
   C. Smoking
   D. Eating

10. Which health team member is most likely to assess the person's need for mouth care?
    A. Speech-language pathologist
    B. Nursing assistant
    C. Physical therapist
    D. Occupational therapist

11. Which child has increased risk for baby bottle tooth decay?
    A. Child drinks formula from a baby bottle.
    B. Baby is being breast-fed.
    C. 1-year old child is bottle-fed.
    D. Baby is put to bed with a bottle.

12. Which method of oral hygiene would you use for a 3-month old baby?
    A. Gently brush with a soft toothbrush.
    B. Use a sponge swab and a smear of toothpaste.
    C. Use a clean damp washcloth and wipe the gums.
    D. Gently massage the gums with your fingertip.

13. According to the American Dental Association, teeth are flossed
    A. When teeth cannot be brushed
    B. Once or twice a week
    C. At least once a day
    D. When food is caught between teeth

14. Sponge swabs are used for
    A. Persons with sore, tender mouths
    B. Cleaning dentures
    C. Oral care on children
    D. Oral care on elderly people

15. What is the rationale for using Standard Precautions and the Bloodborne Pathogen Standard when giving oral hygiene?
    A. Mouth care creates aerosol droplets.
    B. Bad breath indicates presence of microbes.
    C. Gums may bleed during mouth care.
    D. Teeth and dentures are considered aseptic.

16. When the person is able to perform oral hygiene in bed, you arrange the items on
    A. The over-bed table
    B. The bedside table
    C. The sink counter
    D. The bed

17. When you are brushing the person's teeth, which of these steps would you use?
    A. Let the person rinse the mouth with water.
    B. Use a sponge swab to clean the teeth.
    C. Wipe the gums with a damp gauze.
    D. Floss the teeth that are easily reached.

18. What is the most serious complication of using a sponge swab to clean the mouth of an unconscious person?
    A. The sponge swab is uncomfortable in the person's mouth.
    B. The person could bite down on the swab stick.
    C. The person could choke on the foam pad if it comes off.
    D. The sponge swab does not remove plaque as well as a toothbrush.

19. You are assigned to assist person perform oral hygiene? Which action would you perform?
    A. Position the person for oral hygiene.
    B. Brush the teeth gently.
    C. Move the floss gently up and down between the person's teeth.
    D. Apply lubricant to the person's lips.

20. Which nursing assistant needs a reminder about the steps to use when flossing a person's teeth?
    A. Nursing Assistant A starts at the lower back tooth on the right side.
    B. Nursing Assistant B holds the floss between the middle fingers.
    C. Nursing Assistant C moves the floss gently up and down between the teeth.
    D. Nursing Assistant D moves to a new section of floss after every second tooth.

21. When providing mouth care for an unconscious person, position the person on his/her side with the head turned well to the side to
    A. Make it easier to brush the teeth
    B. Make the person more comfortable
    C. Prevent or reduce the risk of aspiration
    D. Make it easier for the person to breathe

22. When giving oral hygiene to an unconscious person who wears dentures, you should
    A. Remove the dentures, clean them, and replace them in the mouth.
    B. Remove the dentures; they are not worn when the person is unconscious.
    C. Clean the dentures in the mouth without removing them.
    D. Use a plastic tongue depressor to clean the dentures.

23. Mouth care is given to an unconscious person
    A. After each meal
    B. When AM and PM care is given
    C. At least every 2 hours
    D. Once a day

24. A plastic tongue depressor is used when giving oral hygiene to an unconscious person to
    A. Keep the mouth open.
    B. Clean the teeth.
    C. Clean the tongue.
    D. Prevent aspiration.

25. When cleaning dentures at a sink, line the sink with a towel to
    A. Prevent infections.
    B. Prevent damage to the dentures if they fall.
    C. Dry the dentures.
    D. Clean the dentures.

26. If dentures are not worn after cleaning, store them in
    A. Cool water
    B. Hot water
    C. A soft towel
    D. Soft tissues or a napkin

27. If the person cannot remove the dentures, what would you use to get a good grip on the slippery dentures?
    A. Gloves
    B. Sponge swab
    C. Gauze square
    D. Clean hands

Fill in the Blank

28. Write out the abbreviations.
    A. ADA _____
    B. ID _____

29. List five benefits of good oral hygiene.
    A. _____.
    B. _____
    C. _____.
    D. _____
    E. _____

30. List four circumstances where you would need to perform oral hygiene for the person
    A. _____
    B. _____
    C. _____
    D. _____

31. When giving oral care to an unconscious person, explain what you are doing because you always assume
    _____
    _____.

32. What observations related to oral hygiene should be reported and recorded?
    A. _____
    B. _____
    C. _____
    D. _____
    E. _____
    F. _____

Labeling

33. Look at the figure and answer these questions.

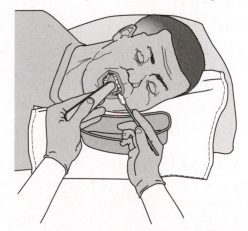

    A. Why is the person positioned on his side?
    _____

    B. What is the purpose of the plastic tongue depressor?
    _____

34. In this figure, what is the staff member using to remove the upper denture?

_____

Why? _____

35. According to the charting sample, what observations were made and what care was performed?

ORAL HYGIENE		
Observations		

Lips	**Gums**	**Mouth and tongue**
☒ Dry, cracked	☐ Bleeding	☐ Mouth or breath odor
☐ Swelling	☐ Swelling	☐ Swelling
☐ Blisters	☐ Redness	☐ Redness
☐ Pain	☐ Pain or irritation	☐ Pain or irritation
☐ Other: _____	☐ Other: _____	☐ Sores
		☐ White patches
Teeth	**Dentures**	☐ Other: _____
☒ Pain	☐ Rough or sharp area(s)	
☐ Loose teeth	☐ Chipped area(s)	
☐ Other: _____	☐ Loose denture(s)	Nurse notified: M. Rhodes, RN

Care Measures	
Oral hygiene	**Denture care**
☒ Teeth brushed	☐ Upper denture
☒ Teeth flossed	☐ Lower denture
☐ Mouth cleaned with sponge swabs	☐ Denture(s) cleaned
☒ Lip lubricant applied	☐ Adhesive applied
	☐ Denture(s) placed in mouth
	☐ Denture(s) soaked in cleaning solution

Optional Learning Exercises

36. What factors cause mouth dryness for an unconscious person?

A. _____

B. _____

C. _____

37. The factors listed above cause crusting on the

_____ and

_____ .

Use the FOCUS ON PRIDE section to complete these statements and then use the critical thinking and discussion questions to develop your ideas.

38. Always check food trays and place settings for

_____ .

Some persons _____ them after meals or wrap them in _____ after eating.

39. When should you give or offer oral hygiene to a person?

_____

Critical Thinking and Discussion Questions

40. You are assisting a person to remove his dentures before he goes to bed. As you are removing the dentures, he begins to cough and choke and reaches out and grabs your hand. Accidentally, the dentures are knocked out of your hand and they fall to the floor and break.
    A. Discuss what you would do.
    B. Discuss methods to prevent this type of incidents from happening.

Fill in the Blank: Key Terms

AM care   Early morning care   Pericare   Uncircumcised

Circumcised   Evening care   Perineal care

Diaphoresis   Morning care   PM care

1. The person is _____ when he has a foreskin covering the head of the penis.

2. Care given at bedtime or PM care is

   _____.

3. _____ is cleaning the genital and anal areas; pericare.

4. Sometimes evening care is called

   _____.

5. Sometimes early morning care is called

   _____.

6. Care given after breakfast is called

   _____

   Hygiene measures are more thorough at this time.

7. Another name for perineal care is

   _____.

8. Another name for AM care is

   _____.

9. Profuse sweating is _____.

10. When the foreskin covering the glans of the penis was surgically removed, the man is _____.

Circle the Best Answer

11. If a person requires help with personal hygiene, you can find out what needs he/she has by
    A. Following the nurse's directions and the care plan
    B. Asking the person about hygiene preferences
    C. Asking other nursing assistants that know the person
    D. Making decisions based on your experience

12. You should help residents with personal hygiene
    A. According to the assignment sheet
    B. Only in the morning
    C. Whenever help is needed
    D. When you have time

13. When giving personal hygiene, you need to remember to protect the person's right to
    A. Privacy and personal choice
    B. Care and security of personal possessions
    C. Activities
    D. Environment

14. Which of these hygiene measures is done before breakfast?
    A. Assisting with washing the face and hand hygiene
    B. Providing back massage or other comfort measures
    C. Assisting with activity by providing range-of-motion exercises
    D. Storing eyeglasses, hearing aids or other devices

15. Which of these is done every time you assist with hygiene measures throughout the day?
    A. Assisting with dressing and hair care
    B. Assisting with elimination
    C. Assisting with activity
    D. Assisting the person change clothes

16. Older persons usually need a complete bath or shower only twice a week because
    A. They are less active.
    B. They are often ill.
    C. They have increased perspiration.
    D. Dry skin often occurs with aging.

17. If a person has dry skin, which of these will help keep it soft?
    A. Soaps
    B. Creams, lotions, and oils
    C. Powders
    D. Deodorants and antiperspirants

18. If a person with dementia resists bathing, you may
    A. Quickly perform the bath and limit the cleaning.
    B. Speak firmly in a loud voice while giving clear instructions.
    C. Try giving the bath during a time of day when the person is calmer.
    D. Have a co-worker hold the person so that you are not harmed.

19. When choosing skin care products for bathing, you should use
    A. A mild, low cost soap or body wash
    B. Products the person prefers, whenever possible
    C. Bath oils that have a light fresh odor
    D. Creams and lotions that moisturize

20. The water temperature for a complete bed bath is usually between 110°F and 115°F (43.3°C and 46.1°C) for adults. For older persons, the temperature
    A. Should be between 110°F and 115°F (43.3°C and 46.1°C)
    B. May need to be lower
    C. Is safer if it is cool to the touch
    D. May need to be warmer

21. When applying powder
    A. Shake or sprinkle the powder directly on the person.
    B. Sprinkle a small amount of powder onto your hands or a cloth.
    C. Apply a thick layer of powder.
    D. You should never put powder on the feet.

22. When helping a bariatric person with hygiene, it is important to
    A. Use only water to prevent dry or irritated skin.
    B. Dry under skin folds to prevent skin breakdown.
    C. Work alone to protect the person's privacy.
    D. Apply a thick layer of powder in skin folds.

23. A complete bed bath is given to persons who
    A. Ask for a complete bath
    B. Are being cared for at home
    C. Are weak from illness or surgery
    D. Are newly admitted to a facility

24. When you are giving a complete bed bath, the bed is made
    A. Only if needed
    B. Before the bath begins
    C. After the bath is completed
    D. After the person gets out of bed

25. Offering the bedpan, urinal, commode, or bathroom is
    A. Done before the bath begins
    B. Done after the bath ends
    C. Not related to bath time
    D. Done to prevent incontinence while bathing

26. During the bed bath, the bath blanket is placed
    A. Over the person after the top linens are removed
    B. Under the top linens
    C. Over the person before top linens are removed
    D. Under the person

27. Do not use soap when washing
    A. The face, ears, and neck
    B. Around the eyes
    C. The abdomen
    D. The perineal area

28. How do you avoid exposing the person when washing the chest?
    A. Keep the bath blanket over the area.
    B. Keep the top linens over the chest.
    C. Place a towel over the chest cross-wise.
    D. Make sure the curtains are closed.

29. Bath water is changed
    A. Every 5 minutes during the bath
    B. When it becomes cool and soapy
    C. Only once during the bath
    D. After washing the face, ears, and neck

30. Which person may respond well to a towel bath?
    A. A person who has dementia
    B. A person who is frequently incontinent
    C. A person who has skin breakdown
    D. A person who needs a partial bath

31. A partial bath involves bathing
    A. The body parts that are soiled
    B. The face, hands, underarms, back, buttocks, and perineal area
    C. The face and hands
    D. The perineal area

32. When giving any type of bath, you should
    A. Wash from the dirtiest to the cleanest areas.
    B. Strive to remove all microbes.
    C. Provide for privacy.
    D. Decide what is best for the person.

33. A tub bath should not last longer than
    A. 10 minutes
    B. 15 minutes
    C. 20 minutes
    D. 30 minutes

34. If a person is weak or unsteady, which equipment should be used to help the person accomplish bathing or showering?
    A. Shower chair
    B. Transfer belt
    C. Wheelchair
    D. Stretcher

35. Which of these would be a time management strategy to use when giving a tub bath or shower?
    A. Take the person to the shower room and then collect your equipment.
    B. Ask a co-worker to give the bath or shower for you.
    C. Ask a co-worker to make the person's bed while you give the bath or shower.
    D. Clean and disinfect the tub or shower before returning the person to his or her room.

36. When assisting with a tub bath or shower, which of these steps is first?
    A. Help the person undress and remove footwear.
    B. Assist or transport the person to the tub or shower room.
    C. Put the occupied sign on the door.
    D. Place a rubber bath math in the tub or on the shower floor.

37. When cleaning the perineal area
    A. Use a liberal amount of mild soap and flush with plenty of water.
    B. Work from the anal area to the urethral area (back to front, bottom to top).
    C. Work from the urethral area to the anal area (front to back, top to bottom).
    D. Work from the dirtiest area to the cleanest area.

38. When gathering equipment for perineal care, you will need
    A. 1 washcloth and toilet paper
    B. 2 washcloths
    C. 3 Washcloths
    D. At least 4 washcloths

39. When giving perineal care to a male, you
    A. Retract the foreskin if he is uncircumcised.
    B. Wash from the scrotum to the tip of the penis.
    C. Use 1 bag bath for the entire procedure.
    D. Leave the foreskin retracted after finishing the care.

Matching

Match the skin care product with the benefit or the problem that may occur if you use the product.

A. Soaps   D. Powders
B. Bath oils   E. Deodorants and
C. Creams and lotions   antiperspirants

40. _____ Absorbs moisture and prevents friction
41. _____ Makes showers and tubs slippery
42. _____ Protects skin from the drying effect of air and evaporation
43. _____ Excessive amounts can cause caking and crusts that can irritate the skin
44. _____ Masks and controls body odors or reduces perspiration
45. _____ Tends to dry and irritate skin
46. _____ Keeps skin soft and prevents drying of skin
47. _____ Removes dirt, dead skin, skin oil, some microbes, and perspiration

Fill in the Blank

48. Write out the abbreviations.
    A. ID _____
    B. C _____
    C. F _____

49. The _____ must be intact to prevent microbes from entering the body and causing an
    _____.

50. The religion of East Indian Hindus requires at least _____ a day.

51. Some Hindus believe that bathing is _____ after a meal.

52. When following the rules for bathing in Box 24-2 p 354, you protect the skin by following these rules:
    A. Rinse _____
    B. Pat _____
    C. Dry _____
    D. Bathe _____

53. What methods can be used to measure the water temperature for a bed bath?
    A. _____
    B. _____

54. When you place a person's hand in the basin during the bed bath, you may have the person _____ the hands and fingers.

55. When assisting with partial baths, most people need help with washing the _____.

56. A tub bath can cause a person to feel _____, especially if the person has been on bedrest.

57. When the shower room has more than 1 stall or cabinet, you must protect the person's right to
    _____.
    What can you do to protect this right?
    A. _____
    B. _____

58. When giving a tub bath or shower, you use safety measures to protect the person from
    _____,
    _____, and
    _____.

59. When you are assisting a person with perineal care, what terms may help the person understand what you are going to do? _____
    _____

60. What observations made while assisting with hygiene should be reported at once?
    A. _____
    B. _____
    C. _____
    D. _____
    E. _____

Labeling

61. In this figure, explain what the staff member is doing.
    _____

    Why is the towel positioned vertically on the person?
    _____

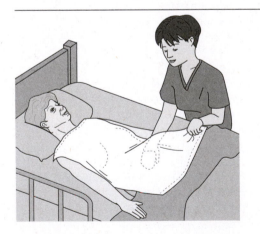

62. Refer to the charting sample below.

SKIN CARE		
Abnormal Skin Observations		

Problems:	**Color:**	**Temperature:**
☐ Blister	☒ Redness	☐ Cold
☐ Non-intact skin (open skin)	☐ Pallor (pale skin)	☐ Cool
☐ Bruise	☐ Gray	☐ Hot
☐ Bleeding	☐ Cyanosis (blue skin)	
☐ Drainage/discharge	☐ Jaundice (yellow skin)	
☐ Swelling		**Moisture:**
☒ Rash	**Texture:**	☐ Dry
☒ Itching	☐ Rough	☐ Moist
☐ Odor	☐ Scaly/flaky	☐ Diaphoresis (sweating)

Nurse notified: J. Anderson, RN

Click to mark affected area(s).

Right   Left   Left   Right

☐ No new skin issues

Bathing

☐ Shower
☐ Tub bath
☒ Complete bed bath
☐ Partial bath
☐ Bag/towel bath
☒ Perineal care

A. What abnormal skin observations were made?

_____

B. What was the location on the person's body?

_____

C. Which hygiene measures were performed?

_____

Optional Learning Exercises

63. Hygiene promotes comfort, safety, and health. Answer these questions about hygiene.

A. What does intact skin prevent? _____

64. What are the benefits of bathing?

A. Cleans _____

B. Also cleans _____

C. Removes _____

D. Bath is _____ and

_____

E. Stimulates _____

F. Exercises _____

G. You can make _____

H. You have time _____

65. When you are bathing a person with dementia, list five communication strategies that you can use.

A. _____

B. _____

C. _____

D. _____

E. _____

66. You are preparing to give perineal care to a person. How many washcloths should you gather?

_____ Why?

_____

_____

_____

67. You are delegated to give an elderly person (Mrs. Johnson) a bath. Before beginning, what information do you need?

A. _____

B. _____

C. _____

D. _____

E. _____

F. _____

G. _____

H. _____

68. As you are bathing Mrs. Johnson, what observations should you make to report and record?

    A. _____

    B. _____

    C. _____

    D. _____

    E. _____

    F. _____

    G. _____

    H. _____

    I. _____

    J. _____

    K. _____

    L. _____

Use the FOCUS ON PRIDE section to complete these statements and then use the critical thinking and discussion question to develop your ideas.

69. You can promote independence and social interaction when you allow

    A. Personal choice of _____

    B. Encourage the person to _____

Critical Thinking and Discussion Question

70. You are assigned to care for an elderly resident who has dementia. His regular shower days are Tuesday and Friday mornings. On Tuesday evening around 8:30 PM, he asks you to help him take a shower. You remind him that he had a shower this morning and that the next shower day is Friday. On Wednesday evening he asks you again to help him with a shower. He is easily re-directed and you help him get ready for bed. On Thursday evening around 8:00 PM, you find him partially undressed and he is attempting to get into the shower.

    A. What do you think is happening with this resident?

    B. Why is it important to report this behaviour to the nurse?

25 Grooming

Fill in the Blank: Key Terms

Alopecia
Anticoagulant
Dandruff

Hirsutism
Infestation
Lice

Mite
Pediculosis
Pediculosis capitis

Pediculosis corporis
Pediculosis pubis
Scabies

1. Being in or on a host is an _____.
2. The infestation with wingless insects (lice) that feed on blood is _____.
3. A very small spider-like organism is a _____.
4. _____ is an excessive amount of dry, white flakes from the scalp.
5. The infestation of the body with lice is _____.
6. Hair loss is _____.
7. _____ is the infestation of the pubic hair with lice.
8. Excessive body hair is _____.
9. The infestation of the scalp with lice is _____.
10. Another description of pediculosis is _____.
11. A drug that prevents or slows down blood clotting is an _____.
12. _____ is a skin disorder caused by the female mite.

Circle the Best Answer

13. Hair care, shaving, and nail and foot care are important to many people because these measures affect
    A. Safety and security needs
    B. Love, belonging, and self-esteem needs
    C. Physical needs
    D. Self-actualization needs

14. If you see any signs of lice, you should report it to the nurse because
    A. Lice bites can cause severe contagious infections.
    B. Lice spread to others through clothing, furniture, bed linens, and sexual contact.
    C. Lice can cause the person's hair to permanently fall out.
    D. The lice will cause the hair to mat and tangle.

15. If a person has scabies, what signs or symptoms may be present?
    A. You may see lice that are small and tan to grayish white in color.
    B. The person has a rash and intense itching on fingers, wrists, and underarms.
    C. You may see eggs (nits) attached to the hair shaft.
    D. The person has an excessive amount of dry, white flakes on the scalp.

16. Who chooses how you will brush, comb, and style a person's hair?
    A. The person
    B. You decide.
    C. The nurse tells you.
    D. It is written in the care plan.

17. If long hair becomes matted or tangled, you should
    A. Braid the hair.
    B. Cut the hair to remove the tangles and matting.
    C. Tell the nurse and ask for directions.
    D. Get the family's permission to change the hairstyle.

18. If hair is curly, coarse, and dry, which of these measures could you use?
    A. Braid the hair.
    B. Use a wide-toothed comb.
    C. Comb downwards.
    D. Clip the dry ends.

19. When assisting a person who has small braids
    A. Undo the hair and re-braid it each time it is shampooed.
    B. Leave the braids intact for shampooing.
    C. Undo the braids only at night.
    D. Comb out the braids once a week.

20. If a woman's hair is done by the beautician in long-term care
    A. Wash her hair only once a week.
    B. Shampoo her hair on the day she goes to the beautician.
    C. Have her wear a shower cap during the tub bath or shower.
    D. Wash her hair each time she gets a shower or tub bath.

21. If a person has limited range of motion in the neck, he or she is not shampooed
    A. At the sink or on a stretcher
    B. In the shower
    C. During a tub bath
    D. In bed

22. Which of these observations, noted while shampooing, should be reported to the nurse?
    A. Hair has been dyed and permed
    B. Amount of time it took to shampoo
    C. Hair is matted or tangled
    D. Amount of hair on the head

23. If a person receives anticoagulants and needs shaving
    A. Use an electric razor.
    B. Use disposable safety razors.
    C. It must be done by the nurse or barber.
    D. It should be done only during the shower or bath.

24. When using safety razors (blade razors)
    A. The same razor can be used for several persons until it becomes dull.
    B. Use the resident's own razor as many times as possible.
    C. Discard the disposable razor or razor blade in the sharps container.
    D. Be careful when shaving a person who takes anticoagulants.

25. Why is an electric razor used for shaving a person with dementia?
    A. The person usually bleeds easily.
    B. The person may resist or move suddenly.
    C. It is faster than using a safety razor.
    D. The skin is tender and sensitive.

26. When shaving a person with a safety razor, wear gloves
    A. To protect the person from infections
    B. To prevent contact with blood
    C. To apply shaving cream
    D. To maintain sterile technique

27. When caring for a mustache and beard, what should you do?
    A. Trim the beard when you notice it is too long.
    B. Shampoo the beard when you shampoo the hair.
    C. Shave off the mustache if it interferes with eating.
    D. Wash and comb the mustache or beard daily.

28. You can cut or trim toenails
    A. Whenever you have the time
    B. On any person that is assigned to you
    C. If agency policy allows you to trim toenails
    D. If the person tells you to cut them

29. When caring for the fingernails or toenails, which action would you use?
    A. Shape the nails with an emery board or nail file.
    B. Clean under the nails with a scrub brush.
    C. Clip the nails in a curved shape to match the toe.
    D. Cut the nails with small scissors.

Fill in the Blank

30. Write out the abbreviations.
    A. C _____
    B. F _____
    C. ID _____

31. When you brush and comb the hair, you should report and record
    A. _____
    B. _____
    C. _____
    D. _____
    E. _____
    F. _____
    G. _____
    H. _____

32. If you give hair care to a person in bed after a linen change, collect falling hair by _____
    _____.

33. It may help to prevent tangled and matted hair when you brush and comb small sections of the hair, starting at the _____.

34. If hair is curly, coarse, and dry, special measures are needed. You should
    A. Use a _____
    B. Start at _____
    C. Work _____,
       lift and _____
    D. Wet _____
       or apply _____

35. You can protect the person's eyes during shampooing by asking the person to hold a _____
    _____.

36. What delegation guidelines do you need when shaving a person?
    A. _____
    B. _____
    C. _____
    D. _____
    E. _____
    F. _____
    G. _____
    H. _____

37. What should be reported *at once* when you are shaving a person?
    A. _____
    B. _____
    C. _____
    D. _____

38. When you are shaving the face and underarms with a safety razor, shave in the direction of the
    _____.

39. When shaving legs with a safety razor, shave
    _____.

40. When using an electric shaver, shave
    _____.

41. What delegation guidelines do you need when giving a person nail and foot care?

    A. _____

    B. _____

    C. _____

    D. _____

    E. _____

    F. _____

    G. _____

    H. _____

42. When you are delegated to give nail and foot care, what do you report and record?

    A. _____

    B. _____

    C. _____

    D. _____

    E. _____

    F. _____

43. Foot care for persons with diabetes or poor circulation is provided by _____

    or _____.

Optional Learning Exercises

44. You are caring for a person who is receiving cancer treatments. What effect could this treatment have on the person's hair? _____

    _____

45. Dandruff not only occurs on the scalp, but also may involve the _____.

46. Brushing the hair increases _____ to the scalp. It also brings _____ along the hair shaft.

47. Why do older persons usually have dry hair?

    _____

48. What water temperature is usually used when shampooing the hair?

    _____

49. How can the beard be softened before shaving?

    _____

    _____

50. After shaving, why do some people apply after-shave or lotion?

    A. Lotion _____

    B. After-shave _____

51. Injuries to the feet of a person with poor circulation are serious because poor circulation prolongs

    _____.

Use the FOCUS ON PRIDE section to complete these statements and then use the critical thinking and discussion question to develop your ideas.

52. Grooming promotes _____, _____, and _____. Clean hair and nails help _____ well-being.

53. When a person allows family members to assist with giving personal care, this promotes

    _____.

54. If you cut a person's hair or shave a mustache or beard without permission, you have violated the person's right to be free from

    _____.

Critical Thinking and Discussion Question

55. You are assigned to help residents with morning hygiene and grooming. Resident A is usually alert, cheerful and talkative and she is very particular about how her hair is combed, how her make-up is applied and the appearance of her nails. This morning when you offer to assist her with grooming, she seems tired and irritable. She turns away, refuses to acknowledge you and mumbles, "Leave me alone." Resident B has mild dementia and usually looks quite disheveled. He never wants your help with grooming. He doesn't like to change his clothes and he usually pushes your hand away if you try comb his hair or offer to file his nails. Both residents have refused your offers to help with hygiene. Discuss the difference between these two residents and discuss what you would do.

26 Dressing and Undressing

Fill in the Blank: Key Terms

affected side   garment   unaffected side   under-garment

1. An item of clothing is a _____
2. The side of the body opposite the affected side; strong or "good" side is the _____ side.
3. The side of the body with weakness from illness or injury; weak side is the _____ side.
4. An item of clothing worn next to the skin under clothing is an _____

Circle the Best Answer

5. When changing clothing, remove the clothing from
   A. The weak side first
   B. The lower limbs first
   C. The right side last
   D. The strong side first

6. What do you need to obtain before you assist a person who is lying in bed to undress?
   A. Washcloth
   B. Deodorant or antiperspirant
   C. Gloves
   D. Bath blanket

7. You are helping a person who is lying in bed to undress. Which position do you place the person in first?
   A. Prone
   B. Sidelying
   C. Supine
   D. Trendelenburg

8. When you are undressing a person, you use good body mechanics when you
   A. Lower the bed rail on the person's weak side
   B. Position the person in a supine position
   C. Raise the bed to a good working level
   D. Turn the person away from you

9. To provide warmth and privacy when assisting a person to undress you
   A. Keep the top sheets in place
   B. Cover the person with a bath blanket
   C. Close the curtains
   D. Close the door

10. To assist a person with Alzheimer's to get dressed, what is the best strategy?
    A. Have him put on the same clothes everyday
    B. Take him to the closet and show him how to select clothes
    C. Stack clothes in the order they are to be put on
    D. Put the clothes you want him to wear in an obvious place

11. You are assisting a person to remove a pullover garment. Which action do you perform first?
    A. Remove the garment from the strong side
    B. Bring the garment over the person's head
    C. Undo any buttons, zippers, snaps, or ties
    D. Remove the garment from the weak side

12. You ask a co-worker to assist you in dressing a person. What is the main role of the co-worker?
    A. To help turn and position the person
    B. To select the person's clothing
    C. To undress the person
    D. To check the care plan for details

13. You are assisting a person to put on a garment that opens in the front. The person is lying in bed and cannot raise the head and shoulders. What would you do?
    A. Turn the person away from you
    B. Put the garment on so the opening is in the back
    C. Use the bed mechanism to lower the head of the bed
    D. Cover the person with an extra bath blanket

14. When changing the gown of a person with an IV
    A. Temporarily turn off the IV and later tell the nurse
    B. Lay the IV bag on the bed and remove the gown
    C. Slide the gathered sleeve over the tubing, hand, arm, and IV site
    D. Disconnect the IV where the tubing connects with the bag

15. When you have finished changing the gown of a person with an IV, you should
    A. Restart the pump
    B. Reconnect the IV
    C. Ask the nurse to check the flow rate
    D. Check the flow rate

16. In which circumstance, could you change the patient's gown without notifying the nurse?
    A. Patient has an IV that is attached to a pump and is wearing a standard gown
    B. Patient has an IV that is attached to the pump, the bag is empty, and he is being discharged
    C. Patient has an IV that is attached to a pump and is wearing a gown with snap fasteners
    D. Patient has an IV that is not attached to a pump, but there is blood in the tubing and on the gown

Fill in the Blank

17. Write out the abbreviations.
    A. ID _____
    B. IV _____

18. List three questions you can ask to promote personal choice and independence
    A. _____
    B. _____
    C. _____

19. When assisting people with dressing and undressing, what rules should be followed?
    A. _____
    B. _____
    C. _____
    D. _____
    E. _____
    F. _____
    G. _____
    H. _____

20. According to Alzheimer's and related Dementias Education and Referral Center (ADEAR), what are six strategies that are useful when assisting people with dementia to get dressed?
    A. _____
    B. _____
    C. _____
    D. _____
    E. _____
    F. _____

21. What delegation guidelines do you need when assisting a person to dress or undress?
    A. _____
    B. _____
    C. _____
    D. _____
    E. _____
    F. _____

22. What observations do you need to report and record after assisting a person to dress or undress
    A. _____
    B. _____
    C. _____
    D. _____

23. When undressing a person who cannot raise the head and shoulders, what should you do?
    A. _____
    B. _____
    C. _____
    D. _____
    E. _____

24. When dressing a person who cannot raise the hips and buttocks off the bed, what should you do?
    A. _____
    B. _____
    C. _____
    D. _____
    E. _____

25. Before changing a person's hospital gown who has an IV, what information do you need from the nurse and the care plan?
    A. _____
    B. _____

26. The nursing assistant has correctly performed the steps of assisting a person who had a stroke to remove his gown. Based on the figure, which side is the person's affected (weak) side?

Optional Learning Exercises

Use the FOCUS ON PRIDE section to complete these statements and then use the critical thinking and discussion question to develop your ideas.

27. Appearance affects _____. Garments should be _____, not wrinkled, and comfortable. Dress the person in a way that promotes _____ and_____
    _____.

Critical Thinking and Discussion Question

28. You are assigned to assist an elderly resident with daily hygiene and grooming. He performs most of the care by himself, which includes, bathing, dental hygiene and grooming. For the past week, he puts his dirty clothes, (including his underwear) back on. You informed the nurse who instructed you to "just keep trying" to get him to wear clean clothes. Discuss this situation:
    A. What do you think about this elderly resident's choices?
    B. What are the main reasons for trying to get him to wear clean clothes?
    C. What could you do?

27 Urinary Needs

Fill in the Blank: Key Terms

Dysuria
Enuresis
Functional incontinence
Groin
Hematuria

Mixed incontinence
Nocturia
Oliguria
Over-flow incontinence
Polyuria

Reflex incontinence
Stress incontinence
Transient incontinence
Urge incontinence
Urinary frequency

Urinary incontinence
Urinary retention
Urinary urgency
Urination
Voiding

1. Where the thigh and abdomen meet is called the
   _____.

2. The production of abnormally large amounts of urine
   is _____.

3. _____ is the combination of
   stress incontinence and urge incontinence.

4. _____ is the loss of bladder
   control.

5. Frequent urination at night is
   _____.

6. The loss of small amounts of urine that leak from a
   bladder that is always full is
   _____.

7. The involuntary loss or leakage of urine during sleep
   or bedwetting is _____.

8. _____ occurs when the
   person has bladder control but cannot use the toilet in
   time.

9. The process of emptying urine from the bladder is
   voiding or _____.

10. Blood in the urine is _____.

11. Voiding at frequent intervals is _____.

12. When urine leaks during exercise and certain
    movements that cause pressure on the bladder, it is
    called _____.

13. Another word for urination is _____.

14. _____ is the need to void at
    once.

15. The loss of urine in response to a sudden, urgent need
    to void is _____.

16. Painful or difficult urination is
    _____.

17. The loss of urine at predictable intervals when the
    bladder is full is _____.

18. A scant amount of urine, usually less than 500 mL in
    24 hours, is _____.

19. _____ is temporary
    or occasional incontinence that is reversed when the
    cause is treated.

20. The inability to void is _____.

Circle the Best Answer

21. Solid wastes are removed from the body by the
    A. Digestive system
    B. Urinary system
    C. Blood
    D. Integumentary system

22. How much urine does a healthy adult excrete in a day.
    A. 500 mL   C. 1500 mL
    B. 1000 mL   D. 2000 mL

23. Which voiding pattern is typical for most people?
    A. After bathing, eating and exercise
    B. In the morning and in the evening
    C. Bedtime, after sleep, and before meals
    D. Goes only when there is complete privacy

24. If the person has difficulty starting the urine stream, it
    may help to
    A. Play music on the TV
    B. Provide perineal care
    C. Use a stainless steel bedpan
    D. Run water in a nearby sink

25. The urine may be bright yellow if the person eats
    A. Asparagus
    B. Carrots or sweet potatoes
    C. Beets or blackberries
    D. Rhubarb

26. If you are caring for an infant, which of these
    observations should be reported to the nurse at once?
    A. The infant has had a wet diaper 4 times in 3 hours.
    B. The infant has not had a wet diaper for several
       hours.
    C. The urine in the diaper is pale yellow.
    D. The urine in the diaper has a faint odor.

27. When you are getting ready to give a person the
    bedpan, you should
    A. Raise the head of the bed slightly for the person's
       comfort
    B. Position the person in the Fowler's position
    C. Warm the bedpan using hot water
    D. Place the bed in a flat position

28. A urinal is usually
    A. Hung on the bed rails
    B. Placed on the over-bed table
    C. Put on the bedside stand
    D. Kept on the floor under the bed

29. If a man is unable to stand and handle a urinal to void, you should
    A. Tell the nurse
    B. Ask a male co-worker to help the man
    C. Place and hold the urinal for him
    D. Pad the bed with incontinence pads

30. A commode chair is used when
    A. The person is unable to stand and pivot
    B. The person is not allowed to get out of bed
    C. The person needs to be in the normal position for elimination
    D. The bathroom is being used by another person

31. When you place a commode over the toilet
    A. Attach a transfer belt to the commode
    B. Stay in the room with the person
    C. Lock the wheels
    D. Make sure the container is in place

32. When you do not answer call lights quickly or do not position the call light within the person's reach, it contributes to
    A. Over-flow incontinence
    B. Mixed incontinence
    C. Reflex incontinence
    D. Functional incontinence

33. You are caring for an incontinent person who often wets right after you have changed the clothes and bedding. It would be correct if you
    A. Wait 15 to 30 minutes before changing the person each time
    B. Place extra waterproof under-pads over the wet bedding
    C. Talk to the nurse at once if you find yourself becoming impatient
    D. Tell the person that you can only change the linens once a shift

34. When a person has dementia, what measures may help keep the person clean and dry?
    A. Tell the person to use the call light when he or she needs to void.
    B. Decrease fluid intake at breakfast, lunch time and bedtime.
    C. Observe for signs that the person may need to void, such as pulling at the clothing.
    D. Remove any incontinence garments and seat the person on a commode.

35. Which nursing assistant needs a communication reminder related to assisting people with incontinence products?
    A. Nursing Assistant A asks, "Would you like to try a different size of incontinence briefs."
    B. Nursing Assistant B offers, "I want to help you change your wet underwear."
    C. Nursing Assistant C says, "Don't be embarrassed, an adult diaper will keep you dry."
    D. Nursing Assistant D says, "If the incontinence pad is uncomfortable, let me know."

36. When applying an incontinence product, you should
    A. Apply a new one when the old one has a strong odor
    B. Weigh the used product to determine the urine output
    C. Mark the date, time, and your initials on the new product
    D. Clean the skin by rubbing it with dry paper towels

37. The goal of bladder training is
    A. To keep the person dry
    B. To control urination
    C. To prevent skin breakdown
    D. To prevent infection

38. When you are assisting the person with habit training to have normal elimination
    A. Help the person to the bathroom every 15 or 20 minutes
    B. Voiding is scheduled at regular times to match the person's voiding habits
    C. Make sure the person drinks at least 1000 mL each shift
    D. Tell the person he or she can void twice a shift

39. When you assist with bladder training for a person with a catheter
    A. Empty the drainage bag every hour
    B. At first, clamp the catheter for 1 hour
    C. At first, clamp the catheter for 3 to 4 hours
    D. Give the person 15 to 20 minutes to start voiding

Fill in the Blank

40. Write out the abbreviations.
    A. BM _____
    B. mL _____
    C. OAB _____
    D. UI _____
    E. UTI _____

41. What substances increase urine production?
    A. _____
    B. _____
    C. _____
    D. _____

42. A normal position for voiding for women is _____. For men, a normal position is _____.

43. What can you do to mask urination sounds?
    A. _____
    B. _____
    C. _____

44. Fracture pans are used for persons
    A. _____
    B. _____
    C. _____
    D. _____
    E. _____
    F. _____
    G. _____

45. A bariatric bedpan is placed with the _____ end under the buttocks.

46. When a person voids in a bedpan or urinal, what observations about the urine are important?
    A. _____
    B. _____
    C. _____
    D. _____
    E. _____

47. You should report complaints of _____, _____, or _____ when the person is voiding.

48. When you are handling bedpans, urinals, and commodes and their contents, you should follow _____ and _____.

49. When you are delegated to provide a urinal, what guidelines should you follow?
    A. _____
    B. _____
    C. _____
    D. _____
    E. _____
    F. _____
    G. _____
    H. _____

50. When you transfer a person to a commode from bed, you must practice safe transfer procedures and use a _____ and _____ the wheels.

51. Name risk factors and causes of incontinence related to
    A. Women _____
    B. Men _____
    C. Age _____
    D. Over-weight _____
    E. Smoking _____
    F. Diabetes _____

52. How are these related to transient incontinence?
    A. Alcohol _____
    B. Bladder irritation caused by _____
    C. Caffeine _____
    D. Constipation or fecal impaction _____
    E. Increased fluid intake _____
    F. Urinary tract infection _____

53. When you are delegated to apply incontinence products, what information do you need from the nurse and care plan?
    A. _____
    B. _____
    C. _____
    D. _____
    E. _____
    F. _____

54. What observations should you report and record when you are delegated to apply incontinence products?
    A. _____
    B. _____
    C. _____
    D. _____
    E. _____
    F. _____
    G. _____

55. When you provide perineal care after a person is incontinent, what do you need to do?
    A. _____
    B. _____
    C. _____
    D. _____
    E. _____
    F. _____

56. The catheter is clamped for 1 hour at first and, over time, for 3 to 4 hours when _____ is being done.

Optional Learning Exercises

57. When a person eats a diet high in salt, it causes the body to _____. When this happens, how does it affect urine output?
    _____

58. You would ask the nurse to observe urine that looks or smells _____.

59. A fracture pan can be used with older persons who have fragile bones from _____ or painful joints from _____.

60. Covering the lap and legs of a person using a commode provides _____ and promotes _____.

61. What would you do if you are caring for an incontinent person and you become short-tempered and impatient? _____. What rights are you protecting when you do this? _____

62. When using incontinence products, it is important to use the correct size. If the product is too large, _____. If it is too small, the product will cause _____.

63. When bladder training is being done, the person needs to
    A. _____
    B. _____
    C. _____

Use the FOCUS ON PRIDE section to complete these statements and then use the critical thinking and discussion question to develop your ideas.

64. If you notice a person is uncomfortable talking about urinary elimination, what can you do put the person at ease?

    A. _____

    B. _____

    C. _____

65. Urine-filled devices in the person's room do not respect the person's right to _____.

Critical Thinking and Discussion Question

66. You are recently hired at a long-term care center. You observe that Nursing Assistant A, who has worked there a long time, is leaving the residents on the commode or the bedpan for prolonged periods without checking on them. You answer a call light and the resident asks you for help because Nursing Assistant A, "put me on the bedpan a long time ago and never came back". When you mention the incident to A, she says, "I told the person to call when she was finished. I believe that people need their privacy." What would you do?

Crossword

Fill in the crossword by answering the clues below with words from this list:

Dysuria	Hematuria	Nocturia	Polyuria
Frequency	Incontinence	Oliguria	Urgency

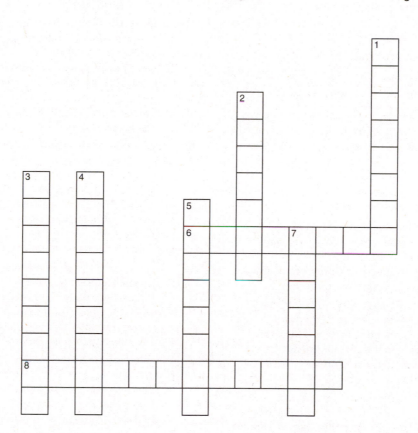

Across

6. Scant amount of urine, usually less than 500 mL in 24 hours
8. Inability to control loss of urine from bladder

Down

1. Production of abnormally large amount of urine
2. Painful or difficult urination
3. Blood in the urine
4. Voiding at frequent intervals
5. Frequent urination at night
7. Need to void immediately

28 Urinary Catheters

Fill in the Blank: Key Terms

Catheter   Condom catheter   Indwelling catheter   Straight catheter

Catheterization   Foley catheter   Retention catheter   Supra-pubic catheter

1. A soft sheath that slides over the penis and is used to drain urine is a _____.

2. A Foley or indwelling catheter is also called a _____.

3. The process of inserting a catheter is _____.

4. A catheter left in the bladder so urine drains constantly into a drainage bag is called a retention, Foley, or _____.

5. A _____ is a tube used to drain or inject fluid through a body opening.

6. A catheter that drains the bladder and then is removed is a _____.

7. An indwelling or retention catheter is also called a _____.

8. A _____ is surgically inserted into the bladder through an incision above (supra) the pubis bone (pubic).

Circle the Best Answer

9. Which person is most likely to have a catheter?
   A. Person who is going to have surgery today
   B. Person who can't walk to the bathroom
   C. Person who has frequent episodes of incontinence
   D. Person who has a urinary tract infection

10. When securing the drainage tubing, you should
    A. Clip the tubing to the person's gown
    B. Pin the tubing so that it is tight and straight
    C. Secure the tubing to the bottom linens
    D. Attach the tubing to the bed rails

11. When cleaning a catheter, you should
    A. Wipe the entire catheter and the tubing
    B. Disconnect the tubing from the drainage bag
    C. Clean from the meatus down the catheter about 4 inches
    D. Wash the catheter by wiping up and down the tubing

12. The drainage bag from a catheter should be attached to the
    A. Bed frame
    B. Bottom linens
    C. Person's gown
    D. Bed rail

13. If a catheter is accidentally disconnected from the drainage bag, you should tell the nurse at once and then
    A. Clean downwards starting at the meatus, and down the catheter for 4 inches
    B. Clamp the catheter to prevent leakage and get permission to remove it
    C. Wipe the connecting ends of the tube and catheter with clean antiseptic wipes
    D. Discard the drainage bag, get a new bag and attach it to the catheter

14. If a person uses a leg drainage bag, it
    A. Is switched to a drainage bag when the person is in bed
    B. Is attached to the clothing with tape or safety pins
    C. Is attached to the bed rail when the person is in bed
    D. Can be worn 24 hours a day, but must be frequently emptied

15. A leg bag needs to be emptied more often than a drainage bag because
    A. It holds less than 1000 mL and the drainage bag holds about 2000 mL
    B. It is more likely to leak than the drainage bag
    C. It holds about 250 mL and the drainage bag holds 1000 mL
    D. It interferes with walking if it is full

16. When you empty a drainage bag, you
    A. Disconnect the bag from the tubing
    B. Clamp the catheter to prevent leakage
    C. Open the clamp on the drain and let urine drain into a graduate
    D. Take the bag into the bathroom to empty it

17. When removing an indwelling catheter, a syringe is needed to
    A. Remove water in the balloon
    B. Instill water into the drainage bag
    C. Flush the catheter with water
    D. Clean the perineal area after removing the catheter

18. A condom catheter is changed
    A. Daily after perineal care
    B. Once or twice a week on bath days
    C. When the adhesive wears out
    D. When a leg bag is switched to a large drainage bag

19. When applying a condom catheter
    A. Apply elastic tape in a spiral around the penis
    B. Make sure the catheter tip is flush with the head of the penis
    C. Apply adhesive tape securely in a snug circle around the penis
    D. Clean the penis and reapply condom every shift

20. When working with urinary drainage systems, which equipment would be considered sterile?
    A. Plug and cap
    B. Graduate cylinder
    C. Outside of connection tubing
    D. Drainage bag

Fill in the Blank

21. Even though catheters create a risk of urinary tract infections, they are used to
    A. _____
    B. _____
    C. _____
    D. _____
    E. _____
    F. _____

22. When a catheter is inserted after a person voids and then removed, it is used to measure the
    _____.

23. A catheter is secured to the inner thigh or the man's abdomen to prevent
    _____.

24. When a person has a catheter, what observations should you report and record?
    A. _____
    B. _____
    C. _____
    D. _____
    E. _____
    F. _____
    G. _____
    H. _____

25. When you give catheter care, clean the catheter about _____ inches. Clean _____ from the meatus with _____ stroke.

26. What happens if a drainage bag is higher than the bladder? _____ This can cause
    _____.

27. Name two things you could do to make a person with a catheter feel less embarrassed and more comfortable when visitors are coming.
    A. _____
    B. _____

28. When you are allowed to remove a catheter, what information is needed from the nurse?
    A. _____
    B. _____
    C. _____
    D. _____
    E. _____
    F. _____

29. Do not apply a condom catheter if the penis is
    _____, _____, or shows signs of _____.

30. What type of tape is used to apply a condom catheter?
    _____ Why?
    _____
    What can happen if you use the wrong tape?
    _____

Optional Learning Exercises

31. What can happen if microbes enter a closed drainage system? _____

32. What are the signs and symptoms of a urinary tract infection that must be reported at once to the nurse?
    A. _____
    B. _____
    C. _____
    D. _____
    E. _____
    F. _____

Labeling

33. Mark the places you would secure the catheter and drainage bag.

34. Mark the places you would secure the catheter.

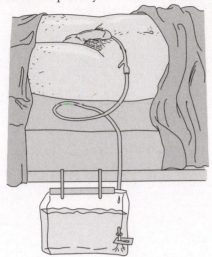

35. Why is it important to secure the catheters and drainage tubing as shown in the drawings?

_____

_____

Use the FOCUS ON PRIDE section to complete these statements and then use the critical thinking and discussion question to develop your ideas.

36. When you are careful handling and caring for catheters, you decrease the risk of _____ for the person.

37. When you need to transfer a person from the bed to the chair or move a drainage bag to the other side of the bed, list four things that you should do.

   A. _____
   B. _____
   C. _____
   D. _____

Critical Thinking and Discussion Question

38. The risk for urinary tract infection (UTI) increases when a person has a catheter. UTI can be life-threatening, especially for older people. There are many actions that you can perform to help prevent infection for people that must wear catheters. For example, using a clean area of the washcloth for each stroke during catheter care. Name at least six other actions that you could do.

29 Bowel Needs

Fill in the Blank: Key Terms

Colostomy	Diarrhea	Feces	Ostomy	Stool
Constipation	Enema	Flatulence	Peristalsis	Suppository
Defecation	Fecal impaction	Flatus	Stoma	
Dehydration	Fecal incontinence	Ileostomy		

1. A surgically created opening that connects an internal organ to the body's surface is a stoma or

   _____.

2. The process of excreting feces from the rectum through the anus is a bowel movement or

   _____.

3. The excessive formation of gas in the stomach and intestines is _____.

4. A _____ is a cone-shaped solid drug that is inserted into a body opening.

5. The frequent passage of liquid stools is

   _____.

6. _____ is the prolonged retention and buildup of feces in the rectum.

7. _____ is the excessive loss of water from tissues.

8. Gas or air passed through the anus is

   _____.

9. The introduction of fluid into the rectum and lower colon is an _____.

10. Excreted feces is _____.

11. A surgically created opening between the colon and the body's surface is a _____.

12. _____ is the alternating contraction and relaxation of intestinal muscles.

13. The passage of a hard, dry stool is

    _____.

14. _____ is the inability to control the passage of feces and gas through the anus.

15. A surgically created opening seen on the body's surface is an ostomy or a _____.

16. The semi-solid mass of waste products in the colon is

    _____.

17. A surgically created opening between the ileum and the body's surface is an _____.

Circle the Best Answer

18. Which bowel movement pattern might be considered abnormal for an adult?
    A. Every day
    B. Every 2 to 3 days
    C. 2 or 3 times a day
    D. 6 or 8 times a day

19. Bleeding in the stomach and small intestines causes stool to be
    A. Brown   C. Red
    B. Black   D. Clay-colored

20. The characteristic odor of stool is caused by
    A. Poor personal hygiene
    B. Poor nutrition
    C. Bacterial action in the intestines
    D. Lack of fluid intake

21. When you observe stool that is abnormal
    A. Ask the nurse to observe the stool
    B. Report your observation and discard the stool
    C. Ask the person if the stool is normal for him or her
    D. Record your observations after giving care

22. Which of these could interfere with defecation?
    A. Relaxing with a book or newspaper
    B. Eating a diet with high-fiber foods
    C. Having others present in a semi-private room
    D. Drinking 6 to 8 glasses of water daily

23. For a person who must stay in bed, which factor is most likely to be contributing to irregular elimination and constipation?
    A. Poor diet   C. Inactivity
    B. Poor fluid intake D. Lack of privacy

24. Which of these would provide safety for the person during bowel elimination?
    A. Make sure the bedpan is warm.
    B. Place the call light and toilet paper within reach.
    C. Provide privacy by closing the door
    D. Allow enough time for defecation.

25. Constipation can be relieved by
    A. Eating a low-fiber diet
    B. Increasing activity
    C. Decreasing fluids
    D. Delaying defecation

26. A person tries several times to have a bowel movement and cannot. Liquid feces seep from the anus. This may mean he has
    A. Diarrhea   C. Fecal impaction
    B. Constipation   D. Fecal incontinence

27. When a fecal impaction is present, it is relieved by
    A. Changing the person's diet
    B. Giving more fluids
    C. Removing the fecal mass with a gloved finger
    D. Increasing the activity of the person

28. When checking for and removing a fecal impaction, which vital sign is the most important to take?
    A. Temperature
    B. Pulse
    C. Respirations
    D. Blood pressure

29. What is the most important reason to give good skin care when a person has diarrhea?
    A. To prevent noxious odors
    B. To prevent skin breakdown
    C. To prevent the spread of microbes
    D. To prevent fluid loss

30. Why is diarrhea very serious in older persons?
    A. It causes skin breakdown.
    B. It causes odors.
    C. It can cause dehydration and death.
    D. It decreases activity.

31. If a person with diarrhea has *C. difficile*, you should
    A. Wear sterile gloves and gown
    B. Practice Standard Precautions and contact precautions
    C. Restrict all visitors from visiting the person
    D. Use alcohol hand rubs to clean your hands

32. When fecal incontinence occurs, which nursing action is your responsibility?
    A. Reviewing diet and medications as contributing factors
    B. Designing an individualized bowel training program
    C. Assessing when the person needs help with elimination
    D. Changing incontinence products to keep garments and linens clean

33. If flatus is not expelled, the person may complain of
    A. Abdominal cramping or pain
    B. Diarrhea
    C. Fecal incontinence
    D. Nausea

34. Which action could you take to help the person expel flatus?
    A. Assist the person to walk
    B. Encourage the person to eat vegetables
    C. Offer the person extra fluids
    D. Gently massage the person's abdomen

35. Which observation would be most useful to the nurse who must plan a bowel training program for a person?
    A. The amount and appearance of the stool the person expels
    B. The person's response to perineal care following fecal incontinence
    C. The usual time of day the person has a bowel movement
    D. The type of foods and fluids that cause flatus for the person

36. When the nurse delegates you to prepare a soapsuds enema for an adult, mix
    A. 2 teaspoons of salt in 1000 mL of tap water
    B. 3 to 5 mL of castile soap in 500 to 1000 mL of tap water
    C. 2 mL of mild dish soap in 200 mL of tap water
    D. Mineral oil with sterile water

37. When you give a cleansing enema, it should be given to the person
    A. Over 5 to 6 minutes
    B. Over 30 minutes
    C. Over 10 to 15 minutes
    D. Over 20 minutes

38. The person receiving an enema is usually placed in a
    A. Supine position
    B. Prone position
    C. Semi-Fowler's position
    D. Left side-lying or Sims' position

39. Which nursing assistant needs a reminder about preparing and giving cleansing enemas for adults?
    A. Nursing Assistant A prepares the solution at 110°F
    B. Nursing Assistant B inserts the tubing 2 to 4 inches into the rectum
    C. Nursing Assistant C holds the solution container about 12 inches above the bed
    D. Nursing Assistant D lubricates the enema tip before inserting it into the rectum

40. When the doctor orders enemas until clear, what would you do?
    A. Give 1 enema using a clear fluid
    B. Stop giving enemas when the return is clear
    C. Ask the nurse how many enemas to give
    D. Use clear tap water for repeated enemas

41. If you are giving an enema and the person complains of cramping
    A. Tell the person that cramps are normal and continue the enema
    B. Clamp the tube until the cramping subsides
    C. Discontinue the enema immediately and tell the nurse
    D. Raise the bag higher to increase the flow rate

42. If you are giving a cleansing enema to a child, which solution is correct?
    A. Soap suds enema.
    B. Saline enema.
    C. Small-volume enema.
    D. Tap water enema.

43. When giving a small-volume enema, do not release pressure on the bottle because
    A. It will cause cramping if pressure is released
    B. The fluid will leak from the rectum
    C. Solution will be drawn back into the bottle
    D. It will cause flatulence

44. When giving a small-volume enema to an adult
    A. Place the person in the prone position
    B. Insert the enema tip 2 inches into the rectum
    C. Heat the solution to 105°F
    D. Clamp the tubing if cramping occurs

45. An oil-retention enema is given to
    A. Cleanse the bowel to prepare for surgery
    B. Regulate the person who is receiving bowel training
    C. Relieve flatulence
    D. Soften the feces and lubricate the rectum

46. If you feel resistance when you are giving an enema
    A. Lubricate the tube more thoroughly
    B. Push more firmly to insert the tube
    C. Stop tube insertion
    D. Ask the person to take a deep breath and relax

47. You are assigned to give skin care for several people who have ostomies. Which person is most likely to have skin irritation if you fail to give good care?
    A. Person has a permanent colostomy
    B. Person has temporary colostomy
    C. Person has ileostomy
    D. Person's stoma bleeds slightly

48. A person with an ostomy pouch is worried that the pouch will cause a bulge under her clothing. What could you do to help?
    A. Assist her to empty the pouch whenever it is ⅓ to ½ full
    B. Suggest that she wear a snug pair of blue jeans to keep the bulge flattened
    C. Make a small slit at the top of the pouch, so that flatus does not cause ballooning
    D. Recommend that she wear an extra-large flowing dress that is loose at the waist

49. A person with an ostomy requests that you change the pouch after every bowel movement. What is the best rationale for notifying the nurse about the person's request?
    A. The person will run out of pouches and supplies
    B. The care plan indicates that it should be changed once a day
    C. Frequent pouch changes are damaging to the skin
    D. Stool is continuously being expelled in small amounts

50. The person has an ostomy and would like to shower with the pouch off. When is best time to assist the person with the shower?
    A. Before breakfast
    B. Before going to bed
    C. After lunch
    D. After exercise

51. After a new ostomy pouch has been applied, when can you assist the person to take a bath or a shower?
    A. 15 to 20 minutes after pouch application
    B. 1 to 2 hours after the new pouch has been applied
    C. Later in the day, towards bedtime
    D. The day after the pouch has been applied

Fill in the Blank

52. Write out the abbreviations
    A. BM _____
    B. CMS _____
    C. GI _____
    D. ID _____
    E. IV _____
    F. mL _____
    G. SSE _____

53. When observing stool, what should be reported to the nurse?
    A. _____
    B. _____
    C. _____
    D. _____
    E. _____
    F. _____
    G. _____
    H. _____
    I. _____

54. What 3 food groups are high in fiber?
    A. _____
    B. _____
    C. _____

55. Name 6 gas-forming foods.
    A. _____
    B. _____
    C. _____
    D. _____
    E. _____
    F. _____

56. Drinking warm fluids such as coffee, tea, hot cider, and warm water will increase _____.

57. If you are delegated to remove a fecal impaction, what observations should you report and record?
    A. _____
    B. _____
    C. _____
    D. _____
    E. _____

58. When checking and removing impactions, the vagus nerve may be stimulated. Why is this dangerous?
    _____

59. How will dehydration affect these?
    A. Skin is _____.
    B. Urine is _____.
    C. Blood pressure is _____.
    D. Pulse and respirations are _____.

60. Flatulence may be caused when a person _____ while eating and drinking.

61. When a nurse inserts a suppository, how soon would you expect the person to defecate?
    _____

62. Before giving an enema, make sure that
    A. Your state _____
    B. The procedure _____
    C. You have the necessary _____ and _____
    D. You review the _____ with the nurse.
    E. A nurse is available to _____ _____ and to supervise you

63. After giving an enema, what should be reported and recorded?

    A. _____
    B. _____
    C. _____
    D. _____
    E. _____
    F. _____
    G. _____

64. Because it is likely you will have contact with stool while giving an enema, you should follow _____ and _____.

65. How can cramping be prevented during an enema?

    A. _____
    B. _____

66. How long does it usually take for a tap water, saline, or soapsuds enema to take effect? _____

67. A small-volume enema is usually given for _____.

68. A person should retain a small-volume enema _____.

69. When you start to insert the tube to give an enema, ask the person to _____.

70. What can you place in the ostomy pouch to prevent odors? _____

71. Showers and baths are delayed 1 or 2 hours after applying a new pouch to allow _____.

72. Why can tap water enemas be dangerous? _____

    How many tap water enemas can be given? _____
    Why? _____

73. Compare small-volume enemas and oil-retention enemas.

    A. Small-volume enemas _____ the rectum. This causes _____.
       Oil-retention enemas are given to relieve _____.

    B. Small-volume enemas take effect in about _____ minutes.
       Oil-retention enemas should be retained for at least _____ minutes.

74. What would you expect if you touched a person's stoma while cleaning the surrounding skin? _____

Labeling

Answer questions 75 to 77 using these figures.

75. Name the four colostomies shown.

    A. _____
    B. _____
    C. _____
    D. _____

76. Why does would a sigmoid colostomy have the most solid and formed stool? _____

77. Which type of colostomy is usually a temporary colostomy? _____

Answer questions 78 to 80 using this figure.

78. What type of ostomy is shown? _____

79. What part of the bowel has been removed? _____

80. Will the stool from the ostomy be liquid or formed? _____

Optional Learning Exercises

81. You are caring for Mr. Evans, who is in a semi-private room. His roommate has a large family and many visitors. Mr. Evans has not had a bowel movement in 3 days, even though he is eating well and taking medications to assist elimination. What could be a reason he has not had a bowel movement?

_____

_____

_____

82. Mrs. Weller usually has a bowel movement after breakfast. What are some activities that may assist her to defecate more easily?

_____

_____

83. The nurse tells you to make sure Mr. Johnson eats the high-fiber foods in his diet to assist in his elimination. What foods are high in fiber?

_____

_____

84. Mrs. Shaffer tells you she cannot digest fruits and vegetables and she refuses to eat them. With her permission, what may be added to her cereal and prune juice to provide fiber?

_____

85. You offer Mr. Murphy _____ of water each day to promote normal bowel elimination.

86. Mr. Hernandez has been taking an antibiotic to treat his pneumonia and he has developed diarrhea. You think he may have diarrhea because

_____.

87. You are caring for 83-year-old Mrs. Chen and you helped her to the bathroom 30 minutes ago where she had a bowel movement. When you enter her room to make her bed, she tells you she needs to use the bathroom for a bowel movement. You know that older people _____

_____

Use the FOCUS ON PRIDE section to complete these statements and then use the critical thinking and discussion question to develop your ideas.

88. If your state allows a nursing assistant to insert suppositories, you may be allowed to insert them in persons who _____. You are not allowed to give a suppository for _____.

89. When the person needs to have a bowel elimination, you can provide comfort and privacy when you

A. _____

B. _____

C. _____

D. _____

E. _____

F. _____

G. _____

Critical Thinking and Discussion Question

90. You overhear a co-worker, who also happens to be your friend, tell a resident to "go ahead and just pee or have a bowel movement in the bed". You have cared for this resident and she is often incontinent, and she will also pull off dry and clean incontinence pants whenever she feels like it. You know that your co-worker is frustrated. What would you do?

Fill in the Blank: Key Terms

Anorexia   Calorie   Dysphagia   Nutrition
Aspiration   Cholesterol   Nutrient

1. A soft, waxy substance found in the bloodstream and all body cells is _____.

2. The amount of energy produced from the burning of food by the body is a _____.

3. The loss of appetite is _____.

4. The many processes involved in the ingestion, digestion, absorption, and use of food and fluids by the body is _____.

5. A substance that is ingested, digested, absorbed, and used by the body is a

   _____.

6. _____ is difficulty or discomfort in swallowing.

7. The breathing of fluid, food, vomitus, or an object into the lungs is _____.

Circle the Best Answer

8. Which task could you perform to contribute to the requirements set by the Center for Medicare and Medicaid Services (CMS) for assessment of the resident's nutritional status?
   A. Ask the person if his/her drugs are causing dry mouth or nausea
   B. Find out about factors that affect eating and nutrition
   C. Obtain and report the resident's height and weight
   D. Observe the person for signs and symptoms of fluid imbalance

9. Body fuel for energy is found in
   A. Vitamins
   B. Minerals
   C. Fats, proteins, and carbohydrates
   D. Water

10. A person is ordering food at a restaurant. Which food choice is aligned with the recommendations from MyPlate?
    A. French fries with catsup
    B. Steamed vegetable plate
    C. Double meat cheeseburger
    D. Orange soda with ice

11. The amount needed from each food group in MyPlate depends on
    A. The cultural and religious preferences of the person
    B. The age, sex, and physical activity of the person
    C. The likes and dislikes of the person
    D. The budget available to the person

12. Whole grains in the grain group include
    A. Bulgur, oatmeal, and brown rice
    B. White flour and white rice
    C. Snack crackers and rice noodles
    D. Biscuits and cookies

13. When choosing from the protein food group, foods that may have a higher risk for heart disease are
    A. Seafood, such as trout, salmon or herring
    B. Nuts, such as almonds, walnuts or pistachios
    C. Legumes, such as soybeans, pinto beans or chickpeas
    D. Meats that are processed, such as deli meats and hot dogs

14. Which food is in one of the food groups recommended by MyPlate?
    A. Yogurt   C. Brown sugar
    B. Butter   D. Olive oil

15. An example of moderate physical activity recommended by the USDA is
    A. Bicycling at less than 10 miles per hour
    B. Freestyle swimming laps
    C. Chopping wood
    D. Running and jogging at 5 miles per hour

16. Which nutrient is especially important for children, because of tissue growth?
    A. Carbohydrates   C. Vitamins
    B. Fats   D. Protein

17. Which vitamin is important for wound healing?
    A. Vitamin K   C. Vitamin A
    B. Vitamin C   D. Vitamin B_{12}

18. Which food represents the type of food that a person with a limited income is most likely to buy?
    A. Chicken   C. Lettuce
    B. Bread   D. Cheese

19. When people buy cheaper foods, the diet may lack
    A. Fats   C. Vitamins
    B. Starch   D. Sugars

20. Appetite can be stimulated by
    A. Increasing fluid intake
    B. Increasing portion size
    C. Controlling odors
    D. Talking about food

21. During illness
    A. Appetite for carbohydrate food increases
    B. Fewer nutrients and calories are needed
    C. Nutritional needs increase to heal tissue
    D. The person will prefer protein foods

22. Which physiologic change is expected in older adults?
    A. Increased sensitivity to smells and odors
    B. Decreased secretion of digestive juices
    C. Decreased interest in food and fluids
    D. Increased need for calories for tissue repair

23. Requirements for food served in nursing centers are made by
    A. The doctor
    B. The nurse
    C. Food and Drug Administration (FDA)
    D. Centers for Medicare & Medicaid Services (CMS)

24. Which of these are requirements for food served in long-term care centers?
    A. The center provides needed adaptive equipment and utensils
    B. The person's diet should include whatever he/she wants to eat
    C. All food is served at room temperature and all liquids must be chilled
    D. People with diabetes must receive 3 meals a day and unlimited snacks

25. A general diet
    A. Is ordered for persons with chronic health problems
    B. Has no dietary limits or restrictions
    C. May have restricted amounts of sodium
    D. Includes meat, dairy, and produce, but no desserts

26. How much sodium is required each day?
    A. 2300 mg   C. 5000 mg
    B. 3000 mg   D. 1000 mg

27. When the body tissues swell with water, what organ has to work harder?
    A. Kidneys   C. Heart
    B. Liver   D. Lungs

28. Which snack item should be offered to a person on a sodium-controlled diet?
    A. Bag of mini-pretzels
    B. Sardines on crackers
    C. Tomato juice and celery sticks
    D. Pear and plum slices

29. A person may be given a mechanical soft diet because
    A. The person is over-weight
    B. The person has dental problems
    C. The person has diarrhea
    D. The person has constipation

30. A person is on a fiber-and residue-restricted diet. Which food item needs to be removed from the tray?
    A. Raw plum   C. White toast
    B. Apple juice   D. Plain pasta

31. A person who has serious burns would receive a
    A. Sodium-controlled diet
    B. Fat-controlled diet
    C. High-calorie diet
    D. High-protein diet

32. When a person has dysphagia, the thickness of the food is determined by the
    A. Person   C. Family
    B. Chef   D. Speech therapist

33. Which of these may be a sign of a swallowing problem (dysphagia)?
    A. Has frequent episodes of diarrhea
    B. Prefers to eat foods that are sweet or salty
    C. There is excessive drooling of saliva
    D. Eats well in the morning, but refuses dinner

34. When assisting a person who is on aspiration precautions, you can help to prevent aspiration while the person is eating by placing him or her in
    A. A Semi-Fowler's position
    B. An upright a position
    C. The side-lying position
    D. The supine position

35. When residents are served meals in a family dining program
    A. They serve themselves as at home
    B. The person can eat any time the buffet is open
    C. Food is available in a common area refrigerator
    D. Food is served as in a restaurant

36. Which of the following needs to be done before the person is served a meal?
    A. Give complete personal care.
    B. Change all linens.
    C. Check the person's position.
    D. Ask if the visitors want food.

37. What can you do to provide comfort during meals?
    A. Ask visitors to minimize noise and distractions
    B. Make sure dentures, eyeglasses, or hearing aids are in place
    C. Suggest different foods if the person doesn't like what is served
    D. Give complete personal hygiene and a linen change

38. What should you do if a food tray has not been served within 15 minutes?
    A. Re-check the food temperatures.
    B. Serve the tray immediately.
    C. Throw the food away.
    D. Serve only the cold items on the tray.

39. How can you make sure the food tray is complete?
    A. Ask the person being served.
    B. Ask the nurse.
    C. Call the dietary department.
    D. Check items on the tray with the dietary card.

40. If you become impatient while feeding a resident with dementia, you should
    A. Take a break
    B. Give finger foods
    C. Talk to the nurse
    D. Feed the person later

41. When you are feeding a person, you should
    A. Allow the person to assist by holding his/her own coffee cup
    B. Give the person a fork and knife to assist with cutting the food
    C. Feed the person in a private area to maintain confidentiality
    D. Use a teaspoon because it is less likely to cause injury

42. When feeding a person, liquid foods are given
    A. Only at the start of feeding
    B. During the meal, alternating with solid foods
    C. At the end of the meal, when all solids have been eaten
    D. Only if the person has difficulty swallowing

43. When re-heating cooked foods, it should be heated
    A. To 105°F
    B. To 165°F
    C. According to agency policy
    D. To room temperature

44. You are assisting a person in a home setting. The person asks you to re-heat leftover food so that she can eat if for lunch. Which question would you ask to help prevent foodborne illness?
    A. What type of leftover food would you like to eat?
    B. How long have the leftovers been in the refrigerator?
    C. How hot do you like your food?
    D. What time would you like to eat?

Fill in the Blank

45. Write out the abbreviations.
    A. CMS_____
    B. F _____
    C. FDA _____
    D. GI _____
    E. ID _____
    F. mg _____
    G. NPO _____
    H. oz _____
    I. USDA _____

46. How many calories are in each of these?
    A. 1 gram of fat _____
    B. 1 gram of protein _____
    C. 1 gram of carbohydrate _____

Use the Dietary Guidelines for Americans, to answer questions 47 to 48.

47. What are the three main purposes of *Dietary Guidelines for Americans*?
    A. _____
    B. _____
    C. _____

48. The *Dietary Guidelines* focus on
    A. _____
    B. _____
    C. _____

Questions 49 to 53 relate to MyPlate.

49. What are the 5 food groups in MyPlate?
    A. _____
    B. _____
    C. _____
    D. _____
    E. _____

50. When using MyPlate, calories are balanced by
    A. _____
    B. _____

51. When making food choices, which foods are increased in the diet?
    A. _____
    B. _____
    C. _____

52. Which mineral is supplied by the fruit group?
    _____

53. Which food group or groups has the following health benefits?
    A. Builds and maintains bone mass throughout life
    _____
    B. Provide B vitamins and vitamin E
    _____
    C. May prevent constipation
    _____
    D. May reduce risk of kidney stones _____
    or _____
    E. May prevent birth defects
    _____
    F. May help lower calorie intake _____
    or _____
    G. Provides nutrients needed for health and body maintenance _____

54. What is the most important nutrient for tissue growth and repair? _____

55. If dietary fat is not needed by the body, it is stored as
    _____.

56. What is the function of each of these nutrients?
    A. Protein _____
    B. Carbohydrates _____
    C. Fats _____
    D. Vitamins _____
    E. Minerals _____
    F. Water _____

57. Which vitamins can be stored by the body?
    _____

58. Which vitamins must be ingested daily?
    _____

59. What vitamin is important for these functions? *Formation of substances that hold tissues together; healthy blood vessels, skin, gums, bones, and teeth; wound healing; prevention of bleeding; resistance to infection*
    _____

60. Which mineral is needed for red blood cell formation?
    _____

61. Which mineral is necessary for nerve function, muscle contraction and heart function?
    _____

62. Identify at least three food sources for calcium.
    A. _____
    B. _____
    C. _____

63. Older persons need _____ calories than younger people do.

64. Why do the diets of some older people lack protein?
    _____

65. What foods are included in a clear-liquid diet?
    _____
    _____
    _____

66. When the person receives a full-liquid diet, it will include all of the foods on the clear-liquid diet as well as these foods: _____
    _____

67. If a person has poorly fitted dentures and has chewing problems, the doctor may order a
    _____ diet.

68. A person who is constipated and has other GI disorders may receive a _____ diet. The foods in this diet increase the
    _____
    to stimulate _____.

69. If a person is receiving a high-calorie diet, the calorie intake is _____ daily.

70. If you are feeding a person a dysphagia diet, what observations should be reported to the nurse immediately?
    A. _____, _____, or
    _____ during or after meal
    B. _____ or
    _____

71. Which type of dining program would be best for a person who is mildly confused?
    _____

72. What can be done to promote comfort when preparing residents for meals?
    A. _____
    B. _____
    C. _____
    D. _____
    E. _____
    F. _____

73. When you are delegated to serve meal trays, what information do you need from the nurse or care plan?
    A. _____
    B. _____
    C. _____
    D. _____
    E. _____
    F. _____
    G. _____

74. When you are serving meal trays, you make sure the right person gets the right tray by
    A. _____
    B. _____

75. When you are feeding a person, the spoon should be filled _____.

76. Why is it important to sit facing the person when you feed him or her?
    A. _____
    B. _____
    C. _____

77. What should be reported after you have fed a person?
    A. _____
    B. _____
    C. _____
    D. _____

78. Explain each of the concepts below that are recommended by the USDA to keep food safe.
    A. Clean _____
    _____
    B. Separate _____
    _____
    C. Cook _____
    _____
    D. Chill _____
    _____

79. The safe temperature to keep foods at are
    A. Cold foods _____
    B. Hot foods _____
    C. The danger zone for foods is
    _____ for more than
    _____ hours or
    _____ hour if temperature is
    warmer than 90°F
    D. Keep the refrigerator at _____
    or below. Keep the freezer at _____
    or below.

Optional Learning Exercises

80. This is a person's food intake for one day. Place the foods in the correct food groups on MyPlate.

BREAKFAST
¾ cup Orange juice
1 cup Oatmeal
2 slices Toast
¼ cup Milk
2 cups Black coffee

LUNCH
1 cup Tomato soup
Grilled cheese sandwich
½ cup Applesauce
Can of regular soda
Candy bar

DINNER
2–4 oz. Pork chops
Baked potato/butter
¼ cup Green beans
2 Brownies
2 cups Black coffee

SNACKS
1 Apple
1 4-ounce bag Potato chips
⅓ cup Nuts
Can of regular soda
½ cup Ice cream

A. Grains _____

_____

B. Vegetables _____

_____

C. Fruits _____

_____

D. Dairy _____

_____

E. Proteins _____

_____

F. Oils _____

_____

G. Other_____

_____

Figures

81. Based on the food label. _____ What is the serving size? _____ How many servings are in the container? _____ How many calories are in one serving? _____ How many calories would the person get if he/she ate all of the food in the container? _____

Nutrition Facts

8 servings per container

Serving size   2/3 cup (55 g)

Amount per serving

Calories   230

		% Daily Value*
Total Fat 8 g		**10%**
Saturated Fat 1 g		**5%**
Trans Fat 0 g		
Cholesterol 0 mg		**0%**
Sodium 160 mg		**7%**
Total Carbohydrate 37 g		**13%**
Dietary Fiber 4 g		**14%**
Total Sugars 12 g		
Includes 10 g Added Sugars		**20%**
Protein 3 g		
Vitamin D 2 mcg		10%
Calcium 260 mg		20%
Iron 8 mg		45%
Potassium 240 mg		6%

* The % Daily Value (DV) tells you how much a nutrient in a serving of food contributes to a daily diet. 2,000 calories a day is used for general nutrition advice.

(Label from U.S. Food and Drug Administration, 2016.)

82. Label the plate in the figure with numbers so that you can describe the location of food to a blind person. What would you tell a visually impaired person who asks you where to find these food items on the plate?

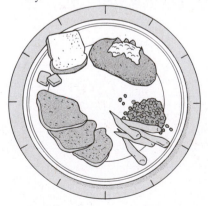

A. Bread _____

B. Baked potato _____

C. Vegetables _____

D. Meat _____

83. After reading the nutritional information in this chapter, compare your own dietary habits to the MyPlate recommendations. What changes could you make to improve your own nutrition?

_____

_____

_____

Use the FOCUS ON PRIDE section to complete these statements.

84. When you respect the person's likes and dislikes of food or complaints about the food, it meets the right to _____.

85. When family members bring food to a resident, it is important that you tell _____. The food must not interfere with the _____.

Critical Thinking and Discussion Question

86. Think about a meal tray that you have seen being served in a hospital or nursing care center.
    A. If you had to eat that type of food, how would that food compare to what you normally eat?
    B. Think about people who have to eat institutional food every day for every meal. What could you talk about as you are feeding them or assisting them to eat?
    C. What can health care staff do to help patients and residents who miss familiar foods?

31 Fluid Needs

Fill in the Blank: Key Terms

Dehydration   Electrolyte   Hydration   Output
Edema   Graduate   Intake

1. Having an adequate amount of water in body tissues is _____.

2. _____ is the amount of fluid taken in.

3. A decrease in the amount of water in body tissues is

_____.

4. The amount of fluid lost is _____.

5. A _____ is a calibrated container used to measure fluid.

6. _____ is the swelling of body tissues with water.

7. Minerals dissolved in water are _____.

Circle the Best Answer

8. If fluid intake exceeds fluid output, the person will
   A. Have edema (swelling) in the tissues
   B. Be dehydrated
   C. Have vomiting and diarrhea
   D. Have increased urinary output

9. How much fluid is needed every day for normal fluid balance?
   A. 1500 mL
   B. 1000 to 1500 mL
   C. 2000 to 2500 mL
   D. 3000 to 4000 mL

10. In the morning, as you are helping a person to get out of bed, you notice that he is heavily perspiring, and his pajamas and linens are damp with sweat. What would you do first?
    A. Help the person shower
    B. Tell the nurse
    C. Give the person drinking water
    D. Change the linens

11. The nurse tells you the person is likely to be dehydrated and directs you to get a urine sample. What would you expect to see when you obtain the urine?
    A. Moderate amount of normal urine
    B. Large amount or pale straw-colored urine
    C. Small amount of urine with blood
    D. Scant amount of dark amber urine

12. The person's blood pressure is low and the pulse and respirations are high. You would report these findings to the nurse, because the person might have
    A. Over-hydration
    B. Edema
    C. Dehydration
    D. Low electrolytes

13. Which person is most likely to have increased fluid requirements?
    A. Person who works as a nursing assistant
    B. Elderly person with nocturia
    C. Child who just woke up
    D. Woman who is breastfeeding

14. Which person is most likely to have an order to "encourage fluids"?
    A. Person who has kidney stones
    B. Person who has urinary retention
    C. Person who has kidney failure
    D. Person who has trouble swallowing

15. A person who is mildly confused is NPO for a procedure keeps asking you, visitors and others to get him a glass of water. What should you do?
    A. Remind him and others that he can have water after the procedure
    B. Place NPO signs above the bed, on the door and in the bathroom
    C. Tell the nurse that the person is having difficulties complying with NPO
    D. Help the person with oral hygiene and get him a few ice chips

16. During your shift a person drank 350 mL at breakfast, 390 mL at lunch, 225 mL as a snack, and 400 mL of water. What is the total fluid intake for your shift?
    A. 1315 mL   C. 1350 mL
    B. 1325 mL   D. 1365 mL

17. A person voided two times during your shift—350 mL and 150 mL. He vomited once—100 mL. There was 125 mL in his wound drainage container. What was the total output for your shift?
    A. 705 mL   C. 825 mL
    B. 725 mL   D. 855 mL

18. If the person you are caring for has an order for restricted fluids, which of these should you do?
    A. Offer a variety of liquids.
    B. Thicken all fluids.
    C. Remove the water mug or keep it out of sight.
    D. Do not allow the person to swallow any liquids during oral hygiene.

19. Which nursing assistant needs a reminder about what is counted in I&O records?
    A. Nursing Assistant A measures milk, water, coffee, and tea
    B. Nursing Assistant B records mashed potatoes and creamed vegetables
    C. Nursing Assistant C adds amounts of soups and gelatin
    D. Nursing Assistant D includes ice cream, custard, and pudding

20. When you are measuring I&O, you need to know that 1 ounce equals
    A. 10 mL
    B. 30 mL
    C. 100 mL
    D. 500 mL
21. When you are using the graduate to measure output, you read the amount by
    A. Holding the graduate and looking down into the container
    B. Holding the graduate steadily while looking at the fluid level
    C. Placing the graduate at eye level to read it
    D. Setting the graduate on the floor and reading it
22. When I&O is ordered, which of the following is included in the measurement?
    A. Mucous
    B. Solid stool
    C. Blood on a bandage
    D. Vomitus
23. When delegated to provide drinking water, what information do you need from the nurse and the care plan?
    A. What size of mug to use
    B. If a person can have ice
    C. If the person is able to hold the mug
    D. How often to refill the mug

Fill in the Blank

24. Write out the abbreviations.
    A. I&O _____
    B. IV _____
    C. mL _____
    D. NPO _____
    E. oz _____
25. Why is it important to offer water often to older persons? _____
26. When you give oral hygiene to a person who is receiving nothing by mouth, the person must not _____.
27. What information do you need when you are delegated to measure intake and output?
    A. _____
    B. _____
    C. _____
    D. _____
    E. _____

28. When you are providing drinking water, list four questions that you could ask the person about ice in the water and the drinking mug.
    A. _____
    B. _____
    C. _____
    D. _____

Table Activity

29. Complete the table below by writing in the correct equivalent amounts in mL

Unit	Equivalent amount in mL
1 cubic centimeter	
1 teaspoon	
1 tablespoon	
1 ounce	
1 cup	
1 pint	
1 quart	
1 liter	

30. Examine the illustration of the urinal below. How much urine is in the urinal?

Labeling

31. Enter the information below on the Intake and Output record. Total amounts for the 8-hour and 24-hour periods. Amounts in the ( ), for example (whole bowl), to indicate how much the person ate or drank. (Use 2300–0700, 0700–1500, and 1500–2300 as 8-hour periods.)

FLUID INTAKE AND OUTPUT FLOW SHEET
DATE

RECORD TOTALS IN PATIENT'S MEDICAL RECORD		DIET/FLUID ORDERS	
Water glass	240 mL	Gelatin	120 mL
Juice glass	120 mL	Ice cream	90 mL
Milk carton	240 mL	Broth/strained soup	180 mL
Coffee cup	240 mL	Styrofoam cup	180 mL
Soft drink can	360 mL	Water mug	1000 mL
Tea glass	180 mL	Ice chips	½ amount of mL in cup

			INTAKE				OUTPUT		
	TIME	ORAL	TYPE & AMOUNT	TIME	IV	ENTERAL	TIME	SOURCE	AMOUNT
2300-0700		FLUIDS							
		MUG/OTHER							
			8-HOUR SUB-TOTAL				**8-HOUR SUB-TOTAL**		
0700-1500		BREAKFAST							
		SNACK							
		LUNCH							
		SNACK							
		MUG/OTHER							
			8-HOUR SUB-TOTAL				**8-HOUR SUB-TOTAL**		
1500-2300		DINNER							
		SNACK							
		MUG/OTHER							
			8-HOUR SUB-TOTAL				**8-HOUR SUB-TOTAL**		
			24-HOUR TOTAL				**24-HOUR TOTAL**		

0200	Voided	300 mL
0600	Voided	500 mL
0615	Water	240 mL
0730	**Breakfast**	
	Orange juice	(whole glass)
	Milk	(1/2 carton)
	Coffee	(1 cup)
0800	Voided	300 mL
1130	**Lunch**	
	Soup	(whole bowl)
	Milk	(1/2 carton)
	Tea	(1 cup)
	Jello	(1 serving)
1330	Voided	450 mL
1430	Water	240 mL
1530	Vomited	50 mL
1730	**Dinner**	
	Soup	(whole bowl)
	Tea	(1 cup)
	Juice	(whole glass)
	Ice cream	(all)
1830	Vomited	100 mL
1845	Water	240 mL
1915	Voided	500 mL
2000	Milk	(1 carton)
2015	Voided	300 mL
2230	Voided	200 mL

Optional Learning Exercises

Use the FOCUS ON PRIDE section to complete these statements and then use the critical thinking and discussion questions to develop your ideas.

32. What are three of your responsibilities that promote good fluid intake?
    A. _____
    B. _____
    C. _____

Critical Thinking and Discussion Questions

33. Review the case of Caruso v Pine Manor Nursing Center, Ill., 1989, in the FOCUS ON PRIDE section of Chapter 31.
    A. What factors do you think may have contributed to Mr. Caruso's dehydration?
    B. If you had been a nursing assistant that had taken care of Mr. Caruso, what could you have done that might have prevented his death?

Fill in the Blank: Key Terms

Aspiration
Enteral nutrition
Flow rate
Gastrostomy tube

Gavage
Intravenous (IV)
    therapy
Jejunostomy tube

Naso-enteral tube
Naso-gastric (NG)
    tube
Parenteral nutrition

Percutaneous
    endoscopic
    gastrostomy (PEG)
    tube

Regurgitation

1. Giving nutrients into the gastro-intestinal (GI) tract through a feeding tube is _____ _____.

2. A _____ is a tube inserted through a surgically created opening in the stomach.

3. _____ is the backward flow of stomach contents into the mouth.

4. A _____ is a feeding tube inserted into a surgically created opening in the jejunum of the small intestine.

5. The process of giving a tube feeding is called _____.

6. The _____ is the number of drops per minute.

7. _____ is breathing fluid, food, vomitus, or an object into the lungs.

8. Giving nutrients through a catheter inserted into a vein is _____.

9. _____ is giving fluids through a needle or catheter inserted into a vein.

10. A feeding tube inserted through the nose into the stomach is a _____.

11. A _____ is a feeding tube inserted into the stomach through a small incision made through the skin.

12. A feeding tube inserted through the nose into the small bowel is a _____.

Circle the Best Answer

13. The nurse instructs you to do a syringe feeding on a patient. What is the most important thing to do before you start the task?
    A. Make sure that the nurse is available to answer your questions
    B. Ask the nurse about the type of formula and the rate
    C. Locate the correct equipment for the procedure
    D. Know if your state allows you to do the procedure

14. Which of these is used for short-term nutritional support?
    A. Naso-gastric tube
    B. Gastrostomy tube
    C. Jejunostomy tube
    D. PEG tube

15. The nurse instructs you to warm the formula for a tube feeding. What would you do?
    A. Take formula out of the refrigerator about 4 hours before the feeding
    B. Take formula out of the refrigerator about 30 minutes before the feeding
    C. Warm refrigerated formula in the microwave for several minutes
    D. Obtain an unopened can that has been stored at room temperature

16. Which person is mostly likely to need frequent cleaning of the nose and nostrils as a comfort measure related to a feeding tube?
    A. Has a jejunostomy tube
    B. Has a gastrostomy tube
    C. Has a PEG tube
    D. Has a naso-enteral tube

17. A major risk with nasogastric tube feedings is
    A. Nausea
    B. Complaints of flatulence
    C. Aspiration
    D. Elevated temperature

18. If a person is receiving a tube feeding, which sign/symptom should you immediately report?
    A. Fatigue   C. Loss of appetite
    B. Respiratory distress   D. Feeling of hunger

19. You can help to prevent regurgitation when a person is receiving gavage when you
    A. Position the person in a left side-lying position
    B. Maintain Fowler's or semi-Fowler's position after the feeding
    C. Assist the person to ambulate in the hallway
    D. Offer the person extra water or other clear fluid

20. When a person is receiving nutrition through a tube, oral hygiene is needed because
    A. It stimulates peristalsis to aid digestion
    B. It decreases dry mouth, dry lips, and sore throat
    C. Formula feedings increase risk for dental caries
    D. Tube feedings give the person bad breath

21. Which task can you perform if allowed by your state and agency?
    A. Insert a feeding tube
    B. Check tube for placement
    C. Remove a nasogastric tube
    D. Check for residual stomach contents

22. You see a new and recently graduated nurse preparing to administer formula feeding through an IV line. What would you do?
    A. Observe for signs and symptoms of distress
    B. Assist by positioning the patient and obtaining a pump
    C. Offer to provide frequent oral hygiene and other basic needs
    D. Tell her to stop and immediately find the charge nurse

23. A person is receiving IV therapy; the drip rate seems to be very rapid. What should you do?
    A. Adjust the flow too slow it down
    B. Tell the nurse about your observations
    C. Try changing the position of the person's arm
    D. Change the IV bag when it is empty

24. You notice that the person's IV has stopped flowing and the IV site is cool and puffy. What would you do first?
    A. Tell the person to keep the arm straight
    B. Ask the person if there is pain or itching
    C. Raise the height of the IV bag
    D. Tell the nurse about the site and the IV

Fill in the Blank

25. Write out the abbreviations.
    A. GI _____
    B. gtt _____
    C. gtt/min _____
    D. IV _____
    E. mL _____
    F. mL/hr _____
    G. NG _____
    H. NPO _____
    I. oz _____
    J. PEG _____
    K. TPN _____

26. Gastrostomy, jejunostomy, and PEG tubes are used for long-term support, usually longer than

    _____.

27. Identify 11 common causes of difficulties with ingesting, chewing, or swallowing food that result in poor nutrition. People with these problems may require enteral nutrition through a feeding tube.
    A. _____
    B. _____
    C. _____
    D. _____
    E. _____
    F. _____
    G. _____
    H. _____
    I. _____
    J. _____
    K. _____

28. Formula is given through a feeding tube at room temperature because cold fluids cause

    _____.

29. When a person has a formula feeding, you can demonstrate good teamwork and time management if you remind the nurse when the

    _____.

30. Coughing, sneezing, vomiting, suctioning, and poor positioning can move a tube out of place and are common causes of _____.

31. What can the nursing assistant do to assist the nurse in preventing regurgitation and aspiration?
    A. _____
    B. _____
    C. _____

32. What comfort measures will help a person with a feeding tube who has a dry mouth?
    A. _____
    B. _____
    C. _____

33. The nose and nostrils are cleaned every 4 to 8 hours because a feeding tube can _____ and

    _____.

34. You are caring for a person who is receiving tube feedings. List 12 observations that need to be reported to the nurse that could be related to the enteral therapy.
    A. _____
    B. _____
    C. _____
    D. _____
    E. _____
    F. _____
    G. _____
    H. _____
    I. _____
    J. _____
    K. _____
    L. _____

35. You are walking by a room and you hear the alarm of an IV pump. You immediately notify the nurse. Name 4 problems that could be causing the pump to alarm.
    A. _____
    B. _____
    C. _____
    D. _____

36. You are assisting a person who has an IV to move and turn in bed. List 2 things that you must do, related to IV bag and IV tubing.
    A. _____
    B. _____

37. When caring for a person who is receiving IV therapy, what signs and symptoms of complications may occur at the IV site?

A. _____

B. _____

C. _____

D. _____

E. _____

F. _____

Optional Learning Exercises

38. What type of feeding tube would each of these persons probably have in place?

A. The nurse tells you Mr. S is expected to have a feeding tube to his stomach for 2 to 3 weeks.

_____

B. Mrs. G. has had a feeding tube inserted into her stomach for 9 months. _____ or

_____

C. The nurse tells you to observe Mr. H. for irritation of his nose and nostrils when you give care.

_____ or

_____

D. The nurse tells you that Mrs. K. is at great risk for regurgitation from her feeding tube.

_____ or _____

39. When you are assisting with tube feedings, why do you turn the lights on in a dark room before beginning?

_____

_____

40. You are caring for a person receiving continuous tube feeding. You note that the formula was hung 7¾ hours ago, so you tell the nurse. Why did you report this to the nurse?

_____

_____

41. Why are older persons more at risk for regurgitation and aspiration?

A. _____

B. _____

42. What would you do if a person with a feeding tube asks you for something to eat or drink?

_____ Why?

_____

_____

43. Mrs. H. has a feeding tube in her nose. Answer these questions about caring for her nose and nostrils.

A. How often should the nose and nostrils be cleaned?

_____

B. How is the tube secured to the nose?

_____

C. Why is the tube secured to the person's garment at the shoulder?

_____

_____

D. What are 2 ways the tube can be secured at the shoulder?

i. _____

ii. _____

44. If a person is receiving TPN, how will you assist the nurse?

A. _____

B. _____

C. _____

45. How can you check the flow rate of an IV?

_____

46. What would you tell the RN at once when you check the flow rate?

A. _____

B. _____

C. _____

D. _____

Use the FOCUS ON PRIDE section to complete these statements and then use the critical thinking and discussion question to develop your ideas.

47. A person with an IV needs a shower. The nurse may have you apply a_____, _____, or

_____.

48. A person receiving IV therapy needs to move from the bed to the chair. You must plan the move to avoid

_____.

Critical Thinking and Discussion Question

49. The nurse is very busy, so she tells you how to change the setting on the person's IV pump. You have watched how it is done and the task seems simple and the nurse's instructions are clear, but you were told in orientation that nursing assistants are not allowed to alter the settings on the pump. What would you do?

33 Vital Signs

Fill in the Blank: Key Terms

Afebrile
Apical-radial pulse
Blood pressure
Body temperature
Bradycardia

Diastole
Diastolic pressure
Febrile
Fever
Hypertension

Hypotension
Pulse
Pulse deficit
Pulse rate
Respiration

Sphygmomanometer
Stethoscope
Systole
Systolic pressure
Tachycardia

Thermometer
Vital signs

1. _____ means with a fever.

2. A rapid heart rate is _____. The heart rate is over 100 beats per minute.

3. The _____ is taking the apical and radial pulse at the same time.

4. An instrument used to listen to the sounds produced by the heart, lungs, and other body organs is a

   _____

5. Low blood pressure is called _____.

6. The _____ is the number of heartbeats or pulses felt in 1 minute.

7. The amount of heat in the body that is a balance between the amount of heat produced and amount lost by the body is the _____.

8. _____ is the period of heart muscle contraction; the heart is pumping blood.

9. High blood pressure is called

   _____

10. The cuff and measuring device used to measure blood pressure is a _____.

11. The beat of the heart felt at an artery as a wave of blood passes through the artery is the

    _____

12. Without a fever is _____.

13. Temperature, pulse, respirations, and blood pressure are _____; pulse oximetry and pain are included in some agencies.

14. _____ is a slow heart rate; the rate is less than 60 beats per minute.

15. The amount of force it takes to pump blood out of the heart into the arterial circulation is the

    _____

16. The period when the heart is at rest is

    _____

17. The difference between the apical and radial pulse rates is the _____.

18. _____ is the amount of force exerted against the walls of an artery by the blood.

19. Breathing air into and out of the lungs is

    _____

20. _____ is the pressure in the arteries when the heart is at rest.

21. Elevated body temperature is

    _____.

22. A _____ is a device used to measure temperature.

Circle the Best Answer

23. Persons in nursing centers usually have vital signs measured
    A. Once a shift   C. Once a month
    B. Every 4 hours   D. Weekly

24. Unless otherwise ordered, take vital signs when the person
    A. Is lying or sitting
    B. Has been walking or exercising
    C. Has just finished eating
    D. Is getting ready to take a shower or tub bath

25. Body temperature is lower in the
    A. Afternoon   C. Evening
    B. Morning   D. Night

26. If you are taking vital signs on a person with dementia, it may be better if
    A. You have a co-worker hold the person so he or she does not move
    B. The vital signs are taken when the person is asleep
    C. Pulse and respirations are done; temperature and blood pressure are done later
    D. You ask the nurse to take the vital signs

27. What should you do if a person asks about their vital sign measurements?
    A. You can tell the person the measurements if center policy allows.
    B. Tell the nurse that the person wants to know the measurements.
    C. Tell the person you cannot tell them this information.
    D. This information is private and cannot be shared.

28. If you take a rectal temperature, the normal range of the temperature would be
    A. 96.6°F to 98.6°F (35.9°C to 37.0°C)
    B. 97.6°F to 99.6°F (36.5°C to 37.5°C)
    C. 98.6°F to 100.6°F (37.0°C to 38.1°C)
    D. 98.6°F to 101°F (37°C to 38.3°C)

29. If you are taking the temperature of an older person, you would expect the temperature to be
    A. Lower than the normal range
    B. Higher than the normal range
    C. About in the middle of the normal range
    D. The same as in a younger adult

30. For a 1-year old child with an ear infection, which equipment would you use to ensure safety and to get the most accurate temperature?
    A. Tympanic thermometer with probe cover
    B. Glass mercury thermometer with a red stem
    C. Digital thermometer at the axillary site
    D. Electronic probe with a red stem

31. To read a glass thermometer you should hold it at the
    A. Stem above eye level and look up to read it
    B. Tip and bring it to eye level to read it
    C. Stem and bring it to eye level to read it
    D. Tip at waist level and look down to read it

32. If you are preparing to take an oral temperature, ask the person not to
    A. Eat, drink, smoke, or chew gum for at least 15 to 20 minutes
    B. Shower or bathe right before the temperature is taken
    C. Exercise for 30 minutes before
    D. Eat, drink, or smoke for at least 5 to 10 minutes

33. An electronic thermometer is inserted into the rectum
    A. 1 inch   C. ½ inch
    B. 2 inches   D. 3 inches

34. When taking a temperature for persons who are confused and resist care, the best choice would be to
    A. Take a rectal temperature
    B. Use a glass oral thermometer
    C. Take an axillary temperature
    D. Use a tympanic or temporal artery thermometer

35. Which site is most commonly used to check the pulse?
    A. Carotid   C. Radial
    B. Brachial   D. Popliteal

36. Which site is used to take a pulse during cardiopulmonary resuscitation (CPR)?
    A. Carotid   C. Femoral
    B. Temporal   D. Radial

37. When using a stethoscope, you can help to prevent infection by
    A. Covering the ear-pieces and diaphragm with a disposable plastic cover
    B. Wiping the ear-pieces and diaphragm with antiseptic wipes before and after use
    C. Soaking and washing the stethoscope in a disinfectant solution
    D. Placing a clean paper towel between the person's skin and the diaphragm

38. A pulse rate of 120 beats per minute would be considered
    A. Bradycardia   C. Tachycardia
    B. Bounding   D. Irregular

39. You counted 40 heartbeats in 30 seconds. What is the person's pulse rate?
    A. 40 beats per minute   C. 70 beats per minute
    B. 60 beats per minute   D. 80 beats per minute

40. The nurse tells you that the person's pulse was thready on the previous shift. What is the nurse describing about the pulse?
    A. Force   C. Rhythm
    B. Rate   D. Deficit

41. When taking the radial pulse, place
    A. The thumb over the pulse site
    B. The index finger on the middle of the wrist
    C. Two fingers on the thumb side of the wrist
    D. The stethoscope on the chest wall

42. You may count the radial pulse for 30 seconds and multiple by 2 if
    A. The pulse is easy to locate
    B. You lose count after 30 seconds
    C. The pulse is regular
    D. The person is restless

43. The apical pulse is taken
    A. For a full minute
    B. For 2 minutes if there is a pulse deficit
    C. For 15 seconds and multiplied by 4
    D. For 30 seconds and multiplied by 2

44. An apical pulse of 72 is recorded as
    A. Pulse 72   C. 72Ap
    B. 72 – Apical pulse   D. P 72

45. An apical-radial pulse is taken by
    A. Taking the radial pulse for 1 minute and then taking the apical pulse for 1 minute
    B. Subtracting the apical pulse from the radial pulse
    C. Having one staff member take the apical pulse and a second staff member take the radial pulse at the same time
    D. Having 2 staff members take the apical pulse at the same time; than the 2 staff members take the radial pulse at the same time

46. A pedal pulse is found
    A. By listening with a stethoscope
    B. Over a foot bone
    C. On the thumb side of the wrist
    D. At the apex of the heart, just to the left of the sternum

47. When counting respirations, the best way is to
    A. Place your hand on the person's chest and watch the chest rise and fall
    B. Keep your fingers on the pulse site while you are counting the respirations
    C. Tell the person to breathe normally so you can count the respirations
    D. Use the stethoscope to hear the respirations clearly and count for 1 full minute

48. Each respiration involves
    A. 1 inhalation
    B. 1 exhalation
    C. 1 inhalation and 1 exhalation
    D. Counting for 30 seconds and multiplying by 2

49. The blood pressure may be higher in older persons because
    A. They have orthostatic hypotension
    B. Their diet is higher in sodium
    C. Blood pressure increases with age
    D. They are usually over-weight

50. The blood pressure may not be taken in the left arm
    A. If person has a dialysis access site in the left arm
    B. If the person has been sleeping on his left side
    C. If the person is very obese and both arms are large
    D. If the person plays sports and he is left-handed

51. You will find out the size of blood pressure cuff needed
    A. By asking the nurse
    B. By measuring the person's arm
    C. By looking at the equipment
    D. By asking the person

52. When taking a blood pressure with an aneroid manometer, you place the stethoscope diaphragm
    A. Over the radial artery on the thumb side of the wrist
    B. Over the brachial artery at the inner aspect of the elbow
    C. Over the carotid during cardiopulmonary resuscitation
    D. Over the apical pulse site just left of the sternum

53. When getting ready to take the blood pressure, position the person's arm
    A. Beside the body
    B. Level with the heart
    C. Below the level of the heart
    D. Abducted from the body

54. The blood pressure cuff is inflated _____ beyond the point where you last felt the radial pulse.
    A. 10 mm Hg   C. 30 mm Hg
    B. 20 mm Hg   D. 40 mm Hg

Fill in the Blank

55. Write out the abbreviations.
    A. BP _____
    B. C _____
    C. F _____
    D. Hg _____
    E. ID _____
    F. IV _____
    G. mm _____
    H. mm Hg _____
    J. TPR _____

56. Vital signs are taken when the person takes drugs that affect the _____ or _____ systems.

57. When vital signs are taken, report to the nurse at once if
    A. _____
    B. _____

58. Sites for measuring temperature are the
    A. _____
    B. _____
    C. _____
    D. _____
    E. _____

59. Which site has the highest normal range temperature?
    _____

60. Which site has the lowest baseline temperature?
    _____

61. If a glass thermometer breaks, _____ at once because it may contain _____, which is a _____.

62. When you read a Fahrenheit thermometer, the short lines mean _____.

63. List how long the glass thermometer remains in place for these sites.
    A. Oral _____ or as required by center policy
    B. Rectal _____ or as required by center policy
    C. Axillary _____ or as required by center policy

64. When taking an oral temperature, place the tip of the thermometer _____.

65. When taking an axillary temperature, the axilla must be _____.

66. Tympanic membrane and temporal artery thermometers are used for confused persons because they are _____.

67. When using an electronic thermometer, what does the color of the probe mean?
    A. Blue _____
    B. Red _____

68. When you take a rectal temperature, you _____ the tip of the thermometer or the end of the covered probe before inserting it into the rectum.

69. When taking a tympanic membrane temperature on an adult, pull up and back on the ear to _____.

70. The adult pulse rate is between
_____ beats per minute.

71. List words used to describe:
A. Forceful pulse _____
B. Hard-to-feel pulse _____

72. If a pulse is irregular, count the pulse for
_____.

73. When you take a pulse, what observations should be reported and recorded?
A. _____
B. _____
C. _____
D. _____
E. _____

74. Do not use your thumb to take a pulse because
_____.

75. When taking an apical pulse, each *lub-dub* sound is counted as _____.

76. The apical pulse rate is never less than the
_____.

77. The nurse may mark the skin with an X where the
_____ is found.

78. A healthy adult has _____ respirations per minute.

79. What observations should be reported and recorded when counting respirations?
A. _____
B. _____
C. _____
D. _____
E. _____
F. _____

80. One respiration is counted for each _____
_____.

81. Respirations are counted for _____
_____ if they are abnormal or irregular.

82. Blood pressure is controlled by
A. _____
B. _____
C. _____

83. Report blood pressures that have these readings.
A. Systolic over _____;
systolic below _____
B. Diastolic over _____;
diastolic below _____

84. Let the person rest for _____ before taking the blood pressure.

85. When you are taking a blood pressure, the person should be in a _____
or _____ position.
Sometimes, the doctor orders blood pressure in the
_____ position.

86. When listening to the blood pressure, the first sound you hear is the _____
pressure and the point where the sound disappears is the _____ pressure.

Optional Learning Exercises

Taking Temperatures

87. You prepare to take Mr. Harrison's temperature with a glass thermometer. When you take the thermometer from the container, it reads 97.8 °F. What should you do? _____

88. If the thermometer registers between 2 short lines, record the temperature to the _____.

Taking Pulses and Respirations

89. You are assigned to take Mrs. Sanchez's pulse and respirations. You note that the pulse rate and respirations are regular, so you take each one for
_____. When you complete counting the pulse, you keep your
_____ and count respirations. This is done so that Mrs. Sanchez will _____.

90. When you finish counting Mrs. Sanchez's pulse and respirations, your numbers are pulse 36 and respirations 9. What numbers should be recorded?
Pulse _____
Respirations _____ Why?
_____
_____

91. The nurse tells you to take an apical-radial pulse on Mrs. Hellman. Why do you ask a co-worker to help you? _____

92. How long is an apical-radial pulse counted?
_____ After you have taken the apical-radial pulse, how do you find the pulse deficit? _____
_____

Taking Blood Pressures

93. You are assigned to take Mr. Hardaway's blood pressure. You know that he goes for dialysis 3 times a week. What do you need to know before you take his blood pressure? _____
_____
Why? _____
_____

94. When you inflate the cuff, you cannot feel the pulse after you pump the cuff to 130 mm Hg. How high will you inflate the cuff to take his blood pressure?

_____

95. You should deflate the cuff at an even rate of _____ per second.

Labeling

96. Fill in the drawings so that the thermometers read correctly.

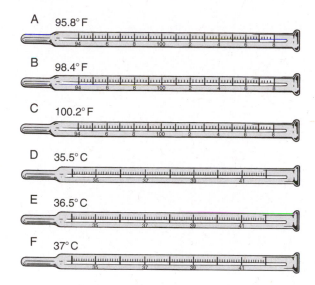

A   95.8° F

B   98.4° F

C   100.2° F

D   35.5° C

E   36.5° C

F   37° C

97. Name the pulse sites shown.

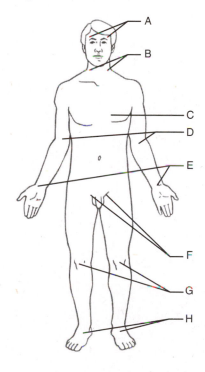

A. _____
B. _____
C. _____
D. _____
E. _____
F. _____
G. _____
H. _____
I. Which pulse is used during cardiopulmonary resuscitation (CPR)? _____
J. Which pulse is most commonly taken?

_____

K. Which pulse is used when placing the stethoscope to take the blood pressure? _____
L. Which pulse is found with a stethoscope?

_____

98. Fill in the drawings so that the dials show the correct blood pressures.

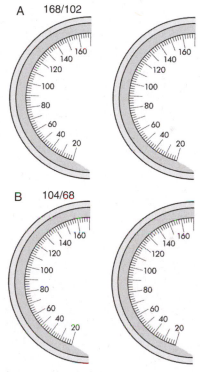

A   168/102

B   104/68

99. Which step, for taking a blood pressure, is depicted in the figure?

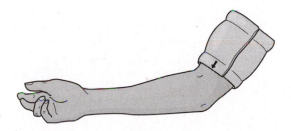

Use the FOCUS ON PRIDE section to complete these statements.

100. If the person is on Transmission-Based Precautions, the isolation cart with the vital sign equipment must be _____

101. A friend is in the nursing assistants' program with you. She is unable to master the skill of taking a blood pressure using a stethoscope and an aneroid manometer. Suggest ways to help her.

34 Exercise and Activity

Fill in the Blank: Key Terms

Abduction
Adduction
Ambulation
Atrophy
Bed rest
Contracture

Deconditioning
Dorsiflexion
Extension
External rotation
Flexion
Footdrop

Hyperextension
Internal rotation
Opposition
Orthostatic
  hypotension
Orthotic

Plantar flexion
Postural hypotension
Pronation
Range of motion
  (ROM)
Rotation

Supination
Syncope

1. Touching the opposite finger with the thumb is
_____.

2. The foot is bent down at the ankle when
_____ is present.

3. A brief loss of consciousness or fainting is
_____.

4. Bending a body part is
_____.

5. Moving a body part away from the mid-line of the
body is _____.

6. _____ is
the movement of a joint to the extent possible without
causing pain.

7. Turning the joint outward is _____.

8. A drop in blood pressure when the person suddenly
stands up is postural hypotension or
_____.

9. _____ occurs when
moving a body part toward the mid-line of the body.

10. Turning the joint upward is called
_____.

11. Bending the toes and foot up at the ankle is
_____.

12. Excessive straightening of a body part is
_____.

13. A decrease in size or a wasting away of tissue is
_____.

14. Turning the joint is
_____.

15. _____ is straightening
of a body part.

16. _____ is another name
for orthostatic hypotension.

17. _____ is permanent
plantar flexion; the foot falls down at the ankle.

18. The act of walking is
_____.

19. _____ is turning the
joint downward.

20. The loss of muscle strength from inactivity is
_____.

21. _____ is turning the
joint inward.

22. The lack of joint mobility caused by abnormal
shortening of a muscle is a
_____.

23. An _____ is
used to support a muscle, promote a certain motion,
or correct a deformity.

24. Restricting a person to bed and limiting activity for
health reasons is _____.

Circle the Best Answer

25. Which complication of bedrest will result in loss of
function and deformity of the joint?
A. Contracture
B. Pressure injury
C. Blood clot
D. Postural hypotension

26. If a contracture develops
A. It will require extra range-of-motion exercises to
correct it
B. Good body alignment and positioning will relieve
the complication
C. The contracted muscle is fixed into position and
cannot stretch
D. It will resolve as soon as the person is able to walk
and exercise

27. When you are caring for a person who has orthostatic
hypotension, you should
A. Raise the head of the bed slowly to Fowler's
position
B. Have the person stand up and pause while the
dizziness passes
C. Keep the bed flat when getting the person out of
bed
D. Have the person slowly walk around to decrease
dizziness

28. Which nursing care prevents complications from
bedrest?
A. Using the Fowler's position
B. Taking frequent vital signs
C. Maintaining good body alignment
D. Encouraging deconditioning

29. If a person sitting on the edge of the bed complains of weakness, dizziness, or spots before the eyes, you should
    A. Assist the person to slowly stand
    B. Help the person to sit in a chair or walk around
    C. Have the person return to the Fowler's position
    D. Tell the person that the symptoms are a normal response

30. Bed-boards are used to
    A. Maintain alignment by preventing the mattress from sagging
    B. Prevent plantar flexion that can lead to footdrop
    C. Keep the hips abducted
    D. Keep the weight of top linens off the feet

31. Which equipment do you need to obtain in order to position the person and prevent plantar flexion?
    A. Foot-board
    B. Bed cradle
    C. Foam rubber sponge
    D. Abduction wedge

32. To prevent the hips and legs from turning outward, you can use
    A. Bed cradles
    B. Hip abduction wedges
    C. Trochanter rolls
    D. Splints

33. Which action would be the best to help the person to exercise?
    A. Give the person a schedule of activities
    B. Talk about the benefits of exercise
    C. Encourage the person to use a trapeze to move
    D. Leave the person alone to do self-care

34. When you move the person's joints through the range of motion, you are preforming
    A. Active range-of-motion
    B. Activities of daily living
    C. Active-assistive range-of-motion
    D. Passive range-of-motion

35. A nursing assistant can perform range-of-motion exercises on the _____ only if allowed by center policy.
    A. Shoulder
    B. Neck
    C. Hip
    D. Knee

36. With the nurse's approval, which play activity would be the best for a child who needs shoulder ROM?
    A. Pretending to fly like a bird
    B. Drawing a picture of a bird
    C. Making a bird out of clay
    D. Playing a video game with birds

37. Pronation and supination would be included in ROM for which body part?
    A. Forearms
    B. Elbows
    C. Knees
    D. Fingers

38. Which of these joints can be adducted and abducted?
    A. Neck
    B. Hip
    C. Forearm
    D. Knee

39. When you help a person who is weak and unsteady to walk, you should
    A. Apply a gait (transfer) belt
    B. Have the person lean on furniture for balance
    C. Put the person in a wheelchair
    D. Get the person a pair of crutches

40. When the person is walking with crutches, the person should wear
    A. Soft slippers on the feet
    B. Clothes that fit well
    C. Clothes that are padded
    D. Exercise pants

41. When walking with a cane, it is held
    A. On the strong side of the body
    B. On the weak side of the body
    C. In the right hand
    D. On the left side of the body

42. When a person is using a walker, it is
    A. Picked up and moved 1 to 2 inches in front of the person
    B. Moved forward with a rocking motion
    C. Moved first on the left side and then on the right
    D. Pushed and moved 6 to 8 inches in front of the person's feet

43. When you are caring for a person who wears a brace, it is important to immediately report
    A. How far the person can walk without assistance
    B. Progress the person has made in independently donning the brace
    C. The amount of mobility in joints when doing range-of-motion exercises
    D. Any redness or signs of skin breakdown when you remove the brace

Fill in the Blank

44. Write out the abbreviations.
    A. ADL _____
    B. ID _____
    C. PROM _____
    D. ROM _____

45. You assist the nurse in promoting _____ and _____ for all persons to the extent possible.

46. Bedrest is ordered to
    A. _____
    B. _____
    C. _____
    D. _____

47. The nurse tells you the resident is on bedrest, but can use the bathroom for elimination. This type of bedrest is _____.

48. When a person is moved from lying or sitting to a standing position, the blood pressure may _____. This is called _____.

49. Supportive devices such as bed-boards are used to _____ and _____ the person in a certain position.

50. When you use a foot-board, the soles of the feet are _____ against it to prevent _____.

51. A trochanter roll is placed along the body to prevent the hips and legs from _____.

52. Hand rolls or grips prevent

_____ of the thumb, fingers, and wrists.

53. A splint is used to keep these joints in their normal positions.
    A. _____
    B. _____
    C. _____
    D. _____
    E. _____
    F. _____

54. Bed cradles are used because the weight of top linens can cause _____ and

_____.

55. A trapeze bar allows the person to lift the

_____

off the bed. It also allows the person to

_____

and _____ in bed.

56. When a person does exercises with some help, they are doing _____ range-of-motion exercises.

57. When range-of-motion exercises are done, what should be reported or recorded?
    A. _____
    B. _____
    C. _____
    D. _____
    E. _____

58. When performing range-of-motion exercises, each movement should be repeated _____ times or the _____.

59. List the safety measures to follow when performing range-of-motion exercises.
    A. _____
    B. _____
    C. _____
    D. _____
    E. _____
    F. _____
    G. _____
    H. _____
    I. _____

60. When you help a person to walk, you should walk to the _____ and

_____ the person. Provide support with the _____.

61. Many people prefer a walker because it gives more support than a _____.

Optional Learning Exercises

62. What kind of range of motion would be used with each of these residents?
    A. The resident needs complete care for bathing, grooming, and feeding.

    _____

    B. The resident takes part in many activities in the center. She walks to most activities independently.

    _____

    C. The resident has weakness on his left side. He is able to feed himself but needs help with bathing and dressing.

    _____

63. As you plan to help a person out of bed, you are concerned about orthostatic hypotension. To make sure the person is able to stand and get up safely, you plan to take the blood pressure, pulse, and respirations several times. When would you take the blood pressure?
    A. _____
    B. _____
    C. _____
    D. _____
    E. _____

64. When doing range-of-motion exercises, you should ask the person if he or she
    A. _____
    B. _____
    C. _____

65. When you are going to assist a person to ambulate, you can promote comfort and reduce fears when you explain
    A. _____
    B. _____
    C. _____
    D. _____
    E. _____

66. When you help a person to walk, what observations are reported and recorded?
    A. _____
    B. _____
    C. _____
    D. _____
    E. _____

67. When using a cane, the person walks as follows:
    A. Step A: _____
    B. Step B: _____
    C. Step C: _____

68. What should be immediately reported if observed when a brace is removed? _____

_____

Use the FOCUS ON PRIDE section to complete these statements.

69. You can promote activity, exercise, and well-being when you

    A. _____

    B. _____

    C. _____

    D. _____

70. If an elderly person can slowly ambulate, pushing him or her in a wheelchair to the dining room is contributing to that person's deconditioning. What other examples can you think of that contribute to deconditioning?

Labeling

71. ROM exercises for the _____ joint are shown in these drawings. Name the movements shown in each drawing.

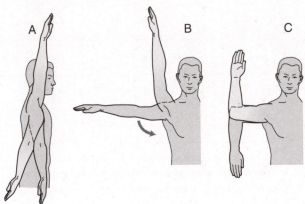

    A. _____

    B. _____

    C. _____

72. ROM exercises for the _____ are shown in these drawings. Name the movements shown in each drawing.

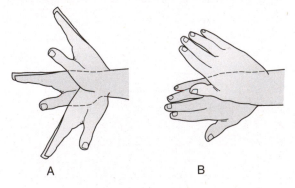

    A. _____

    B. _____

73. ROM exercises for the _____ are shown in these drawings. Name the movements shown in each drawing.

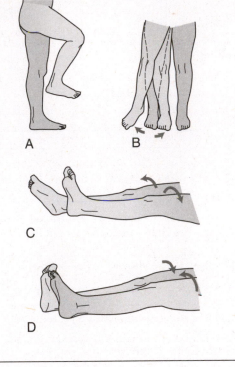

    A. _____

    B. _____

    C. _____

    D. _____

Crossword

Fill in the crossword by answering the clues below with the words from this list:

Abduction	Flexion	Rotation	Plantar flexion
Adduction	Hyperextension	Internal rotation	Pronation
Extension	Dorsiflexion	External rotation	Supination

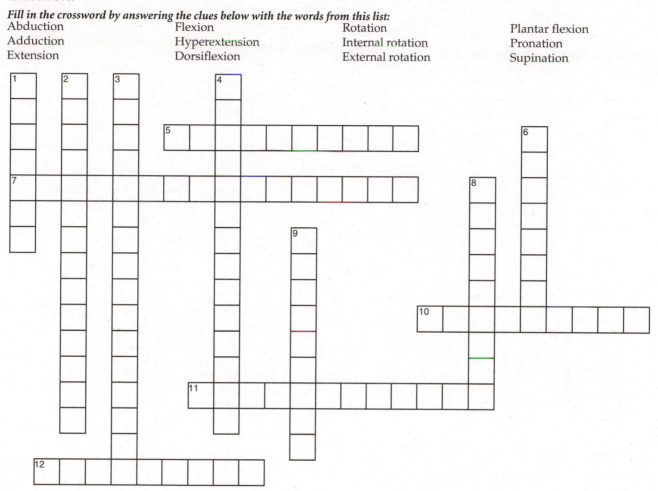

Across

5. Turning the joint upward
7. Turning the joint inward
10. Straightening a body part
11. Bending the toes and foot up at the ankle
12. Turning the joint downward

Down

1. Bending a body part
2. Bending the foot down at the ankle
3. Turning the joint outward
4. Excessive straightening of a body part
6. Turning the joint
8. Moving a body part away from the midline of the body
9. Moving a body part toward the midline of the body

35 Comfort, Rest, and Sleep

Fill in the Blank: Key Terms

Acute pain	Discomfort	Pain	Relaxation	Sleepwalking
Chronic pain	Distraction	Phantom pain	Rest	
Circadian rhythm	Guided imagery	Radiating pain	Sleep	
Comfort	Insomnia	Referred pain	Sleep deprivation	

1. The amount and quality of sleep are not adequate when _____ occurs.

2. To hurt, ache or be sore is _____.

3. _____ is pain that is felt suddenly from injury, disease, trauma, or surgery.

4. _____ is a way to focus a person's attention on something unrelated to the pain.

5. _____ is a state of unconsciousness, reduced voluntary muscle activity, and lowered metabolism.

6. Pain lasting longer than 12 weeks is _____. It is constant or occurs off and on.

7. _____ is to be free from mental or physical stress.

8. _____ is a state of well-being. The person has no physical or emotional pain and is calm and at peace.

9. To be calm, at ease, and relaxed is to _____. The person is free of anxiety and stress.

10. Creating and focusing on an image is _____.

11. Pain from a body part that is felt in another body part is _____.

12. _____ is a chronic condition in which the person cannot sleep or stay asleep all night.

13. The day-night cycle or body rhythm is also called _____. This daily rhythm is based on a 24-hour cycle.

14. _____ is felt at the site of tissue damage and spreads to other areas.

15. To ache, hurt, or be sore is _____. It is also called pain.

16. Pain felt in a body part that is no longer there is _____.

17. When the person leaves the bed and walks about while sleeping, he or she is _____.

Circle the Best Answer

18. When you explain what to expect, this helps to reduce
    A. Attention
    B. Anxiety
    C. Pain
    D. Insomnia

19. Which question indicates that you want the person to be comfortable?
    A. "What do you want to drink for lunch?"
    B. "Did you have a nice visit with your family?"
    C. "What time do you like to go to bed?"
    D. "Should I adjust your pillow?"

20. Which question, related to pain, is a surveyor most likely to ask you?
    A. "What would you do to restore a person's well-being?"
    B. "What kind of medications are given for pain?"
    C. "What are the signs and symptoms of pain?"
    D. "How would you teach a person to relax?"

21. Rest and sleep are needed to
    A. Restore well-being and energy
    B. Prevent anxiety
    C. Increase muscle strength
    D. Prevent pain

22. CMS requirements related to comfort, rest, and sleep include
    A. Only two people in a room
    B. Bright lighting in all areas
    C. Room temperature between 65°F and 71°F
    D. Adequate ventilation and room humidity

23. When a person complains of pain or discomfort
    A. You rely on what the person says about the pain or discomfort
    B. It must be carefully measured to determine if the person has pain
    C. You should compare the person's pain to others' pain
    D. You can tell if the person has pain by the way he or she acts

24. When a person complains of pain that is nearby an area of tissue damage, which kind of pain is the person describing?
    A. Acute
    B. Chronic
    C. Radiating
    D. Phantom

25. If the person thinks that pain is a sign of weakness, which behavior is he or she most likely to display?
    A. Cries quietly and softly
    B. Enjoys being pampered
    C. Denies or ignores pain
    D. Seeks support from others

26. A stoic reaction to pain is most likely to be related to
    A. Illness
    B. Culture
    C. Anxiety
    D. Attention

27. When a person has anxiety, the person
    A. May feel increased pain
    B. Will usually feel less pain
    C. May deny having pain
    D. Will usually refuse pain medication

28. When you ask a person, to rate the pain on a pain scale of 0 to 10, you are asking the person to
    A. Describe the pain
    B. Tell you the location of the pain
    C. Tell you the onset and duration of the pain
    D. Explain the intensity of the pain

29. A child may deal with pain by
    A. Restricting play or school activities
    B. Describing pain to an adult
    C. Asking for pain medications
    D. Concentrating on reading or playing quietly

30. Older persons may ignore new pain because they
    A. Cannot verbally communicate pain
    B. May think it is related to a known health problem
    C. Have increased anxiety
    D. Are used to being in pain

31. When a person tells you he or she has pain when coughing or deep breathing, this is
    A. A factor causing pain
    B. A measurement of the onset of pain
    C. Words used to describe the pain
    D. The location of the pain

32. A distraction measure to promote comfort and relieve pain may be
    A. Asking the person to focus on an image
    B. Learning to breathe deeply and slowly
    C. Listening to music or playing games
    D. Contracting and relaxing muscle groups

33. If the nurse has given a person pain medication, it is best if you
    A. Give the person a bath
    B. Walk the person according to the care plan
    C. Wait 30 minutes before giving care
    D. Give care before the medication makes the person sleepy

34. Which time of day is pain most likely to seem worse for the person?
    A. Upon waking   C. Late afternoon
    B. Just before meals   D. Nighttime

35. You can promote comfort and help relieve pain when you
    A. Perform passive range-of-motion exercises
    B. Provide blankets for warmth and to prevent chilling
    C. Make sure the person ambulates every 2 hours
    D. Keep the person in the supine position

36. Lotion is used for back massage because it
    A. Stimulates circulation
    B. Heals any skin breakdown
    C. Reduces friction during the massage
    D. Refreshes the skin

37. Which condition could be a dangerous contraindication for giving a back massage?
    A. Sleep deprivation   C. Arthritis
    B. Lung disorder   D. Insomnia

38. The best position for a back massage is
    A. Prone position
    B. Supine position
    C. Semi-Fowler's position
    D. Fowler's position

39. When giving a back massage, the strokes
    A. Start at the shoulders and go up towards the neck
    B. Are circular over the buttocks and up and down on the arms
    C. Start at the lower back and go up to the shoulders
    D. Are continued for at least 10 minutes

40. Which action promotes rest?
    A. Helping with elimination needs
    B. Making sure the person feels happy
    C. Allowing the person to sleep through breakfast
    D. Giving care whenever you have extra time

41. When caring for an ill or injured person, you know the person may need more rest. You can help the person to get rest by making sure you
    A. Provide range-of-motion exercises on a set schedule
    B. Provide rest periods during or after a procedure
    C. Give complete hygiene and grooming measures
    D. Spend time talking with the person to distract him or her

42. Which of these occurs during sleep?
    A. The person cannot respond to stimuli.
    B. Metabolism is reduced during sleep.
    C. Vital signs are higher.
    D. Arm or leg movements are voluntary

43. If you are thinking about taking a night shift job, you should consider your own
    A. Circadian rhythm
    B. Bedtime rituals
    C. Ability to relax
    D. Preference for job tasks

44. An elderly resident who frequently gets up at 3:00 am and comes to the nursing station to visit with the staff is likely to be having
    A. Sleepwalking   C. Disorientation
    B. Agitation   D. Insomnia

45. Which food would help to induce sleep if given as a snack before bedtime?
    A. Apple slices   C. Tomato juice
    B. Low-fat milk   D. Chocolate cookie

46. Which age-group requires the least amount of sleep?
    A. Newborns
    B. Pre-schoolers
    C. Teenagers
    D. Adults, including the elderly

47. Which person is most likely to have an increased need for sleep?
    A. Person who started a new exercise program
    B. Person who was seriously injured in a car accident
    C. Person who started an extreme weight loss diet
    D. Person who was transferred to night shift

48. An increase in vital signs is expected when a person is
    A. Napping during the day
    B. Experiencing insomnia
    C. Sleeping soundly
    D. Having acute pain

49. Which pain report is the most serious and requires that the nurse be immediately notified?
    A. Person is having referred pain that is felt in the left arm and shoulder
    B. Person is having phantom pain that is felt in the amputated leg
    C. Person is having chronic pain related to joint stiffness and arthritis
    D. Person is having radiating pain that starts in the lower back and goes to buttocks

50. Persons who are ill, in pain, or receiving hospital care are at risk for
    A. Sleep deprivation
    B. Sleepwalking
    C. Insomnia
    D. Over sedation

51. If a person has decreased reasoning; red, puffy eyes; and coordination problems, report this to the nurse because the person
    A. Is having a reaction to sleeping medications
    B. Has signs and symptoms of sleep disorders
    C. May be having episodes of uncontrolled pain
    D. May need an increase in sleeping pills

52. Which of these measures help to promote sleep?
    A. Provide extra blankets and turn down the room temperatures
    B. Help persons to void or make sure incontinent persons are clean and dry.
    C. Follow bedtime routines to make sure everyone is in bed at the scheduled time
    D. Offer everyone a cup of coffee or tea with crackers at bedtime.

53. When a person with Alzheimer's disease wanders at night, you can assist her by
    A. Giving her a cup of coffee or tea
    B. Turning on the TV in the room to distract her
    C. Being calm and quiet and helping her back to her room
    D. Explaining to her that it is night and she needs to go to bed

54. Which nursing measures would be best to promote sleep for a 9-year old child is having trouble falling asleep in the strange hospital environment?
    A. Hold the child and rock her
    B. Help her take a warm bath
    C. Darken the room and close the door
    D. Read a favorite story to her

Fill in the Blank

55. CMS have requirements about the person's room. List the requirements that relate to each of these.
    A. Suspended curtain _____
    B. Linens _____
    C. Bed _____
    D. Room temperature _____
    E. Persons in room _____

56. Name the type of pain described.
    A. A person with an amputated leg may still sense leg pain. _____
    B. There is tissue damage. The pain decreases with healing. _____
    C. Pain from a heart attack is often felt in the left chest, left jaw, left shoulder, and left arm. _____
    D. The pain remains for a long time. Common causes are arthritis and cancer. _____
    E. Person has gallbladder disease, but experiences pain in the right shoulder _____

57. Older persons may ignore or deny new pain because
    A. _____
    B. _____

58. In persons with dementia, pain may be signaled by changes _____.

59. When gathering information about a person in pain, you can use a scale of 1 to 10. Which end of the scale is the most severe pain? _____

60. What happens to vital signs when the person has acute pain? _____

61. What happens to vital signs when the person has chronic pain? _____

62. When the person uses words such as *aching, knifelike,* or *sore* to describe pain, what do you report to the nurse? _____

63. What body responses that you can see or measure (objective signs) may mean the person has pain?
    A. _____
    B. _____
    C. _____
    D. _____
    E. _____

64. What changes in these behaviors may be symptoms of pain?
    A. Affected body part _____
    B. Body position _____

65. List nursing measures to promote comfort and relieve pain related to these clues.
    A. Position of the person _____
    B. Linens _____
    C. Blankets _____
    D. Pain medications _____
    E. Family members _____

66. If a person is receiving strong pain medication or sedatives, what safety measures are important?
    A. _____
    B. _____
    C. _____
    D. _____

67. When giving a back massage, what is the effect of
    A. Fast movements _____
    B. Slow movements _____

68. When you are delegated to give a back massage, what observations should you report and record?
    A. _____
    B. _____
    C. _____
    D. _____

69. When you explain the procedure before performing it, you may help a person to rest better because you met the need for _____.

70. A clean, neat, and uncluttered room can promote rest by meeting _____ needs.

71. The mind and body rest, the body saves energy, and body functions slow during
    _____.

72. If work hours change, it can affect the normal _____ cycle or _____ rhythm.

73. Alcohol tends to cause _____ and sleep However, after drinking alcohol the person may _____ and have difficulty falling back to sleep.

74. List six questions you could ask the person to see if he or she needs additional nursing measures to promote comfort.
    A. _____
    B. _____
    C. _____
    D. _____
    E. _____
    F. _____

75. A person reports pain. List the 8 things that the nurse needs to know about the person's pain.
    A. _____
    B. _____
    C. _____
    D. _____
    E. _____
    F. _____
    G. _____
    H. _____

Optional Learning Exercises

76. You are caring for 2 residents who both have arthritis. Mr. Forman tells you this is the first time he has had any health problems. Mrs. Wegman tells you she has had several surgeries and has had 3 children. Who is likely to be more anxious about the pain and to be unable to handle the pain well, Mr. Forman or Mrs. Wegman?
    _____ Why? _____
    _____

77. Mr. Forman tells you his pain seems much worse at night. What could be the reason for this reaction?
    _____
    _____

78. You are caring for Mrs. Reynolds. She tells you she misses her children who have moved to another state. Today, Mrs. Reynolds is complaining of pain in her abdomen. In spite of providing nursing comfort measures, she still rates her pain at a 7. What is a possible reason that Mrs. Reynolds is not getting relief of her pain? _____
    _____

79. When a person is ill, how do these affect sleep?
    A. Treatments and therapies _____.
    B. Care devices such as traction or a cast
    _____.
    C. Emotions that affect sleep include
    _____.

80. Certain foods affect sleep. Tell how these foods affect sleep and list foods that contain the substances.
    A. Caffeine _____ sleep. It is found in
    _____
    _____.
    B. Trytophan _____ sleep. It is found in _____.

Labeling

81. Complete the Wong-Baker FACES scale by writing the number and the description of the pain under each face.

(From Hockenberry MJ and others: *Wong's nursing care of infants and children*, ed 10, St Louis, 2015, Mosby.)

Use the FOCUS ON PRIDE section to complete these statements.

82. When you are caring for persons who have pain, what is your responsibility?

A. Report _____ and

_____ .

B. Report what the person _____

and what you _____ .

83. It is important to report signs and symptoms of pain because the nurse uses this information to

_____ .

84. Avoid making _____ about the person's pain.

Critical Thinking and Discussion Question

85. You are assigned to help a person with hygiene and ADLs in a home setting. You notice that the person frequently complains of pain when certain family members are present. You suspect that the person may enjoy the extra attention and pampering from family members. What would you do?

Fill in the Blank: Key Terms

Admission   Discharge   Transfer

1. Moving the person to another health care setting or moving the person to a new room within the agency is a_____

2. The official entry of a person into a health care setting is _____.

3. _____ occurs with the official departure of a person from a health care setting.

Circle the Best Answer

4. The nurse has instructed you to assist with the admission of a person to the health care facility. Which information do you need to get from the nurse?
   A. Reason for admission and anticipated length of stay
   B. What to say about who gives care and how care is given
   C. If the person if being separated from family and friends
   D. How the person will move about: walk, wheelchair, or stretcher

5. Which event would most likely be viewed as a happy time for the person?
   A. Admission from home to a long-term care facility
   B. Discharge from the hospital to the home setting
   C. Transfer from a hospital to a rehabilitation center
   D. Transfer from a long-term care facility to the hospital

6. When a person with dementia is admitted to a nursing center, which response is most likely to occur?
   A. Sudden onset of depression
   B. An increase in confusion
   C. An interest in the environment
   D. A display of aggression

7. If a person being admitted is arriving by stretcher, you should
   A. Raise the bed to the level of the stretcher
   B. Place the stretcher perpendicular to the bed
   C. Raise the head of the bed to Fowler's position
   D. Assist the person to get off of the stretcher

8. The nurse asks you to get the weight on a newly admitted person. Which information do you need to get from the nurse?
   A. Where to record the weight
   B. What the person should wear
   C. Person's normal weight
   D. What type of scale to use

9. What would you do first if the nurse tells you to get the person's weight using a wheelchair scale?
   A. Weigh the person in the wheelchair
   B. Weigh the wheelchair
   C. Subtract the weight of wheelchair
   D. Add the weight of the person

10. You measure a person's height using the standing scale and obtain a reading of 61 inches. You must record the height in feet and inches. What will you record?
    A. 5 ft   C. 5 ft 11 in
    B. 5 ft 1 in   D. 6 ft 1 in

11. When weighing a resident, have the person
    A. Wear socks and shoes and a bathrobe
    B. Remove regular clothes and wear a gown or sleepwear
    C. Wear regular street clothes
    D. Remove clothing after weighing and then weigh the clothes

12. A chair scale is used when a person
    A. Cannot transfer from a wheelchair
    B. Cannot stand
    C. Can sit with support
    D. Is in the supine position

13. When a person cannot stand on the scale to have his or her height measured
    A. Ask the person or the family the height of the person at the last known measurement
    B. Have the person sit in a chair and use a tape measure from head to toe to measure the person
    C. Position the person in supine position, if allowed, and measure with a tape measure
    D. Have the person roll to the side and hold the rail while you spread the measure tape along the person's back.

14. A person is being moved to a new room. Which action would you use to show support and reassurance?
    A. Promise to come and visit the person
    B. Introduce the person to the staff and roommates
    C. Pat the person on the head and say, "You're okay."
    D. Sit with the person until the end of your shift

15. You are transferring a person. Which statement typifies your reporting responsibilities to the receiving nurse?
    A. "The person is difficult to take care of and she is argumentative."
    B. "The person is being transferred because her condition has changed."
    C. "The person is being transferred after a disagreement with a roommate."
    D. "The person vomited a small amount during the transfer."

16. If a person wishes to leave the center without the doctor's permission, you should
    A. Tell the person this is not allowed
    B. Prevent the person from leaving
    C. Tell the nurse at once
    D. Try to convince the person to stay

17. When you are assisting a person who is being discharged, which task is your responsibility?
    A. Give the prescriptions to the person or family
    B. Check the clothing and personal belongings lists
    C. Give the valuables to the person or the family
    D. Provide discharge and follow-up instructions

Fill in the Blank

18. Write out the abbreviations.
    A. ft _____
    B. ID _____
    C. in _____
    D. lb _____

19. Based on standards established by Centers for Medicare & Medicaid Services, list 5 reasons for transfers and discharges from a long-term care center.
    A. _____.
    B. _____
    C. _____.
    D. _____
    E. _____.

20. When you are delegated to assist with admissions, transfers, or discharges, what information do you need from the nurse?
    A. _____
    B. _____
    C. _____
    D. _____
    E. _____
    F. _____
    G. _____
    H. _____
    I. _____
    J. _____

21. When a person is being admitted, what identifying information is obtained?
    A. _____
    B. _____
    C. _____

22. During admission, what is the person given to allow the staff to identify the person? _____ and _____

23. In which health care setting is the person likely to have a photo ID taken? _____

24. When you are asked to admit a person, what can you do to make a good first impression?
    A. _____
    B. _____
    C. _____
    D. _____
    E. _____

25. Why is it important to have a person void before being weighed? _____

26. What is done to the balance scale before having the person step on it?
    A. _____
    B. _____
    C. _____

27. When measuring a person in the supine position, the ruler is placed _____.

28. When you transfer or discharge a person, tell the nurse when the person is ready, so that the nurse can
    A. _____
    B. _____
    C. _____
    D. _____

29. When you assist with a discharge, you should report and record
    A. _____
    B. _____
    C. _____
    D. _____
    E. _____
    F. _____

Optional Learning Exercises

Answer the questions about the following person and situation: Rosa Romirez, 65, had a stroke (CVA) last week and is being admitted to a rehabilitation unit in the nursing care center where you work.

30. Since you know Mrs. Romirez is arriving by wheelchair, you leave the bed _____ and _____ the bed to its _____.

31. The nurse instructs you to collect the necessary equipment to admit a new person. You collect
    A. _____
    B. _____
    C. _____
    D. _____
    E. _____
    F. _____
    G. _____
    H. _____
    I. _____
    J. _____

32. When Mrs. Romirez arrives with her husband, it may help them feel more comfortable if you offer them _____.

33. You greet Mrs. Romirez by name and ask her if a certain _____.

34. Mrs. Romirez has some weakness on her left side and cannot stand alone but can safely transfer from the

wheelchair to chairs or the bed. The nurse tells you to weigh Mrs. Romirez with the _____ scale.

When you arrive at work one day, you are told Mrs. Romirez is being transferred to another nursing unit and you are asked to assist. Answer these questions about transferring her.

35. When you transport Mrs. Romirez in a wheelchair, she is covered with a _____.

36. What items are taken with Mrs. Romirez to the new unit? _____

37. What information is recorded and reported about the transfer?

    A. _____
    B. _____
    C. _____
    D. _____
    E. _____
    F. _____
    G. _____

Several weeks later, you are sent to the nursing unit where Mrs. Romirez is living and find she is going home. Answer these questions about her discharge.

38. Mrs. Romirez tells you she and her family have been taught about her _____, _____, _____, _____, and _____.

39. Good communication skills should be used when assisting with the discharge. When Mrs. Romirez and her family leave, you should _____.

Use the FOCUS ON PRIDE section to complete these statements and then use the critical thinking and discussion question to develop your ideas.

40. When you admit, transfer, or discharge a person, it is your professional responsibility to help the person adjust by

    A. _____
    B. _____
    C. _____
    D. _____
    E. _____

41. List 5 ways that you can show care and concern for the family if the person needs privacy during the admission process.

    A. _____
    B. _____
    C. _____
    D. _____
    E. _____

Critical Thinking and Discussion Question

42. A resident who is newly admitted to a long-term care facility is quiet and seems depressed. She frequently sits by herself and looks out the window. When you ask how she is doing, she says, "I was watching to see if my daughter is coming to take me home." What would you do?

Fill in the Blank: Key Terms

Dorsal recumbent position
Genupectoral position
Horizontal recumbent position
Knee-chest position
Laryngeal mirror
Lithotomy position
Nasal speculum
Ophthalmoscope
Otoscope
Percussion hammer
Tuning fork
Vaginal speculum

1. An instrument vibrated to test hearing is a

   _____.

2. In the _____, the woman lies on her back with her hips at the edge of the exam table, her knees are flexed, her hips are externally rotated, and her feet are in stirrups.

3. The supine position with the legs together is called the _____.

4. An _____ is a lighted instrument used to examine the external ear and the eardrum (tympanic membrane).

5. A _____ is an instrument used to open the vagina for examination of the vagina and the cervix.

6. When a person kneels and rests the body on the knees and chest, the head is turned to one side, the arms are above the head or flexed at the elbows, the back is straight, and the body is flexed about 90 degrees at the hip, the person is in the _____.

7. A _____ is an instrument used to tap body parts to test reflexes.

8. An instrument used to examine the mouth, teeth, and throat is called a _____.

9. An instrument used to examine the inside of the nose is a _____.

10. The dorsal recumbent position is also called the

    _____.

11. An _____ is a lighted instrument used to examine the internal structures of the eye.

12. Another name for knee-chest position is _____.

Circle the Best Answer

13. In nursing centers, residents have a physical examination
    A. Only when the person is admitted
    B. Once a month
    C. At least once a year
    D. Only when the person is ill

14. If a person is having a physical examination, which task would be your responsibility?
    A. Restrain a person who is confused or struggling
    B. Ask if the person wants a same gender examiner
    C. Explain why the examination is being done
    D. Position and drape the person

15. When the doctor is examining the person's mouth, teeth, and throat, you may be asked to hand him or her the
    A. Ophthalmoscope   C. Tuning fork
    B. Percussion hammer   D. Laryngeal mirror

16. Which piece of equipment is most essential in providing privacy for a person having a physical examination?
    A. Towel
    B. Waterproof under-pad
    C. Drape
    D. Undergarments

17. When a child is examined
    A. Parents should leave during painful procedures
    B. Parents are allowed to be present
    C. Parents must assist if they stay in the room
    D. Parents can stay if the examiner has questions

18. It is important to have a person empty the bladder before an examination because
    A. An empty bladder allows the examiner to feel the abdominal organs
    B. A full bladder may cause the person to be incontinent
    C. A urine specimen is always collected before an examination
    D. A full bladder will cause the person to have intense pain

19. Which action would promote safety during an exam?
    A. Tell the person how to put on the gown
    B. Have an extra bath blanket
    C. Screen the person or close the door
    D. Stay with the person

20. After you have taken the person to the exam room and positioned the person, you should
    A. Put on the call light for the examiner
    B. Leave the room so the person has privacy
    C. Go to the examiner to report that the person is ready
    D. Open the door to alert the examiner

21. When the abdomen, chest, and breasts are to be examined, you will place the person in the
    A. Lithotomy position
    B. Sims' position
    C. Dorsal recumbent position
    D. Knee-chest position

22. If a person is asked to stand on the floor during an exam, you should
    A. Assist the person to put on shoes
    B. Place paper towels on the floor
    C. Place a clean sheet on the floor
    D. Wipe the floor with antiseptic cleaner

Fill in the Blank

23. Physical exams are done to:
    A. _____
    B. _____
    C. _____

24. List the equipment you need to collect when the ears are being examined.
    A. _____
    B. _____

25. What equipment is needed to examine the eyes?
    A. _____
    B. _____

26. When the nose, mouth, and throat are being examined, you should collect
    A. _____
    B. _____
    C. _____
    D. _____

27. What concerns may the person have about the physical examination?
    A. _____
    B. _____
    C. _____

28. When the examiner is a man and the person being examined is female, who else should be in the examination room? _____ Why?
    _____

29. After the examination is completed, you make sure the exam room _____.

30. When you are delegated the job of preparing a person for an exam, what information do you need from the nurse and the care plan?
    A. _____
    B. _____
    C. _____
    D. _____
    E. _____
    F. _____

31. When you are delegated the job of preparing a person for an exam, why do you need the following information?
    A. The time of the examination. _____

    B. What are 2 reasons it would be helpful to know which examinations will be done?
    _____

C. What equipment will you need if you are assigned to take vital signs? _____
_____

32. You are a female nursing assistant assisting a male examiner with an examination of a female resident. The nurse tells you to stay in the exam room during the entire procedure. Why is this important to the examiner and to the woman?

_____

Labeling

Look at the instruments and answer the questions.

33. Name the instruments.

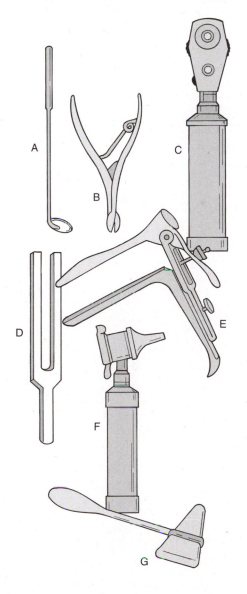

A. _____
B. _____
C. _____
D. _____
E. _____

F. _____

G. _____

34. Which instrument is used to examine the nose?

_____

35. When the eye is examined, the examiner uses the

_____.

36. If a person has a sore throat, the examiner will look at the throat with the _____.

37. The reflexes are examined by using the _____.

Look at the positions and answer these questions.

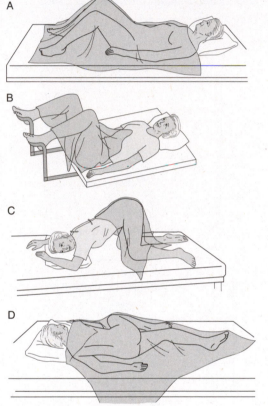

38. Name the positions.

A. _____

B. _____

C. _____

D. _____

39. Which positions may be used when a rectal examination is done?

A. _____

B. _____

40. When the abdomen, chest, and breasts are examined, the person is placed in _____.

41. The _____ position is used for a vaginal exam.

Use the FOCUS ON PRIDE section to complete these statements and then use the critical thinking and discussion questions to develop your ideas.

42. Fears about the exam affect the person's well-being. Common fears are

A. _____

B. _____

C. _____

D. _____

43. What could you do to ease a person's fears about examination?

A. _____

B. _____

C. _____

Critical Thinking and Discussion Questions

44. A nursing assistant that you work with tells you to check out her social media posting. In the posting she describes helping an examiner with a vaginal examination. She does not reveal any names or dates but gives explicit details about the examiner's findings and observations. Discuss this situation, from two different viewpoints:

A. The nursing assistant who posted

B. The unnamed person who had the vaginal examination

C. What would you do if your friends and co-workers told you they are posting stories about work on social media?

38 Collecting and Testing Specimens

Fill in the Blank: Key Terms

Acetone	Glucosuria	Hematuria	Ketone	Melena
Glucometer	Hematoma	Hemoptysis	Ketone body	Sputum

1. Bloody sputum is _____.

2. Ketone or acetone is also called _____.

3. A black, tarry stool is _____.

4. _____ is sugar in the urine.

5. _____ is mucus from the respiratory system that is expectorated through the mouth.

6. _____ is a substance that appears in urine from the rapid breakdown of fat for energy.

7. Another name for ketone or ketone body is _____.

8. A device for measuring blood glucose is a _____.

9. _____ is blood in the urine.

10. A swelling that contains blood is a _____.

Circle the Best Answer

11. The nurse asks you to do an occult blood test on a stool specimen. In addition to the test kit, which piece of equipment do you need to obtain?
    A. Glucometer
    B. Tongue blades
    C. Gauze sponges
    D. Lancet

12. When you would you apply the label to the specimen container for a midstream urine specimen?
    A. At the nurses' station in the presence of the nurse
    B. Before the specimen is collected in the presence of the person
    C. After putting the specimen container in the biohazard bag
    D. After the specimen is collected in the presence of the person

13. When you are collecting a specimen, which part of the collection system can you touch with your nonsterile gloved hand?
    A. It depends on the type of specimen you are collecting
    B. The inside of the lid
    C. The inside of the container
    D. The outside of the biohazard bag

14. In which circumstance would you need to wear a respirator when collecting the specimen?
    A. Sputum specimen from a person who might have tuberculosis
    B. Random urine specimen from a person who might have a urinary tract infection
    C. Stool specimen from a person who might have infectious diarrhea
    D. Blood glucose from a person who might have acquired immunodeficiency syndrome

15. A random urine specimen is collected
    A. First thing in the morning
    B. After meals
    C. At any time
    D. At bedtime

16. When a person is collecting a random urine specimen, you remind the person to put the toilet paper in
    A. The toilet
    B. The specimen container
    C. The specimen pan
    D. The bedpan

17. When obtaining a midstream specimen, the perineal area is cleaned to
    A. Remove all microbes from the perineal area
    B. Reduce the number of microbes in the urethral area
    C. Follow Standard Precautions and the Bloodborne Pathogen Standard
    D. Reduce infection during specimen collection

18. When collecting a midstream specimen, what would you do?
    A. Collect the entire amount of urine voided just before bedtime.
    B. Collect about 4 oz (120 mL) of urine from the first morning void.
    C. Have the person void, then stop, position the sterile specimen cup and void into the cup.
    D. Collect several specimens and add them to the specimen cup, until the cup is filled.

19. When collecting a 24-hour urine specimen, the urine is kept
    A. Chilled on ice or refrigerated during the entire time
    B. At room temperature in the bathroom
    C. In a sterile container at the nurses' station
    D. In a drainage collection bag at the bedside

20. A 24-hour urine specimen collection is started
    A. At the beginning of a shift
    B. After a meal
    C. At night
    D. After the person voids and that urine is discarded

21. At the end of 24-hour specimen collection
    A. The person voids and that urine is saved
    B. Write down any missed or spilled urine
    C. Record the amount of urine collected
    D. The person voids and that urine is discarded

22. When a urine specimen is needed from infants or very young children, it is obtained by
    A. Inserting a straight catheter
    B. Using a collection bag applied over the urethra
    C. Having the parent hold the child on a potty chair until the child voids
    D. Applying a diaper and then squeezing the urine out of the diaper

23. A child may be able to void for a specimen if you give the child fluids
    A. 5 to 10 minutes before the test
    B. 30 minutes before the test
    C. 1 hour before the test
    D. While you are obtaining the specimen
24. When you test urine with a reagent strip, it is important that you
    A. Follow the manufacturer's instructions
    B. Use a sterile urine specimen
    C. Wear sterile gloves
    D. Make sure the urine is cold
25. When you are assigned to strain a person's urine, you
    A. Have the person void directly into the strainer and then measure the urine
    B. Collect all urine and save it so that it can be sent to the laboratory
    C. Have the person void into the voiding device and then pour the urine through the strainer
    D. Discard the strainer if it contains stones and obtain a new one for the next voiding
26. If a warm stool specimen is required, it is
    A. Placed in an insulated container
    B. Stored on the nursing unit until the end of the shift
    C. Tested at once on the nursing unit
    D. Taken at once to the laboratory or the storage area
27. When collecting a stool specimen, ask the person to
    A. Void and have a bowel movement in a bedpan
    B. Use only a bedpan or commode to collect the specimen
    C. Urinate into the toilet and collect the stool in the specimen pan
    D. Place the toilet tissue in the bedpan, commode, or specimen pan with the stool
28. When collecting the stool specimen
    A. Pour it into the specimen container and use a tongue blade to collect remaining stool from collection device
    B. Use your gloved hand to obtain a specimen, place the stool in the container, remove gloves and perform hand hygiene
    C. Use a tongue blade to take about 2 tablespoons of stool from the middle of the formed stool
    D. Use a tongue blade to scoop the entire stool specimen from the collection device into the specimen container
29. When you test a stool specimen for occult blood
    A. It must be sent to the laboratory
    B. The specimen must be sterile
    C. You will need to test the entire stool specimen
    D. Use a tongue blade to make a thin smear of stool on the test card
30. A sputum specimen is more easily collected
    A. Upon awakening   C. At bedtime
    B. After eating   D. After activity
31. Before obtaining a sputum specimen, ask the person to
    A. Rinse the mouth with clear water
    B. Brush the teeth and use mouthwash
    C. Cough and discard the first sputum expectorated
    D. Walk around for a short time to stimulate secretions
32. Postural drainage is used when collecting a sputum specimen to
    A. Collect sterile specimens
    B. Make the sputum specimen more liquid
    C. Stimulate coughing
    D. Help secretions drain by gravity
33. If a sputum specimen is needed from an infant or small child, you may assist the nurse by
    A. Positioning the child for postural drainage
    B. Holding the child's head and arms still
    C. Positioning the sputum specimen cup near the child's mouth
    D. Explaining the procedure to the child
34. If you are delegated to do blood glucose testing, the most common site for testing is
    A. The earlobe
    B. A fingertip
    C. The forearm
    D. The abdomen
35. It is important to do glucose testing at correct times because
    A. The results are needed before certain drugs are given
    B. The results determine how much the person is allowed to eat
    C. A low blood glucose in the morning is a danger sign
    D. It must be done at a time when the person is not sleeping

Fill in the Blank

36. Write out the abbreviations.
    A. BM _____
    B. ID _____
    C. I&O _____
    D. mL _____
    E. oz _____
    F. U/A _____
37. When collecting urine specimens, what observations are reported and recorded?
    A. _____
    B. _____
    C. _____
    D. _____
    E. _____
    F. _____
38. How much urine is collected for a random urine specimen? _____
39. When collecting a midstream urine specimen, the person may not be able to stop voiding. If so, you will pass _____.

40. When you are obtaining a midstream specimen from a female, spread the labia with your thumb and index finger with your _____ hand.

41. When cleaning the female perineum for a midstream specimen, clean from _____.

42. When cleaning the male perineum for a midstream specimen, clean the penis starting _____.

43. What information is marked on the room and bathroom container labels for a 24-hour urine collection? _____

44. Urine pH measures if the urine is _____ or _____.

45. When you use reagent strips, you read the strip by comparing it to the _____.

46. When you strain urine, you are looking for stones that can develop in the _____.

47. The strainer is placed in the specimen container if any _____appear.

48. Stool specimens are studied and checked for
    A. _____
    B. _____
    C. _____
    D. _____
    E. _____

49. After collecting a stool specimen, place the labeled container in a _____.

50. When you are delegated to collect a stool specimen, what observations are reported and recorded?
    A. _____
    B. _____
    C. _____
    D. _____
    E. _____

51. When stools are black and tarry, there is bleeding in the _____.

52. Blood in the stool that is hidden is called _____.

53. Mouthwash is not used before a sputum specimen is collected because it _____.

54. When you are delegated to collect a sputum specimen, report and record
    A. _____
    B. _____
    C. _____
    D. _____
    E. _____
    F. _____
    G. _____
    H. _____
    I. _____

55. When you are assisting a person to collect a sputum specimen, ask the person to take 2 or 3 _____ and _____ the sputum.

56. Why do you avoid swollen, bruised, cyanotic, or calloused sites when testing for blood glucose? _____

57. Why do you avoid the center, fleshy part of the fingertip when you make a skin puncture? _____

58. When you test for blood glucose, what should you report and record?
    A. _____
    B. _____
    C. _____
    D. _____
    E. _____
    F. _____
    G. _____

Optional Learning Exercises

59. If you are collecting a midstream specimen, what should you do if it is hard for the person to stop the stream of urine? _____

60. You are caring for a person who is having a 24-hour urine specimen test. He tells you he forgot to save a specimen an hour ago. What should you do and why? _____

61. What is normal pH for urine? _____ What can cause changes in the normal pH? _____

62. When the body cannot use sugar for energy, it uses fat. When this happens _____ appear in the urine.

63. Why is privacy important when collecting a sputum specimen? _____

Use the FOCUS ON PRIDE section to complete these statements.

64. When collecting a specimen, you are responsible to correctly _____ the person.

65. When collecting specimens, you respect the person's right to privacy when you
    A. _____
    B. _____
    C. _____

Critical Thinking and Discussion Questions

66. The nurse instructed you to get a midstream urine specimen from an older overweight woman. You explained how to collect the specimen, but she was not able to spread the labia and clean and maintain the hand position. You tried to assist her, but cleaning and maintaining the hand position was still not achieved.
    A. What would you tell the nurse?
    B. Why is it important to report this to the nurse?

Crossword

Fill in the crossword by answering the clues below with the words from this list:

Calculi   Expectorated   Midstream   Postural   Specimens
Dysuria   Labia   Occult   Random   Suctioning

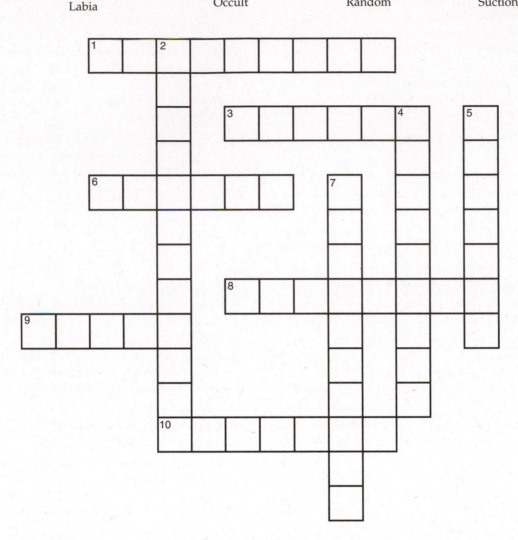

Across

1. Samples
3. Urine specimen that can be collected at any time
6. Hidden, as in blood in stool
8. Drainage position with head lower than body used to cause fluid to flow downward
9. Folds of tissue on each side of the vagina
10. Pain when urinating

Down

2. Expelled, as in sputum through the mouth
4. Urine specimen that is collected after the person starts to void
5. Stones that develop in kidneys, ureters, or bladder
7. Removal of sputum from the trachea with a machine

39 The Person Having Surgery

Fill in the Blank: Key Terms

Anesthesia	Embolus	Local anesthesia	Regional anesthesia	Thrombus
Antiseptic	Emergency surgery	Post-operative	Sedation	Urgent surgery
Elective surgery	General anesthesia	Pre-operative	Surgical site infection	

1. The loss of consciousness and all feeling or sensation is_____.

2. _____ is surgery done by choice to improve the person's life or well-being.

3. A blood clot is called a _____.

4. _____ is the loss of feeling or sensation produced by a drug.

5. An _____ is a blood clot that travels through the vascular system until it lodges in a blood vessel.

6. _____ is before surgery.

7. _____ is surgery needed for the person's health. It is done soon to prevent further damage or disease.

8. _____ is after surgery.

9. The loss of feeling or sensation in a large area of the body is _____.

10. Surgery done immediately to save life or function is _____.

11. _____ is the loss of feeling or sensation in a small area.

12. A state of quiet, calmness, or sleep produced by a drug is _____.

13. A chemical applied to the skin to prevent the growth and reproduction of microbes is an _____.

14. An infection that occurs after surgery in the body part where the surgery took place is a _____.

Circle the Best Answer

15. A surgery that can be delayed for a few days is
    A. Emergency surgery
    B. Elective surgery
    C. Urgent surgery
    D. Out-patient surgery

16. When a serious motor vehicle accident occurs, the person often requires
    A. Elective surgery
    B. Emergency surgery
    C. General anesthesia
    D. Urgent surgery

17. When a person tells you about fears and concerns before surgery, you should
    A. Explain that the surgeon is very skilled
    B. Tell the person not to worry
    C. Show warmth, sensitivity, and caring
    D. Change the subject and talk about something else

18. When a patient asks you about test results or the diagnosis
    A. Answer the questions honestly
    B. Tell the person you will get the nurse
    C. Say that information is not available to you
    D. Explain that you do not know but will find out

19. Which nursing assistant needs a reminder about the roles and responsibilities of caring for a surgical patient?
    A. Nursing Assistant A explains the care that she will give to the person.
    B. Nursing Assistant B provides pre-operative care with skill and ease.
    C. Nursing Assistant C tells the person about her own experience with surgery.
    D. Nursing Assistant D reports a request to see the clergy to the nurse.

20. How often are deep-breathing and coughing exercises done after surgery?
    A. Once a shift
    B. Every 1 or 2 hours when the person is awake
    C. Every 4 hours
    D. Every 2 hours for the first 48 hours after surgery

21. How is a child prepared for surgery?
    A. The parents are responsible for explaining the surgery to the child.
    B. A doll may be used to show the site of the surgery.
    C. Children are told an imaginary story about the surgery.
    D. The child is introduced to another child who had the same surgery.

22. If blood loss is expected during surgery, which test is done pre-operatively?
    A. Type and crossmatch
    B. Complete blood count
    C. Urinalysis
    D. Electrocardiogram

23. A person is NPO for 6 to 8 hours before surgery to reduce
    A. Breathing problems after surgery
    B. Pain post-operatively
    C. Diarrhea and flatulence post-operatively
    D. Vomiting and aspiration during and after surgery

24. Cleansing enemas may be ordered before surgery to
    A. Prevent contamination of the abdominal cavity during surgery
    B. Prevent incontinence during and after surgery
    C. Prevent infectious diarrhea after surgery
    D. Prevent abdominal pain and constipation after surgery

25. The person being prepared for surgery needs to void
    A. Right before going to the operating room
    B. The morning of surgery
    C. Before the nurse gives the pre-operative drugs
    D. Before an enema is given

26. Make-up, nail polish, and fake nails are removed before surgery because
    A. These artificial substances are sources of infection
    B. It reduces the number of microbes on the body
    C. Skin, lips, and nail beds are observed for color during and after surgery
    D. A baseline appearance needs to be established before surgery

27. When preparing a child for surgery, it is important to report
    A. A dry mouth   C. Any missing teeth
    B. Any loose teeth   D. Last oral hygiene

28. If a person is allowed to wear a wedding ring during surgery, you should
    A. Record this information on the chart
    B. Secure it according to agency policy
    C. Make sure it fits well and will not come off
    D. Put a clean glove on the person's hand

29. Which task are you most likely to be assigned related to the pre-operative skin preparation for a person who will have surgery in the perineal area?
    A. Clean the perineum and surrounding area with antiseptic
    B. Use a razor and carefully shave away the pubic hair
    C. Mark the surgical site with a waterproof ink pen
    D. Assist the person to take a shower with special soap

30. A patient says, "You may think I am stupid but, I didn't really understand what the surgeon said about the risks and complications." What would you do?
    A. Check to see if the surgical consent was signed by the patient
    B. Report the patient's concerns to the nurse
    C. Call the surgeon and explain what the person said
    D. Reassure the patient that the surgeon is experienced

31. Pre-operative medications are given
    A. After the person gets up to void
    B. At a time specified by the checklist
    C. Before the person takes a shower
    D. After the person is assisted to the stretcher

32. After you are delegated to assist with the pre-operative checklist, it must be completed
    A. Before the nurse gives the pre-operative drugs
    B. Before the consent form is signed and completed
    C. Just before the patient leaves the unit for surgery
    D. The night before the surgery

33. Which pre-operative action helps to reduce the incidence of surgical site infection?
    A. Assisting with a complete bath with special cleanser
    B. Helping the person to follow NPO instructions
    C. Removing, cleaning and storing dentures
    D. Correctly applying anti-embolic stockings

34. You are assigned to prepare the room for a person who will soon be transferred from PACU. Which equipment will you obtain?
    A. Kidney basin   C. Gauze sponges
    B. Elastic bandage   D. Extra pillow

35. When you prepare a room for a person to return from surgery
    A. Raise the head of the bed and the side rails
    B. Put the bed in the lowest position
    C. Raise the bed for a transfer from a stretcher
    D. Make the bed using sterile sheets and blankets

36. You may be assigned to take the vital signs after surgery. They are usually measured
    A. Once a shift
    B. Every 15 minutes until the person is stable
    C. Every 2 hours
    D. Every 5 minutes for the first hour

37. Post-operatively, the person is positioned
    A. In the supine position
    B. To allow for easy and comfortable breathing
    C. In Fowler's position
    D. To allow for easy turning and repositioning

38. Coughing and deep-breathing exercises are done after surgery to
    A. Prevent hemorrhage and hypovolemia
    B. Prevent pneumonia and atelectasis
    C. Decrease pain and discomfort
    D. Prevent nausea and vomiting

39. Leg exercises are important to prevent
    A. Pneumonia and atelectasis
    B. Thrombus and embolus (blood clots)
    C. Pain at the surgical site
    D. Low blood pressure

40. Leg exercises are done
    A. At least every 1 to 2 hours while the person is awake
    B. Once in the morning and once in the evening
    C. When the person has leg cramps or discomfort
    D. After the person begins to independently ambulate

41. Elastic stockings are used to
    A. Prevent weakness and discomfort in the legs
    B. Prevent hypertension and dizziness
    C. Promote blood return to the heart and prevent blood clots
    D. Give support to the legs when ambulation begins

42. When applying elastic stockings, you should have the person
    A. Lie in a supine position
    B. Sit in a chair with legs at a 90-degree angle
    C. In Fowler's position
    D. Walk around the room first

43. When applying elastic bandages
    A. Start at the proximal part of the extremity
    B. Completely cover the fingers or toes
    C. Use a figure-eight pattern
    D. Expose the fingers and toes if possible

44. When you assist a person to walk after surgery, you first measure
    A. The person's temperature
    B. The blood pressure and pulse
    C. The distance from the bed to the door
    D. The person's weight

45. If a person is NPO after surgery, important personal hygiene is
    A. Frequent oral hygiene
    B. Giving ice chips frequently
    C. Offering sips of cool water
    D. Giving a complete bed bath

46. It is important to report the time and amount of the first voiding after surgery because the person must void
    A. Within 2 hours after surgery
    B. During the first 24 hours after surgery
    C. Within 8 hours after surgery
    D. At least 1000 mL within the first 4 hours after surgery

Fill in the Blank

47. Write out the abbreviations.
    A. AE _____
    B. ASC _____
    C. CBC _____
    D. ECG _____
    E. EKG _____
    F. ID _____
    G. IV _____
    H. NG _____
    I. NPO _____
    J. OR _____
    K. PACU _____
    L. Pre-op _____
    M. Post-op _____
    N. SCD _____
    O. SSI _____
    P. TED _____

48. If a person has out-patient, 1-day, or ambulatory surgery, the person is admitted in the morning and _____.

49. Before surgery, special personal care is done. Describe the care given and the reasons it is important.
    A. Baths _____
    _____
    B. Removing make-up, nail polish, and fake nails
    _____
    _____
    C. Hair care _____
    _____
    D. Oral hygiene _____
    _____

50. Some people do not like being seen without their dentures. How can you promote dignity and self-esteem when dentures must be removed before surgery? _____

51. When you are delegated to apply elastic stockings, what information do you need from the nurse?
    A. _____
    B. _____
    C. _____

52. Which vital signs are recorded on the pre-operative checklist? _____
    _____

53. After the pre-operative drugs are given, the person is not allowed _____
    _____.

54. When a person returns to the room after surgery, how often are vital signs usually measured?
    A. _____
    B. _____
    C. _____
    D. _____

55. What post-operative observations of the vital signs should be reported to the nurse?
    A. Temperature _____
    B. Pulse
        i. _____
        ii. _____
        iii. _____
        iv. _____
    C. Respirations
        i. _____
        ii. _____
        iii. _____
        iv. _____
        v. _____
        vi. _____
        vii. _____
    D. Blood pressure _____

56. You may be able to turn a person who has had surgery by yourself when the person's condition _____.

57. Why are older persons at risk for respiratory complications?
    A. _____
    B. _____
    C. _____

58. Leg exercises are done at least every _____.
    These exercises are done _____ times.

59. Describe four leg exercises that are done post-operatively to promote venous blood flow and to prevent thrombi.

    A. _____

    B. _____

    C. _____

    D. _____

60. When you apply elastic stockings, you avoid twists because they can _____. Creases and wrinkles can cause _____.

61. When you apply elastic bandages, what observations are reported and recorded?

    A. _____

    B. _____

    C. _____

    D. _____

    E. _____

    F. _____

    G. _____

    H. _____

62. What is the purpose of sequential compression devices?

    _____

63. Why would it be important to make sure that the device is plugged in and functioning?

    _____

    _____

64. Early ambulation prevents

    A. _____

    B. _____

    C. _____

    D. _____

    E. _____

Optional Learning Exercises

Mr. Shafer is an 82-year-old man admitted for knee replacement surgery. Answer the questions about Mr. Shafer and his pre-operative care.

65. This surgery is done by choice and is an

    _____ surgery.

66. When you are in the room, you listen quietly while Mr. Shafer talks about his fears and concerns. By sitting quietly and showing concern for his feelings, you can assist in Mr. Shafer's

    _____ care.

67. The nurse teaches Mr. Shafer about what to expect. What pre-operative topics will the nurse cover?

    A. _____

    B. _____

    C. _____

    D. _____

    E. _____

    F. _____

    G. _____

    H. _____

    I. _____

    J. _____

68. The nurse tells you she will give Mr. Shafer his pre-operative drugs in 10 minutes. What should you do?

    _____

Mrs. Johnson is a 70-year-old woman who is scheduled for abdominal surgery. Answer these questions about her care.

69. The nurse tells you she is busy and asks you to have Mrs. Johnson sign the surgery consent. What should you do? _____

    _____

70. Mrs. Johnson returns to her room 2 hours after the surgery is completed. You know she is transported to her room when

    A. _____

    B. _____

    C. _____

71. How is the room prepared for Mrs. Johnson's return?

    A. _____

    B. _____

    C. _____

72. You are caring for Mrs. Johnson 3 days after her surgery. She tells you she has not had a bowel movement since before surgery. You know that one reason for constipation can be drugs given for

    _____.

Matching

Instructions: Match the post-operative complication with the observation that is most likely to signal the complication.

Complication	Observation
73. _____ Pneumonia	a. Increased temperature
74. _____ Hypovolemic shock	b. Cannot void
75. _____ Thrombus	c. Weak rapid pulse
76. _____ Urinary retention	d. Shortness of breath
77. _____ Wound infection	e. Discomfort and swelling in calf

Labeling

78. Describe the correct application of an elastic bandage as depicted in the figure.

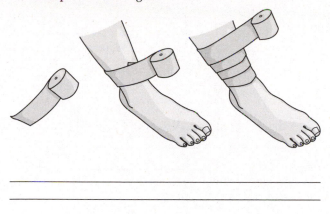

_____

_____

_____

_____

_____

Use the FOCUS ON PRIDE section to complete these statements and then use the critical thinking and discussion questions to develop your ideas.

79. How can you ease a person's fears and concerns when he or she has surgery?

A. _____

B. _____

C. _____

D. _____

80. What questions can you answer when caring for a person having surgery? _____

_____

_____

81. When you are delegated to take post-operative vital signs, what should you report at once to the nurse?

A. _____

B. _____

C. _____

Critical Thinking and Discussion Questions

82. You and the nurse are very busy. You are assigned to assist the nurse with three patients who need post-operative care.

Patient A had surgery on her leg two days ago. Today the surgical site is red and painful. The drainage has a foul odor. She appears flushed and her skin is hot to the touch.

Patient B had abdominal surgery this morning. She is confused and disoriented. Her skin is pale and cool. Her abdomen is distended and she says it hurts.

Patient C had surgery for a broken wrist this morning. She says the pain was relieved by the pain medication. She tells you she is "ready to eat and drink something, take a brief nap and go home as soon as possible."

A. Which patient needs attention from you and the nurse first?

B. Discuss your decision and what you think might be happening to each patient.

Fill in the Blank: Key Terms

Abrasion
Arterial ulcer
Chronic wound
Circulatory ulcer
Diabetic foot ulcer

Excoriation
Incision
Laceration
Penetrating wound
Puncture wound

Purulent drainage
Sanguineous
  drainage
Serosanguineous
  drainage

Serous drainage
Skin tear
Stasis ulcer
Ulcer
Vascular ulcer

Venous ulcer
Wound

1. A _____ is a break or rip in the skin that separates the epidermis from underlying tissues.

2. An open wound with clean, straight edges, usually intentional from a sharp instrument, is an _____.

3. A shallow or deep crater-like sore of the skin or mucous membrane is an _____.

4. _____ is thick green, yellow, or brown drainage.

5. A _____ is a break in the skin or mucous membrane.

6. An _____ is a partial-thickness wound caused by the scraping away or rubbing of the skin.

7. A _____ is an open wound on the foot caused by complications from diabetes.

8. Thin, watery drainage that is blood-tinged is called _____.

9. An open sore on the lower legs or feet caused by decreased blood flow through arteries or veins is a _____.

10. A _____ is an open wound with torn tissues and jagged edges.

11. An _____ is an open wound on the lower legs and feet caused by poor arterial blood flow.

12. Clear, watery fluid is _____.

13. A _____ is a wound that does not heal easily.

14. An open sore on the lower legs or feet caused by poor blood flow through the veins is a _____; stasis ulcer.

15. An open wound made by a sharp object is a _____. The entry of the skin and underlying tissues may be intentional or unintentional.

16. A _____ is an open wound that breaks the skin and enters a body area, organ, or cavity.

17. A circulatory ulcer is also called a _____.

18. A _____ is another name for a venous ulcer.

19. Bloody drainage is called _____.

20. _____ is the loss of epidermis caused by scratching or when skin rubs against skin, clothing, or other materials.

Circle the Best Answer

21. When you inspect a resident's elbow, you find some of the skin is rubbed away. You would report this to the nurse as
    A. A laceration
    B. An abrasion
    C. An ulcer
    D. An incision

22. A resident's arm was caught on the chair and the tissue was torn with jagged edges. This is a
    A. Puncture wound
    B. Abrasion
    C. Penetrating wound
    D. Laceration

23. Which person has the greatest risk for skin tears?
    A. The person is obese and requires help with bathing.
    B. The person is thin, confused and requires total help to move.
    C. The person needs help to eat and drink.
    D. The person has altered mental awareness but is ambulatory

24. Applying lotion will help to prevent skin breakdown or skin tears because it may prevent
    A. Loss of fatty layer
    B. Thinning of the skin
    C. Dryness of the skin
    D. Excoriation of the skin

25. Ulcers of the feet and legs are caused by
    A. Poor hygiene and poor nutrition
    B. Decreased blood flow through arteries or veins
    C. Walking on concrete or paved surfaces
    D. Obesity and lack of exercise

26. A measure to prevent venous (stasis) ulcers is
    A. Secure the person's socks tightly in place
    B. Remind the person not to sit with the legs crossed
    C. Dry the skin vigorously to stimulate circulation
    D. Massage the legs and feet after bathing

27. Which action would be best for the prevention of arterial ulcers?
    A. Encourage the person to wear warm socks
    B. Support the person's efforts to stop smoking
    C. Assist the person to stand up and walk
    D. Help to the person to prepare for rest and sleep

28. It is important to check the feet of a person with diabetes every day because
    A. The person may not feel an injury to the foot
    B. The person can't check his or her own feet
    C. Good hygiene is difficult for people with diabetes
    D. People with diabetes have poor nutrition

29. A person with diabetes should
    A. Apply cream or petroleum jelly to toes
    B. Use a heating pad to stimulate circulation
    C. Wear athletic or walking shoes
    D. Soak feet in water to keep skin moisturized

30. When would signs and symptoms of inflammation: redness, swelling, heat or warmth, and pain be considered normal and expected?
    A. During phase 1 of wound healing
    B. During phase 3 of wound healing
    C. Recently discovered diabetic foot ulcer
    D. Skin tear that is not healing

31. What would be your role in caring for a patient with a surgical wound that is supposed to heal by first intention?
    A. Take vital signs frequently as directed by the nurse
    B. Alert the nurse if the sutures or staples are not intact
    C. Alert the nurse when the infected wound drainage is excessive
    D. Give emotional support to the person for prolonged wound healing

32. A sign of hemorrhage is
    A. Dressings that are soaked with blood
    B. Warmth at the surgical site
    C. An increase in the blood pressure
    D. Watery drainage from the wound

33. If you observe signs of shock or hemorrhage, you should
    A. Report it to the nurse at once
    B. Place the person in the Fowler's position
    C. Record your observations on the flow sheet
    D. Hold pressure on the wound site

34. The nurse tells you to make sure that the patient supports her abdominal wound when she coughs. This done to protect against
    A. Contamination   C. Scarring
    B. Infection   D. Dehiscence

35. Which type of drainage would be reported immediately, because it indicates hemorrhage?
    A. Thick purulent drainage
    B. Watery serosanguineous drainage
    C. Clear thin serous drainage
    D. Bright red sanguineous drainage

36. How would you remove an old soiled dressing from a wound?
    A. Don sterile gloves and grasp the center of the dressing
    B. Perform hand hygiene and use forceps to grasp edge of the dressing
    C. Don clean non-sterile gloves, grasp dressing edge and gently lift
    D. Pour sterile water on the dressing and then pull it off

37. Plastic and paper tape may be used to secure a dressing
    A. Because they allow movement of the body part
    B. When the dressing must be changed frequently
    C. If the person is allergic to adhesive tape
    D. Because they stick well to the skin

38. If you care for a person who has Montgomery straps to secure a dressing, you should
    A. Replace the cloth ties when you give care
    B. Tell the nurse if the tape strips need to be replaced
    C. Replace the tape strips each time you give care
    D. Re-tie the cloth ties when you re-position the person

39. If you are assigned to change a dressing, what information do you need?
    A. What kind of medication the person receives
    B. The person's medical diagnosis
    C. How long to wait for pain medication to take effect
    D. When the dressing was last changed

40. What can you do to make the person more comfortable when changing a dressing?
    A. Talk about topics that are not related to the wound
    B. Remove tape by pulling it toward the wound
    C. Encourage the person to look at the wound and ask questions
    D. Tell the person that the wound site is normal and healing

41. You are very gentle as you remove an old dressing, but removal causes a tiny skin tear. The person says, "Don't worry dear, my skin tears easily. The nurses always just smooth it down and cover it." What should you do?
    A. Do as the person suggests
    B. Report the incident to the nurse
    C. Gently clean it with an antiseptic
    D. Document what the person told you to do

42. What is the purpose of a binder?
    A. To prevent infection which would delay healing
    B. To reduce drainage and prevent bleeding
    C. To reduce swelling, promote comfort, and prevent injury
    D. To limit movements that may cause wound dehiscence

43. A binder should be applied
    A. With firm, even pressure over the area
    B. And secured with cloth straps
    C. Very loosely to allow breathing and movement
    D. During AM care and removed during PM care

44. Which food would you encourage an elderly person to order and eat because it contains the nutrient that is most important for wound healing?
    A. Oatmeal with cinnamon
    B. Orange and apple slices
    C. Tossed salad with croutons
    D. Grilled chicken breast

Fill in the Blank

45. Write out the abbreviations.
    A. GI _____
    B. PPE _____

46. What are common causes of skin tears?
    A. _____
    B. _____
    C. _____
    D. _____
    E. _____
    F. _____
    G. _____
    H. _____

47. List ways to prevent skin tears in the following:
    A. Keep the person hydrated by _____
    _____.
    B. What kind of clothing would be helpful? _____
    _____
    C. Nail care of the person _____
    _____.
    D. Lift and turn the person with an _____
    _____.
    E. Support the arms and legs _____
    _____.
    F. Pad _____.
    G. Keep your fingernails _____
    and _____. Do not wear rings with
    _____.

48. Skin tears are portals _____.

49. When the person has circulatory ulcers, report any
    _____.

50. You are caring for a person with a disease that affects venous circulation. You notice her toenails are long and sharp. You should _____
    _____.

51. What 2 diseases are common causes of circulatory ulcers?
    _____

52. When a person has diabetes, what complications can occur with the following?
    A. Nerves—person does not feel
    _____ and can develop
    _____ or _____
    and not feel or recognize the problems.

B. Blood vessels—blood flow _____.
   What can occur? _____

53. Explain what can happen if a person with diabetes has these foot problems.
    A. Athlete's foot _____
    B. Ingrown toenails _____
    C. Hammer toes _____
    D. Dry and cracked skin _____

54. With first intention healing, the wound edges are held together with _____.

55. Second intention healing is used for
    _____
    wounds. Because healing takes longer, the threat of
    _____ is great.

56. If you suspect a person has external hemorrhage, where would you check for drainage?
    _____

57. What should you do if you find a person's wound has dehiscence or evisceration? _____
    _____

58. What observations would you make about wound appearance?
    A. _____
    B. _____
    C. _____
    D. _____
    E. _____

59. When you are delegated to change a dressing, what should you do if the old dressings stick to the wound?
    _____

60. List four types of drainage that you might observe at a wound site.
    A. _____
    B. _____
    C. _____
    D. _____

61. What is the purpose of a transparent dressing?
    _____

62. When large amounts of drainage are expected, the doctor inserts a _____ into the wound.

63. Name two closed drainage systems that prevent microbes from entering a wound.
    _____

64. When you are changing a nonsterile dressing, why do you need 2 pairs of gloves?
    _____
    _____

65. Before applying tape, what are two questions that you would ask?
    A. _____
    B. _____

66. When taping a dressing in place, the tape should not encircle the entire body part because _____ _____.

67. When delegated to apply dressings, list what observations should be reported and recorded.
    A. _____
    B. _____
    C. _____
    D. _____
    E. _____
    F. _____
    G. _____
    H. _____
    I. _____
    J. _____
    K. _____
    L. _____

Optional Learning Exercises

You are assigned to care for Mrs. Stevens. She is 87 years old and has diabetes and high blood pressure. She walks with difficulty and spends most of her day sitting in her chair. She is somewhat over-weight and tells you she had a knee replacement 5 years ago and had phlebitis after surgery. The nurse tells you to watch carefully for signs of circulatory ulcers.

68. Identify seven risk factors that Mrs. Stevens has that place her at risk for circulatory ulcers.
    A. _____
    B. _____
    C. _____
    D. _____
    E. _____
    F. _____
    G. _____

Mr. Hawkins, age 74, was in an automobile accident and has a wound on his leg that is large and open. It has become infected and he is being treated with antibiotics. When you are talking with him, he tells you he has smoked for 55 years and has poor circulation in his legs. He lives alone and generally eats takeout foods or eats cereal when he is at home.

69. Why is he receiving antibiotics?
    _____

70. What side effect of the antibiotics can cause a problem that could interfere with healing? _____
    _____

71. Identify four factors that increase Mr. Hawkins' risk for complications.
    A. _____
    B. _____
    C. _____
    D. _____

72. What is missing in Mr. Hawkins' diet that is needed to help in healing the wound?
    _____

73. When a wound is infected and has poor circulation, the wound may be left open at first and then closed later. This type of wound healing is called healing through _____. This type of healing combines _____ and _____ intention healing.

You are assisting the nurse with wound care. Mr. Wendel has a drain in his wound that is attached to suction.

74. How does the nurse find out the amount of drainage from Mr. Wendel's wound? _____
    _____

Use the FOCUS ON PRIDE section to complete these statements and then use the critical thinking and discussion question to develop your ideas.

75. When you are giving care, you are responsible to protect the person's safety and well-being. What are your responsibilities regarding wound care in these situations?
    A. If you are careless during a transfer, you can cause a _____.
    B. If you rush during a bath, you may not notice a _____ between skin folds on a bariatric person.
    C. If you do not apply shoes properly on a diabetic person, _____ can develop.

76. To promote comfort and interaction with family and friends for a person with a wound, you may
    A. _____
    B. _____
    C. _____
    D. _____
    E. _____

Critical Thinking and Discussion Question

77. Review the care measures in Box 40-3 (p 621) and discuss your professional responsibilities in helping people with diabetes take good care of their feet.

41 Pressure Injuries

Fill in the Blank: Key Terms

Avoidable pressure injury
Bedfast
Bony prominence
Chairfast

Colonized
Epidermal stripping
Eschar
Intact skin

Pressure point
Pressure injury
Shear
Skin breakdown

Slough
Unavoidable pressure
injury

1. Normal skin and skin layers without damage or breaks is _____.

2. _____ is the presence of bacteria on the wound surface or in wound tissue; the person does not have signs and symptoms of an infection.

3. Dead tissue that is shed from the skin is _____ _____.

4. A pressure injury that develops from the improper use of the nursing process is an

   _____.

5. A _____ is an area where the bone sticks out or projects from the flat surface of the body.

6. Thick, leathery dead tissue that may be loose or adhered to the skin is _____.

7. Another name for bony prominence is _____ _____.

8. _____ occurs when layers of the skin rub against each other; when the skin remains in place and underlying tissues move and stretch and tear underlying capillaries and blood vessels causing tissue damage.

9. _____ means confined to bed.

10. An _____ is a pressure injury that occurs despite efforts to prevent one through proper use of the nursing process.

11. Localized damage to the skin and/or underlying tissue, usually over a bony prominence, resulting from pressure or pressure in combination with shear is a

    _____.

12. _____ means confined to a chair.

13. Removing the epidermis as tape is removed from the skin is _____.

14. Changes or damage to intact skin is _____ _____.

Circle the Best Answer

15. Which piece of equipment is most likely to provide a surface that is involved in a pressure injury?
    A. Commode chair
    B. Mattress
    C. Blood pressure cuff
    D. Mechanical lift

16. A pressure injury occurs because
    A. Dizziness causes the person to stumble and fall
    B. Sharp edges can cause skin lacerations
    C. Pressure or pressure with shearing occurs
    D. Repositioning is done too frequently

17. Older and disabled persons are at great risk for pressure injuries because they have
    A. Acute illnesses that are not properly treated
    B. Physical needs that cannot be met
    C. Thin and fragile skin that is easily injured
    D. Lost interest in performing daily hygiene

18. Which person has the greatest risk factor for a pressure injury?
    A. Often paces back and forth, and nursing assistant has to redirect
    B. Frequently slumps in bed and is pulled up by nursing assistant
    C. Continually asks nursing assistant for help with hygienic care
    D. Repeatedly asks nursing assistant for help to go to the bathroom

19. The first sign of a pressure injury in an area may be
    A. Reddened skin over a bony prominence
    B. Small wound that is pink and moist
    C. A skin flap over a bony prominence
    D. Exposed tissue and some drainage

20. A resident keeps sliding down in bed. The nurse tells you to raise the head of the bed no more than 30 degrees. This position will prevent tissue damage caused by
    A. Pressure over hard surfaces
    B. Shearing forces
    C. Poor body mechanics
    D. Moisture on skin surfaces

21. In children and infants, pressure injuries commonly occur
    A. Over bony areas such as the hips
    B. Underneath the breasts
    C. Between abdominal folds
    D. On the back of the head

22. The nurse tells you that the person has a Kennedy terminal injury. Which action is the nurse most likely to ask you to perform?
    A. Increase turning frequency to every 30 minutes to relieve pressure
    B. Give comfort measures because death will occur in 2 to 3 days
    C. Assist the person to drink extra fluids and eat high protein foods
    D. Avoid using soap because person is having an allergic reaction

23. A Stage 3 pressure injury would have
    A. Intact skin with redness over a bony prominence
    B. Exposed subcutaneous fat and slough
    C. Full-thickness skin and tissue loss
    D. A blister or shallow injury

24. The most common site for a pressure injury is the
    A. Elbow   C. Thighs
    B. Sacrum   D. Ears

25. When following a re-positioning schedule, the person should be re-positioned
    A. Every 15 minutes
    B. Every 60 minutes
    C. Every 2 hours
    D. According to the individualized plan

26. Which factor increases friction when moving people in the bed?
    A. Decreased ability to sense pain
    B. Supine position and flat surface
    C. Pillow placement to prevent skin on skin contact
    D. Moisture on the skin and bed linens

27. Bed cradles are used to
    A. Position the person in good body alignment
    B. Prevent pressure on the legs, feet, and toes
    C. Keep the heels off the bed
    D. Distribute body weight evenly

28. Some special beds allow
    A. The person to move around easily
    B. Changes in where pressure is placed on the body
    C. 1 staff member to move the person every 2 hours
    D. Automatic and correct alignment of body position

Fill in the Blank

29. Write out the abbreviations.
    A. CMS _____
    B. NPIAP _____

30. Name the stage of pressure injury described in each of these.
    A. The skin is gone and subcutaneous fat may be exposed. _____
    B. Non-blanchable erythema of intact skin. _____
    C. Muscle, tendon, and bone are exposed and damaged. Eschar may be present. _____
    D. The wound is pink or red and moist. It may involve a broken or intact blister. Fat and deeper tissues are not visible. _____

31. You can help prevent shearing by raising the head of the bed only _____. The care plan tells you
    A. _____
    B. _____
    C. _____

32. Explain how the following conditions place a person at risk for pressure injuries.
    A. Urinary or fecal incontinence _____
       _____
    B. Poor nutrition _____
       _____
    C. Limited mental awareness _____
       _____
    D. Circulatory problems _____
       _____
    E. Have weight loss or are very thin _____
       _____

33. Explain how these protective devices help prevent pressure injuries.
    A. Bed cradle prevents pressure on _____
       _____.
    B. Heel and elbow protectors promote _____
       _____ and reduce
       _____ and _____.
    C. Heel and foot elevators raise _____
       _____.
    D. Gel or fluid-filled pads have _____
       _____.
    E. Special beds are particularly useful for patients who have _____ injuries.

34. According to the CMS, infection is present in Stages _____ of pressure injuries.

Labeling

Answer questions 35 and 36 using the following illustration.

35. Name this position. _____

36. Place an "X" on each of the 5 pressure points. Name the bony point for each one.
    A. _____
    B. _____
    C. _____
    D. _____
    E. _____

Answer questions 37 and 38 using the following illustration.

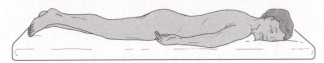

37. Name this position. _____

38. Place an "X" on each of the 10 pressure points. Name the bony point for each one.

A. _____
B. _____
C. _____
D. _____
E. _____
F. _____
G. _____
H. _____
I. _____
J. _____

Answer questions 39 and 40 using the following illustration.

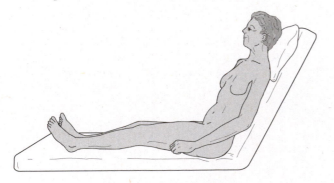

39. Name this position. _____

40. Place an "X" on each of the 10 pressure points. Name the bony point for each one.

A. _____
B. _____
C. _____
D. _____
E. _____
F. _____
G. _____
H. _____
I. _____
J. _____

Answer questions 41 and 42 using the following illustration.

41. Name this position.
_____

42. Place an "X" on each of the 6 pressure points. Name the bony point for each one.

A. _____
B. _____
C. _____
D. _____
E. _____
F. _____

Answer questions 43 and 44 using the following illustration.

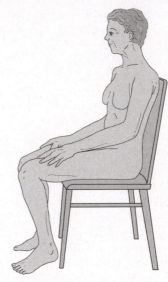

43. Name this position. _____

44. Place an "X" on each of the 5 pressure points. Name the bony point for each one.

A. _____
B. _____
C. _____
D. _____
E. _____

45. Examine the documentation sample below and answers the following questions.

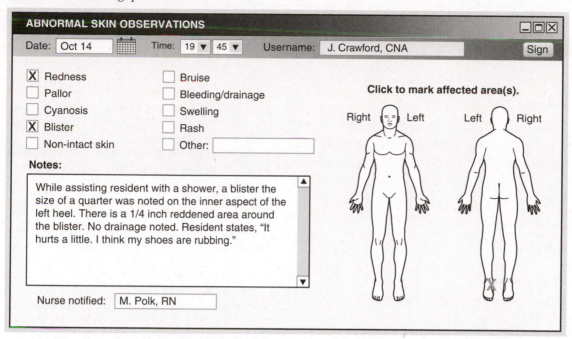

ABNORMAL SKIN OBSERVATIONS

Date: Oct 14   Time: 19 ▼ 45 ▼   Username: J. Crawford, CNA   Sign

[X] Redness   [ ] Bruise
[ ] Pallor   [ ] Bleeding/drainage
[ ] Cyanosis   [ ] Swelling
[X] Blister   [ ] Rash
[ ] Non-intact skin [ ] Other: _____

Notes:

While assisting resident with a shower, a blister the size of a quarter was noted on the inner aspect of the left heel. There is a 1/4 inch reddened area around the blister. No drainage noted. Resident states, "It hurts a little. I think my shoes are rubbing."

Nurse notified: M. Polk, RN

Click to mark affected area(s).

Right   Left   Left   Right

A. The nursing assistant observed a problem with the patient's skin. Which body part was affected?

_____

B. How did the nursing assistant describe the area?

_____

C. What did the resident say about the wound?

_____

Optional Learning Exercises

46. The _____ requires that nursing centers identify persons at risk for pressure injuries.

47. How quickly can a person develop a pressure injury after the onset of pressure? _____

48. When handling, moving, and positioning a person, it is important to follow the _____

_____

in the person's care plan.
   A. How often should a bedfast person be re-positioned? _____
   B. How often should a chairfast person be re-positioned? _____
   C. Why would a person be re-positioned more frequently (as often as every 15 minutes)?

_____

49. What are 2 ways pressure injuries can occur on the ears?
   A. _____
   B. _____

50. If you are interviewed during a survey, what questions may be asked about pressure injuries?
   A. _____
   B. _____
   C. _____
   D. _____
   E. _____

Use the FOCUS ON PRIDE section to complete these statements.

51. When you observe and report skin problems to the nurse, it can prevent _____.

52. When you speak up for your patients and residents, this is called being an _____.

Critical Thinking and Discussion Question

53. Discuss reasons why the nursing assistant may be the first member of the health care team to notice a problem with a person's skin.

Fill in the Blank: Key Terms

Compress   Cyanosis   Pack
Constrict   Dilate

1. A bluish color is _____.
2. _____ means to narrow.
3. A treatment that involves wrapping a body part with a wet or dry application is a _____.
4. A _____ is a soft pad applied over a body area.
5. _____ means to expand or open wider.

Circle the Best Answer

6. Which person is most likely to have an order for a heat application?
   A. Person reports straining back muscles after bending forward
   B. Pregnant woman would like relief from mild abdominal cramps
   C. Older person with metal wrist implant reports mild swelling
   D. Older confused person has swelling in knee and lower leg

7. You apply a warm moist pack to a person's arm according to the nurse's instructions. Which observation would be considered normal and expected?
   A. Skin is pale and numb
   B. Skin is warm and red
   C. Skin is moist and painful
   D. Skin is hot and blistered

8. When heat is applied to the skin
   A. Blood vessels in the area dilate
   B. Tissues have less oxygen
   C. Blood flow decreases
   D. Skin and muscle constrict

9. If heat is applied for too long, blood vessels constrict. Which observation would accompany the constriction?
   A. Skin becomes excessively red
   B. Skin becomes pale and damaged
   C. Skin becomes thin and fragile
   D. Skin becomes moist with sweat

10. Moist heat applications should have cooler temperatures than dry heat applications because
    A. Dry heat penetrates more deeply
    B. Dry heat cannot cause burns
    C. Heat penetrates deeper with a moist application
    D. Moist heat has a slower effect than dry heat

11. You applied a heat application to a person's leg and you must frequently check it. Which action represents the best time management?
    A. Help a person in the next room to take a shower
    B. Make the person's bed and straighten the room
    C. Tell the nurse that you are busy for the next 5 minutes
    D. Tell the person to push the call bell in 5 minutes

12. The care plan states that the person receives a heat application of 110°F. As a nursing assistant you know that you should
    A. Measure the temperature carefully before applying heat to the person
    B. Not apply an application that is above 106° F
    C. Ask the person if the application is too warm
    D. Apply the application and remind the person not to remove it

13. Heat and cold applications are applied for no longer than
    A. 15 to 20 minutes   C. 1 hour
    B. 30 to 45 minutes   D. 2 hours

14. When a hot or cold application is in place, you should check the area
    A. Every 5 minutes
    B. Every 15 to 20 minutes
    C. About every 30 minutes
    D. Once an hour

15. When hot compresses are in place, you may apply an aquathermia pad over the compress
    A. To keep the compress wet
    B. To protect the area from injury
    C. To measure the temperature of the compress
    D. To maintain the correct temperature of the compress

16. A hot soak is applied
    A. By putting the body part into water
    B. By applying a soft pad to a body part
    C. And is covered with plastic wrap
    D. When the water temperature cools down

17. When giving a sitz bath
    A. Check the person often to assess for weakness, fainting, or fatigue
    B. Keep the door open so you can see the person from the hallway
    C. Give privacy by closing the door and leaving the person alone
    D. Make sure the water temperature is hot and deep enough to sit in

18. When you use an aquathermia pad
    A. Wrap the pad in a moist towel and place it over the body part
    B. Instruct the person how to use the temperature setting key
    C. Place the pad underneath the person's body part
    D. Check the hoses for kinks and bubbles; water must flow freely

19. Which condition would commonly be treated with an ice pack application?
    A. Has a sprained ankle
    B. Has hypothermia
    C. Has a headache
    D. Has a sore throat

20. When a cold application is applied, the numbing effect helps to
    A. Reduce or relieve pain in the part
    B. Constrict blood vessels
    C. Decrease blood flow
    D. Cool the body part

21. Which of these cold applications is moist?
    A. Ice bag   C. Ice glove
    B. Ice collar   D. Cold compress

22. You should remove the cold application if
    A. The skin is red, moist and cool to the touch
    B. The person says the area feels numb and pain has decreased
    C. The skin appears pale, white, gray, or bluish in color
    D. The person is slightly chilled and asks for another blanket

23. When a person has hypothermia, which piece of equipment is the nurse most likely to ask you to obtain?
    A. Ice glove   C. Aquathermia pad
    B. Sitz bath   D. Warming blanket

Fill in the Blank

24. Write out the abbreviations.
    A. F _____
    B. C _____

25. What are the effects of heat applications?
    A. _____
    B. _____
    C. _____
    D. _____
    E. _____

26. In applying heat or cold applications for infants or children, crying can communicate
    _____

27. What are the advantages of dry heat applications?
    A. _____
    B. _____

28. Give an example of a dry heat application.
    _____

29. When the nurse delegates you to prepare a warm soak, what is the correct temperature range?
    _____

30. When you are giving a sitz bath, what observations should be reported to the nurse?
    _____

31. List three questions that you should ask the person when you are applying heat or cold.
    A. _____
    B. _____
    C. _____

32. Name five uses for cold applications.
    A. _____
    B. _____
    C. _____
    D. _____
    E. _____

33. When you prepare an ice bag, ice collar, or ice glove remove the excess air by
    _____.

34. When a cooling blanket is being used, _____ are checked often.

35. How can you manage your time to stay in or near the person's room during a heat or cold application?
    A. _____
    B. _____
    C. _____
    D. _____
    E. _____
    F. _____

Optional Learning Exercises

Situation: The nurse instructs you to apply a cold pack to a resident who has twisted her ankle. Use the information you learned in this chapter to answer these questions about carrying out this treatment.

36. What is the purpose of the cold application for this injury? _____
    _____

37. What can you use to make a cool dry application to the ankle if no commercial packs are available?
    _____

38. Why do you squeeze the application tightly after filling it with ice?
    _____

39. How will you protect the person's skin?

40. How often do you check the application?

_____

41. When you check the area where the cold pack was applied, what signs and symptoms should be reported?

A. _____

B. _____

C. _____

D. _____

E. _____

F. _____

G. _____

42. What should you do if any of these signs or symptoms are present?

_____

43. How long should you leave the application in place?

_____

44. What happens if you leave the cold pack in place for too long?

_____

Table Activity

45. Instructions: Complete the table below by filling in the missing temperature or temperature ranges

Heat and Cold Temperature Ranges

Temperature	Fahrenheit (F) Range	Centigrade (C) Range
Hot		37°C to 41°C
Warm		34°C to 37°C
Tepid	80°F to 92°F	26°C to 34°C
Cool	65°F to 79°F	
Cold		10°C to 18°C

Use the FOCUS ON PRIDE section to complete these statements and then use the critical thinking and discussion question to develop your ideas.

46. When applying heat or cold, you must allow time for

A. _____

B. _____

C. _____

D. _____

E. _____

47. When applying heat and cold, harm and legal action can result if you

A. _____

B. _____

C. _____

D. _____

E. _____

F. _____

G. _____

Critical Thinking and Discussion Question

48. You are assigned to assist a person in the home setting with hygienic care and activities of daily living. The person asks you to prepare a hot water bottle and place it on her stomach. You tell her that this is not in her care plan, but she says, "Please get it for me. I have been doing this since I was a little girl and it makes me feel so much better." What would you do?

43 Oxygen Needs

Fill in the Blank: Key Terms

Allergy
Apnea
Atelectasis
Biot's respirations
Bradypnea

Cheyne-Stokes
  respirations
Cyanosis
Dyspnea
Hemoptysis
Hyperventilation

Hypoventilation
Hypoxemia
Hypoxia
Kussmaul
  respirations
Orthopnea

Orthopneic position
Oxygen
  concentration
Pollutant
Pulse oximetry
Respiratory arrest

Respiratory
  depression
Sputum
Tachypnea

1. _____ are respirations that are rapid and deep followed by 10 to 30 seconds of apnea.

2. Bloody sputum is called _____.

3. Rapid breathing where respirations are usually greater than 20 per minute is called

   _____.

4. An _____ is a sensitivity to a substance that causes the body to react with signs and symptoms.

5. Difficult, labored, or painful breathing is

   _____.

6. Mucus from the respiratory system that is expectorated through the mouth is

   _____.

7. Being able to breathe deeply and comfortably only while sitting is _____.

8. Respirations that are less than 12 per minute is slow breathing or _____.

9. A reduced amount of oxygen in the blood is

   _____.

10. _____ describes slow, weak respirations that occur at a rate of fewer than 12 per minute.

11. The lack or absence of breathing is

    _____.

12. _____ is a pattern of respirations that is rapid and deeper than normal.

13. A harmful chemical or substance in the air or water is a

    _____.

14. _____ are respirations that gradually increase in rate and depth and then become shallow and slow. Breathing may stop for 10 to 20 seconds.

15. The _____ is sitting up and leaning over a table to breathe.

16. When breathing stops, it is _____.

17. Very deep and rapid respirations (can occur with diabetic acidosis) are _____.

18. _____ is the amount (percentage) of hemoglobin containing oxygen.

19. When cells do not have enough oxygen, it is called

    _____.

20. Respirations that are slow, shallow, and sometimes irregular is _____.

21. The collapse of a portion of the lung is _____

    _____.

22. _____ is a bluish color to the skin, lips, mucous membrane, and nail beds.

23. _____ measures the oxygen concentration in arterial blood.

Circle the Best Answer

24. With aging, the respiratory muscles weaken. This increases an elderly person's risk to develop
    A. Tachypnea
    B. Hemoptysis
    C. Allergic reactions
    D. Pneumonia

25. Oxygen needs increase when
    A. The person grows older
    B. Pain medications are taken
    C. The person has fever
    D. After the person has eaten

26. Respiratory depression or arrest can occur when
    A. The person exercises too strenuously
    B. Iron and vitamins are excluded from the diet
    C. Morphine is taken in excessively large doses
    D. The person smokes or uses tobacco products

27. Restlessness is one of the early signs of
    A. Hypoxia
    B. Apnea
    C. Hyperventilation
    D. Bradypnea

28. Which of these is a sign of hypoxia?
    A. Sputum production
    B. Decrease in pulse rate
    C. Apprehension and anxiety
    D. Red, flushed skin

29. If a pulse oximeter is being used on a person with tremors or poor circulation in the extremities, which of these sites would be best to use?
    A. A toe
    B. A finger
    C. Palm of the hand
    D. An earlobe

30. You are delegated to place a pulse oximeter on a person. Which information would you report to the nurse?
    A. How to use the equipment
    B. Pulse rate below the alarm limit
    C. The person's normal SpO$_2$ range
    D. Type of tape used to secure the oximeter

31. When a person has breathing difficulties, it is usually easier for the person to breathe
    A. In the supine position
    B. Lying on one side for long periods
    C. In the semi-Fowler's or Fowler's position
    D. In the prone position

32. Deep-breathing and coughing exercises
    A. Help prevent pneumonia and atelectasis
    B. Decrease pain after surgery or injury
    C. Are not performed if the person uses oxygen
    D. Can cause lung collapse if performed incorrectly

33. When assisting with coughing and deep breathing, you ask the person to
    A. Inhale through the mouth
    B. Hold the breath for 30 seconds
    C. Exhale slowly through pursed lips
    D. Repeat the exercise 1 or 2 times

34. The goal when using an incentive spirometer is to
    A. Teach the person how to use oxygen
    B. Increase the number of respirations
    C. Improve lung function and prevent complications
    D. Help the person stop smoking

35. If a person is receiving oxygen, you may
    A. Set the flow rate
    B. Adjust the flow rate
    C. Set up the system
    D. Turn on the oxygen

36. If you are caring for a person with oxygen therapy, which action is part of your responsibility?
    A. Remove the person's mask for eating and drinking
    B. Stop the oxygen if the person wants to walk
    C. Tell the person if the rate is too high or too low
    D. Check for skin irritation from the oxygen device

37. You are caring for a person who uses oxygen in the home setting. He requests that you place an electric space heater close to the bed for warmth. What should you do?
    A. Tell the person that the space heater is too dangerous
    B. Place the heater 10 feet from the oxygen and tell the nurse
    C. Turn off the oxygen whenever the heater is running
    D. Turn off the heater whenever you leave the house

38. If a person receives oxygen through a nasal cannula, it is important to look for irritation
    A. On the nose, ears, and cheekbones
    B. Under the mask
    C. In the throat
    D. In the oral cavity

39. If you are delegated to set up for oxygen administration, which action is part of your responsibility?
    A. Determine which device and tubing are needed
    B. Attach the flowmeter to the wall outlet or tank
    C. Apply the oxygen device to the person
    D. Ask the person if the oxygen is helping

40. If you are near a person receiving oxygen, which of these should you report?
    A. The humidifier is creating water vapor.
    B. The humidifier has water in it.
    C. The humidifier is bubbling.
    D. The humidifier has a low water level.

Fill in the Blank

41. Write out the meaning of the abbreviations.
    A. CO$_2$ _____
    B. ID _____
    C. L/min _____
    D. O$_2$ _____
    E. RBC _____
    F. SpO$_2$ _____

42. Indicate how these factors change with aging and affect the person's oxygen needs.
    A. Respiratory muscles _____
    B. Lung tissue _____
    C. Strength for coughing _____

43. Identify four diseases are related to smoking.
    A. _____
    B. _____
    C. _____
    D. _____

44. How does alcohol increase the risk of aspiration?
    It depresses the _____, reduces the _____, and increases _____.

45. What terms can be used to describe sputum when reporting and recording?
    A. Color: _____
    B. Odor: _____
    C. Consistency: _____
    D. Hemoptysis: _____

46. The normal range for oxygen concentration is _____.

47. If you are caring for a person with a pulse oximeter, what observations should be reported and recorded?
    A. _____
    B. _____
    C. _____
    D. _____
    E. _____
    F. _____

48. If a pulse oximeter is in place, what should be reported at once to the nurse?
    A. SpO$_2$ _____
    B. Pulse rate _____
    C. Signs and symptoms of _____
    _____

49. If a person has difficulty breathing, he or she may prefer a position where the person is sitting
    _____.
    This position is called _____.

50. If a person has a productive cough, what respiratory hygiene and cough etiquette should be taught?
    A. Cover _____.
    B. Use _____.
    C. Dispose of tissues _____.
    D. Wash _____.

51. If a person is using an incentive spirometer, how long is the breath held to keep the piston floating?
    _____

52. What observations should be reported after a person uses an incentive spirometer?
    A. _____
    B. _____
    C. _____
    D. _____

53. When a person wears a mask to receive oxygen, what should you do when the person needs to eat?
    _____
    How will the person receive oxygen during the meal?
    _____

54. Oxygen is humidified because otherwise it will
    _____.

Optional Learning Exercises

Situation: You are caring for Mr. R., age 84, who has chronic obstructive pulmonary disease. Answer questions 55 and 56 about caring for Mr. R.

55. What position would make it easier for Mr. R. to breathe when he is in bed?
    _____
    _____

56. How can you increase his comfort when he is sitting up?
    _____
    What is this position called?
    _____

Situation: Mrs. F. is receiving oxygen through a nasal cannula at 2 L/min. Her respirations are unlabored at 16 per minute unless she is walking about or doing personal care. Then her respirations are 28 and dyspneic. Answer questions 57 to 60 about her care.

57. Why is there no humidifier with the oxygen setup for Mrs. F.?
    _____

58. Where should you check for signs of irritation from the cannula? _____
    _____

59. You should make sure there are _____ in the tubing and that Mrs. F. does not _____ of the tubing.

60. What are the abnormal respirations that Mrs. F has with activity called?
    _____

Use the FOCUS ON PRIDE section to complete these statements and then use the critical thinking and discussion question to develop your ideas.

61. When you remind the person or visitors not to smoke when NO SMOKING signs are used, you are protecting the person's right to a _____.

62. You do not adjust the oxygen flow rate unless allowed by your _____ and _____ and instructed _____.

Critical Thinking and Discussion Question

63. You are caring for a person in the home setting. He uses oxygen occasionally. You catch him smoking while the oxygen is on. When you remind him about the "no smoking" rule for safety, he just smiles and tells you he forgets, because, "I've smoked all my life, but just lately started to need this oxygen. I'll try to remember." What should you do?

Crossword

Fill in the crossword puzzle by answering the clues below with the words from this list:

Apnea	Bradypnea	Dyspnea	Hypoventilation	Orthopnea
Biot's	Cheyne-Stokes	Hyperventilation	Kussmaul	Tachypnea

Across

9. Respirations are rapid and deeper than normal
10. Rapid and deep respirations followed by 10 to 30 seconds of apnea; occur with nervous disorders

Down

1. Respirations gradually increase in rate and depth; common when death is near
2. Respirations are 20 or more per minute
3. Respirations are slow, shallow, and sometimes irregular
4. Very deep and rapid respirations; signal diabetic coma
5. Difficult, labored, or painful breathing
6. Breathing deeply and comfortably only when sitting
7. Lack or absence of breathing
8. Respirations are fewer than 12 per minute

Fill in the Blank: Key Terms

Hemothorax   Patent   Suction

Intubation   Pleural effusion   Tracheostomy

Mechanical ventilation   Pneumothorax

1. The escape and collection of fluid in the pleural space is _____.

2. _____ is blood in the pleural space.

3. A _____ is a surgically created opening into the trachea.

4. _____ is the process of withdrawing or sucking up fluid.

5. Inserting an artificial airway is _____.

6. _____ is air in the pleural space.

7. _____ is using a machine to move air into and out of the lungs.

8. _____ is open or unblocked.

Circle the Best Answer

9. When caring for a person with an artificial airway, you should tell the nurse at once if
   A. The airway interferes with speaking
   B. The person needs frequent oral hygiene
   C. The airway comes out or is dislodged
   D. The person feels as if he or she is gagging

10. Because a person with an endotracheal tube (ET) cannot speak, it is important to
    A. Never ask questions
    B. Speak clearly and loudly
    C. Always keep the call light within reach
    D. Use simple language during your explanations

11. For a person with an ET tube, which piece of equipment will the nurse ask you to obtain to assist the person with communication?
    A. Headphones   C. Hearing aide
    B. Paper and pencil   D. Self-help device

12. The nurse asks you to assist in changing the ties that secure the outer cannula in place. Which action will you perform?
    A. Cut the soiled ties and then assist the nurse to insert clean ties
    B. Hold the outer cannula in place until the nurse secures the new ties
    C. Clean the inner and outer cannulas, while the nurse inserts the new ties
    D. Remove the soiled ties; clean the stoma and cannulas; replace the ties

13. The stoma or tube must be
    A. Covered when shaving
    B. Covered with plastic when outdoors
    C. Covered with a loose gauze dressing when bathing
    D. Uncovered when the person goes swimming

14. If you are assisting with tracheostomy care, you may be delegated to
    A. Remove the ties and wash them
    B. Suction the tube before and after meals
    C. Clean the stoma to prevent infection
    D. Remove the inner and outer cannulas to clean them

15. Which position would you use, when the nurse asks you to position the person for suctioning?
    A. Prone position with head turned to the side
    B. Semi-Fowler's position with head turned to the side
    C. Supine position with head elevated on small pillow
    D. Dorsal recumbent with head in a neutral position

16. Suctioning is done
    A. When the morning hygiene is completed
    B. When respiratory distress is observed
    C. When the person starts coughing
    D. When the person wants suctioning

17. When the alarm sounds on a machine used for mechanical ventilation, you should first
    A. Report to the nurse at once
    B. Re-set the alarms
    C. Re-assure the person that the alarm is normal
    D. Check to see if the tube is attached to the ventilator

18. When caring for a person with chest tubes, tell the nurse at once if
    A. The person is reluctant to do the deep-breathing exercises
    B. There is a small amount of drainage in the chest tube
    C. The bubbling in the drainage system has increased
    D. The person indicates that there is a need for suctioning

19. Petrolatum gauze is kept at the bedside of a person with chest tubes to
    A. Cover the insertion site if the chest tube comes out
    B. Lubricate the site of the chest tube
    C. Protect the skin around the chest tube
    D. Cover the insertion site to prevent drainage

Fill in the Blank

20. Write out the meaning of the abbreviations.
    A. CO_2 _____
    B. ET _____
    C. O_2 _____
    D. RT _____

21. When assisting with suctioning, tell the nurse if there is
    A. A decrease in _____ to less than _____
    B. Irregular _____ rhythm
    C. An increase or decrease in _____
    D. Signs and symptoms of altered _____
    E. Decrease in oxygen _____

22. What are the 3 parts of a tracheostomy tube?
    A. _____
    B. _____
    C. _____

23. Which part of the tracheostomy tube is removed for cleaning and mucus removal? _____

24. Which part of the tracheostomy tube is not removed? _____

25. Why is the obturator kept at the bedside? _____

26. A suction cycle takes no more than _____ seconds. The cycle involves
    A. _____
    B. _____
    C. _____

27. Before, during, and after suctioning, what is checked and observed?
    A. _____
    B. _____
    C. _____
    D. _____

28. When a person has mechanical ventilation, what should you do when you enter the room? _____
    _____

29. What should you do each time you leave the room of a person with mechanical ventilation? _____
    _____

30. If chest tubes are in place, what should be reported to the nurse at once?
    A. _____
    B. _____
    C. _____
    D. _____
    E. _____
    F. _____

Optional Learning Exercises

31. If you are caring for a person with a tracheostomy, why is the tracheostomy covered when the person is outdoors? _____ ; _____

32. If a person with a tracheostomy is outdoors, what is used to cover the tracheostomy? _____
    _____

33. What is done to protect the stoma in the following situations?
    A. Showers _____
    B. Shaving _____
    C. Shampooing _____

34. The stoma is never covered with _____
    _____
    Why? _____
    _____

35. What do you need to check before using an Ambu bag attached to oxygen? _____

36. If a person has mechanical ventilation, where do you find a plan for communication? _____
    Why is it important for everyone to use the same signals for communication? _____
    _____

37. If a person has chest tubes, why is it important to prevent kinks in the tubing? _____
    _____

38. Which step of tracheostomy care is depicted in the figure? _____
    _____
    _____

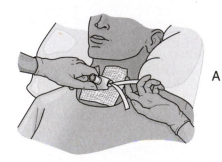

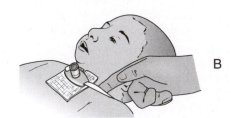

Use the FOCUS ON PRIDE section to complete these statements and then use the critical thinking and discussion question to develop your ideas.

39. It is important to report signs and symptoms that a person needs suctioning because the airway must be clear for _____ .

40. When a person has an ET tube, you can provide social support by

    A. _____

    B. _____

    C. _____

    D. _____

    E. _____

Critical Thinking and Discussion Question

41. You are caring for a woman who has a tracheostomy; she is currently living in a long-term care facility. Her daughter says, "Mom was always very chatty and social before having the tracheostomy, but now she can't talk like she used to. She's so withdrawn. I wished we could do something to help her." Discuss ways that the health care team could assist this person and her family.

45 Rehabilitation Needs

Fill in the Blank: Key Terms

Activities of daily
 living

Disability
Prosthesis

Rehabilitation
Restorative aide

Restorative nursing
 care

1. A nursing assistant with special training in restorative nursing and rehabilitation skills is a

   _____.

2. _____ are activities usually done during a normal day in a person's life.

3. An artificial replacement for a missing body part is a

   _____.

4. Care that helps persons regain their health and strength for safe and independent living is

   _____.

5. A _____ is any lost, absent, or impaired physical or mental function.

6. The process of restoring the disabled person to the highest possible level of physical, psychological, social, and economic functioning is

   _____.

Circle the Best Answer

7. Which person is acting to fulfill one of the goals of rehabilitation?
   A. Athlete is training to improve his endurance
   B. Person takes prescribed antibiotics as directed
   C. Person does physical therapy exercises after knee surgery
   D. Older person practices yoga for better balance and strength

8. Restorative nursing programs include measures that promote
   A. Self-care, elimination, and positioning
   B. Giving total care to persons who are incapacitated
   C. Curing disease and restoring normal function
   D. Good nursing care for rapid post-surgical recovery

9. Which question is a surveyor most likely to ask you about caring for people with rehabilitation needs?
   A. What kinds of rehabilitation programs are offered?
   B. How long does it take for people to complete therapy?
   C. How much do you for the person when you assist with hygiene?
   D. Have you experienced hostility when caring for people with disabilities?

10. You are assisting with rehabilitation and restorative care, which action would you perform during mealtime?
    A. Put the food tray in front of person and let him figure how to eat
    B. Cut the food into small pieces and put assistive eating devices within reach
    C. Suggest that eating should be done in the dining room for socialization
    D. Feed the person with a spoon, give him sips of fluid, and wipe his face

11. Which of these would be most helpful for a person receiving rehabilitative care?
    A. Give the person pity or sympathy when tasks are difficult
    B. Remind the person not to try new skills or those that are difficult
    C. Give praise when even a little progress is made
    D. Tell the person to do the task like he normally would

12. Good alignment, turning and re-positioning, and range-of-motion exercises, address which aspect of rehabilitation and restorative care?
    A. Psychological   C. Social
    B. Economic   D. Physical

13. Rehabilitation begins
    A. After the person has recovered
    B. When the person first seeks health care
    C. When the person asks for help
    D. When a discharge date has been set

14. Adaptive (assistive) devices help to meet the goal of
    A. Recovering all former abilities
    B. Achieving independence in self-care
    C. Living alone in own home
    D. Using services provided by others

15. The occupational therapist is preparing to teach the person about assistive devices for cooking. The nurse suggests that you accompany the therapist. What is your role?
    A. Give the person emotional support while learning these new skills
    B. Listen to the therapist; you should use the same words when guiding the person
    C. Help the therapist to physically and emotionally control the person as needed
    D. Do whatever the therapist tells you to do during the teaching session

16. You are caring for a person who has dysphagia. Which information do you need to get from the nurse and the care plan?
    A. Limitations of mobility
    B. Type of assistive device
    C. Type of diet
    D. Method of communication

17. A person who has had a joint replacement would receive
    A. Spinal cord rehabilitation
    B. Amputee rehabilitation
    C. Orthopedic rehabilitation
    D. Stroke rehabilitation

18. The care plan indicates use of a picture board to communicate with a person who has a speech disorder, but when you try to use it, he gets angry and yells. What would you do?
    A. Try a different method of communicating that does not include the board
    B. Recognize that he is frustrated; remain calm, talk to the nurse as needed
    C. Don't let the person control you; tell him that anger is not necessary
    D. Be polite, ignore the angry outburst and continue attempts to use the board

19. You are part of the home health team for a rehabilitation patient, which action could you perform to contribute to the person's safety?
    A. Help the person to install an automatic garage door opener
    B. Teach the person how to use the grab bars in the bathroom
    C. Determine where handrails are needed indoors and outdoors
    D. Make sure that there is a flashlight on the bedside table

Fill in the Blank

20. Write out the meaning of the abbreviations.
    A. ADL _____
    B. ROM _____

21. The three goals of rehabilitation are to
    A. _____
    B. _____
    C. _____

22. In long-term care, residents may have progressive illnesses. Goals for them are to
    A. _____
    B. _____

23. A person with health problems or a disability needs to adjust in these four areas.
    A. _____
    B. _____
    C. _____
    D. _____

24. Rehabilitation takes longer in which age-group? _____ What are reasons?
    A. Changes affect _____.
    B. Chronic _____.
    C. Risk for _____.

25. What are some adaptive (assistive) devices that will assist in self-feeding?
    A. _____
    B. _____
    C. _____

26. The goal for a prosthesis is for the device to
    _____.

27. When you are assisting with rehabilitation and restorative care, why should you practice the task that the person must perform? _____
    _____

28. When assisting with rehabilitation and restorative care, what complications can be prevented if you report early signs and symptoms? _____
    _____

29. The key team member of the rehabilitation team is the _____. Other members are
    A. _____
    B. _____
    C. _____
    D. _____

30. Which rehabilitation program would help a person with
    A. Severe vision problems: _____
    B. Chronic obstructive pulmonary disease: _____
    C. Severe burns: _____
    D. Traumatic brain injury: _____
    E. A fractured leg: _____

31. Name seven things that you can do to promote the person's quality of life.
    A. _____
    B. _____
    C. _____
    D. _____
    E. _____
    F. _____
    G. _____

Optional Learning Exercises

Mrs. Mercer is 82 years old. She is a resident in a rehabilitation unit because she had a stroke that has caused weakness on her left side. Although she is right-handed, she needs to learn to use several adaptive (assistive) devices as she re-learns ways to carry out ADLs. She often becomes angry or depressed. Answer the following questions about Mrs. Mercer and her care.

NOTE: Some of these questions will require information contained in other chapters.

32. Mrs. Mercer is having difficulty with controlling urinary and bowel elimination. What would be the goal of her care for these problems?

_____ Her plan

of care would include programs for _____.

33. What should you do to prepare Mrs. Mercer's food at meal time so she can feed herself? *(Chapter 30)*

_____

_____

34. Mrs. Mercer can brush her teeth but needs help getting prepared. What should you do to get her ready to brush her teeth? *(Chapter 23)*

_____

35. Why does she need help at mealtime and to brush her teeth? *(Chapters 23 and 30)* _____

_____

36. Mrs. Mercer needs help to get in and out of bed. When helping her to transfer, you remember to position the chair on her _____ side. *(Chapter 20)*

37. When Mrs. Mercer becomes discouraged because progress is slow, how can you help her? You can stress _____ and focus on _____.

Use the FOCUS ON PRIDE section to complete these statements and then use the critical thinking and discussion question to develop your ideas.

38. If a nursing assistant is being considered for promotion to a restorative aide position, list three qualities that are considered.

A. _____

B. _____

C. _____

39. List seven things you can do to promote independence when a person is receiving rehabilitation and restorative care.

A. _____

B. _____

C. _____

D. _____

E. _____

F. _____

G. _____

Critical Thinking and Discussion Question

40. You are working on a busy long-term care unit. You see another nursing assistant pushing one of the residents to the dining room in a wheelchair. You know that part of the rehabilitation goal for that resident is to encourage ambulation. Discuss reasons that may have caused the nursing assistant to use the wheelchair.

Fill in the Blank: Key Terms

Aphasia	Cerumen	Hearing loss	Tinnitus
Blindness	Deafness	Low vision	Vertigo
Braille	Expressive aphasia	Mixed aphasia	Wernicke's aphasia
Broca's aphasia	Global aphasia	Receptive aphasia	

1. _____ is a touch reading and writing system that uses raised dots for each letter of the alphabet.

2. Another name for receptive aphasia is _____.

3. Another name for earwax is _____.

4. _____ is dizziness.

5. A ringing, roaring, hissing, or buzzing sound in the ears is _____.

6. The total or partial loss of the ability to use or understand language is _____.

7. _____ is not being able to hear the normal range of sounds associated with normal hearing.

8. _____ is difficulty expressing or sending out thoughts through speech or writing; motor aphasia, Broca's aphasia.

9. Eyesight that cannot be corrected with eyeglasses, contact lenses, medicine, or surgery is

_____.

10. Difficulty understanding language is _____; also called Wernicke's aphasia.

11. A hearing loss in which it is impossible for the person to understand speech through hearing alone is

_____.

12. Another name for expressive aphasia is

_____.

13. _____ is difficulty expressing or sending out thoughts and difficulty understanding language; mixed aphasia.

14. The absence of sight is _____.

15. Another name for global aphasia is _____.

Circle the Best Answer

16. Which ear problem would be the easiest to resolve?
    A. Cerumen in the ear canal
    B. Tinnitus related to ear infection
    C. Risk for falling related to vertigo
    D. Loss of hearing related to aging

17. If a person has chronic otitis media, the person may develop
    A. Vertigo
    B. Permanent hearing loss
    C. Sore throat
    D. Nausea and vomiting

18. If an infant or young child has otitis media, what you would expect to observe?
    A. The child pulls or tugs at the ear
    B. The child sleeps more than usual
    C. The child is frightened by normal sounds
    D. The child turns the better ear towards sounds

19. How would you know a person with dementia has otitis media?
    A. The person would report dizziness
    B. You can barely hear the person speak
    C. You notice behavioral changes
    D. The person would have tinnitus

20. If you are caring for a person who has Meniere's disease, what is the most important consideration?
    A. Risk for falls
    B. Difficulty with hearing
    C. Dietary restrictions
    D. Avoidance of flashing lights

21. Which of these is a preventable cause of hearing loss?
    A. Aging
    B. Heredity and genetics
    C. Exposure to loud sounds
    D. Birth defects

22. Which nursing assistant needs a reminder about communicating with a person with a hearing loss?
    A. Nursing Assistant A lightly touches the person's arm
    B. Nursing Assistant B speaks as loudly as possible
    C. Nursing Assistant C faces the person when speaking.
    D. Nursing Assistant D use gestures and facial expressions to give clues.

23. A child with normal hearing begins to babble in a speech-like way at
    A. Birth to 3 months   C. 4 to 6 months
    B. 7 months to 1 year   D. 1 to 2 years

24. A person with a hearing loss
    A. Can understand by attentive listening
    B. Is usually very irritable
    C. Often has drainage from the ears
    D. May deny a hearing loss

25. When you are caring for a person with a hearing aid, report to the nurse
    A. When turning the hearing aid off at night
    B. If a new battery is inserted
    C. If the hearing aid is lost or damaged
    D. When removing the battery at night

26. If a person has expressive aphasia, he or she
    A. Would not understand simple language
    B. Would give incorrect answers to questions
    C. Would have difficulty hearing what was said
    D. Might put words in the wrong order

27. An effective measure to develop communication with a speech-impaired person is to
    A. Speak in a child-like way
    B. Ask the questions to which you know the answer
    C. Give complete and detailed instructions
    D. Make sure the TV and radio is turned on

28. Cataracts most commonly are caused by
    A. Aging   C. Poor diet
    B. Injury   D. Surgery

29. For a person who had eye surgery for cataracts, the care includes
    A. Removing the eye shield or patch for naps and at night
    B. Having the person cover both eyes during a shower or shampoo
    C. Reminding the person not to rub or press on the affected eye
    D. Placing the over-bed table on the operative side

30. After cataract surgery, report to the nurse at once if
    A. The person complains of eye pain
    B. The person can't see well enough to read
    C. The person tries to wear their old glasses
    D. The person asks for help with basic needs

31. For a person with advanced age-related macular degeneration (AMD), which activity is he or she most likely to need your assistance?
    A. Standing up   C. Reading a menu
    B. Brushing teeth   D. Getting dressed

32. Which of these measures can reduce the risk of AMD?
    A. Wearing sunglasses in bright light
    B. Eating a diet high in green leafy vegetables and fish
    C. Controlling diabetes as directed by doctor
    D. Having regular eye examinations

33. Diabetic retinopathy is the result of
    A. Taking too much insulin
    B. Damage to tiny blood vessels in the retina
    C. Trauma that causes clouding of the lens
    D. Increased pressure in the eye

34. When a person has glaucoma, he or she may have difficulty seeing objects
    A. That are far away
    B. In the peripheral vision
    C. Directly in front
    D. That are brightly colored

35. Which group has the greatest risk for glaucoma?
    A. Everyone over 60 years of age
    B. Caucasians and Asians over 40 years of age
    C. Younger persons with diabetic retinopathy
    D. Those who need corrective glasses or lens

36. A person who is legally blind
    A. Is totally unable to see anything including light
    B. Had normal vision at birth and became blind later in life
    C. Can see light at 200 feet, but cannot discern clear details
    D. Sees at 20 feet what a person with normal vision sees at 200 feet.

37. When you enter the room of a blind person, you should first
    A. Touch the person to let him or her know you are there
    B. Speak loudly to make sure the person knows you are there
    C. Make sure the lights are bright and the walkways are cleared
    D. Identify yourself and give your name, title, and reason for being there

38. When a person is blind, you should
    A. Give extensive and detailed explanations for your actions
    B. Avoid embarrassing words such as "see," "look," or "read"
    C. Offer your arm to assist the person to move about
    D. Perform most of the hygienic care for the person

39. When you assist a blind person to walk, it is best if you
    A. Walk slightly behind the person and put your arm around the person's waist
    B. Walk slightly ahead with the person holding your arm just above the elbow
    C. Grasp the person's arm firmly to guide the way
    D. Walk very slowly to allow the person to take small steps

40. If a blind person uses a cane, you can assist by
    A. Grasping the person by the arm holding the cane
    B. Coming up behind the person and grasping his or her elbow
    C. Storing the cane so it is out of the way
    D. Asking if you can assist before trying to help

41. If a blind person uses a guide dog, it is correct to
    A. Take the person by the arm on the side opposite from the dog
    B. Avoid distracting a guide dog by petting or feeding the dog
    C. Give the dog commands to avoid dangers
    D. Greet, praise and pet the dog and compliment performance

42. Eyeglasses should be cleaned with
    A. Warm water   C. Detergent
    B. Hot water   D. Paper towels

43. When cleaning an ocular prosthesis, you should
    A. Wash the artificial eye with mild soap and warm water
    B. Wash the eyelid and eyelashes with sterile water
    C. Dry the artificial eye before inserting it in the socket
    D. Use sterile technique throughout the entire procedure

Fill in the Blank

44. Write out the abbreviations.
    A. AMD _____
    B. ASL _____
    C. ADA _____

45. Otitis media often begins with _____
    _____.

46. If a person has chronic otitis media, it can cause permanent _____.

47. For a person who has Meniere's disease, list five safety practices.
    A. _____
    B. _____
    C. _____
    D. _____
    E. _____

48. Name four examples of noises that can cause hearing loss.
    A. _____
    B. _____
    C. _____
    D. _____

49. List four problems that could occur with a hearing loss.
    A. _____
    B. _____
    C. _____
    D. _____

50. Identify nine symptoms of hearing loss.
    A. _____
    B. _____
    C. _____
    D. _____
    E. _____
    F. _____
    G. _____
    H. _____
    I. _____

51. If a woman is speaking to a hearing-impaired person, why should she adjust the pitch of her voice?
    _____
    _____

52. Why is it important for a person with a hearing loss to see your face when you are speaking to the person?
    _____
    _____

53. What are three common causes of speech disorders?
    A. _____
    B. _____
    C. _____

54. If a person has apraxia, the brain _____
    _____.

55. Measures you can use to communicate with a speech-impaired person are
    A. Listen, and give _____.
    B. Repeat _____.
    C. Write down _____.
    D. Allow the person _____.
    E. Watch _____.

56. When a person has expressive aphasia, the person knows what _____
    _____.

57. When a person has receptive aphasia, the person has trouble _____.

58. Symptoms of glaucoma include
    A. Peripheral _____
    B. Blurred _____
    C. Halos _____

59. Drugs and surgery are used with glaucoma to
    _____.

60. Most cataracts are caused by _____.
    Other risk factors are
    A. _____
    B. _____
    C. _____
    D. _____
    E. _____

61. When you are caring for a person after cataract surgery, an eye shield is worn as directed, and is worn for _____.

62. When assisting a blind or visually impaired person, list seven things that can be done to provide a consistent meal-time setting.
    A. _____
    B. _____
    C. _____
    D. _____
    E. _____
    F. _____
    G. _____

63. A person with age-related macular degeneration (AMD) would develop a blind spot _____
    _____.

64. For people who have diabetes, there is an increased risk for which eye disorder? _____.

65. How can a person with low vision use a computer as an adaptive device?
    A. _____
    B. _____

66. The legally blind person sees at 20 feet what a person with normal vision sees at

    _____.

67. When you orient a person to the room, why do you let the person move about the room?

    _____

Optional Learning Exercises

Mr. Herman is an 85-year-old man with a hearing loss that has developed as he has gotten older. Answer these questions about his care.

68. Two nursing assistants, a male and a female, are caring for Mr. Herman. They notice that he answers questions asked by the male nursing assistant more quickly. What is the likely reason for this?

    _____

    _____

69. The nursing assistants have found that Mr. Herman is alert and oriented. They are surprised when Joan, another nursing assistant, tells them he is "senile." Why would Joan make this statement?

    _____

70. Mr. Herman says he is too tired to go to the game room for a party. He says no one likes him. What are some reasons for his actions and statements?
    A. Tired because

    _____

    B. No one likes him

    _____

71. When giving care, the nursing assistant turns off the TV and radio in Mr. Herman's room. Why is this done? _____

You are caring for Mrs. Sanchez, who is legally blind because of glaucoma. Answer the questions about her care.

72 When you enter the room, you notice that Mrs. Sanchez is looking at her mail with a magnifying glass. How is this possible since you thought she was blind? _____

    _____

73. When you enter the room, Mrs. Sanchez asks you to adjust the blinds. Why? _____

74. When you are helping Mrs. Sanchez to move about the room, you are careful to tell her where furniture is located. Why? _____

    _____

Use the FOCUS ON PRIDE section to complete these statements and then use the critical thinking and discussion questions to develop your ideas.

75. When you are referring to a person who has speech, hearing, or vision problems, he or she should be

    referred to by _____, not by the

    _____

76. Braille signs for areas with public access are required by the _____.

Critical Thinking and Discussion Questions

77. A resident in a long-term care center has a hearing aid that she cannot independently use or maintain. She is pleasant and cooperative, but mildly confused. Sometimes she removes the hearing aid and then misplaces it. On other days, she wears it all day long without problems. Today, she has removed the hearing aid several times and you found it among the bed linens, on the bathroom sink and on her roommate's bedside table. You tell the nurse, who instructs you to store it in the case for today. Later, the daughter visits and she is upset because the resident is not wearing the hearing aid.

    Discuss this situation:
    A. What are the issues for the staff?
    B. Why is the daughter upset?
    C. What could the staff do?

78. For the four American sign examples, identify the meaning of each sign.

    A. _____
    B. _____
    C. _____
    D. _____

Fill in the Blank: Key Terms

Benign tumor   Cancer   Metastasis   Stomatitis
Biopsy   Malignant tumor   Mole   Tumor

1. A _____ is a tumor that invades and destroys nearby tissue and can spread to other body parts.

2. Inflammation of the mouth is _____.

3. A tumor that does not spread to other body parts is a _____.

4. A new growth of abnormal cells that may be benign or malignant is a _____.

5. The spread of cancer to other body parts is _____.

6. Another name for a malignant tumor is _____.

7. A _____ is a brown, tan, or black spot on the skin that is flat or raised and round or oval.

8. A _____ is a procedure in which a piece of tissue is removed for testing.

Circle the Best Answer

9. Leukemia is the most common cancer that occurs in children. What would be an early sign/symptom?
   A. Seizures   C. Weight loss
   B. Fatigue   D. Black colored mole

10. Which person is performing an action that represents a risk factor for cancer?
    A. Applying sunscreen   C. Eating an apple
    B. Smoking a cigarette   D. Drinking a soda

11. Surgery is done to
    A. Cure or control the cancer
    B. Kill the cancer cells
    C. Shrink the tumor
    D. Block hormone production

12. When you care for a person receiving radiation therapy, you might expect the person to
    A. Have pain related to the therapy
    B. Need extra rest related to fatigue
    C. Be at risk for bleeding and infections
    D. Have flu-like symptoms

13. Chemotherapy involves
    A. X-ray beams aimed at the tumor
    B. Local radiation to kill the tumor
    C. Therapies that spare normal cells
    D. Giving drugs that kill cells

14. While caring for a person receiving chemotherapy, she tells you she is upset because her hair is falling out. You
    A. Know that hair often falls out after chemotherapy
    B. Tell her this is a symptom of her disease
    C. Should report this to the nurse at once
    D. Change the subject so she will not be so upset

15. When hormone therapy is used to treat cancer, a woman may experience
    A. Stomatitis and alopecia
    B. Flu-like symptoms
    C. Hot flashes, and loss of sexual desire
    D. Burns and skin breakdown

16. Complementary and alternative medicine treatment includes
    A. Drugs or surgeries to remove hormone sources in the body
    B. Massage therapy, herbal products, and spiritual healing
    C. Implanting of radiation implants
    D. Giving blood-forming stem cells

17. A person with cancer may complain of constipation because of
    A. Side effects of pain-relief drugs
    B. Loss of muscle tone
    C. Fluid loss to the tumor
    D. Inability to digest fiber

18. When a person has cancer and expresses anger, fear, and depression, you can help most by
    A. Telling the person not to worry or get upset
    B. Giving the person privacy and time alone
    C. Being there when needed and listening to the person
    D. Changing the subject to distract the person

19. For which activity of daily living, is a person with celiac disease most likely to require assistance?
    A. Toileting   C. Bathing
    B. Ambulating   D. Dressing

20. Which action would you perform when caring for a person who has AIDS?
    A. Assist the nurse to isolate the person using respiratory precautions
    B. Encourage self-care, so that you don't get infected
    C. Assist with daily hygiene; avoid irritating soaps
    D. Double bag all linen and mark with a biohazard label

21. To protect yourself from HIV and AIDS, you should
    A. Avoid body fluids, such as urine, sputum and saliva when giving care
    B. Wear filter mask, gloves, gown, and shoe covers for routine care
    C. Follow Standard Precautions and the Bloodborne Pathogen Standard
    D. Always use the sterile technique when giving any care

22. Shingles is caused by the same virus that causes
    A. HIV
    B. Measles
    C. Chicken pox
    D. Mumps

Fill in the Blank

23. Write out the abbreviations.
    A. AIDS _____
    B. CDC _____
    C. HIV _____
    D. STD _____
    E. TB _____

24. Cancer is the _____ most common cause of death in the United States.

25. The three goals of cancer treatment are
    A. _____
    B. _____
    C. _____

26. The signs and symptoms of colon cancer are
    A. _____
    B. _____
    C. _____
    D. _____
    E. _____
    F. _____
    G. _____
    H. _____

27. When radiation therapy is used, _____ cells and _____ cells are both destroyed.

28. List seven skin changes that are side effects of radiation therapy.
    A. _____
    B. _____
    C. _____
    D. _____
    E. _____
    F. _____
    G. _____

29. When chemotherapy is used, it affects _____ cells and _____ cells.

30. For a person who is receiving chemotherapy, list six side effects that might occur.
    A. _____
    B. _____
    C. _____
    D. _____
    E. _____

31. Immunotherapy treats cancer by _____

32. Complementary and alternative medicine (CAM) is sometimes used with standard cancer treatment. List seven treatments.
    A. _____
    B. _____
    C. _____
    D. _____
    E. _____
    F. _____
    G. _____

33. When a person has an autoimmune disorder, it means the _____ system attacks the _____.

34. List three treatment goals for autoimmune disorders.
    A. _____
    B. _____
    C. _____

35. Acquired immunodeficiency syndrome (AIDS) is caused by a _____ that attacks the _____.

36. How is human immunodeficiency virus (HIV) mainly transmitted?
    A. _____
    B. _____

37. When caring for a person with HIV, the main threat to health care workers is from _____.

38. Identify three groups of people who are at risk for developing shingles.
    A. _____
    B. _____
    C. _____

Optional Learning Exercises

Mrs. Myers is a 62 year old who is having chemotherapy to treat cancer. She has not been eating well and complains of feeling very tired. When you assist her with personal care, you notice a large amount of hair on her pillow. Answer these questions about Mrs. Myers and her care.

39. Mrs. Myers may not be eating well because the chemotherapy _____ the gastro-intestinal tract and causes _____.

_____, _____,

and _____.

40. She may also have _____,
which is called stomatitis. You can help to relieve the
discomfort from this side effect when you provide

_____.

41. What is causing Mrs. Myers to lose her hair?
_____ This
condition is called _____.

*Use the FOCUS ON PRIDE section to complete these statements
and then use the critical thinking and discussion question to
develop your ideas.*

42. If you work on an oncology unit, staff and patients
value a person who is _____,

_____, _____,

and _____.

43. When you work closely with oncology patients and
families, you must protect the person's privacy and
rights and avoid crossing _____.

Critical Thinking and Discussion Question

44. You are caring for an older woman who was recently
diagnosed with breast cancer. The nurse tells you
that the woman is also HIV positive. You don gloves,
before picking up soiled items and then discard the
gloves and wash your hands after you are finished.
The woman seems upset and remarks, "I have cancer.
It's not contagious you know that don't you? Why are
you wearing gloves and why do you keep washing
your hands?" What should you say and do?

Fill in the Blank: Key Terms

Amputation	Closed fracture	Fracture	Open fracture	Quadriplegia
Arthritis	Comminuted fracture	Gangrene	Paralysis	Simple fracture
Arthroplasty	Compound fracture	Hemiplegia	Paraplegia	Tetraplegia

1. An open fracture is also called a
   _____.

2. Another name for quadriplegia is
   _____.

3. The removal of all or part of an extremity is
   _____.

4. A _____ is when the bone is broken but the skin is intact.

5. _____ is paralysis and loss of sensory function in the arms, legs, and trunk. It can also be called tetraplegia.

6. Paralysis on one side of the body is
   _____.

7. Joint inflammation is
   _____.

8. A closed fracture can also be called
   _____.

9. A _____ is a broken bone.

10. An _____ occurs when the broken bone has come through the skin. It is also called a compound fracture.

11. An _____ is the surgical replacement of a joint.

12. Paralysis and loss of sensory function in the legs is
    _____.

13. A condition in which there is death of tissue is
    _____.

14. _____ is loss of motor function, loss of sensation, or both.

15. A _____ occurs when a bone is shattered or broken into three or more pieces.

Circle the Best Answer

16. If a person has stroke-like symptoms that last a few minutes, it means that
    A. The person has had a transient ischemic attack (TIA)
    B. It is not a dangerous situation since it was temporary
    C. The person needs to lie down and rest
    D. The person should make an appointment with his or her doctor

17. Which risk factor for stroke could be modified or controlled?
    A. Male gender
    B. Age over 55 years
    C. Family history for heart disease
    D. High cholesterol

18. When a person has right-sided "neglect" after a stroke, which action would you perform?
    A. Assist the person to wash the left side of the face
    B. Approach the person on the right side
    C. Perform range of motion exercises on the right side
    D. Point out food items on the left side of the plate

19. When you are caring for a person who has had a stroke, the call light
    A. Is positioned near the person's head
    B. Is placed on the weak side of the body
    C. Is placed on the strong side of the body
    D. Is given to a family member to use for the person

20. A safety concern for a person with Parkinson's disease would be
    A. Changes in speech
    B. Swallowing problems
    C. A mask-like expression
    D. Emotional changes

21. For a person with multiple sclerosis (MS), what is the main safety concern?
    A. Risk for falls
    B. Prone to infections
    C. Risk for aspiration
    D. Problems with breathing

22. As amyotrophic lateral sclerosis (ALS) progresses, the person is
    A. Confused and disoriented
    B. Able to walk with some assistance
    C. Incontinent of bladder and bowel functions
    D. Unable to move the arms, legs, and body

23. If a person is in a vegetative state after traumatic brain injury, you will
    A. Assist with meals by spoon feeding small portions
    B. Gently wake the person up and explain care
    C. Encourage the person to participate in self-care
    D. Perform total hygienic care for the person

24. A person who has paraplegia from a spinal cord injury, which action are you most likely to perform?
    A. Comb the person's hair
    B. Cut food into bite-sized pieces
    C. Lock the wheelchair prior to transfer
    D. Assist the person to button his shirt

25. Which person is most likely to require the application of elastic stockings to prevent thrombi?
    A. Person who had a stroke
    B. Person who has osteoarthritis
    C. Person who has a comminuted wrist fracture
    D. Person who has multiple sclerosis

26. Autonomic hyperreflexia occurs in a person who has
    A. Recent traumatic brain injury
    B. Paralysis above the mid-thoracic level
    C. Stroke caused by cerebral hemorrhage
    D. Advanced amyotrophic lateral sclerosis

27. If you are caring for a person with autonomic hyperreflexia, report to the nurse at once if
    A. The person reports a throbbing headache
    B. The blood pressure is low
    C. The person has pain below the level of the injury
    D. The person has the urge to urinate

28. If a person is at risk for autonomic hyperreflexia, it is best if only the nurse
    A. Gives basic hygienic and daily care
    B. Makes sure the catheter is draining properly
    C. Checks for fecal impactions or gives an enema
    D. Re-positions the person at least every 2 hours

29. In caring for a person with rheumatoid arthritis, which task would be part of your responsibility?
    A. Identifying exercise activities that have low risk for joint stress
    B. Applying heat or cold applications according to the care plan
    C. Teaching the person how to use a cane or a walker
    D. Telling the person to eat low calorie foods

30. When you are caring for a person with arthritis, which of these would be most helpful to the person?
    A. Encourage the person to stay in bed and to take frequent naps
    B. Keep the room cool and well ventilated at all times.
    C. Help the person to use good body mechanics and good posture
    D. Tell the person to talk to the doctor about joint replacement surgery

31. When caring for a person who has had a total hip replacement, which action would you perform?
    A. Have a soft plush chair for the person to sit on
    B. Perform full range of motion on the affected side
    C. Remind the person not to cross his or her legs
    D. Place a low commode chair close to the bed

32. Which person requires gentle handling because of an increased risk for fractures?
    A. Has an amputated limb
    B. Had traumatic brain injury
    C. Has osteoporosis
    D. Had a stroke

33. Which person is displaying a sign or symptom of a fracture?
    A. Has full range of motion in the affected limb
    B. Has bruising and color change in the affected area
    C. Has tremors and pill rolling movements in the area
    D. Has sudden weakness and numbness in the affected limb

34. When a closed reduction is done, the person is less likely to have problems with
    A. Infection   C. Dysfunction
    B. Pain   D. Swelling

35. When a person has a newly applied plaster cast, it will dry in
    A. 2 to 4 hours   C. 24 to 48 hours
    B. 3 to 4 days   D. 12 to 24 hours

36. You can prevent flat spots on a cast by
    A. Positioning the cast on a hard, flat surface
    B. Supporting the entire cast with pillows
    C. Grasping the edge of the cast with your fingertips
    D. Covering the cast with a blanket

37. If a person complains of numbness in a limb that has a cast, you should
    A. Move the limb to relieve the numbness
    B. Re-position the limb to decrease pressure
    C. Gently rub the exposed toes or fingers
    D. Tell the nurse at once

38. When giving care to a person in traction, you should
    A. Put bottom linens on the bed from the top down
    B. Remove the weights while you are giving care
    C. Turn the person from side to side to give care
    D. Assist the person to use the commode chair when needed

39. After surgery to repair a hip fracture, the operated leg should be
    A. Abducted at all times
    B. Adducted at all times
    C. Massaged every 4 hours
    D. Positioned to maintain external rotation

40. When you assist a person to get up in a chair after hip surgery
    A. Place the chair at the foot of the bed
    B. Place the chair on the unaffected side
    C. Have a low, soft comfortable chair for the person to use
    D. Encourage the person to briefly stand on the affected leg

41. If a person complains of pain in the amputated part
    A. Report this to the nurse at once
    B. Be calm; the person is probably confused
    C. Re-assure the person that this is a normal reaction
    D. Remind the person that body part is gone

Fill in the Blank

42. Write out the abbreviations.
    A. ADL _____
    B. ALS _____
    C. CVA _____
    D. JA _____
    E. MS _____
    F. RA _____
    G. ROM _____
    H. TBI _____
    I. TIA _____
    J. AD _____

43. List five warning signs of stroke.
    A. _____
    B. _____
    C. _____
    D. _____
    E. _____

44. Name four signs and symptoms of Parkinson's disease.
    A. _____
    B. _____
    C. _____
    D. _____

45. A person with Parkinson's disease will receive
    A. Drugs to control _____
    B. Exercise and physical therapy to help _____
    C. Therapy for speech and _____
    D. Safety measures to prevent _____

46. Multiple sclerosis (MS) may present in many ways.
    A. When symptoms disappear, the person is in

       _____.

    B. When symptoms flare up, the person is in a

       _____.

47. What effect does amyotrophic lateral sclerosis have on
    A. Mind, intelligence, memory _____
    B. Senses _____
    C. Bowel and bladder functions _____
    D. Nerve cells for voluntary movement _____

48. When traumatic brain injury occurs
    A. Brain tissue is _____
    B. Bleeding can be in the _____ or

       _____

    C. Spinal cord injuries are _____

49. _____ are the major cause of head injuries in newborns.

50. When caring for a person with paralysis, you must check the person often if he or she is unable to use

    _____.

51. Range-of-motion exercises are important when caring for a person with paralysis because they will maintain

    _____ and prevent

    _____.

52. A person with a spinal cord injury, reports blurred vision and a headache. You notice that the urinary catheter tube is kinked. You immediately notify the nurse because the person is having signs or symptoms of _____.

53. If you are caring for a person with arthritis, what are the benefits of these treatments?
    A. Drugs _____
    B. Heat _____
    C. Exercise _____
    D. Rest and joint care _____

54. How do these assistive devices help a person with arthritis?
    A. Canes and walkers _____
    B. Splints _____
    C. Adaptive and self-help devices _____

55. When caring for a person who had a hip replacement, what instructions are given to the person to protect the hip?
    A. Positioning legs _____
    B. To sit _____
    C. To bend _____
    D. To reach _____
    E. Toileting _____
    F. Sleeping _____

56. List six risk factors for developing osteoporosis.
    A. _____
    B. _____
    C. _____
    D. _____
    E. _____
    F. _____

57. Calcium is lost from bone if it does not _____. What happens to the bone when calcium is lost?

    _____

58. What joints are exercised to help prevent osteoporosis?
    _____

    What types of exercise are used for these joints?

    _____

59. When a person has cast on a fracture, what do these symptoms mean?
    A. Pain _____
    B. Odor _____
    C. Numbness _____
    D. Cool skin _____
    E. Hot skin _____

60. When caring for a person in traction, what would you do in these situations?
    A. Rope is frayed. _____
    B. Some joints should receive exercise. _____
    C. Person needs positioning. _____
    D. Redness, drainage, and odor are noted at the pin site. _____
    E. Person complains of numbness.

       _____

61. How should the fractured hip be supported in these situations?
    A. Prevent external rotation _____
    B. Keep leg abducted _____

62. When turning and positioning a person after hip surgery, usually the person is not positioned on

    _____.

63. If the person has an internal fixation device, the operative leg is not elevated when sitting in a chair because _____.

64. What disease is a common cause of vascular changes that can lead to an amputation? _____

65. Phantom pain after an amputation may occur for a _____ or for _____.

Optional Learning Exercises

You are caring for Mrs. Huber, who has had a stroke. The next 5 questions relate to Mrs. Huber and her care. The care plan gives the following instructions; explain the reason for these instructions.

66. Position Mrs. Huber in a side-lying position.

_____

67. Approach Mrs. Huber from the unaffected side.

_____

68. Mrs. Huber is given a dysphagia diet.

_____

69. Elastic stockings are applied as part of her care.

_____

70. Range-of-motion exercises are given.

_____

You are caring for 2 persons who have arthritis. Read the information about each of them and answer the 2 questions about these persons.

- *Mr. Miller is 78 years old. He worked in construction for many years, where he did heavy physical work. He complains about pain in his hips and right knee. His fingers are deformed by arthritis and interfere with good range of motion.*
- *Mrs. Haxton is 40 years old. She has swelling, warmth, and tenderness in her wrists, several finger joints on both hands, and both knees. She tells you that she has had arthritis for about 10 years and it "comes and goes." At present, Mrs. Haxton has a temperature of 100.2°F and she states she is tired and does not feel well.*

71. Which type of arthritis does Mr. Miller have? _____ His job may have caused _____.

72. Mrs. Haxton probably has _____ arthritis. She complains of not feeling well because the arthritis affects _____ as well as the joints.

Use the FOCUS ON PRIDE section to complete this statement and then use the critical thinking and discussion questions to develop your ideas.

73. List four ways to promote independence when caring for persons with neurologic or musculo-skeletal disorders.
    A. _____
    B. _____
    C. _____
    D. _____

Critical Thinking and Discussion Questions

74. You are assigned to care for a person who had a stroke. The nurse tells you that he has hemiplegia on the right-side and will need assistance with most ADLs during the day. He is alert and he appears to understand your explanations and instructions. After you finish helping him with morning hygiene, you ensure that the call bell is within reach and the side rails are in place according to the care plan. You complete a safety check of the room before leaving. Thirty minutes later, you come back to check on him and he is attempting to climb over the side rails. You successfully help him get repositioned in the bed.
    A. What do you think caused the person to try and climb over the siderails?
    B. Why would you report this incident to the nurse?

Fill in the Blank: Key Terms

Apnea   Congenital   Hypertension   Pneumonia
Arrhythmia   Dysrhythmia   Lymphedema   Sleep apnea

1. An inflammation and infection of lung tissue is
   _____.

2. An abnormal heart rhythm is _____.

3. Pauses in breathing that occur during sleep is
   _____.

4. The lack or absence of breathing is _____.

5. _____ means to be born
   with a condition.

6. _____ is another name
   for dysrhythmia.

7. A buildup of lymph in the tissues causing edema is
   _____.

8. Another name for hypertension is
   _____.

Circle the Best Answer

9. When you see a large amount of bright red blood
   around a surgical wound site, you immediately the
   notify nurse because bright red blood signals bleeding
   from
   A. A capillary   C. An artery
   B. A vein   D. A venule

10. Which component of the blood picks up oxygen and
    releases carbon dioxide?
    A. Plasma   C. Platelets
    B. Hemoglobin   D. White blood cells

11. If you are caring for an infant who has a congenital
    heart defect, what might you observe about the
    infant's skin?
    A. Face and upper body are red
    B. Skin is dry and flaky
    C. Skin has a yellowish tint
    D. Lips and skin have a bluish tint

12. Which breakfast item could potentially contribute to
    plaque formation and atherosclerosis?
    A. Coffee   C. Oatmeal
    B. Orange juice   D. Bacon

13. Hypertension (high blood pressure) would be a
    reading of
    A. 120/70   C. 140/90
    B. 100/60   D. 130/60

14. A risk factor for hypertension that cannot be modified
    or changed is
    A. Stress   C. Age
    B. Being over-weight   D. Lack of exercise

15. The most common cause of coronary artery disease is
    A. Lack of exercise   C. Family history
    B. Atherosclerosis   D. Stress

16. For a person who needs cardiac rehabilitation, which
    action is part of your responsibilities?
    A. Develop an exercise training program for the
       person
    B. Teach the person about the heart condition
    C. Ensure the person maintains strict bedrest
    D. Help the person select foods from a heart healthy
       menu

17. If a person has angina pain, it will usually be
    relieved by
    A. Resting for 3 to 15 minutes
    B. Taking an aspirin or pain reliever
    C. Using oxygen therapy
    D. Getting up and walking for exercise

18. If a person takes a nitroglycerin tablet for angina, you
    should
    A. Give them a large glass of water to swallow the
       pill
    B. Take the pills back to the nurses' station
    C. Make sure the nurse is told a pill was taken
    D. Encourage the person to walk around the room

19. A person is admitted to the long-term care facility
    and has a high risk for myocardial infarction. Which
    equipment is the nurse most likely to ask you to
    obtain?
    A. Oxygen tank and nasal cannula
    B. Continuous positive airway pressure (CPAP)
       device
    C. Cart with items for airborne precautions
    D. Elastic compression stockings

20. If a person complains of pain or numbness in the
    back, neck, jaw, or stomach, you should tell the nurse
    at once because the person
    A. Is having an angina attack
    B. May be having a stroke
    C. May be having a myocardial infarction
    D. Has symptoms of chronic obstructive pulmonary
       disease

21. When pulmonary edema secondary to heart failure occurs, what are you most likely to observe?
    A. Dyspnea, cough, pink sputum, and gurgling sounds
    B. Irregular pulse and a low blood pressure
    C. Hot, red, dry skin with chills and fever
    D. Sneezing, coughing, and stuffy or runny nose

22. An older person with heart failure is at risk for
    A. Contractures
    B. Skin breakdown
    C. Fractures
    D. Urinary tract infections

23. In a home setting, you are assigned to care for a person who has a pacemaker. Which task will you perform related to the pacemaker?
    A. Test the battery function and change it as needed
    B. Check the lead wires to make sure they are intact and not frayed or kinked
    C. Assist the person to check the function of the pacemaker via phone or internet
    D. Clean the pacemaker according to the manufacturer's instructions

24. The most important risk factor for chronic obstructive pulmonary disease (COPD) is
    A. Family history
    B. Respiratory infections
    C. Cigarette smoking
    D. Exercise

25. When a person has COPD, it interferes with
    A. Oxygen (O_2) and carbon dioxide (CO_2) exchange in the lungs
    B. Blood flow to the heart
    C. The function of the kidneys and bladder
    D. Heart rhythm and the strength of the contractions

26. If a person has chronic bronchitis, a common symptom is
    A. Wheezing and tightening in the chest
    B. Shortness of breath on exertion
    C. A smoker's cough that produces a lot of mucus
    D. A high temperature for several days

27. In caring for a person with asthma, what information do you need to get from the nurse and the care plan?
    A. What the person is allergic to
    B. The setting for the oxygen level
    C. The amount of fluid allowed
    D. How often to reposition the person

28. For a person who has sleep apnea, which action will you perform?
    A. Wake the person every time you hear loud snoring or gasping
    B. Position the person in a high-Fowler's position for sleep and rest
    C. Check to see if the continuous positive airway pressure device is working
    D. Encourage the person to taking several naps during the day

29. If an older person has influenza, he or she may
    A. Have a body temperature below normal
    B. Have chest pain and a hacking cough
    C. Feel very thirsty and hungry
    D. Have no symptoms of illness

30. Which of these symptoms is more likely to be from a cold rather than the flu?
    A. Stuffy nose
    B. High fever (100°F to 102°F)
    C. Fatigue for 2 to 3 weeks
    D. Bronchitis or pneumonia

31. Which person needs Standard Precautions and airborne precautions?
    A. Person has emphysema and is unwilling to stop smoking
    B. Person is admitted for asthma, probably allergy induced
    C. Person was recently diagnosed with tuberculosis
    D. Person has chronic bronchitis

32. When a person has pneumonia, fluid intake is increased to
    A. Decrease the amount of bacteria in the lungs
    B. Dilute medication given to treat the disease
    C. Thin secretions and help reduce fever
    D. Decrease inflammation of the breathing passages

33. Breathing is easier for a person with pneumonia when the person is positioned in
    A. Semi-Fowler's position
    B. Side-lying position
    C. Supine position
    D. A soft chair

34. When a person has lymphedema, it is important that you
    A. Never use an affected arm to take a blood pressure
    B. Keep the affected arm or leg elevated at all times
    C. Keep the person on strict bedrest
    D. Restrict fluid intake

Fill in the Blank

35. Write out the abbreviations.
    A. CAD _____
    B. CDC _____
    C. CHF _____
    D. CO_2 _____
    E. COPD _____
    F. IV _____
    G. MI _____
    H. mm Hg _____
    I. O_2 _____
    J. RBC _____
    K. TB _____
    L. WBC _____

36. Name four risk factors for hypertension that cannot be changed.
    A. _____
    B. _____
    C. _____
    D. _____

37. The most common cause of coronary artery disease (CAD) is _____. When this occurs, _____ collects on the _____.

38. When a person has CAD, list four life-style changes that are needed.
    A. _____
    B. _____
    C. _____
    D. _____

39. Identify six activities or other factors that can cause angina.
    A. _____
    B. _____
    C. _____
    D. _____
    E. _____
    F. _____

40. Where are nitroglycerin tablets kept?
    _____

41. List five descriptions of chest pain that indicate myocardial infarction.
    A. _____
    B. _____
    C. _____
    D. _____
    E. _____

42. List three goals of cardiac rehabilitation after a myocardial infarction.
    A. _____
    B. _____
    C. _____

43. Older persons with heart failure are at risk for skin breakdown because of
    A. _____
    B. _____
    C. _____

44. How can you help to prevent skin breakdown in older persons with heart failure?
    _____

45. Dysrhythmias are caused by changes in the heart's
    _____.

46. Name four changes that occur in the lungs when a person has chronic obstructive pulmonary disease (COPD).
    A. _____
    B. _____
    C. _____
    D. _____

47. If a person has bronchitis or emphysema, the person must stop _____.

48. List nine signs and symptoms of sleep apnea.
    A. _____
    B. _____
    C. _____
    D. _____
    E. _____
    F. _____
    G. _____
    H. _____
    I. _____

49. A common complication of influenza is
    _____.

50. List nine signs and symptoms that may be present if a person has active tuberculosis (TB).
    A. _____
    B. _____
    C. _____
    D. _____
    E. _____
    F. _____
    G. _____
    H. _____
    I. _____

51. Why does TB sometimes become active as a person ages? _____

52. List four treatment goals for lymphedema.
    A. _____
    B. _____
    C. _____
    D. _____

53. Lymphoma is cancer involving cells in the
    _____.

Matching
Match the symptom listed with disorders of coronary artery disease.

A. Angina
B. Myocardial infarction
C. Heart failure

54. _____ Chest pain occurs with exertion.

55. _____ Blood flow to the heart is suddenly blocked.

56. _____ Blood backs up into the venous system.

57. _____ Fluid in the lungs.

58. _____ Rest and nitroglycerin often relieves the symptoms.

59. _____ Breaks out in a cold sweat.

Match the respiratory disorder with the related symptom.

A. Chronic bronchitis

B. Emphysema

C. Asthma

60. _____ Person develops a barrel chest.

61. _____ Mucus and inflamed breathing passages obstruct airflow.

62. _____ Alveoli become less elastic.

63. _____ Sudden attacks can be mild or severe.

64. _____ The most common symptom is often a smoker's cough

65. _____ Normal O_2 and CO_2 exchange cannot occur in affected alveoli.

66. _____ Allergies and air pollutants are common causes.

Optional Learning Exercises

67. A parent with a congenital heart defect is at risk for having a child with one. What are other risk factors that may cause a congenital heart defect?

A. _____

B. _____

C. _____

D. _____

E. _____

68. Older persons may not have typical symptoms of flu. List five symptoms that signal flu in an older person.

A. _____

B. _____

C. _____

D. _____

E. _____

Use the FOCUS ON PRIDE section to complete these statements and then use the critical thinking and discussion question to develop your ideas.

69. When a person makes unhealthy choices, such as smoking, the health team

A. Teaches the person the _____ and encourages _____

B. Cannot force _____

C. Must be sure the person understands the

_____

70. Color-coded wristbands communicate _____ or _____.

71. If a color-coded bracelet says "limb alert" or "forbidden extremity," it means that an arm must not be used for

A. _____

B. _____

C. _____

Critical Thinking and Discussion Questions

72. In the table below, check all of the factors that apply to you. In the section of "factors you can change," select two or three that apply to you and answer the following questions.

A. I'd like to change factor _____,
   because_____

B. Three things that I could do to begin to change
   factor_____ include
   a. _____
   b. _____
   c. _____

C. Three things that I could do to begin to change
   factor_____ include
   a. _____
   b. _____
   c. _____

D. Three things that I could do to begin to change
   factor_____ include
   a. _____
   b. _____
   c. _____

	Cardiovascular Disorders—Risk Factors
	Factors You *Cannot* Change
	• Age—45 years or older for men; 55 years or older for women
	• Biological sex—risk increases for women after menopause; having diabetes increases the risk more in women than in men
	• Race—African-Americans are at greater risk
	• Family history—tends to run in families
	Factors You *Can* Change
	• Being over-weight
	• Stress
	• Smoking and tobacco use
	• Poor diet—high in fat, salt, sugar, and cholesterol
	• Excessive alcohol
	• Lack of exercise
	• Not getting enough sleep
	• High blood pressure
	• Unhealthy blood cholesterol levels
	• Diabetes

Fill in the Blank: Key Terms

Acid reflux	Heartburn	Hypoglycemia	Vomitus
Emesis	Hyperglycemia	Jaundice	

1. High sugar in the blood is

   _____.

2. _____ is food and/or fluids that are expelled from the stomach through the mouth.

3. Low sugar in the blood is

   _____.

4. Another word for vomitus is

   _____.

5. _____ is yellowish color of the skin or whites of the eyes.

6. A burning sensation in the chest and sometimes the throat is _____.

7. Another term for heartburn is _____.

Circle the Best Answer

8. You are caring a resident who has gastro-esophageal reflux disease (GERD). Which request from the resident should be reported to the nurse?
   A. Resident wants to frequently eat a small snack
   B. Resident wants to sit in the dayroom after lunch
   C. Resident wants to wear loose elastic-waist pants
   D. Resident wants fried chicken and french fries for dinner

9. Aspirated vomitus
   A. Can lead to shock
   B. Can obstruct an airway
   C. Contains blood
   D. Causes a hiatal hernia

10. If vomitus looks like coffee grounds, you should report at once to the nurse because
    A. There could be bleeding in the gastrointestinal tract
    B. The person may need a change in diet
    C. This indicates an infection in the stomach
    D. The person may have swallowed a foreign object

11. A person with diverticular disease had surgery for the diseased portion of the bowel. Which procedure checklist are you most likely to follow in the care of this person?
    A. Checking for and removing a fecal impaction
    B. Giving a small volume enema
    C. Assisting the person to empty an ostomy pouch
    D. Emptying a urinary drainage bag

12. In the care of a person with ulcerative colitis, you plan to spend extra time with which task?
    A. Frequently measuring emesis and cleaning the kidney basin
    B. Helping the person to clean up after frequent diarrheal episodes
    C. Reminding the person not to lie down after eating or drinking
    D. Donning and doffing personal protective equipment for isolation precautions

13. Which activity is most likely to precede a "gallbladder attack"?
    A. Eating a meal   C. Lying down
    B. Overexertion   D. Smoking

14. Which lifestyle modification is part of the treatment for hepatitis?
    A. Increasing exercise
    B. Smoking cessation
    C. Abstaining from alcohol
    D. Eating a high protein diet

15. A person with cirrhosis needs good skin care because of symptoms caused by the disease process. What care measure will you use?
    A. Cleanse with cold water
    B. Apply lotion
    C. Report sweating
    D. Check for incontinence

16. Which person needs to be assisted to ambulate for exercise as part of the treatment for diabetes?
    A. A 17-year-old adolescent has just taken insulin for type 1 diabetes
    B. An obese 50-year-old woman with hypertension has type 2 diabetes
    C. A 26-year-old woman is pregnant and has gestational diabetes
    D. An underweight 45-year-old woman with dizziness has type 2 diabetes

17. A person with diabetes has thirst, frequent urination, a flushed face and rapid, deep, and labored respirations. Which action is the most important?
    A. Provide plenty of clear fluids
    B. Assist the person to the bathroom
    C. Count the respiratory rate
    D. Report your observations to the nurse

Fill in the Blank

18. Write out the meaning of the abbreviations.
    A. BMs _____
    B. GERD _____
    C. GI _____
    D. IBD _____
    E. I&O _____

19. What life-style changes may be needed for a person with GERD?
    A. _____
    B. _____
    C. _____
    D. _____
    E. _____

20. What measures will help the person who is vomiting?
    A. Turn _____.
    B. Place _____.
    C. Move _____.
    D. Provide _____.
    E. Eliminate _____.

21. Risk factors related to diverticular disease are
    A. Diet _____
    B. Weight _____

22. A gallbladder attack often occurs suddenly after
    _____.

23. List the characteristics of the types of hepatitis.
    A. Hepatitis A is spread by the
       _____ route.
    B. Hepatitis B is present in the
       _____ of infected persons.
    C. Hepatitis C can be transmitted in ways similar to
       hepatitis _____.
    D. Hepatitis D is spread by having sex with someone
       who has _____.
    E. Hepatitis E can occur by eating undercooked
       _____.

24. Signs and symptoms of cirrhosis that may occur are
    A. _____
    B. _____
    C. _____
    D. _____
    E. _____
    F. _____
    G. _____
    H. _____
    I. _____

25. A person with _____
    diabetes can be treated with healthy eating, exercise,
    and sometimes oral drugs.

26. A person with _____
    diabetes will be treated with daily insulin therapy as
    well as healthy diet and exercise.

Matching

Match the type of hepatitis with the cause.

A. Hepatitis A
B. Hepatitis B
C. Hepatitis C
D. Hepatitis D
E. Hepatitis E

27. _____ Born to a mother who has hepatitis B
28. _____ Received blood clotting factor before 1987
29. _____ Had unprotected sex with someone who has hepatitis D
30. _____ Oral contact with infected person's feces
31. _____ Drinking contaminated water; more common in Africa, Asia, or Central America

Match the symptom with either hypoglycemia or hyperglycemia.

A. Hypoglycemia
B. Hyperglycemia

32. _____ Trembling, shakiness
33. _____ Sweet breath odor
34. _____ Tingling around the mouth
35. _____ Cold, clammy skin
36. _____ Rapid, deep, and labored respirations
37. _____ Leg cramps
38. _____ Flushed face
39. _____ Frequent urination

Optional Learning Exercises

You are caring for several persons with diabetes. Answer these questions about these persons.

Mr. Jones, a 75-year-old African-American man
Ms. Miller, a 45-year-old white, over-weight woman
Mrs. Thorpe, a 32-year-old pregnant woman
Ms. Hernandez, a 60-year-old Hispanic woman with hypertension
Emily F., a 12-year-old girl who has lost 15 pounds recently without dieting

40. Three of these persons are most likely to have type 2 diabetes. They are
    A. _____
    B. _____
    C. _____

41. The 32-year-old probably has _____
    diabetes. She is at risk for developing
    _____ later in life.

42. The 12-year-old probably has
    _____ diabetes.

43. Which type of diabetes develops rapidly?
    _____

44. Mrs. Hernandez has an open wound on her ankle. Why is this wound a concern?

    _____

45. Why is Ms. Miller instructed to decrease her food intake? _____

46. Mr. Jones tells you he feels shaky, dizzy, and has a headache when he misses a meal. He probably is experiencing

    _____.

47. Why does Emily F. take a snack with her when she goes to school? _____

    _____

Use the FOCUS ON PRIDE section to complete these statements and then use the critical thinking and discussion question to develop your ideas.

48. Understanding health problems allows you to safely

    _____.

49. Health care workers are at risk for exposure to the hepatitis B virus through _____,

    _____, and

    _____.

Critical Thinking and Discussion Question

50. Health care workers are at risk for hepatitis. In addition to getting the vaccine for hepatitis B, what can you do to protect yourself and others from getting hepatitis?

Fill in the Blank: Key Terms

Dialysis	Hematuria	Pyuria	Urostomy
Dysuria	Oliguria	Urinary diversion	

1. Scant urine is _____.

2. Difficult or painful urination is _____.

3. _____ is a surgically created opening that connects to the urinary tract.

4. The process of removing waste products from the blood is _____.

5. A surgically created pathway for urine to leave the body is a _____.

6. Blood in the urine is _____.

7. _____ is pus in the urine.

Circle the Best Answer

8. Which task is your responsibility in the prevention of urinary tract infections (UTIs) among elderly residents in a long-term care center?
   A. Administer antibiotics as prescribed for UTIs
   B. Use sterile technique to insert indwelling catheters
   C. Give drinking water to those who are not on fluid restrictions
   D. Ensure that equipment for urologic examinations is sterile

9. Women have a higher risk for urinary tract infections because
   A. Female hormones affect immunity
   B. The urethra is shorter in the female
   C. The vagina harbors bacteria
   D. Menstrual blood is contaminated

10. If a person has a UTI, the care plan will include
    A. Restricting fluid intake
    B. Assisting with frequent ambulation
    C. Straining the urine
    D. Assisting with proper perineal care

11. If a man has prostate enlargement, he will probably
    A. Have a urinary diversion
    B. Have frequent voiding at night
    C. Have severe back pain
    D. Have chronic renal failure

12. After surgery to correct benign prostatic hyperplasia (BPH), the care plan may include
    A. A balanced diet to prevent constipation
    B. Increased activity with an exercise plan
    C. Restricted fluid intake
    D. Care of the surgical incision

13. When caring for a person with a urinary diversion, the pouch is changed
    A. Every shift
    B. Every 3 to 4 hours
    C. After showers or bathing
    D. Every 5 to 7 days or if it leaks

14. If you are caring for a person with kidney stones, your care will include
    A. Restricting fluids
    B. Maintaining strict bedrest
    C. Straining all urine
    D. Maintaining a strict diet

15. When you care for a person with acute renal failure, the care plan will include
    A. Increasing fluid intake to 2000 to 3000 mL per day
    B. Measuring and recording urine output
    C. Making sure the person does not drink any fluids
    D. Measuring weight every week

16. Which food item causes you to check with the nurse before giving the meal tray to a person with chronic renal failure?
    A. Beef steak
    B. Green beans
    C. Whole wheat roll
    D. Tomato slices

17. If a person has chronic renal failure, which of these would be included in the care plan?
    A. Frequently check the linens for moisture
    B. Daily routine of moderate aerobic exercise
    C. Measures to prevent itching
    D. Frequent bathing with soap

18. During perineal care, you notice a gray vaginal discharge and with an odor. The woman reports itching and painful urination. Which care measure is the most important?
    A. Make sure she has clean underwear
    B. Assist her with a sitz bath
    C. Obtain clean perineal pads for her
    D. Inform the nurse about your observations

Fill in the Blank

19. Write out the meaning of the abbreviations.
    A. BPH _____
    B. CKD _____
    C. mL _____
    D. STD _____
    E. STI _____
    F. TURP _____
    G. UTI _____
    H. AIDS _____
    I. HIV _____
    J. HPV _____

20. After a transurethral resection of the prostate (TURP), the person's care plan may include
    A. _____
    B. _____
    C. _____
    D. _____
    E. _____
21. A person with kidney stones needs to drink 2000 to 3000 mL of fluid a day to help _____.
22. When acute renal failure occurs, the onset is _____ in a few days or less.
23. Acute renal failure may be _____; whereas chronic renal failure has no cure.
24. You may need to assist a person in chronic renal failure with nutritional needs. List what the care plan is likely to include for the following:
    A. Diet _____
    B. Fluids _____
25. Sexually transmitted diseases are transmitted by
    _____.
26. Using _____ prevents the spread of STDs.
27. When caring for a person with an STD, you should follow _____ and _____.

Matching

Match the sexually transmitted disease with the disease characteristics. Use Box 51-4 (p 768) to complete the matching.
A. Herpes
B. Low-risk HPV
C. Gonorrhea
D. Chlamydia
E. Syphilis
F. Trichomoniasis
G. HIV/AIDS
H. High-risk HPV

28. _____ Virus stays in the body for life; repeated outbreaks are common
29. _____ Causes genital warts
30. _____ Yellow-green or gray vaginal discharge
31. _____ Can cause various cancers
32. _____ Men have pain on urination and a penile discharge
33. _____ White blood cells are destroyed
34. _____ Painless sores develop first on genitals
35. _____ Occurs in cervix, rectum or throat in women; urethra, rectum or throat in men

Optional Learning Exercises

You give home care to Mrs. Eunice Weber twice a week. She is 92 years old and lives alone. She has severe osteoporosis and uses a walker to move about in her home. She receives Meals on Wheels and spends most of the day sitting on the sofa. She has periods of incontinence or dribbling because of poor bladder control. When you arrive to care for her today, she tells you she is not feeling well. She tells you it burns when she urinates. When she needs to urinate, the urge comes on suddenly and she often does not get to the toilet in time. Answer these questions about Mrs. Weber.

36. You should tell the _____ because these symptoms may mean Mrs. Weber has _____.
37. When the feeling to urinate comes on suddenly, it is called _____.
38. How does Mrs. Weber's immobility affect the following?
    A. Fluid intake _____ _____
    B. Perineal care _____ _____
39. Why does gender increase Mrs. Weber's risk for urinary tract infections? _____
40. The doctor will probably order _____ to treat the condition.
41. The care plan will probably include "Encourage fluids to _____ per day."

Two weeks later you notice that Mrs. Weber has chills. When you take her temperature, it is 102°F. She tells you she has been vomiting since yesterday. You observe her urine and see that it is very cloudy.

42. You report these symptoms to the nurse, because it can indicate Mrs. Weber now has _____. This means the infection has moved from the _____ to the _____.

Use the FOCUS ON PRIDE section to complete these statements.

43. Proper _____ care can prevent UTIs.
44. When a person has a urinary or reproductive disorder, you protect the person's rights and give respect when you give information only to _____.

Critical Thinking and Discussion Question

45. Poor fluid intake, healthcare-associated infections related to urinary catheters and poor hygiene are mentioned as causes of urinary tract infections. Based on previous chapters that you have studied, what skills and knowledge can you use in the prevention of urinary tract infections?

52   Mental Health Disorders

Fill in the Blank: Key Terms

Addiction
Alcoholism
Anxiety
Compulsion
Defense mechanism
Delusion

Delusion of grandeur
Delusion of
   persecution
Detoxification
Drug addiction
Flashback

Hallucination
Mental health
Mental health
   disorder
Mental illness
Obsession

Panic
Personality
Phobia
Psychiatric disorder
Psychosis
Stress

Stressor
Suicide
Suicide contagion
Withdrawal syndrome

1. A feeling of worry, nervousness, or fear about an event or situation is _____.

2. Alcohol dependence that involves craving, loss of control, physical dependence, and tolerance is

   _____.

3. When a person has an exaggerated belief about one's own importance, wealth, power, or talents, it is called

   _____.

4. A _____ is a serious illnesses that can affect a person's thinking, mood, behavior, function, and ability to relate to others; mental illness, psychiatric disorder

5. A _____ is an event or factor that causes stress.

6. _____ is the strong urge or craving to use the substance and cannot stop using; tolerance develops.

7. A frequent, upsetting and unwanted thought, idea, or an image is an _____.

8. The response or change in the body caused by any emotional, psychological, physical, social, or economic factor is _____.

9. A _____ is an intense fear of something that has little or no real danger.

10. A false belief is a _____.

11. Mental _____ is another name for a mental health disorder.

12. A state of severe mental impairment is _____.

13. A _____ is seeing, hearing, feeling or tasting things that are not real.

14. An overwhelming urge to repeat certain rituals, acts or behaviors is a _____.

15. _____ involves a person's emotional, psychological, and social well-being.

16. The set of attitudes, values, behaviors, and traits of a person is _____.

17. _____ is a false belief that one is being mistreated, abused, or harassed.

18. An intense and sudden feeling of fear, anxiety, or dread is _____.

19. _____ is another name for mental health disorder, or mental illness.

20. A _____ is an unconscious reaction that blocks unpleasant or threatening feelings.

21. _____ occurs with exposure to suicide or suicidal behaviors within one's family, or peer group, or media reports of suicide.

22. Reliving the trauma in thoughts during the day and in nightmares during sleep is _____.

23. The physical and mental response after stopping or severely reducing the use of a substance that was used regularly is _____.

24. The process of removing a toxic substance from the body is _____.

25. To end one's life on purpose is called _____.

26. _____ is a chronic disease involving substance seeking behaviors and use that is compulsive and hard to control despite the harmful effects

Circle the Best Answer

27. Which person is displaying an early warning sign of a mental health disorder?
    A. Teenager likes to sleep in late on the weekends
    B. College student feels anxious about finding a job
    C. Middle-aged adult likes to have a drink with friends after work
    D. Older adult pulls away from friends and usual activities

28. Which person has a risk factor for mental health disorders that is modifiable?
    A. Person's father and grandfather had bipolar disorder
    B. Person sustained a traumatic brain injury during childhood
    C. Person drinks alcohol and smokes marijuana
    D. Person has cancer that is not responding to chemotherapy

29. For which circumstance would anxiety be considered a normal and helpful reaction to stress?
    A. Person can't sleep because work deadlines are looming
    B. Student needs to study for a final examination

C. Building is on fire and the person can't find the exit
D. Child refuses to go to school because of bullying

30. An unhealthy coping mechanism would be
A. Talking about the problem
B. Playing music
C. Over-eating
D. Exercising

31. A student fails a test and blames a friend for not being a better study partner. Which defense mechanism is the student using?
A. Conversion
B. Projection
C. Repression
D. Displacement

32. When a person has a panic attack, you
A. Know that the person cannot function
B. Ask the person what you can do to help
C. Tell the person to listen to you, not the voices
D. Call for help and don't let the person leave

33. When a person washes his or her hands over and over, it may be a sign of
A. Schizophrenia
B. Hallucinations
C. Anorexia nervosa
D. Obsessive-compulsive disorder

34. A young child who was abused has post-traumatic stress disorder. Which sign/symptom would the child display?
A. Does many tasks at once without getting tired
B. Sits for hours without moving or responding
C. Hears the abuser's voice and answers
D. Acts out the traumatic event during play

35. A person you are caring for tells you he is the president of the United States. Which psychotic feature is he displaying?
A. Disorganized speech
B. Delusion of persecution
C. Hallucination
D. Delusion of grandeur

36. A person in the manic phase of bipolar disorder may be at risk for
A. Immobility
B. Constipation
C. Pressure injuries
D. Exhaustion

37. A safety risk of depression is that the person
A. May be very sad
B. Has thoughts of suicide and death
C. Has depressed body functions
D. Cannot concentrate

38. Depression may be overlooked in older persons because it may be mistaken for a
A. Reproductive disorder
B. Cardiac disorder
C. Cognitive disorder
D. Respiratory disorder

39. A person with an antisocial personality may
A. Be suspicious and distrust others
B. Have emotional highs and lows
C. See, hear, or feel something that is not real
D. Have no regard for the safety of others

40. Among teenagers, which substance is most commonly abused?
A. Stimulants
B. Hallucinogens
C. Marijuana
D. Alcohol

41. When alcohol is ingested, it will
A. Stimulate alertness and agitation
B. Cause drowsiness and reduce anxiety
C. Cause hallucinations and delusions
D. Stimulate hyperactivity and anger

42. Older persons have more risks for injury when drinking alcohol because they
A. Have slower reaction times
B. Have more experience with alcohol
C. Have memory loss
D. Have problems concentrating

43. When a person uses drugs over a period of time, a sign of addiction is
A. Using two or three substances once or twice a month
B. Taking larger amounts of the substance to get the same effect
C. Using the substance occasionally in a social setting
D. Taking the substance if a friend says the experience is safe

44. When a young woman eats large amounts of food and then purges the body, she has
A. Anorexia nervosa
B. Binge-eating disorder
C. Substance abuse disorder
D. Bulimia nervosa

45. If a person mentions suicide, you
A. Watch for psychosis
B. Take the person seriously
C. Change the topic of conversation
D. Disregard the attention-seeking behavior

Fill in the Blank

46. Write out the meaning of the abbreviations.
A. BPD _____
B. CDC _____
C. GAD _____
D. OCD _____
E. PTSD _____
F. AIDS _____
G. HIV _____

47. List eight risk factors for mental health disorders.
A. _____
B. _____
C. _____
D. _____
E. _____
F. _____
G. _____
H. _____

48. Name the defense mechanism being used in these situations.
    A. After a heart attack a man continues to smoke.
    _____

    B. A man does not like his boss. He buys the boss an expensive Christmas present. _____
    _____

    C. A girl complains of a stomach-ache so she will not have to read aloud at school. _____
    D. A child is angry with his teacher. He hits his brother.
    _____

    E. A woman misses work frequently and is often late. She gets a bad evaluation. She says that the boss does not like her. _____
    _____

49. Identify the phobia in each example.
    A. _____ Being afraid of strangers
    B. _____ Fear of pain or seeing others in pain
    C. _____ Being trapped in an enclosed area
    D. _____ Fear of darkness

50. During a _____, the person may lose touch with reality and believe the trauma is happening all over again. This occurs when the person has _____.

51. Below are examples of problems that occur with schizophrenia. Identify each one.
    A. A woman says that voices told her to set fire to her apartment. _____
    B. A man believes that others can hear his thoughts on the radio. _____
    C. A woman tells you she owns three mansions and is the governor of California. _____

Optional Learning Exercises

52. Mr. Johnson is very worried about his surgery tomorrow. You notice that he is talking very fast and sweating. You give him directions to collect a urine specimen. Five minutes later, he turns on his call light to ask you to repeat the directions. He tells you he is using the toilet "all the time" because he has diarrhea and frequent urination. The nurse tells you all of these things are signs and symptoms of _____.

53. You are assigned to care for Mrs. Grand, a new resident. She is getting ready to go to the dining room. You assist her to get dressed and she tells you she wants to wash her hands before going to the dining room. She goes to the bathroom and washes her hands for several minutes. As she leaves the room, she stops to turn off the light. Then she tells you she must wash her hands again. She repeats washing her hands and turning the lights on and off 4 or 5 times. You report this to the nurse, who tells you Mrs. Grand has _____.

Use the FOCUS ON PRIDE section to complete these statements and then use the critical thinking and discussion questions to develop your ideas.

54. When caring for a person with mental illness, the team must react quickly to_____.

55. When caring for a person with a mental illness, you can take pride in working as a team when you_____ when a team member calls for help.

Critical Thinking and Discussion Question

56. When you first begin to care for persons who have mental health disorders, you may feel a little anxious. How can you use this "normal" feeling of anxiety to improve your abilities and skills to care for people with mental health disorders?

53 Confusion and Dementia

Fill in the Blank: Key Terms

Cognitive function   Delirium   Dementia   Hallucination   Sundowning
Confusion   Delusion   Elopement   Paranoia

1. _____ occurs when a person leaves the agency without staff knowledge.

2. A false belief is a _____.

3. Seeing, hearing, smelling, or feeling something that is not real is a _____.

4. Increased signs, symptoms, and behavior of AD during hours of darkness is _____.

5. _____ is a state of sudden, severe confusion and rapid changes in brain function.

6. The loss of cognitive function that interferes with daily life and activities is _____.

7. _____ is a mental state of being disoriented to person, place, situation, or identity.

8. _____ involves memory, thinking, reasoning, ability to understand, judgment, and behavior.

9. _____ is a disorder of the mind; the person has false beliefs and suspicions about a person or situation.

Circle the Best Answer

10. Which activity has safety implications related to changes in the nervous system that occur with aging?
    A. Driving a car
    B. Talking with friends
    C. Attending a party
    D. Petting a dog

11. Which sign/symptom would be considered a normal nervous system change related to aging?
    A. Inability to walk
    B. Depression
    C. Loss of appetite
    D. Change of sleep pattern

12. What is the primary difference between dementia and delirium?
    A. Rapidity of onset
    B. Level of confusion
    C. Ability to make judgments
    D. Degree of memory loss

13. When a person is confused, it is helpful if you
    A. Repeat the date and time as often as necessary
    B. Change the routine each day to stimulate the person
    C. Keep the drapes pulled during the day
    D. Avoid talking too much to the person

14. Vision and hearing decrease with confusion, so you should
    A. Speak in a loud voice
    B. Write out directions to the person
    C. Face the person and speak clearly
    D. Stand by a window, so the person can see you

15. Dementia can be treated if it is caused by
    A. Abnormal protein deposits
    B. Vitamin deficiency
    C. Stroke
    D. Alzheimer's disease

16. Which reminder are you most likely to give to a person who has a mild cognitive disorder?
    A. To put on his underpants before he puts on his trousers
    B. To put toothpaste on the toothbrush before brushing
    C. To call his daughter about a scheduled appointment
    D. To ask for a snack if he is hungry in between meals

17. The most common type of permanent dementia in older persons is
    A. Alzheimer's disease
    B. Dementia
    C. Depression
    D. Delirium

18. People with dementia can have signs and symptoms that are similar to
    A. Depression
    B. Schizophrenia
    C. Heart disease
    D. Diabetes

19. Which behavior is an example of the most common early symptom of Alzheimer's disease (AD)?
    A. Person gets very upset and yells at you when you put his shoes in the closet
    B. Person can't remember the instructions that you just gave him about the call bell
    C. Person is lethargic, difficult to arouse, and you can't understand his garbled speech
    D. Person becomes confused and agitated in the early evening just before sunset.

20. You are caring for a person with mild AD; which action will you use?
    A. Coach step-by-step for donning and buttoning shirt
    B. Perform perineal care for incontinence of bowel and bladder
    C. Allow more time to complete daily tasks, such as showering
    D. Introduce friends and family by name every time they visit

21. You are caring for a person with moderate AD, which action will you use?
    A. Help person to locate a personal item that he misplaced
    B. Consistently use the same routine with morning hygiene
    C. Reassure person that family is handling his finances
    D. Monitor for seizure activity and report findings to the nurse

22. You are caring for a person with severe AD, which action will you use?
    A. Wait patiently if he has trouble organizing his thoughts
    B. Tell him to focus on your voice when he has auditory hallucinations
    C. Be kind and matter of fact when he directs profanity towards you
    D. Explain what you are doing even though he can't communicate

23. A person with Alzheimer's needs home care. A sign on the inside of the front door of the home says, "STOP." You know that you must use care measures that address
    A. Catastrophic reactions
    B. Wandering
    C. Paranoia
    D. Sundowning

24. When a person with AD has symptoms of sundowning, which measure could you try to reduce the agitation?
    A. Offer fluids and a snack
    B. Tell the person to calm down
    C. Have the person join a social group
    D. Put the person in quiet dark room

25. When you assist a person with AD to wear prescribed glasses or hearing aids, it helps to prevent
    A. Wandering
    B. Sundowning
    C. Hallucinations
    D. Paranoia

26. If a person with AD seems afraid or is worried about money, you should
    A. Change the conversation to a pleasant topic
    B. Tell the person that everything is okay
    C. Report the concern to the nurse
    D. Assume the person has paranoia

27. The television is loud, people are laughing and talking, and you are asking the person to select several items off the dinner menu. This stimuli could overwhelm the person and cause
    A. Depression
    B. Catastrophic reactions
    C. Feelings of abandonment
    D. Wandering

28. A caregiver may cause agitation and aggression by
    A. Talking very slowly and using simple language
    B. Selecting activities that are interesting to the person
    C. Encouraging activity early in the day
    D. Expecting the person to complete care quickly

29. When you wish to communicate with the person who has AD or other dementias, you should
    A. Make eye contact to get the person's attention
    B. Give a simple, direct order such as "Sit down and eat"
    C. Ask several open-ended questions
    D. Play soft music in the background

30. If a person with AD frequently rubs his or her genitals, the nurse may tell you to
    A. Inform the person that the behavior is not acceptable
    B. Make sure the person has good hygiene to prevent itching
    C. Isolate the person in a private room with the door closed
    D. Ignore the behavior because the disease causes it

31. What should you do when a person repeats the same motions or repeats the same words over and over?
    A. Remind the person to stop the repeating.
    B. Report this to the nurse immediately.
    C. Distract the person with music or picture books.
    D. Ask the person why he is repeating himself

32. A person with AD is encouraged to take part in therapies and activities that
    A. Help the person to achieve a previous level of function
    B. Help the person to feel useful, worthwhile, and active
    C. Give family caregivers respite from repetitive behaviors
    D. Improve physical problems such as incontinence and contractures

33. You are assigned to work in a memory care unit. You must be particularly mindful of which principle?
    A. Confidentiality
    B. Professionalism
    C. Least restrictive approach
    D. Standard precautions

34. A person with AD no longer stays in a secured unit when
    A. The condition improves
    B. The family requests a move to another unit
    C. The person cannot sit or walk
    D. Aggressive behaviors disrupt the unit

35. A family who cares for a person with dementia at home
    A. Is encouraged to be with the person at all times
    B. May feel guilty, angry, and upset
    C. Generally does not need any help from others
    D. Should not place the person in a long-term care facility

Fill in the Blank

36. Write out the meaning of the abbreviations.
    A. AD _____
    B. ADL _____
    C. CMS _____
    D. NIA _____

37. Cognitive functioning involves
    A. _____
    B. _____
    C. _____
    D. _____
    E. _____
    F. _____

38. What senses decrease with changes in the nervous system from aging?
    A. _____
    B. _____
    C. _____
    D. _____
    E. _____

39. Some early warning signs of dementia affect these areas. Explain or give an example for each one.
    A. Memory _____
    B. Common tasks _____
    C. Language _____
    D. Judgment _____

40. What substances can cause treatable dementia?
    A. _____
    B. _____

41. _____ is a mental health disorder that could be mistake for dementia.

42. With delirium, the onset is _____. It often lasts for about _____. It may take _____ for normal mental function to return.

43. In Alzheimer's disease (AD) there is a slow, steady decline in mental functions, including
    A. _____
    B. _____
    C. _____

44. Certain behaviors are common with AD. Name the behavior for each of these examples.
    A. The person becomes more anxious, confused, or restless during the night. _____
    B. The person sits in a chair and folds the same napkin over and over. _____
    C. The person begins to scream and cry when a visitor asks many questions. _____
    D. The person walks away from home and cannot find the way back home. _____
    E. The person begins to get upset when a set routine for ADL is changed. _____
    F. The person tells you he sees his dog sitting in the room but you do not see anything. _____
    G. You frequently find the person looking for lost items in a wastebasket. _____
    H. The person tries to hug and kiss other residents of the facility. _____

Optional Learning Exercises

You are caring for Mr. Harris, a 78-year-old who is confused. You know there are ways to help a person to be more oriented. Answer these questions about ways to help a confused person.

45. How can you help to orient Mr. Harris every time you are in contact with him? _____

46. What are ways you can help to orient Mr. Harris to time?
    A. _____
    B. _____

47. What are ways you can maintain the day-night cycle?
    A. _____
    B. _____
    C. _____

You are caring for Mrs. Matthews, an 82-year-old resident. The nurse tells you she lived with her daughter for the last 2 years but the family is now concerned for her safety. She left the home when the temperature was 35°F and was found 2 miles away, wearing a light sweater. On another occasion, she turned on the gas stove and could not remember how to turn it off. Sometimes, she does not recognize her daughter and resists getting a bath or changing clothes. Since admission to the care facility, she repeatedly tells everyone she must leave to go to her birthday party. She brushes her arms and legs and tells you "bugs" are crawling on her. Answer these questions about Mrs. Matthews and her care.

48. What is the most important reason that Mrs. Matthews is living in a special care unit in the nursing facility?
    _____

49. Mrs. Matthews is diagnosed with _____ stage AD. What activities would indicate she is in this stage?
    A. _____
    B. _____
    C. _____
    D. _____
    E. _____

50. The nurse may encourage Mrs. Matthews's daughter to join a _____ group. How can this be helpful to the daughter?
    A. _____
    B. _____
    C. _____

Use the FOCUS ON PRIDE section to complete these statements and then use the critical thinking and discussion questions to develop your ideas.

51. You demonstrate personal and professional responsibility when you treat each person as unique, with his or her own _____.

52. You show that you respect the rights of a person when you keep personal items _____. It is important to protect the person's belongings from _____ or _____.

53. You help to maintain independence for a person with AD by maintaining the person's _____ when giving ADLs.

Critical Thinking and Discussion Questions

54. Review Focus on Pride: Ethics and Laws. There is an example of a licensed nursing assistant (LNA) reacting to a person who threw a food tray on the floor. The LNA was reprimanded by the Board of Nursing.
  A. Speculate about the circumstances that may have caused the LNA to react in such an unprofessional manner.
  B. What could the LNA have done to prevent the reaction?

Fill in the Blank: Key Terms

Birth defect
Developmental disabilities

Disability
Inherited

Intellectual disability
Spastic

1. _____ involves severe limits in intellectual function and adaptive behavior occurring before age 18.

2. A problem that develops during pregnancy, often during the first 3 months; it may involve a body structure or function is a _____.

3. _____ means the uncontrolled contractions of skeletal muscles.

4. That which is passed down from parents to children is _____.

5. A severe and chronic disability that involves a mental or physical impairment or both is a _____.

6. Any lost, absent, or impaired physical or mental function is a _____.

Circle the Best Answer

7. Which observation would you report to the nurse, because it could be a warning sign of intellectual or developmental disability in an infant?
   A. Likes to suck his thumb
   B. Cries when he is hungry
   C. Has delayed crawling
   D. Needs frequent diaper change

8. Which comment by a pregnant teenager would you report to nurse for follow-up to decrease the risk of intellectual disability for the unborn child?
   A. "I'm hungry; I'm going to eat pizza."
   B. "I am so tired I sleep all of the time."
   C. "Do I look fat? I think I am getting fat."
   D. "I am going to get so drunk this weekend."

9. The nurse tells you that the person has an IQ score of about 70. Which action would you use?
   A. Use a spoon to feed the person
   B. Perform all hygienic care for person
   C. Assist the person to walk to the bathroom
   D. Repeat instructions using simple language

10. In caring for a person with an intellectual disability and significant limit in social skills, which action would you use?
    A. Patiently remind about the rules
    B. Assist with the use of the phone
    C. Assist the person to get dressed
    D. Help the person to read the menu

11. Which action are you most likely to use when assisting a person with Down syndrome with morning hygiene?
    A. Explain tasks using step-by-step instructions
    B. Tell the person to take a shower
    C. Ask the person how you can assist
    D. Perform perineal care for the person

12. You are caring for a child with Down syndrome; you watch for
    A. Confusion and wandering behaviors
    B. Bruising or bleeding when brushing the teeth
    C. Signs/symptoms of ear or respiratory infections
    D. Seizure activity with urinary incontinence

13. You are caring for a child with Fragile X syndrome. Which care measure is specific to this disorder?
    A. Skin is fragile; use mild soap and wash gently
    B. Joints are loose; avoid over-extending joints
    C. Fats are not well digested; check frequently for diarrheal stools
    D. Hearing loss is common; face the person when speaking

14. In caring for a person with autism, check with the nurse before
    A. Touching the person
    B. Entering the person's room
    C. Talking to the person
    D. Smiling at the person

15. Which approach will the health care team use in the care of a person with autism?
    A. Coach the person through every task
    B. Offer opportunities to explore new activities
    C. Allow the person to do whatever he/she wants to do
    D. Maintain daily routines and schedules

16. Cerebral palsy is primarily considered to be a
    A. Communication disorder
    B. Movement disorder
    C. Cognition disorder
    D. Sensory disorder

17. When a person has spastic cerebral palsy, what would you expect to observe?
    A. Constant slow weaving or writhing motions
    B. Intense muscles with jerking motions
    C. Muscle flaccidity with weak movements
    D. Stiff muscles and awkward movements

18. The nurse tells you that the person has spina bifida; myelomeningocele type. What care measure will you plan to perform?
    A. Spoon feed during meals and give fluids in between meals
    B. Frequently check for bowel and bladder incontinence
    C. Assist with frequent oral hygiene and encourage fluids
    D. Assist with ambulation in the hallway three times per shift

19. For a child with hydrocephalus, you would pay special attention to skin care
    A. In the perineal area
    B. On the back of the head
    C. On the back of the heels
    D. Under the arms

20. Which behavior would you expect to see in a child who has fetal alcohol syndrome?
    A. Hyperactivity
    B. Lethargy
    C. Unresponsiveness
    D. Hypoactivity

Fill in the Blank

21. Write out the abbreviations.
    A. ADA _____
    B. CP _____
    C. DS _____
    D. FAS _____
    E. FASDs _____
    F. Fragile X _____
    G. IDD _____
    H. IQ _____
    I. SB _____
    J. ASD _____

22. Intellectual and developmental disabilities (IDDs) affect 3 areas of development. They are
    A. _____
    B. _____
    C. _____

23. List two ways in which genetics can cause or contribute to intellectual disabilities.
    A. _____
    B. _____

24. _____ is an infection that can cause intellectual or developmental disabilities for the child, if the mother has the infection during pregnancy.

25. According to the Arc of the United States, intellectual disabilities involve the condition being present before _____ years of age.

26. The Arc beliefs about sexuality include the rights to
    A. _____
    B. _____
    C. _____
    D. _____
    E. _____
    F. _____
    G. _____
    H. _____
    I. _____
    J. _____
    K. _____

27. If a child has Down syndrome (DS), what features are present in these areas?
    A. Head, ears, mouth _____
    B. Eyes _____
    C. Tongue _____
    D. Nose _____
    E. Hands and fingers _____

28. Persons with Down syndrome and other developmental disabilities need therapy in these areas.
    A. _____
    B. _____
    C. _____
    D. _____
    E. _____

29. The most common type of cerebral palsy is _____.

30. The goal for a person with developmental disabilities is to be _____.

31. For a person who has autism, list eleven behaviors that indicate a difficulty with social skills.
    A. _____
    B. _____
    C. _____
    D. _____
    E. _____
    F. _____
    G. _____
    H. _____
    I. _____
    J. _____
    K. _____

32. Spina bifida is a defect in which the _____, the bones in the _____, or the _____, do not form properly.

33. Which type of spina bifida would cause the problems in each of the examples given?
    A. The person has leg paralysis and a lack of bowel and bladder control. _____
    B. The person may have no symptoms. _____
    C. Nerve damage usually does not occur and surgery corrects the defect. _____

34. If a hydrochephalus is not treated, pressure increases in the head and causes _____ and _____.

Optional Learning Exercises

Mr. Murphy is one of the residents you care for. He has Down syndrome. Answer the 2 questions that relate to this person.

35. Mr. Murphy is 40 years old. As an adult with Down syndrome, he has a risk for which disorder?

    _____

36. Mr. Murphy is encouraged to eat a well-balanced diet and to attend regular exercise classes. Including these in the care plan will help to prevent the problems of _____ and _____.

You care for Mary Reynolds, who has cerebral palsy. Answer the question about Ms. Reynolds.

37. Because Ms. Reynolds remains in bed or a special chair all the time, she is at special risk for _____ because of immobility and incontinence. She needs to be re-positioned at least every _____.

Use the FOCUS ON PRIDE section to complete these statements and then use the critical thinking and discussion questions to develop your ideas.

38. Persons with developmental disabilities have a right to enjoy and maintain a good quality of life. Such a life involves
   A. _____
   B. _____
   C. _____

39. The goal for children with developmental disabilities is independence _____.

40. Signs of abuse of a developmentally disabled person may be
   A. _____
   B. _____
   C. _____
   D. _____
   E. _____

Critical Thinking and Discussion Question

41. You are caring for a person who has Down syndrome. The person is around your age and you have a good working relationship with this person. The person asks you out on a date.
   A. Discuss how this would make you feel.
   B. What would you say to the person?

55 Sexuality

Fill in the Blank: Key Terms

Bisexual   Gay   Heterosexual   Sexual orientation   Transgender
Erectile dysfunction   Gender identity   Sex   Sexuality

1. A person's sense or feelings of being male, female, a combination of male and female, or neither male nor female is _____.

2. _____ describes people who express their sexuality or gender identity in ways that do not fit with their biological sex.

3. The inability of the male to have an erection is_____.

4. _____ is the physical, emotional, social, cultural, and spiritual factors that affect a person's feelings, attitudes, and behaviors about one's gender identity and sexual behavior

5. _____ is the emotional, romantic, and physical attraction to men, women, or both sexes.

6. A person who is attracted to both sexes is_____.

7. A person who is attracted to members of the other sex is _____.

8. A person who is attracted to members of the same sex is _____.

9. The physical interactions between people involving the body and the reproductive organs is_____.

Circle the Best Answer

10. A 4-year-old girl tells you that she wants to wear her pink princess dress. She is expressing her
    A. Heterosexuality
    B. Transgender identity
    C. Bisexuality
    D. Gender identity

11. Which activity suggests that a 3-year-old boy has identified that he is a male and has learned to behave in a certain way?
    A. Wants to go with Dad to fix the truck
    B. Dresses his sister's doll in a party outfit
    C. Shares a cookie with the family dog
    D. Asks his mom to read a story to him

12. What is the greatest risk for a teenage girl who is gay and sexually active?
    A. Sexual aggression
    B. Gender confusion
    C. Sexually transmitted disease
    D. Pregnancy

13. Which routine action done in health care settings denies the person's sexuality?
    A. Expecting all people to put on generic patient gowns
    B. Always covering people when performing hygienic care

C. Assigning people of the same gender to be roommates
D. Allowing people to have personal items at the bedside

14. A woman who is attracted to men is
    A. Transgender   C. Lesbian
    B. Heterosexual   D. Bisexual

15. Diabetes or spinal cord injury may cause
    A. Erectile dysfunction
    B. Menopause
    C. Sexual aggression
    D. Genital soreness and itching

16. Two older women are roommates in a long-term care center. You enter the room and see the two kissing and fondling. What is the best action?
    A. Close the door and inform the nurse so the staff is aware of their need for privacy
    B. Close the door, leave, and later come back and knock before entering
    C. Politely ask them to stop and wait until the nurse comes to speak to them
    D. Firmly, but kindly state that their behavior makes you uncomfortable

17. When older adult couples live in a nursing center, OBRA requires that they
    A. Are allowed to share the same room
    B. Are placed in separate rooms
    C. Are not encouraged to be intimate
    D. Cannot share a bed

18. If a person touches you in the wrong way, you should
    A. Ignore the behavior; the person is not responsible
    B. Lightly slap the hand away and say, "stop"
    C. Politely tell the person not to act that way
    D. Always have another nursing assistant present

Fill in the Blank

19. Sexuality develops when the baby's _____.

20. Children know their own sex at age _____.

21. Which term is considered offensive by gay rights groups? _____.

22. Women who are sexually attracted to other women are called _____.

23. Sexual function may be affected by chronic illnesses such as
    A. _____
    B. _____
    C. _____
    D. _____

24. Which reproductive surgeries may affect sexuality?
    A. Men _____
    B. Women _____

25. Some older people do not have intercourse. They may express their sexual needs or desires by
    _____.

26. What can you do to allow privacy for a person and a partner?
    A. Close _____.
    B. Let the person and partner know _____.
    C. Tell other _____.
    D. Knock _____.

27. Masturbation is a normal _____.

28. If a person becomes sexually aroused, you should allow for _____.

29. What health-related problems may cause a person to touch his or her genitals?
    A. _____ or _____ system disorders
    B. Poor _____
    C. Being _____ or _____ from urine and feces

Optional Learning Exercises

Mr. and Mrs. Davis are 78-year-old residents in a nursing center, where they share a room. They need assistance with ADL but are mentally alert. They are an affectionate couple that cares deeply for each other. Answer this question about meeting their sexuality needs.

30. Mr. Davis has diabetes and high blood pressure. What effect can these disorders have on sexuality?
    _____

Use the FOCUS ON PRIDE section to complete these statements and then use the critical thinking and discussion question to develop your ideas.

31. When you are caring for a person, it is important to get consent before touching _____, _____, or _____.

32. If you touch without consent, you may be accused of _____.

33. Sexuality includes _____, _____, _____, _____, and _____ factors.

34. When giving care, you can promote sexuality when you
    A. _____
    B. _____
    C. _____
    D. _____

Critical Thinking and Discussion Question

35. You are assigned to assist with hygienic care for a person who is dressed as a woman. The person has the physical features and the deep voice of a man. Discuss how you will handle this situation.

56 Caring for Mothers and Babies

Fill in the Blank: Key Terms

Breast-feeding   Episiotomy   Meconium   Postpartum   Umbilical cord
Circumcision   Lochia   Nursing   Prenatal care

1. An _____ is an incision into the perineum.

2. Breast-feeding is also called _____.

3. The time period after childbirth is called _____.

4. _____ is the surgical removal of foreskin from the penis.

5. The vaginal discharge that occurs after childbirth is _____.

6. The structure that carries blood, oxygen, and nutrients from the mother to the fetus is the _____.

7. A dark green to black, tarry bowel movement is _____.

8. Feeding a baby milk from the mother's breast is _____.

9. _____ is the care a woman receives while pregnant.

Circle the Best Answer

10. You lift a newborn by
    A. Grasping the newborn's forearms and pulling upwards
    B. Scooping your dominant hand under the newborn's back and buttocks
    C. Placing your hands under newborn's armpits and lifting upwards
    D. Using both hands to support the head and back; and to support the legs

11. If a baby is lying on a scale, bed, table, or other surface, you should
    A. Place pillows around the baby
    B. Tuck a blanket firmly around the baby
    C. Always keep one hand on the baby
    D. Keep an eye on the baby at all times

12. What do you do when the baby needs to go to sleep?
    A. Dress the baby in a sleepwear that covers the head
    B. Place pillows around the baby for comfort and security
    C. Place the baby on the stomach with head turned to the side
    D. Lay the baby on his or her back on a firm surface

13. You are caring for a mother and baby in a home setting. Which of these crib features would you report to the nurse for follow-up investigation?
    A. The mattress is flush to the crib, without spaces or gaps.
    B. Side rails are fixed and drop-side latches are absent
    C. Crib slats are closely spaced; about 2 inches apart.
    D. Head-board is decorated with a cute cut-out design

14. Which of these should be reported to the nurse at once?
    A. The baby has a rectal temperature of 99.6°F.
    B. The baby has a soft, unformed stool after being breast-fed.
    C. The baby turns his or her head to one side or puts a hand to the ear.
    D. The baby cries when the diaper is wet or when he or she is hungry

15. A breast-fed newborn baby generally nurses
    A. Every 2 to 3 hours
    B. Every 8 to 12 hours
    C. Once an hour for a brief time
    D. On a very strict schedule

16. You are assisting a mother who will breast-feed the infant. What will you place on the bedside table?
    A. Bottle with formula, in case the baby won't take the nipple
    B. Soap for cleaning the breast after feeding is complete
    C. Crackers and cheese; mother may experience hypoglycemia
    D. Milk, water, or juice; mother may get thirsty when breast feeding

17. When the mother is breast-feeding, she should
    A. Position the baby by using a pillow to prop up the baby
    B. Begin by stroking the baby's cheek with her nipple
    C. Nurse from 1 breast at each feeding
    D. Lay the baby on his or her stomach after feeding

18. When preparing bottles for feeding babies, you should
    A. Prepare and then refrigerate bottles that can be used within 24 hours
    B. Sterilize the bottles by boiling them for 20 minutes
    C. Rinse bottles and nipples that have been used only in cool water
    D. Avoid using soap on the equipment; it can cause gastrointestinal irritation

19. When preparing to give a bottle to a baby
    A. It may be used from the refrigerator without heating
    B. Place the bottle under warm running tap water
    C. Take the bottle out of the refrigerator and allow it to warm
    D. Heat the bottle in a microwave oven

20. You are assigned to bottle feed an older baby. How often should you burp the baby?
    A. Every 5 minutes
    B. After every 1/2 to 1 ounce of formula
    C. After every 2 to 3 ounces of formula
    D. When the newborn stops sucking

21. When diapering a baby, report to the nurse if
    A. The stool is soft and unformed
    B. The stool is hard and formed or watery
    C. The diaper is wet 6 to 8 times a day
    D. The baby has 3 stools in 1 day

22. The diaper is changed
    A. When stool is present, usually 1 to 3 times a day
    B. When the diaper is wet, usually 6 to 8 times a day
    C. Before and after feeding and before and after sleep
    D. Before handing the baby to the mother for cuddling

23. Which action will you use for cord care?
    A. Apply petroleum jelly to the cord to keep it moist
    B. Wash with mild soap and pour warm water over the stump
    C. Keep the diaper below the cord to prevent irritation
    D. Gently pull off the cord if it looks ready to fall off

24. Which action would you perform for circumcision care?
    A. Clean the penis at each diaper change
    B. Clean the area with a sterile solution
    C. Apply a snug dressing to the area
    D. Avoid getting the penis wet

25. When giving a bath to a baby, the water should be
    A. Room temperature
    B. 75°F to 80°F
    C. 100°F to 105°F
    D. 110°F to 115°F

26. When a baby is breast-fed, the baby is weighed
    A. Once a day
    B. Before and after each feeding
    C. After every diaper change
    D. Once a week

27. A mother who had a baby 4 weeks ago has a whitish vaginal drainage. You document this finding and know that this
    A. Should be reported to the nurse at once because it's abnormal
    B. Is unusual because her discharge should be pinkish brown in color
    C. Is normal, at this time, after having a baby
    D. Should be reported because she may have an infection

28. Report to the nurse if during the postpartum period the mother
    A. Has occasional emotional reactions
    B. Has a whitish vaginal discharge 12 days after delivery
    C. Complains of leg, abdominal, or perineal pain
    D. Has a menstrual period about 4 weeks after the baby is born

Fill in the Blank

29. Write out the meaning of the abbreviations.
    A. BM _____
    B. C _____
    C. CPSC _____
    D. C-section _____
    E. F _____
    F. SIDS _____
    G. SUID _____

30. You should not place pillows, quilts, or soft toys in the crib because they may cause _____.

31. Babies are not placed on their stomachs for sleep because this position can _____.

32. What signs or symptoms related to each of these may indicate the baby is ill?
    A. Skin color _____
    B. Respirations _____
    C. Eyes _____
    D. Stools _____

33. When a mother is breast-feeding, if the baby finished the last feeding at the right breast, the baby starts the next feeding at the _____ breast.

34. The baby is burped at least twice when breast-feeding. Burping is done
    A. _____
    B. _____

35. Sudden unexpected infant death may occur because of accidental suffocation or _____ in the bed.

36. When taking a pulse on a baby, it is taken
    _____.

37. Why is it important to thoroughly rinse baby bottles, caps, and nipples to remove all soap?
    _____

38. You can prevent having air in the neck of the bottle or in the nipple by _____
    _____.

39. When you are burping a baby, you should support the _____ for the first _____ months.

40. When changing a baby's diaper, what observations should be reported and recorded?
    A. _____
    B. _____
    C. _____
    D. _____

41. When diapering a newborn, what should you do if the baby has an unhealed circumcision or a cord stump still attached? _____

    A. Circumcision _____

    B. Cord stump _____

42. The base of the cord stump is washed with _____ if it is dirty or sticky. The stump heals faster if allowed to _____.

43. When caring for the umbilical cord, you should report the following to the nurse.

    A. _____

    B. _____

    C. _____

    D. _____

44. Petrolatum gauze dressing or jelly is applied to an unhealed circumcision to

    A. _____

    B. _____

45. To protect an infant during a bath, what safety measures are followed?

    A. Room temperature should be _____

    B. Bath water temperature should be _____

    C. Never leave the baby alone on a _____ or in the_____.

46. What steps are used to wash a baby's head?

    A. _____

    B. _____

    C. _____

    D. _____

    E. _____

47. What signs and symptoms of postpartum complications should be reported to the nurse at once?

    A. _____

    B. _____

    C. _____

    D. _____

    E. _____

    F. _____

    G. _____

    H. _____

    I. _____

    J. _____

    K. _____

Optional Learning Exercises

You are caring for Marilyn Hansen and her newborn son, Samuel, at home. Answer the questions about their care.

48. Ms. Hansen is breast-feeding. What would Ms. Hansen do to encourage Samuel to turn his head and start to suck? _____

49. Ms. Hansen is having difficulty in removing Samuel from her breast. How does she break the suction?

    _____

    _____.

50. What can Ms. Hansen do to prevent drying and cracking of the nipples?

    A. _____

    B. _____

    C. _____

    D. _____

51. When you are changing Samuel's diaper, clean the genital area from _____.

52. Ms. Hansen asks you when the cord stump will fall off. What will you tell her?

    _____.

53. Samuel has been circumcised and Ms. Hansen is concerned because the penis looks red, swollen, and sore. You know that this is _____. However, you should observe the circumcision for

    A. _____ and

    _____

    B. There should be no _____.

54. Ms. Hansen asks whether she should bathe Samuel in the morning or in the evening. You tell her an evening bath might work well because it

    A. _____

    _____

    B. _____

    _____

Use the FOCUS ON PRIDE section to complete these statements and then use the critical thinking and discussion question to develop your ideas.

55. When you return a newborn to the mother, it is your professional responsibility to follow the agency policy for _____.

56. Newborns wear a security bracelet that will signal the agency when he or she is carried _____

    _____.

Critical Thinking and Discussion Question

57. You are assisting a new mother with care of the newborn, but she seems hesitant to try and wants you to do most of the care. What should you do?

Fill in the Blank: Key Terms

Assisted living   Service plan
Medication reminder

1. A _____ is reminding the person to take drugs, observing them being taken as prescribed, and recording that they were taken.

2. A written plan that lists the services needed by the person and who provides them is a

   _____.

3. _____ is a housing option for older persons who need help with activities of daily living but do not need 24-hour nursing care and supervision.

Circle the Best Answer

4. Which person would be the most likely candidate for assisted living?
   A. A person who needs help taking medications
   B. A person who has a feeding tube and tracheostomy
   C. A person who needs total help with all ADLs
   D. A person who has advanced Alzheimer's disease

5. Which feature would be common to all ALRs?
   A. A private patio or balcony
   B. 24-hour room service
   C. Grab bars in the bathroom
   D. A queen-sized bed

6. Which housekeeping measure would help to prevent infection?
   A. Use air fresheners as needed
   B. Clean bathroom surfaces with a disinfectant
   C. Make beds and straighten up the living room
   D. Open bathroom windows for a short time

7. Which of these is included in the Assisted Living Residents' Rights?
   A. May take part in religious, social, community, and other activities
   B. Receive personal care from preferred nursing assistants and nurses
   C. Has a doctor or pharmacist assigned by the facility
   D. Cannot be evicted or asked to vacate if unable to pay for service plan

8. In which area will you need additional training, if you seek employment in an ALR?
   A. Using proper body mechanics
   B. Assisting with daily hygiene
   C. Using service plans
   D. Measuring medications

9. In order for the ALR to meet safety needs in the event of an emergency, residents must be able to
   A. Ambulate independently and help others as needed
   B. Recognize and react appropriately to dangerous situations
   C. Give clear directions to others and follow instructions from the staff
   D. Leave the building with minimal assistance if helped into a wheelchair

10. Which of these services, offered in an ALR, would increase a resident's feeling of safety and security?
    A. A barber and a beauty service
    B. A daily schedule of activities within the ALR
    C. A 24-hour emergency communication system
    D. A common dining room and day area

11. Which care measure would be your responsibility related to meals in an ALR?
    A. Give residents any foods they desire to eat
    B. Take residents out to the restaurants of their choice
    C. Assist residents, as needed, to go to the dining area
    D. Ask residents about their special dietary needs

12. When you assist with housekeeping, you will be expected to
    A. Clean the tub or shower after each use
    B. Put out clean towels every week
    C. Clean the carpet once a month
    D. Dust furniture every day

13. A measure you should follow when handling, preparing, or storing foods is
    A. Empty garbage at least once a week
    B. Wash all pots and pans in a dishwasher
    C. Save or discard left-overs
    D. Use disinfectant to clean appliances, counters, and tables

14. When assisting with laundry, a guideline to follow is
    A. Sort and wash items according to the amount of soil on the items
    B. Wear gloves when handling soiled laundry
    C. Use hot water to wash all items
    D. Use the highest dryer setting to sanitize the items

15. When you assist a person with medication, it may involve
    A. Opening containers for the person who cannot do so
    B. Measuring the medications for the person
    C. Explaining to the person the action of the medication
    D. Preparing a pill organizer for the person each week

16. If a drug error occurs, you should
    A. Tell the person not to do it again
    B. Give the person the correct medication
    C. Report the error to the nurse
    D. Take all medications away from the person

17. Which event represents a drug error?
    A. Taking a tablet from the pill organizer
    B. Taking a drug after getting a medication reminder
    C. Taking a pill from a pre-sorted dose packet
    D. Taking an extra dose of the medication

18. For a resident who is a threat to the health and safety of self or others, what is the best recourse for the ALR?
    A. Assign extra staff to monitor the resident's behavior
    B. Have the resident transferred to a facility that can meet safety needs
    C. Have the resident evicted to prevent injury and accidents
    D. Ask the resident to leave voluntarily within a given time frame

19. A resident who uses self-directed medication management says, "This pill looks different." How would you respond?
    A. "Let's read the label; then you will know what you are taking."
    B. "Let me contact the nurse before you take the pill."
    C. "I'm sure the pharmacist knows to send the right medication."
    D. "Things can look and seem different when you are not at home."

Fill in the Blank

20. Write out the meaning of the abbreviations.
    A. ADL _____
    B. ALR _____

21. When working in an assisted living setting, you should follow _____ when contact with blood, body fluids, secretions, excretions, or potentially contaminated items is likely.

22. Most persons living in ALRs need help with one or more ADL, such as
    A. _____
    B. _____
    C. _____
    D. _____
    E. _____
    F. _____

23. The ALR cannot employ a person with a
    _____.

24. The service plan is a written plan listing
    A. _____
    B. _____
    C. _____

25. The service plan also relates to
    A. _____
    B. _____
    C. _____
    D. _____
    E. _____
    F. _____

26. What 24-hour services are usually provided by the ALR?
    A. _____
    B. _____

27. In which order would you wash cooking equipment, dishes, glassware, and utensils?
    _____

28. If you are assisting the person with taking medications, you should know the 6 rights of drug administration. They are
    A. _____
    B. _____
    C. _____
    D. _____
    E. _____
    F. _____

29. If a person is taking his or her drugs and tells you that a pill looks different, what should you do?
    _____

30. If a person needs a medication reminder, it means reminding _____, observing _____, and recording _____.

31. If you are assisting in drug administration, you should report any drug error to the RN. Errors would include:
    A. _____
    B. _____
    C. _____
    D. _____
    E. _____
    F. _____
    G. _____
    H. _____
    I. _____

32. A resident in the facility has lived there for 2 years and has needed little assistance. He recently had a stroke and now needs care for all of his ADL. Why is he being moved to a nursing facility? _____
    _____

Optional Learning Exercises

You are working in an assisting living facility. What would you do in these situations?

33. Mrs. Jenkins tells you she is expecting an important phone call and wants to eat her lunch in her room. What should you do? _____

_____

34. Mr. Shante asks you to get his medicines ready for him to take. What assistance are you allowed to give after you have received the proper training?
    A. _____
    B. _____
    C. _____
    D. _____
    E. _____
    F. _____
    G. _____
    H. _____

35. When you are assisting Mrs. Clyde with her medicines, you notice 2 of the labels have an expired date. What should you do? _____

_____

36. Mrs. Johnson asks you when the next meeting of the quilting group will be held. She also asks what days the community crafts fair is planned. Where would you direct her to find this information? _____

_____

Use the FOCUS ON PRIDE section to complete these statements and then use the critical thinking and discussion question to develop your ideas.

37. When you are caring for residents in assisted living, your interactions should assure the person and family that you will provide _____.

38. It is important to know your state's laws when you assist with drugs because if you act beyond those limits, you can lose _____ and your ability to work _____.

Critical Thinking and Discussion Question

39. Discuss some of the advantages and disadvantages of working in an ALR.

Fill in the Blank: Key Terms

Anaphylaxis	Convulsion	Hemorrhage	Seizure
Cardiac arrest	Fainting	Hypothermia	Shock
Cardiopulmonary resuscitation (CPR)	First aid	Respiratory arrest	Sudden cardiac arrest
	Frostbite	Resuscitate	

1. Another term for sudden cardiac arrest (SCA) is _____.

2. In _____, breathing stops but the heart action continues for several minutes.

3. The sudden loss of consciousness from an inadequate blood supply to the brain is _____.

4. When the heart stops suddenly and without warning, it is _____ or cardiac arrest.

5. _____ results when there is not enough blood supply to organs and tissues.

6. Emergency care given to an ill or injured person before medical help arrives is _____.

7. Violent and sudden contractions or tremors of muscle groups, caused by abnormal electrical activity in the brain, is a convulsion or _____.

8. _____ is the excessive loss of blood in a short period of time.

9. A life-threatening sensitivity to an antigen is _____.

10. Another term for a seizure is _____.

11. An abnormally low body temperature is _____.

12. _____ is to revive from apparent death or unconsciousness by using emergency measures.

13. _____ is an emergency procedure performed when the heart and breathing stop.

14. _____is an injury to the body caused by freezing of the skin and underlying tissues.

Circle the Best Answer

15. If the nurse instructs you to activate the EMS system, what should you should do?
    A. Tell the operator the victim's name and the family's phone number
    B. Give the operator your name and your employee identification number
    C. Tell the operator your location, include street address and city
    D. Tell the operator to hurry and send someone; then return to help the nurse

16. It is important to restore breathing and circulation quickly because
    A. The person will have a seizure
    B. The person will lose consciousness
    C. Organ damage occurs within minutes
    D. Life-threatening hemorrhage will occur

17. Which set of signs/symptoms causes you to suspect that the person has had sudden cardiac arrest?
    A. Chest pain, jaw pain, and nausea
    B. No pulse, no breathing, and no response
    C. Perspiration, dizziness, and pale skin
    D. Trouble breathing, choking, and wheezing

18. The purpose of chest compressions is to
    A. Deflate the lungs
    B. Increase oxygen in the blood
    C. Force blood through the circulatory system
    D. Help the heart work more effectively

19. In order for chest compressions to be effective, the person must be
    A. In the prone position on any surface
    B. Upright on a soft surface
    C. Supine on a hard, flat surface
    D. In bed in the semi-Fowler's position

20. When giving chest compressions to an adult, depress the sternum
    A. About 1 to 1½ inches   C. At least 2 inches
    B. No more than 1 inch   D. About 3 inches

21. The purpose of the head tilt–chin lift maneuver is to
    A. Make the person more comfortable
    B. Open the airway
    C. Keep the head in alignment
    D. Protect the jaw and teeth

22. Barrier device breathing is used
    A. Whenever possible to avoid contact with body fluids
    B. In order to make a better seal for breathing
    C. When you cannot ventilate through the person's mouth
    D. Only when other methods will not work

23. Mouth-to-mouth-and-nose breathing is used when
    A. The person is semi-conscious
    B. You want to avoid contact with body fluids
    C. Giving rescue breaths to an infant
    D. Chest compressions are not needed

24. If an automated external defibrillator (AED) is available
    A. Use it after other methods have failed
    B. It can be used only by an RN or doctor
    C. Use it as soon as possible
    D. Use it once the person is responsive

25. When an automated external defibrillator (AED) is used, it
    A. Makes the heart beat faster, stronger, and more efficiently
    B. Slows down the heartbeat; then reestablishes a faster rhythm
    C. Stops ventricular fibrillation and restores a regular heartbeat
    D. Replaces chest compressions and rescue breathing

26. You and bystander start CPR at the scene of an automobile accident. When can you stop?
    A. Stop when the EMS arrives
    B. Stop when the bystander tells you to stop
    C. Stop when the person seems dead
    D. Stop when a family member tells you to stop

27. Before starting chest compressions
    A. Make sure the person is breathing
    B. Check carotid pulse for 10 seconds or less
    C. Wait 30 seconds to see if the person responds
    D. Turn the person to the side

28. When CPR is started, you first
    A. Give 30 chest compressions
    B. Give 2 breaths
    C. Look for the defibrillator
    D. Turn the person on his side

29. If the person is not breathing or not breathing adequately, give 2 breaths that
    A. Last about 1 second each
    B. Last about 5 seconds each
    C. Last 5 to 10 seconds each
    D. Last 15 seconds each

30. When performing CPR, chest compressions are at a rate of
    A. 12 to 20 compressions per minute
    B. 15 to 30 compressions per minute
    C. 60 to 80 compressions per minute
    D. 100 to 120 compressions per minute

31. When performing CPR, continue cycles of compressions and breathing
    A. For 5 minutes
    B. For 30 minutes
    C. Until an AED arrives
    D. Until you confirm death

32. The recovery position is used when
    A. Giving chest compressions
    B. Performing mouth-to-mouth breathing
    C. The person is breathing and has a pulse
    D. You are preparing to use an AED

33. When giving CPR to children, the chest compressions
    A. Move the sternum about ⅓ of an inch
    B. Are at least ⅓ the depth of the chest
    C. Are done with your fingertips
    D. Compress the sternum about 2 inches

34. When giving breaths to an infant, you should
    A. Tip the head back as far as possible to open the airway
    B. Pinch the nose closed and breathe through the mouth
    C. Cover the infant's mouth and nose with your mouth
    D. Always use a mouth barrier

35. If a person has swallowed poison, you should
    A. Try to have the person vomit
    B. Give the person something to drink or eat
    C. Contact the Poison Control Center as soon as possible
    D. Ask the person why he swallowed poison

36. Which of these is a sign of internal hemorrhage?
    A. Steady flow of blood from a wound
    B. Pain, shock, vomiting blood, or coughing up blood
    C. Bleeding occurs in bright red spurts
    D. Dried blood at the site of an injury

37. You are at a park; a child gets injured and is bleeding. In which circumstance would you intervene?
    A. Bystander attempts to remove a stick embedded in the skin
    B. Mother places a clean dry towel directly over the wound
    C. Bystander applies direct pressure over the bleeding site
    D. Father talks calmly and quietly to the child

38. For a person who is experiencing the signs and symptoms of shock, which is the best position?
    A. Sitting position in a firm chair with head between legs
    B. Recovery position with a small pillow under the head
    C. High Fowler's position with legs slightly elevated
    D. Supine position with legs elevated 6 to 12 inches

39. Anaphylactic shock occurs because of
    A. Hemorrhage
    B. Allergies
    C. Sudden cardiac arrest
    D. Seizures

40. If you suspect a person has had a stroke, you should
    A. Make the person comfortable
    B. Begin CPR immediately
    C. Activate the EMS system at once
    D. Ask the person to describe what he is feeling

41. If a person has a seizure, which action is most important?
    A. Turn the person on his side
    B. Note the time the seizure started
    C. Put the person into his or her bed
    D. Put something soft between the teeth

42. A group of elderly residents are outside for a picnic. The nurse tells you some of people are showing signs/symptoms of heat-related illness. Which action will the staff take first?
    A. Move everyone to a cooler place
    B. Loosen everyone's tight clothing
    C. Give everyone a cold drink
    D. Spray everyone with a cool mist

43. A person sustains a burn on the forearm. Which action will you take?
    A. Put ice on the burned area
    B. Remove jewelry that is not stuck to the skin
    C. Give the person plenty of fluids
    D. Apply oils or ointments to the burns

Fill in the Blank

44. Write out the abbreviations.
    A. AED _____
    B. CPR _____
    C. EMS _____
    D. RRS _____
    E. SCA _____
    F. VF; V-fib _____

45. If you activate the EMS system, what information should you give to the operator?
    A. _____
    B. _____
    C. _____
    D. _____
    E. _____
    F. _____

46. The 3 major signs of sudden cardiac arrest (SCA) are
    A. _____
    B. _____
    C. _____

47. Rescue breaths are given when there is a _____ but no _____. To give rescue breaths
    A. _____
    B. _____
    C. _____
    D. _____
    E. _____

48. To find the carotid pulse, place 2 fingers on the _____. Slide your fingers down _____.

49. When doing chest compressions, you push _____ and _____ in the center of the chest

50. When performing the head tilt–chin lift maneuver, explain how you tilt the head and lift the chin.
    A. One hand is on the _____.
    B. Pressure is applied to _____ the head back
    C. The _____ is lifted with the fingers of the other hand

51. When you perform mouth-to-mouth breathing, it is likely you will have contact with _____ _____.

52. A bag valve mask is a _____ device. It is squeezed to give _____. It should be connected to an _____.

53. If compressions must be interrupted for any reason (e.g., applying AED), the time should be limited to _____.

54. When performing CPR, a cycle of _____ compressions is followed by _____ breaths.

55. The automated external defibrillator (AED) advises a "shock". What does the nurse say in a loud voice before pushing the SHOCK button? _____ _____.

56. How do you check for a response in an infant? _____

57. For children, start CPR if the child's heart rate is _____.

58. What are the signs and symptoms of a heart attack?
    A. _____
    B. _____
    C. _____
    D. _____
    E. _____
    F. _____

59. What is the best way to stop bleeding from a wound? _____

60. Signs and symptoms of shock include
    A. _____
    B. _____
    C. _____
    D. _____
    E. _____
    F. _____
    G. _____
    H. _____

61. Anaphylaxis is an emergency because the reaction occurs within _____.

62. What are the signs and symptoms of an anaphylactic reaction?
    A. _____
    B. _____
    C. _____
    D. _____
    E. _____
    F. _____
    G. _____
    H. _____
    I. _____
    J. _____
    K. _____

63. Signs of a stroke include sudden
    A. _____
    B. _____
    C. _____
    D. _____
    E. _____

64. How do you protect the person's head when he or she is having a seizure?
    _____

65. For a person with a suspected concussion, what would you do if the person started vomiting?
    _____
    _____

66. For people with suspected hypothermia or frostbite, you would move them into a _____ _____ as soon as possible

67. When giving emergency care for a burn, apply _____ for 10 to15 minutes. Do not put _____ on burns.

Optional Learning Exercises

You are visiting a neighbor and she is washing dishes. As she washes a glass, it shatters and she sustains a deep cut on her wrist. Answer the following questions about how you would respond.

68. Clean rubber gloves are lying on the counter. How can they be useful to you? _____
    _____

69. What materials in the home could be used to place over the wound? _____
    _____

70. Your neighbor is restless and has a rapid and weak pulse. You notice her skin is cold, moist, and pale. These signs indicate she may be in _____.

71. Her wound is still bleeding, and she loses consciousness. What should you do before you continue to give first aid? _____

Use the FOCUS ON PRIDE section to complete these statements and then use the critical thinking and discussion questions to develop your ideas.

72. If a person has an emergency in a public place, you protect the person's right to privacy when you do what you can to _____.

Critical Thinking and Discussion Questions

73. There is an emergency situation with a patient on the unit and you run to help. The charge nurse tells you to continue to care for the other patients, rather than assist with the emergency situation.
    A. Discuss how this would make you feel.
    B. Why would the nurse ask you to continue the care of the other patients?

59 End-of-Life Care

Fill in the Blank: Key Terms

Advance directive   End-of-life care   Post-mortem care   Rigor mortis
Autopsy   Palliative care   Reincarnation   Terminal illness

1. The support and care given during the time surrounding death is _____.

2. The stiffness or rigidity of skeletal muscles that occurs after death is _____.

3. An _____ is a document stating a person's wishes about health care when that person cannot make his or her own decisions.

4. Care of the body after death is _____.

5. An illness or injury from which a person will not likely recover is a _____.

6. _____ is the belief that the spirit or soul is reborn in another human body or in another form of life.

7. The examination of the body after death is an
_____.

8. _____ is care that involves relieving or reducing the intensity of uncomfortable symptoms without producing a cure.

Circle the Best Answer

9. In caring for a person who has a terminal illness, which care measure would be part of your responsibility?
   A. Assisting a person to gather belongings for transfer to a rehabilitation unit
   B. Helping a person to interpret and complete the advanced directive form
   C. Helping a person with hygienic care for comfort and the quality of life
   D. Assisting a person with range-of-motion exercises to increase strength

10. What is the main difference between palliative care and hospice care?
    A. In hospice care, the focus of support is the family
    B. In palliative care, treatment of the disease may continue
    C. In palliative care, the person always remains at home
    D. In hospice care, life-saving measures are taken to prolong life

11. Hospice care
    A. Is given when death is immediately imminent
    B. Usually begins when terminal illness is diagnosed
    C. May occur when a person has less than 6 months to live
    D. Is given until the person recovers from the illness

12. When talking to a dying person, which response is a barrier to communication?
    A. "Would you like to talk? I have time to listen."
    B. "You seem sad. Can I help?"
    C. "Is it okay if I quietly sit with you for a while?"
    D. "I understand what you are going through."

13. Which comment represents a 4-year-old child's understanding of death?
    A. "If grandma dies, she will be gone forever."
    B. "When grandma finishes dying, she's going to play with me."
    C. "If I get sick I might die, but I never get sick, so I won't die."
    D. "I don't think I will die; only old people die and I'm not old."

14. Freedom from pain, suffering, and disability is a view of death attributed to
    A. School-aged children   C. Middle-aged adults
    B. Young adults   D. Older adults

15. In which stage of dying does the person make promises and make "just one more" request?
    A. Acceptance   C. Depression
    B. Anger   D. Bargaining

16. If a dying person begins to talk about worries and concerns, you should
    A. Call a spiritual leader
    B. Tell the nurse
    C. Listen quietly and use touch
    D. Change the subject

17. Care given when a person is dying should be done
    A. To meet the family's expectations
    B. To promote comfort
    C. To keep the person active
    D. To prevent worsening

18. Because vision fails as death approaches, you should
    A. Explain what you are doing
    B. Have the room lit very brightly
    C. Turn off all lights
    D. Keep the eyes covered at all times

19. Hearing is one of the last functions lost, so it is important to
    A. Ask the person questions while giving care
    B. Talk in a loud voice so the person can hear you
    C. Provide re-assurance and explanations about care
    D. Ask the family to be quiet so they do not disturb the person

20. As death nears, oral hygiene is
    A. Given in the morning and in the evening
    B. Given frequently when taking oral fluids is difficult
    C. Given occasionally to avoid disturbing the person
    D. Never given because the person cannot swallow

21. You are giving hygienic care to a person who has been in hospice for several weeks. Which sign/symptom would prompt you to immediately notify the nurse, because death is imminent?
    A. Skin becomes red and warm to the touch
    B. Person reports that pain is getting worse
    C. Person seems more depressed than usual
    D. Respirations become slow and shallow

22. Because of breathing difficulties, the dying person is generally more comfortable in the
    A. Supine position
    B. Trendelenburg's position
    C. Prone position
    D. Semi-Fowler's position

23. When a person is dying, you can help the family by
    A. Allowing family members to stay as long as they wish
    B. Giving privacy, staying away, and delaying care measures
    C. Asking family members to leave so you can give care
    D. Reassuring family members that the person is not in pain

24. If a person has a living will, it may instruct doctors
    A. Not to start measures that will save the person's life
    B. To start CPR whenever necessary
    C. Not to start measures that prolong dying
    D. Never to activate the EMS system for a person

25. If the doctor writes a "Do Not Resuscitate" (DNR) order, it means that
    A. The person will not be resuscitated
    B. The person will be resuscitated if it is an emergency
    C. The doctor will decide whether or not to resuscitate
    D. The RN decides in some situations that resuscitation is needed

26. What is a sign that death is near?
    A. Deep, rapid respirations
    B. Body temperature changes
    C. Muscles tense and contract in spasms
    D. Peristalsis increases

27. When the family wishes to see the body after death, it should
    A. Remain exactly as the person was at death
    B. Be positioned to appear comfortable and natural
    C. Be viewed in a cheerful and well-lit room
    D. Be placed in a semi-Fowler's position

28. In performing post-mortem care, you turn the body and you hear air being expelled from the mouth. How do you interpret this?
    A. The person is still breathing. You must quickly get the nurse.
    B. Decaying tissues are causing bloating of intestinal organs
    C. Cardiopulmonary resuscitation should be initiated
    D. Moving the body has caused trapped air to be expelled.

29. When you are assisting with post-mortem care, you should
    A. Place the body in a side-lying position
    B. Tape all jewelry in place
    C. Gently pull eyelids over the eyes
    D. Dress the person in his or her regular clothing

30. One ID tag from the post-mortem kit is attached to the body, usually the right big toe or ankle. Where is the second ID tag attached?
    A. Person's dentures
    B. Shroud, body bag, or sheet
    C. Opposite toe or ankle
    D. Bag of jewelry and other belongings

Fill in the Blank

31. Write out the abbreviations.
    A. DNR _____
    B. ID _____
    C. OBRA _____

32. It is important to examine your own feelings about death because they will affect _____.

33. When you understand the dying process, you can approach the dying person with _____ _____.

34. Hospice care focuses on these needs of the dying person and families.
    A. _____
    B. _____
    C. _____
    D. _____

35. Religious beliefs strengthen when dying and often provide _____ _____.

36. Adults fear death because they fear
    A. _____ and _____
    B. Dying _____
    C. Invasion _____
    D. _____ and _____ from loved ones
    E. _____ and _____ of those left behind

37. Name the 5 stages of dying.
    A. _____
    B. _____
    C. _____
    D. _____
    E. _____

38. The goals of comfort needs are
    A. _____
    B. _____

39. When caring for a dying person, do not ask questions that need long answers because _____.

40. Because crusting and irritation of the nostrils can occur, you should _____ _____.

41. What kinds of elimination problems can occur in the dying person?
    A. _____ and _____ incontinence
    B. _____
    C. _____ retention

42. The Patient Self-Determination Act and OBRA give 2 rights that affect the rights of a dying person. They are
    A. _____
    B. _____

43. A living will instructs doctors
    A. _____
    B. _____

44. When a person cannot make health care decisions, the authority to do so is given to the person with
    _____.

45. What are the signs that death is near?
    A. _____
    B. _____
    C. _____
    D. _____
    E. _____
    F. _____

46. The signs of death include no _____ _____. The pupils are _____ and _____.

47. When assisting with post-mortem care, what information do you need from the nurse?
    A. _____
    B. _____
    C. _____
    D. _____
    E. _____

Optional Learning Exercises

You are assigned to care for Mrs. Adams, who is dying. Answer the questions regarding this situation.

48. You find Mrs. Adams crying in her room. When you ask her what is wrong, she tells you no one gave her fresh water this morning and she has not had her bath yet. She tells you just to go away. What stage of dying is she displaying? _____

49. Later in the day, Mrs. Adams tells you she can't wait until she is better to go home and plant her garden. She states that she knows the tests done last week were wrong and she will recover quickly from her illness. Now what stage is she displaying?
    _____ Why is she displaying 2 different stages so rapidly? _____

50. A minister comes to visit Mrs. Adams while you are giving care. What should you do?
    _____

51. You are working one night and find Mrs. Adams awake during the night. She asks you to sit with her. She begins to talk about her fears, worries, and anxieties. What are 2 things you can do to convey caring to her?
    _____
    _____

52. Mrs. Adams dies while you are working and the nurse asks you to assist with post-mortem care. As you clean soiled areas, you assist the nurse to turn the body and air is expelled. This occurs because
    _____
    _____.

53. You wear gloves during post-mortem care to protect yourself from _____.

Use the FOCUS ON PRIDE section to complete these statements and then use the critical thinking and discussion questions to develop your ideas.

54. You are giving quality care to a dying person when you
    A. _____
    B. _____
    C. _____
    D. _____

Critical Thinking and Discussion Questions

55. You are assisting in the care of a person who is dying. Initially, the person and the family were grateful for the care, but over the past week, the daughter has become increasingly unhappy and dissatisfied with everything that the staff tries to do. Today as you are doing helping with morning hygiene, the daughter says, "You are being too rough with her!"
    A. What would you do?
    B. What could contribute to the daughter's feelings of dissatisfaction and unhappiness in the past week?

56. Another nursing assistant was with a favorite resident and her family when the woman died. The nursing assistant posted a moving commentary about the last moments of the woman's life and the family's reaction on social media. Several staff members agreed that the woman will be missed and that the posted tribute reflected the staff's affection for the woman. However, the facility administration and the nursing supervisor decide to put the nursing assistant on suspension pending investigation of the incident. Why did the nursing assistant receive such a harsh reprimand?

Fill in the Blank: Key Terms

Discrimination
Job application
Job interview

Reasonable
accommodation

1. When an employer asks a job applicant questions about his or her education and career, it is a

   _____.

2. An agency's official form listing questions that require factual answers from the person seeking employment is a _____.

3. Unjust treatment based on age, race, gender, and other personal qualities is _____.

4. To assist or change a position or workplace to allow an employee to do his or her job despite having a disability is _____.

Circle the Best Answer

5. Displaying good work ethics at your clinical experience site may help you find a job because
   A. You will pass the course
   B. It shows you are ethical
   C. You will get better grades
   D. Students are seen as future employees

6. What is the most important reason to be well-groomed when looking for a job?
   A. Shows you are cooperative and dependable
   B. Shows that you are concerned about first impressions
   C. Shows that you have the needed knowledge and skills
   D. Shows you have values and attitudes that fit with the agency

7. How does an employer know you can perform required job skills?
   A. They request proof of NATCEP completion and check the nursing assistant registry.
   B. They will ask you to give a demonstration of your skills.
   C. You will be asked many questions about performing certain skills.
   D. You will be required to take and pass a written test.

8. During an interview, which question is allowed by the Equal Opportunity Commission?
   A. Which religious holidays would do you observe?
   B. Have you ever had a substance abuse problem?
   C. Who will take care of your children while you are at work?
   D. Tell me about your last job; why did you leave?

9. You are filling out a job application. What information do you need to have about each of your references?
   A. Name, title, address, and phone number
   B. Age, birth date, state of residence
   C. Nature and duration of your relationship
   D. Their qualifications to be your reference

10. You should take a dry run to a job interview to
    A. Show you follow directions well
    B. Show that you are eager to work there
    C. Know how long it takes to get to the agency
    D. Look over the center to see if you want to work there

11. When you are interviewing, it is correct to
    A. Compliment the interviewer's appearance
    B. Look directly at the interviewer
    C. Ask for water if you feel very nervous
    D. Convey animation and energy in your gestures

12. What is a good way to share your list of skills with the interviewer?
    A. Tell the person verbally what you can do
    B. Ask for a list of skills and check the ones you know
    C. Prepare a list of your skills and give it to the interviewer
    D. Tell the interviewer you will send a list as soon as possible

13. What is the most important reason for you to ask questions at the end of the interview?
    A. Demonstrates your interests in taking the job
    B. Helps you to decide if the job is right for you
    C. Shows you have good communication skills
    D. Helps you to anticipate problems related to the job

14. After an interview, it is advised that you
    A. Send a thank you note within 24 hours of the interview
    B. Call the interviewer every day to see if you are being hired
    C. Wait for the employer to contact you
    D. Call one week after the interview to thank the person for the interview

Fill in the Blank

15. Write out the abbreviations.
    A. EEOC _____
    B. NATCEP _____
    C. OBRA _____

16. List 9 places you can find out about jobs.
    A. _____
    B. _____
    C. _____
    D. _____
    E. _____
    F. _____
    G. _____
    H. _____
    I. _____

17. When an employer requests proof of successful NATCEP completion, which items do you need?
    A. _____
    B. _____
    C. _____

18. When a section on a job application does not apply to you, you should _____
    _____.

19. List four reasons that could explain employment gaps.
    A. _____
    B. _____
    C. _____
    D. _____

20. If you lie on a job application, it is _____. If you do this, what can happen? _____
    _____

21. Which items do you need to provide when completing a job application?
    A. _____
    B. _____
    C. _____
    D. _____

22. When you fill out a job application, it is easier to complete if you have a file that contains
    A. _____
    B. _____
    C. _____
    D. _____
    E. _____
    F. _____
    G. _____
    H. _____
    I. _____
    J. _____

Optional Learning Experiences

Applying for a Job in Home Care

23. When the RN is not at the bedside to help you if problems occur, you are expected to be able to
    _____.

24. When you arrive at a person's home on time, you are using _____.
    What temptations should be avoided when you are giving home care? _____
    _____

25. When you shop for a person, what should you accurately report to the person or family? _____
    _____.

26. What questions should you ask if you are interviewing for a job in home care?
    A. _____
    B. _____
    C. _____
    D. _____
    E. _____
    F. _____

Use the FOCUS ON PRIDE section to complete these statements and then use the critical thinking and discussion question to develop your ideas.

27. Application and interview questions must relate to your _____ to do the job.

28. _____, _____, and interview questions help agencies decide if an applicant will meet safety and ethical standards.

Critical Thinking and Discussion Questions

29. A. What type of job setting would be your first preference?
    B. Why is that setting your first choice?
    C. What can you do to seek out that type of job?

Relieving Choking—Adult or Child (Over 1 Year of Age)

Name: _____ Date: _____

Procedure	S	U	Comments

Procedure

1. Asked the person if he or she was choking.
   a. If the person was coughing or talking, stayed with person and encouraged coughing to expel object.   _____ _____ _____
   b. *If the person was unresponsive*, and the cause unknown. Called for help and began CPR.   _____ _____ _____
   c. *If the person nodded "yes" and could not talk*, continued to step 2.   _____ _____ _____
2. Had someone call for help.
   a. *In a public area*, had someone call 911 to activate the EMS system. Sent someone to get an automated external defibrillator (AED).   _____ _____ _____
   b. *In an agency*, had someone call the agency's RRS and sent someone to get the defibrillator (AED).   _____ _____ _____
3. Gave abdominal thrusts.
   a. Stood or knelt behind the person.   _____ _____ _____
   b. Wrapped your arms around the person's waist.   _____ _____ _____
   c. Made fist with 1 hand.   _____ _____ _____
   d. Placed the thumb side of the fist against the abdomen. The fist was slightly above the navel in the middle of the abdomen and well below the end of the sternum (breastbone).   _____ _____ _____
   e. Grasped your fist with your other hand.   _____ _____ _____
   f. Pressed your fist into the abdomen with a quick, upward thrust.
   g. Repeated thrusts until the object was expelled or the person became unresponsive.   _____ _____ _____
4. *If the object was dislodged,* encouraged hospital care. Injuries could occur from abdominal thrusts.   _____ _____ _____
5. *If the person became unresponsive,*
   a. Lowered the person to the floor. Positioned the person supine (lying flat on the back).   _____ _____ _____
   b. Made sure the EMS or RRS was called.   _____ _____ _____
      1) *If alone with a phone*, called while giving care.
      2) *If alone without a phone*, gave about 2 minutes of CPR first. Then called the EMS or RRS.   _____ _____ _____
   c. Started CPR. Did not check for a pulse.
      1) Gave 30 chest compressions.   _____ _____ _____
      2) Opened the airway with the head tilt–chin lift method. Opened the person's mouth wide open. Looked for an object. Removed the object if you saw it and removed it easily.   _____ _____ _____
      3) Gave 2 breaths.   _____ _____ _____
      4) Continued cycles of 30 compressions, followed by 2 breaths. Looked for an object every time you opened the airway.   _____ _____ _____

Procedure—cont'd	S	U	Comments

d) *If choking is relieved*, checked for a response, breathing, and a pulse. (NOTE: Choking is relieved when you feel air move and see the chest rise and fall when giving breaths.)

1) *If no response, no normal breathing, and no pulse—* continued CPR. Used the AED as soon as possible.

2) *If no response and no normal breathing but there was a pulse—*gave rescue breaths. For an adult, gave 1 breath every 5 to 6 seconds. For a child, gave 1 breath every 3 to 5 seconds. Checked for a pulse every 2 minutes. If no pulse, began CPR.

3) *If the person had normal breathing and a pulse—* placed the person in the recovery position if there was no response. Continued to check the person until help arrived. Encouraged hospital care.

Relieving Choking—In the Infant (Less Than 1 Year of Age)

Name: _____ Date: _____

Procedure	S	U	Comments
1. Had someone call for help.			
a. *In a public area,* had someone activate the EMS systems by calling 911. Sent someone to get an AED.	_____	_____	_____
b. *In an agency,* had someone call the agency's RRS and got a defibrillator (AED).	_____	_____	_____
2. Knelt next to the infant. Or sat with the infant in your lap.	_____	_____	_____
3. Exposed the infant's chest and back. Performed this step only if it was done easily.	_____	_____	_____
4. Held the infant face down over your forearm. (Supported your arm on your thigh or lap.) The infant's head was lower than the chest. Supported the head and jaw with your hand.	_____	_____	_____
5. Gave up to 5 forceful back slaps (back blows). Used the heel of your hand. Gave the back slaps between the shoulder blades. (Stopped the back slaps if the object was expelled.)	_____	_____	_____
6. Turned the infant as a unit.			
a. Continued to support the infant's face, jaw, head, neck, and chest with 1 hand.	_____	_____	_____
b. Supported the back and the back of the infant's head with your other hand. Your palm supported the back of the head.	_____	_____	_____
c. Turned the infant as a unit. The infant was in a back-lying position on your forearm. Your forearm rested on your thigh. The infant's head was lower than the chest.	_____	_____	_____
7. Gave up to 5 chest thrusts. The chest thrusts were quick and downward.			
a. Placed 2 fingers in the center of the chest just below the nipple line.	_____	_____	_____
b. Gave chest thrusts at a rate of about 1 every second.	_____	_____	_____
c. Stopped chest thrusts if the object was expelled.	_____	_____	_____
8. Continued giving 5 back slaps followed by 5 chest thrusts until the object was expelled or the infant became unresponsive.	_____	_____	_____
9. *If the infant became unresponsive:*			
a. Sent someone to activate the EMS system or RRS if not already done. If alone, did the following:	_____	_____	_____
1) *If alone with a phone,* called while giving care.	_____	_____	_____
2) If alone without a phone, gave about 2 minutes of CPR first. Then called the EMS or RRS and got an AED.	_____	_____	_____
b. Placed the infant on a firm, flat surface.	_____	_____	_____
c. Started CPR. Did not check for a pulse. Gave 30 compressions.	_____	_____	_____
d. Opened the airway. Used the head tilt–chin lift method. Opened the infant's mouth. Looked for an object. Removed the object if you saw it and could remove it easily. Used your fingers.	_____	_____	_____
e. Gave 2 breaths.	_____	_____	_____
f. Continued cycles of 30 compressions and 2 breaths. Looked for an object. Removed the object if you saw it and could remove it easily. Used your fingers.	_____	_____	_____
g. Continued CPR until help arrived or until choking was relieved.	_____	_____	_____

Using a Fire Extinguisher

Name: _____ Date: _____

Procedure	S	U	Comments
1. Pulled the fire alarm.	____	____	_____
2. Got the nearest fire extinguisher.	____	____	_____
3. Carried it upright.	____	____	_____
4. Took it to the fire.	____	____	_____
5. Followed the word *PASS*.			
a. *P*—for *pull the safety pin*. This unlocked the handle.	____	____	_____
b. *A*—for *aim low*. Directed the hose or nozzle at the base of the fire. Did not try to spray the tops of the flames.	____	____	_____
c. *S*—for *squeeze the lever*. Squeezed or pushed down on the lever, handle, or button to start the stream. Released the lever, handle, or button to stop the stream.	____	____	_____
d. *S*—for *sweep back and forth*. Swept the stream back and forth (side to side) at the base of the fire.	____	____	_____

Using a Transfer/Gait Belt

Name: _____   Date: _____

Procedure	S	U	Comments

Quality of Life
- Knocked before entering the person's room.
- Addressed the person by name.
- Introduced yourself by name and title.
- Explained the procedure before starting and during the procedure.
- Protected the person's rights during the procedure.
- Handled the person gently during the procedure.

Pre-Procedure
1. Saw *Promoting Safety and Comfort: Transfer/Gait Belts.*
2. Practiced hand hygiene.
3. Obtained a transfer/gait belt of the correct type and size.
4. Identified the person. Checked the identification (ID) bracelet against the assignment sheet. Used 2 identifiers. Also called the person by name.
5. Provided for privacy.

Procedure
6. Assisted the person to sitting position.
7. Applied the belt. Held the belt by the buckle. Wrapped the belt around the person's waist over clothing. Did not apply it over bare skin.
    a. *For a belt with a metal buckle:*
        1) Inserted the belt's metal tip into the buckle. Passed the belt through the side with the teeth first.
        2) Brought the belt tip across the front of the buckle. Inserted the tip through the buckle's smooth side.
    b. *For a belt with a quick release buckle,* pushed the belt ends together to secure the buckle.
8. Tightened the belt so it was snug. It did not cause discomfort or impair breathing. You were able to slide your open, flat hand under the belt. Asked about the person's comfort. If the belt was too loose or too tight, adjusted the belt as needed.
9. Made sure that the person's breasts were not caught under the belt.
10. Placed the buckle off-center in the front or off-center in the back for the person's comfort. A quick release buckle was turned around to the back out of the person's reach. The buckle was not over the spine.
11. Tucked any excess strap into the belt.
12. Completed the transfer or ambulation procedure. Grasped the belt from underneath with 2 hands. Or grasped the belt by the handles.

Post-Procedure   S   U   **Comments**

13. Removed the belt after completing the transfer or
    ambulation. The person was not left alone wearing
    the belt.   _____   _____   _____
    a. *For a belt with a metal buckle:*
       1) Brought the belt strap back through the buckle's
          smooth side.   _____   _____   _____
       2) Pulled the belt through the side with the teeth.   _____   _____   _____
    b. *For a belt with a quick release buckle,* pushed inward
       on the quick release buttons.   _____   _____   _____
    c. Removed the belt from the person's waist. Did not
       drag the belt across the waist.   _____   _____   _____
14. Provided for comfort.   _____   _____   _____
15. Placed the call light and other needed items within
    reach.   _____   _____   _____
16. Unscreened the person.   _____   _____   _____
17. Completed a safety check of the room.   _____   _____   _____
18. Returned the transfer/gait belt to its proper place.   _____   _____   _____
19. Practiced hand hygiene.   _____   _____   _____
20. Reported and recorded your observations.   _____   _____   _____

Helping the Falling Person

Name: _____ Date: _____

Procedure	S	U	Comments
1. Stood behind the person with your feet apart. Kept your back straight.	_____	_____	_____
2. Brought the person close to your body as fast as possible. Used the transfer/gait belt. Or wrapped your arms around the person's waist. If necessary, you held the person under the arms.	_____	_____	_____
3. Moved your leg so the person's buttocks rested on it. Moved your leg that is near the person.	_____	_____	_____
4. Lowered the person to the floor. The person slid down your leg to the floor. Bent at your hips and knees as you lowered the person.	_____	_____	_____
5. Called a nurse to check the person. Stayed with the person.	_____	_____	_____
6. Helped the nurse return the person to bed. Asked other staff to help, if needed.	_____	_____	_____

Post-Procedure

	S	U	Comments
7. Provided for comfort.	_____	_____	_____
8. Placed the call light and other needed items within reach.	_____	_____	_____
9. Raised or lowered bed rails. Followed the care plan.	_____	_____	_____
10. Completed a safety check of the room.	_____	_____	_____
11. Practiced hand hygiene.	_____	_____	_____
12. Reported and recorded the following:			
• How the fall occurred	_____	_____	_____
• How far the person walked	_____	_____	_____
• How activity was tolerated before the fall	_____	_____	_____
• Complaints before the fall	_____	_____	_____
• How much help the person needed while walking	_____	_____	_____
13. Completed an incident report.	_____	_____	_____

Applying Restraints

Name: _____   Date: _____

Procedure	S	U	Comments

Quality of Life

- Knocked before entering the person's room.
- Addressed the person by name.
- Introduced yourself by name and title.
- Explained the procedure before starting and during the procedure.
- Protected the person's rights during the procedure.
- Handled the person gently during the procedure.

Pre-Procedure

1. Followed *Delegation Guidelines: Applying Restraints.* Saw *Promoting Safety and Comfort: Safe Restraint Use* and *Applying Restraints.*
2. Collected the following as instructed by the nurse.
   - Correct type and size of restraint
   - Padding for skin and bony areas
   - Bed rail pads or gap protectors (if needed)
3. Practiced hand hygiene.
4. Identified the person. Checked the ID (identification) bracelet against the assignment sheet. Used 2 identifiers. Also called the person by name.
5. Provided for privacy.

Procedure

6. Positioned the person for comfort and good alignment.
7. Placed the bed rail pads or gap protectors (if needed) on the bed if the person was in bed. Followed the manufacturer's instructions.
8. Padded bony areas. Followed the nurse's instructions and the care plan.
9. Read and followed the manufacturer's instructions. Noted the front and back of the restraint.
10. *For limb holders to the wrist:*
    a. Placed the soft or foam part toward the skin.
    b. Secured the holder so it was snug but not tight. Made sure you could slide 1 finger under the holder. Adjusted the straps if the holder was too loose or too tight. Checked for snugness again.
    c. Secured the straps to the movable part of the bed frame out of the person's reach. Used the buckle or quick release knot.
    d. Repeated the following for the other wrist.
       1) Placed the soft or foam part toward the skin.
       2) Secured the restraint so it was snug but not tight. Made sure you could slide 1 finger under the restraint. Adjusted the straps if the restraint was too loose or too tight. Checked for snugness again.
       3) Secured the straps to the movable part of the bed frame out of the person's reach. Used the buckle or quick release knot.
11. *For mitt restraints:*
    a. Cleaned and dried the person's hands.
    b. Inserted the person's hand into the restraint with the palm down.

Procedure—cont'd	S	U	Comments

c. Wrapped the wrist strap around the smallest part of the wrist. Secured the strap with the hook-and-loop or other closure.

d. Secured the restraint to the bed if directed to do so. Secured the straps to the movable part of the bed frame out of the person's reach. Used the buckle or a quick-release tie.

e. Checked for snugness. Slid 1 finger between the restraint and the wrist. Adjusted the straps if the restraint was too loose or too tight. Checked for snugness again.

f. Repeated the following for the other hand.

  1) Inserted the person's hand into the restraint with the palm down.

  2) Wrapped the wrist strap around the smallest part of the wrist. Secured the strap with the hook-and-loop or other closure.

  3) Secured the restraint to the bed if directed to do so. Secured the straps to the movable part of the bed frame out of the person's reach. Used the buckle or a quick-release tie.

  4) Checked for snugness. Slid 1 finger between the restraint and the wrist. Adjusted the straps if the restraint was too loose or too tight. Checked for snugness again.

12. *For a belt restraint:*

  a. Assisted the person to a sitting position.

  b. Applied the restraint.

  c. Removed wrinkles or creases from the front and back.

  d. Brought the ties through the slots in the back.

  e. Positioned the straps at a 45-degree angle between the wheelchair seat and sides. If in bed, helped the person lie down.

  f. Made sure the person was comfortable and in good alignment.

  g. Secured the straps to the movable part of the bed frame. Used the buckle or a quick release knot. The buckle or knot was out of the person's reach. For a wheelchair, criss-crossed and secured the straps.

  h. Checked for snugness. Slid an open hand between the restraint and the person. Adjusted the restraint if it was too loose or too tight. Checked for snugness again.

13. *For a vest restraint:*

  a. Assisted the person to a sitting position. If in a wheelchair:

    1) Person was as far back in the wheelchair as possible.

    2) Buttocks were against the chair back.

  b. Applied the restraint. The "V" neck was in front.

  c. Brought the straps through the slots if the vest criss-crossed.

  d. Ensured that side seams were under the arms. Removed wrinkles in the front and back. Closed the zipper or fastened with other closures.

  e. Positioned the straps at a 45-degree angle between the wheelchair seat and sides. If in bed, helped the person lie down.

  f. Made sure the person was comfortable and in good alignment.

Procedure—cont'd	**S**	**U**	**Comments**

Procedure—cont'd

g. Secured the straps to the movable part of the bed frame at waist level. Used the buckle or a quick release knot. The buckle or knot was out of the person's reach. For a wheelchair, criss-crossed and secured the straps. _____ _____ _____

h. Checked for snugness. Slid an open hand between the restraint and the person. Adjusted the restraint if it was too loose or too tight. Checked for snugness again. _____ _____ _____

14. *For a jacket restraint:*
    a. Assisted the person to a sitting position. If in a wheelchair:
       1) Person was as far back in the wheelchair as possible. _____ _____ _____
       2) Buttocks were against the chair back. _____ _____ _____
    b. Applied the restraint. The jacket opening went in the back. _____ _____ _____
    c. Made sure the side seams were under the arms. Removed wrinkles in the front and back._____
    d. Closed the back with the zipper or other closures. _____ _____ _____
    e. Positioned the straps at a 45-degree angle between the wheelchair seat and sides. If in bed, helped the person lie down. _____ _____ _____
    f. Made sure the person was comfortable and in good alignment. _____ _____ _____
    g. Secured the straps to the movable part of the bed frame at waist level. Used the buckle or quick release knot. The buckle or knot was out of the person's reach. For a wheelchair, criss-crossed and secured the straps. _____ _____ _____
    h. Checked for snugness. Slid an open hand between the restraint and the person. Adjusted the restraint if it was too loose or too tight. Checked for snugness again. _____ _____ _____

15. *For elbow restraints:*
    a. Released the adjustment straps (hook-and-loop). _____ _____ _____
    b. Placed buckles towards the person _____ _____ _____
    c. Wrapped a splint over 1 arm. The splint was centered over the elbow. Opening was towards the inside of the arm.
    d. Secured the splint by following the manufacturer's instructions. Used the clips provided by the manufacturer if secured the splint to a sleeve. _____ _____ _____
    e. Checked for snugness. Slid 2 fingers between the splint and the person's arm. Adjusted the splint if it was too loose or too tight. Checked for snugness again. _____ _____ _____
    f. Repeated for the other arm:
       1) Released the adjustment straps (hook-and-loop). _____ _____ _____
       2) Placed buckles towards the person
       3) Wrapped a splint over 1 arm. The splint was centered over the elbow. Opening was towards the inside of the arm. _____ _____ _____
       4) Secured the splint by following the manufacturer's instructions. Used the clips provided by the manufacturer to secure the splint to the sleeve.
       5) Checked for snugness. Slid 2 fingers between the splint and the person's arm. Adjusted the splint if it was too loose or too tight. Checked for snugness again. _____ _____ _____

Post-Procedure

	S	U	Comments
16. Positioned the person as the nurse directed.	_____	_____	_____
17. Provided for comfort.	_____	_____	_____
18. Placed the call light and other need items within the person's reach.	_____	_____	_____
19. Raised or lowered bed rails. Followed the care plan and the manufacturer's instructions for restraints.	_____	_____	_____
20. Unscreened the person.	_____	_____	_____
21. Completed a safety check of the room.	_____	_____	_____
22. Practiced hand hygiene.	_____	_____	_____

23. Checked the person and the restraint at least every 15 minutes or as often as directed by the nurse and the care plan. Reported and recorded your observations.

	S	U	Comments
a. *For wrist holders, mitt restraints, or elbow splints:* checked the pulse, color, and temperature of restrained parts.	_____	_____	_____
b. *For vest, jacket, or belt restraint:* checked the person's breathing. Made sure the restraint was properly positioned in the front and back. *Released the restraint and called for the nurse at once if the person was not breathing or was having problems breathing.*	_____	_____	_____

24. Did the following at least every 2 hours for at least 10 minutes.

	S	U	Comments
a. Removed or released the restraint.	_____	_____	_____
b. Measured vital signs.	_____	_____	_____
c. Re-positioned the person.	_____	_____	_____
d. Met food, fluid, hygiene, and elimination needs.	_____	_____	_____
e. Gave skin care.	_____	_____	_____
f. Performed ROM exercises or helped the person walk. Followed the care plan.	_____	_____	_____
g. Provided for physical and emotional support.	_____	_____	_____
h. Re-applied the restraint.	_____	_____	_____
25. Completed a safety check of the room.	_____	_____	_____
26. Practiced hand hygiene.	_____	_____	_____
27. Reported and recorded your observations and the care given.	_____	_____	_____

Hand-Washing

Name: _____   Date: _____

Procedure	S	U	Comments
1. Saw *Promoting Safety and Comfort: Hand Hygiene.*	___	___	_____
2. Made sure you had soap, paper towels, an orangewood stick or nail file, and a wastebasket. Collected missing items.	___	___	_____
3. Pushed your watch up your arm 4 to 5 inches. Pushed long uniform sleeves up too.	___	___	_____
4. Stood away from the sink so your clothes did not touch the sink. Stood so the soap and faucet were easy to reach. Did not touch the inside of the sink at any time.	___	___	_____
5. Turned on and adjusted the water until it felt warm.	___	___	_____
6. Wet your wrists and hands. Kept your hands lower than your elbows. Was sure to wet the area 3 to 4 inches above your wrists.	___	___	_____
7. Applied about 1 teaspoon of soap to your hands.	___	___	_____
8. Rubbed your palms together and interlaced your fingers to work up a good lather. Lathered your wrists, hands, and fingers. Kept your hands lower than your elbows. This step should have lasted at least 15 to 20 seconds.	___	___	_____
9. Washed each hand and wrist thoroughly. Cleaned the back of your fingers and between your fingers.	___	___	_____
10. Cleaned under the fingernails. Rubbed your fingernails against your palms.	___	___	_____
11. Cleaned under the fingernails with a nail file or orangewood stick. Did this for the first hand hygiene of the day and when your hands were highly soiled.	___	___	_____
12. Rinsed your wrists, hands, and fingers well. Water flowed from above the wrists to your fingertips.	___	___	_____
13. Repeated steps 7 through 12, if needed.			
a. Applied about 1 teaspoon of soap to your hands.	___	___	_____
b. Rubbed your palms together and interlaced your fingers to work up a good lather. Lathered your wrists, hands, and fingers. Kept your hands lower than your elbows. This step should have lasted at least 15 to 20 seconds.	___	___	_____
c. Washed each hand and wrist thoroughly. Cleaned the back of your fingers and between your fingers.	___	___	_____
d. Cleaned under the fingernails. Rubbed your fingertips against your palms.	___	___	_____
e. Cleaned under the fingernails with a nail file or orangewood stick. Did this for the first hand-washing of the day and when your hands were highly soiled.	___	___	_____
f. Rinsed your wrists, hands, and fingers well. Water flowed from above the wrists to your fingertips.	___	___	_____
14. Dried your fingers, hands, and wrists with clean, dry paper towels. Patted dry starting at your fingertips.	___	___	_____
15. Discarded the paper towels into the wastebasket.	___	___	_____
16. Turned off faucets with clean, dry paper towels. This prevented you from contaminating your hands. Used a clean paper towel for each faucet. Or used knee or foot controls to turn off the faucet.	___	___	_____
17. Discarded the paper towels into the wastebasket.	___	___	_____

Using an Alcohol-Based Hand Sanitizer

Name: _____   Date: _____

Procedure	S	U	Comments
1. Saw *Promoting Safety and Comfort: Hand Hygiene*.	____	____	_____
2. Applied a palmful of an alcohol-based hand sanitizer into a cupped hand.	____	____	_____
3. Rubbed your palms together.	____	____	_____
4. Rubbed the palm of 1 hand over the back of the other. Did the same for the other hand.	____	____	_____
5. Rubbed your palms together with your fingers interlaced.	____	____	_____
6. Interlocked your fingers. Rubbed your fingers back and forth.	____	____	_____
7. Rubbed the thumb of 1 hand into the palm of the other. Did the same for the other thumb.	____	____	_____
8. Rubbed the fingers of 1 hand into the palm of the other hand. Used a circular motion. Did the same for the fingers of the other hand.	____	____	_____
9. Continued rubbing your hands until they were dry.	____	____	_____

Sterile Gloving

Name: _____   Date: _____

Procedure	S	U	Comments
1. Followed *Delegation Guidelines: Assisting With Sterile Procedures.* Saw *Promoting Safety and Comfort:*			
a. *Assisting With Sterile Procedures*	_____	_____	_____
b. *Sterile Gloving*	_____	_____	_____
2. Practiced hand hygiene.	_____	_____	_____
3. Inspected the package of sterile gloves for sterility.			
a. Checked the expiration date.	_____	_____	_____
b. Saw if the package was dry.	_____	_____	_____
c. Checked for tears, holes, punctures, and watermarks.	_____	_____	_____
4. Created a work surface with enough room.	_____	_____	_____
a. Arranged the work surface at waist level and within your vision.	_____	_____	_____
b. Cleaned and dried the work surface.	_____	_____	_____
c. Did not reach over or turn your back on the work surface.	_____	_____	_____
5. Opened the package. Grasped the flaps. Gently peeled them back.	_____	_____	_____
6. Removed the inner package. Placed it on your work surface.	_____	_____	_____
7. Noted the labels on the inner package– *left, right, up,* and *down.*	_____	_____	_____
8. Arranged the inner package for left, right, up, and down. Left glove was on your left. Right glove was on your right. The cuffs were near you, the fingers pointed away from you.	_____	_____	_____
9. Grasped the folded edges of the inner package. Used the thumb and index finger of each hand.	_____	_____	_____
10. Folded back the inner package to expose the gloves. Did not touch or otherwise contaminate the inside package or the gloves. The inside of the inner package was a sterile field.	_____	_____	_____
11. Noted that each glove had a cuff about 2 to 3 inches wide. The cuffs and insides of the gloves were *not sterile.*	_____	_____	_____
12. Put on the right glove if you were right-handed. Put on the left glove if you were left-handed.			
a. Picked up the glove with your other hand. Used your thumb and index and middle fingers.	_____	_____	_____
b. Touched only the cuff and the inside of the glove.	_____	_____	_____
c. Turned the hand to be gloved palm side up.	_____	_____	_____
d. Lifted the cuff up. Slid your fingers and hand into the glove.	_____	_____	_____
e. Pulled the glove up over your hand. If some fingers got stuck, left them that way until the other glove was on. *Did not use your ungloved hand to straighten the glove. Did not let the outside of the glove touch any non-sterile surface.*	_____	_____	_____
f. Left the cuff turned down.	_____	_____	_____
13. Put on the other glove. Used your gloved hand.			
a. Reached under the cuff of the second glove. Used the 4 fingers of your gloved hand. Kept your gloved thumb close to your gloved palm.	_____	_____	_____
b. Put on the second glove. Your gloved hand did not touch the cuff or any surface. Held the thumb of your first gloved hand away from the second gloved palm.	_____	_____	_____

Procedure—cont'd

	S	U	Comments
14. Adjusted each glove with the other hand. The gloves were smooth and comfortable.	_____	_____	_____
15. Slid your fingers under the cuffs to pull them up.	_____	_____	_____
16. Touched only sterile items.	_____	_____	_____
17. Removed and discarded the gloves.	_____	_____	_____
18. Practiced hand hygiene.	_____	_____	_____

Donning and Removing Personal Protective Equipment (PPE)

Name: _____   Date: _____

Procedure	S	U	Comments
1. Followed *Delegation Guidelines: Transmission-Based Precautions*. Saw *Promoting Safety and Comfort:*			
a. *Transmission-Based Precautions*			
b. *Goggles and Face Shields*			
c. *Gloves*			
d. *Donning and Removing PPE*			
2. Removed your watch and all jewelry.			
3. Rolled up uniform sleeves.			
4. Practiced hand hygiene.			
5. Put on a gown.			
a. Held a clean gown out in front of you.			
b. Unfolded the gown. Faced the back of the gown. Did not shake it.			
c. Put your hands and arms through the sleeves.			
d. Made sure the gown covered you from your neck to your knees. It covered your arms to the end of your wrists.			
e. Tied the strings at the back of the neck.			
f. Overlapped the back of the gown. Made sure it covered your uniform. The gown was snug, not loose.			
g. Tied the waist strings. Tied them at the back or the side. Did not tie them in front.			
6. Put on a mask or respirator.			
a. Picked up a mask by its upper ties. Did not touch the part that covered your face.			
b. Placed the mask over your nose and mouth.			
c. Placed the upper strings above your ears. Tied them at the back in the middle of your head.			
d. Tied the lower strings at the back of your neck. The lower part of the mask was under your chin.			
e. Pinched the metal band around your nose. The top of the mask was snug over your nose. If you wore eyeglasses, the mask was snug under the bottom of the eyeglasses.			
f. Made sure the mask was snug over your face and under your chin.			
7. Put on goggles or a face shield (if needed and was not part of the mask).			
a. Placed the device over your face and eyes.			
b. Adjusted the device to fit.			
8. Put on gloves. Made sure the gloves covered the wrists of the gown.			
9. Provided care.			
10. Removed and discarded the PPE. Practiced hand hygiene between each step if your hands became contaminated.			
a. *Method 1: Gloves, goggles, or face shield, gown, mask or respirator.*			
1) Removed and discarded the gloves.			
a) Made sure that glove touched only glove.			
b) Grasped a glove at the palm. Grasped it on the outside.			
c) Pulled the glove down over your hand so it was inside out.			

Procedure—cont'd	S	U	Comments
d) Held the removed glove with your other gloved hand.	___	___	_____
e) Reached inside the other glove. Used the first 2 fingers of the ungloved hand.	___	___	_____
f) Pulled the glove down (inside out) over your hand and the other glove.	___	___	_____
g) Discarded the gloves.	___	___	_____
2) Removed and discarded the goggles or face shield if worn.			
a) Lifted the headband or earpieces from the back. Did not touch the front of the device.	___	___	_____
b) Discarded the device. If re-usable, followed agency policy.	___	___	_____
3) Removed and discarded the gown. Did not touch the outside of the gown.			
a) Untied the neck and then the waist strings.	___	___	_____
b) Pulled the gown down and away from your neck and shoulders. Only touched the inside of the gown.	___	___	_____
c) Turned the gown inside out as it was removed. Held it at the inside shoulder seams and brought your hands together.	___	___	_____
d) Folded or rolled up the gown away from you. Kept it inside out. Did not let the gown touch the floor.	___	___	_____
e) Discarded the gown.	___	___	_____
4) Removed and discarded the mask if worn. (Note: Removed a respirator after leaving the room and closing the door.)			
a) Untied the lower strings of the mask.	___	___	_____
b) Untied the top strings.	___	___	_____
c) Held the top strings. Removed the mask.	___	___	_____
d) Discarded the mask.	___	___	_____
b. *Method 2: Gown and gloves, goggles or face shield, mask or respirator.*			
1) Removed and discarded the gown and gloves.			
a) Grasped the gown in front with your gloved hands. Pulled away from your body so the ties broke. Only touched the outside of the gown.	___	___	_____
b) Folded or rolled the gown inside out into a bundle while removing the gown. Kept it inside-out. Did not let the gown touch the floor.	___	___	_____
c) Peeled off your gloves as you removed the gown. Only touched the inside of the gloves and the gown with your bare hands.	___	___	_____
d) Discarded the gown and gloves.	___	___	_____
2) Removed and discarded the goggles or face shield.			
a) Lifted the headband or earpieces from the back. Did not touch the front of the device.	___	___	_____
b) Discarded the device. If re-usable, followed agency policy.	___	___	_____
3) Removed and discarded the mask if worn. (Note: Removed a respirator after leaving the room and closing the door.)			
a) Untied the lower strings of the mask.	___	___	_____
b) Untied the top strings.	___	___	_____
c) Held the top strings. Removed the mask.	___	___	_____
d) Discarded the mask.	___	___	_____
11. Practiced hand hygiene after removing all PPE.	___	___	_____

Double-Bagging

Name: _____ Date: _____

Procedure	S	U	Comments
1. Asked a co-worker to help you. He or she stood outside the doorway. You were in the room.	_____	_____	_____
2. Placed soiled linen, re-usable items, disposable supplies, and trash in the right containers. Containers were lined with leak-proof biohazard bags. Those were the *dirty (contaminated)* bags.	_____	_____	_____
3. Sealed the *dirty* bags securely.	_____	_____	_____
4. Asked your co-worker to make a wide cuff on a *clean* bag. It was held wide open. The cuff protected the hands from contamination.	_____	_____	_____
5. Placed the *dirty* bag into the *clean* bag. Did not touch the outside of the *clean* bag.	_____	_____	_____
6. Asked your co-worker to seal the *clean* bag. Had the bag labeled with the BIOHAZARD symbol.	_____	_____	_____
7. Repeated the following steps for other *dirty* bags.			
a. Sealed the *dirty* bags securely.	_____	_____	_____
b. Asked your co-worker to make a wide cuff on a *clean* bag. It was held wide open. The cuff protected the hands from contamination.	_____	_____	_____
c. Placed the *dirty* bag into the *clean* bag. Did not touch the outside of the *clean* bag.	_____	_____	_____
d. Asked your co-worker to seal the *clean* bag. Had the bag labeled with the BIOHAZARD symbol.	_____	_____	_____
8. Asked your co-worker to take or send the bags to the appropriate department for disposal, disinfection, or sterilization.	_____	_____	_____

Raising the Person's Head and Shoulders

Name: _____ Date: _____

Quality of Life	S	U	Comments
• Knocked before entering the person's room.	___	___	_____
• Addressed the person by name.	___	___	_____
• Introduced yourself by name and title.	___	___	_____
• Explained the procedure before starting and during the procedure.	___	___	_____
• Protected the person's rights during the procedure.	___	___	_____
• Handled the person gently during the procedure.	___	___	_____

Pre-Procedure

1. Followed *Delegation Guidelines:*
   a. *Moving the Person*   ___ ___ _____
   b. *Moving Persons in Bed*   ___ ___ _____
   Saw *Promoting Safety and Comfort:*
   a. *Moving the Person*   ___ ___ _____
   b. *Preventing Work-Related Injuries*   ___ ___ _____
2. Asked a co-worker to assist if needed.   ___ ___ _____
3. Practiced hand hygiene.   ___ ___ _____
4. Identified the person. Checked the ID (identification) bracelet against the assignment sheet. Used 2 identifiers. Also called the person by name.   ___ ___ _____
5. Provided for privacy.   ___ ___ _____
6. Locked the brakes on bed wheels.   ___ ___ _____
7. Raised the bed for body mechanics. Bed rails were up if used.   ___ ___ _____

Procedure

8. Had your co-worker stand on the other side of the bed. Lowered the bed rails if up.   ___ ___ _____
9. Asked the person to put the near arm behind your near arm and shoulder. His or her hand rested on top of your shoulder. If you were standing on the right side, the person's right hand rested on your right shoulder. The person did the same with your co-worker. The person's left hand rested on your co-worker's left shoulder.   ___ ___ _____
10. Placed your arm nearest to the person under his or her arm. Your hand was on the person's shoulder. Your co-worker did the same.   ___ ___ _____
11. Placed your free arm under the person's neck and shoulders. Your co-worker did the same. Supported the neck.   ___ ___ _____
12. Helped the person rise to a sitting or semi-sitting position on the "count of 3."   ___ ___ _____
13. Used the arm and hand that supported the person's neck and shoulders to give care. Your co-worker supported the person.   ___ ___ _____
14. Helped the person lie down. Provided support with your locked arm. Your co-worker did the same.   ___ ___ _____

Post-Procedure

	S	U	Comments
15. Provided for comfort.			
16. Placed the call light and other needed items within reach.			
17. Lowered the bed to a safe and comfortable level. Followed the care plan.			
18. Raised or lowered bed rails. Followed the care plan.			
19. Unscreened the person.			
20. Completed a safety check of the room.			
21. Practiced hand hygiene.			
22. Reported and recorded your observations.			

Moving the Person Up In Bed

Name: _____   Date: _____

Quality of Life	S	U	Comments
• Knocked before entering the person's room.	_____	_____	_____
• Addressed the person by name.	_____	_____	_____
• Introduced yourself by name and title.	_____	_____	_____
• Explained the procedure before starting and during the procedure.	_____	_____	_____
• Protected the person's rights during the procedure.	_____	_____	_____
• Handled the person gently during the procedure.	_____	_____	_____

Pre-Procedure

1. Followed *Delegation Guidelines:*
   a. *Moving the Person*
   b. *Moving Persons in Bed*
   Saw *Promoting Safety and Comfort:*
   a. *Moving the Person*
   b. *Preventing Work-Related Injuries*
   c. *Moving the Person Up in Bed*
2. Asked a co-worker to help you.
3. Practiced hand hygiene.
4. Identified the person. Checked the ID (identification) bracelet against the assignment sheet. Used 2 identifiers. Also called the person by name.
5. Provided for privacy.
6. Locked brakes on the bed wheels.
7. Raised the bed for body mechanics. Bed rails were up if used.

Procedure

8. Lowered the head of the bed to a level appropriate for the person. It was as flat as possible.
9. Stood on 1 side of the bed. Your co-worker stood on the other side.
10. Lowered the bed rails if up.
11. Removed pillows as directed by the nurse. Placed a pillow upright against the head-board if the person could be without it.
12. Stood with a wide base of support. Pointed the foot near the head of the bed toward the head of the bed. Faced the head of the bed.
13. Bent your hips and knees. Kept your back straight.
14. Placed 1 arm under the person's shoulder and 1 arm under the thighs. Your co-worker did the same. Grasped each other's forearms.
15. Asked the person to grasp the trapeze.
16. Had the person flex both knees.
17. Explained that:
    a. You will count "1, 2, 3."
    b. The move will be on "3."
    c. On "3," the person pushes against the bed with the feet if able. And the person pulls up with the trapeze.
18. Moved the person to the head of the bed on the "count of 3." Shifted your weight from your rear leg to your front leg. Your co-worker did the same.

Procedure—cont'd	**S**	**U**	**Comments**

Procedure—cont'd

19. Repeated the following steps if necessary.
    a. Stood with a wide base of support. Pointed the foot near the head of the bed toward the head of the bed. Faced the head of the bed.
    b. Bent your hips and knees. Kept your back straight.
    c. Placed 1 arm under the person's shoulder and 1 arm under the thighs. Your co-worker did the same. Grasped each other's forearms.
    d. Asked the person to grasp the trapeze.
    e. Had the person flex both knees.
    f. Explained that:
        1) You will count "1, 2, 3."
        2) The move will be on "3."
        3) On "3," the person pushes against the bed with the feet if able. And the person pulls up with the trapeze.
    g. Moved the person to the head of the bed on the "count of 3." Shifted your weight from your rear leg to your front leg. Your co-worker did the same.

Post-Procedure

20. Placed the pillow under the person's head and shoulders. Straightened linens.
21. Positioned the person in good alignment. Raised the head of the bed to a level appropriate for the person.
22. Provided for comfort.
23. Placed the call light and other needed items within reach.
24. Lowered the bed to a safe and comfortable level. Followed the care plan.
25. Raised or lowered bed rails. Followed the care plan.
26. Unscreened the person.
27. Completed a safety check of the room.
28. Practiced hand hygiene.
29. Reported and recorded your observations.

Moving the Person Up in Bed With an Assist Device

Name: _____   Date: _____

	S	U	Comments

Quality of Life
- Knocked before entering the person's room.
- Addressed the person by name.
- Introduced yourself by name and title.
- Explained the procedure before starting and during the procedure.
- Protected the person's rights during the procedure.
- Handled the person gently during the procedure.

Pre-Procedure
1. Followed *Delegation Guidelines:*
   a. *Moving the Person*
   b. *Moving Persons in Bed*
   Saw *Promoting Safety and Comfort:*
   a. *Moving the Person*
   b. *Preventing Work-Related Injuries*
   c. *Moving the Person Up in Bed*
   d. *Moving the Person Up in Bed With an Assist Device*
2. Asked a co-worker to help you.
3. Obtained the needed device
4. Practiced hand hygiene.
5. Identified the person. Checked the ID (identification) bracelet against the assignment sheet. Used 2 identifiers. Also called the person by name.
6. Provided for privacy.
7. Locked brakes on the bed wheels.
8. Raised the bed for body mechanics. Bed rails were up if used.

Procedure
9. Lowered the head of the bed to a level appropriate for the person. It was as flat as possible.
10. Stood on 1 side of the bed. Your co-worker stood on the other side.
11. Lowered the bed rails if up.
12. Removed pillows as directed by the nurse. Placed a pillow upright against the head-board if the person could be without it.
13. Positioned the assistive device.
14. Stood with a wide base of support. Pointed the foot near the head of the bed toward the head of the bed. Faced the head of the bed.
15. Rolled the sides of the assist device up close to the person. (Note: Omitted this step if the device had handles.)
16. Grasped the rolled-up assist device firmly near the person's shoulders and hips. Or grasped it by the handles. Supported the head.
17. Bent your hips and knees.
18. Moved the person up in bed on the "count of 3." Shifted your weight from your rear leg to your front leg.
19. Repeated the following steps if necessary.
   a. Stood with a wide base of support. Pointed the foot near the head of the bed toward the head of the bed. Faced the head of the bed.

Procedure—cont'd

     b. Rolled the sides of the assist device firmly near the person. (Note: Omitted this step if the device had handles.)

     c. Grasped the rolled-up assist device firmly near the person's shoulders and hips. Or grasped it by the handles. Supported the head.

     d. Bent your hips and knees.

     e. Moved the person up in bed on the "count of 3." Shifted your weight from your rear leg to your front leg.

20. Unrolled the assist device. (Note: Omitted this step if the device had handles.) Turned the person to remove the slide sheet if used.

Post-Procedure

21. Placed the pillow under the person's head and shoulders. Straightened linens.
22. Positioned the person in good alignment. Raised the head of the bed to a level appropriate for the person.
23. Provided for comfort.
24. Placed the call light and other needed items within reach.
25. Lowered the bed to a safe and comfortable level. Followed the care plan.
26. Raised or lowered bed rails. Followed the care plan.
27. Unscreened the person.
28. Completed a safety check of the room.
29. Practiced hand hygiene.
30. Reported and recorded your observations.

S   U   Comments

Moving the Person to the Side of the Bed

Name: _____ Date: _____

Quality of Life	S	U	Comments
• Knocked before entering the person's room.	_____	_____	_____
• Addressed the person by name.	_____	_____	_____
• Introduced yourself by name and title.	_____	_____	_____
• Explained the procedure before starting and during the procedure.	_____	_____	_____
• Protected the person's rights during the procedure.	_____	_____	_____
• Handled the person gently during the procedure.	_____	_____	_____

Pre-Procedure

1. Followed *Delegation Guidelines:*
   a. *Moving the Person*   _____ _____ _____
   b. *Moving Persons in Bed*   _____ _____ _____
   Saw *Promoting Safety and Comfort:*
   a. *Moving the Person*   _____ _____ _____
   b. *Preventing Work-Related Injuries*   _____ _____ _____
   c. *Moving the Person to the Side of the Bed*
2. Asked 1 or 2 co-workers to help you if you used an assist device.   _____ _____ _____
3. Obtained a drawsheet.
4. Practiced hand hygiene.   _____ _____ _____
5. Identified the person. Checked the ID (identification) bracelet against the assignment sheet. Used 2 identifiers. Also called the person by name.   _____ _____ _____
6. Provided for privacy.   _____ _____ _____
7. Locked brakes on the bed wheels.   _____ _____ _____
8. Raised the bed for body mechanics. Bed rails were up if used.   _____ _____ _____

Procedure

9. Lowered the head of the bed to a level appropriate for the person. It was as flat as possible.   _____ _____ _____
10. Stood on the side of the bed to which you will move the person.   _____ _____ _____
11. Lowered the bed rail near you if bed rails were used.   _____ _____ _____
12. Removed pillows as directed by the nurse.   _____ _____ _____
13. Crossed the person's arms over the chest.   _____ _____ _____
14. Stood with your feet about 12 inches apart. One foot was in front of the other. Flexed your knees.   _____ _____ _____
15. *Method 1—moving the person in segments:*
    a. Placed your arm under the person's neck and shoulders. Grasped the far shoulder.   _____ _____ _____
    b. Placed your other arm under the mid-back.   _____ _____ _____
    c. Moved the upper part of the person's body toward you. Rocked backward and shifted your weight to your rear leg.   _____ _____ _____
    d. Placed 1 arm under the person's waist and 1 under the thighs.   _____ _____ _____
    e. Rocked backward to move the lower part of the person toward you.   _____ _____ _____
    f. Repeated the procedure for the legs and feet. Your arms were under the person's thighs and calves   _____ _____ _____

Procedure—cont'd   S   U   Comments

16. *Method 2—moving the person with a drawsheet:*
    a. Positioned the drawsheet
    b. Rolled up the drawsheet close to the person.   _____   _____   _____
    c. Grasped the rolled-up drawsheet near the person's
       shoulders and hips. Your co-worker did the same.
       Supported the person's head.   _____   _____   _____
    d. Rocked backward on the "count of 3," moving
       the person toward you. Your co-worker rocked
       backward slightly and then forward toward you
       while keeping the arms straight.   _____   _____   _____
    e. Unrolled the drawsheet. Removed any wrinkles.   _____   _____   _____

Post-Procedure

17. Placed the pillow under the person's head and shoulders.
    Straightened linens.   _____   _____   _____
18. Positioned the person in good alignment.   _____   _____   _____
19. Provided for comfort.   _____   _____   _____
20. Placed the call light and other needed items within reach. _____ _____   _____
21. Lowered the bed to a safe and comfortable level.
    Followed the care plan.   _____   _____   _____
22. Raised or lowered bed rails. Followed the care plan.   _____   _____   _____
23. Unscreened the person.   _____   _____   _____
24. Completed a safety check of the room.   _____   _____   _____
25. Practiced hand hygiene.   _____   _____   _____
26. Reported and recorded your observations.   _____   _____   _____

Turning and Re-Positioning the Person

Name: _____   Date: _____

	S	U	Comments

Quality of Life
- Knocked before entering the person's room.
- Addressed the person by name.
- Introduced yourself by name and title.
- Explained the procedure before starting and during the procedure.
- Protected the person's rights during the procedure.
- Handled the person gently during the procedure.

Pre-Procedure
1. Followed *Delegation Guidelines*:
    a. *Moving the Person*
    b. *Moving Persons in Bed*
    c. *Turning Persons*
    Saw *Promoting Safety and Comfort*:
    a. *Moving the Person*
    b. *Preventing Work-Related Injuries*
    c. *Moving the Person to the Side of the Bed*
    d. *Turning Persons*
2. Practiced hand hygiene.
3. Identified the person. Checked the ID (identification) bracelet against the assignment sheet. Used 2 identifiers. Also called the person by name.
4. Provided for privacy.
5. Locked brakes on the bed wheels.
6. Raised the bed for body mechanics. Bed rails were up if used.

Procedure
7. Lowered the head of the bed to a level appropriate for the person. It was as flat as possible.
8. Stood on the side of the bed opposite to where you will turn the person.
9. Lowered the bed rail.
10. Moved the person to the side near you.
11. Crossed the person's arms over the chest. Crossed the leg near you over the far leg.
12. *Turning the person away from you:*
    a. Stood with a wide base of support. Flexed the knees.
    b. Placed 1 hand on the person's shoulder. Placed the other on the hip near you.
    c. Rolled the person gently away from you toward the raised bed rail.
    d. Shifted your weight from your rear leg to your front leg.
13. *Turning the person toward you:*
    a. Raised the bed rail.
    b. Went to the other side of the bed. Lowered the bed rail.
    c. Stood with a wide base of support. Flexed your knees.
    d. Placed 1 hand on the person's shoulder. Placed the other on the far hip.
    e. Pulled the person toward you gently.

Procedure—cont'd

14. Positioned the person. Followed the nurse's directions and the care plan. The following are common.
    a. Placed a pillow under the head and neck.
    b. Adjusted the shoulder. The person was not on an arm.
    c. Placed a small pillow under the upper hand and arm.
    d. Positioned a pillow against the back.
    e. Flexed the upper knee. Positioned the upper leg in front of the lower leg.
    f. Supported the upper leg and thigh on pillows. Made sure the ankle was supported.

Post-Procedure

15. Provided for comfort.
16. Placed the call light and other needed items within reach.
17. Lowered the bed to a safe and comfortable level appropriate. Followed the care plan.
18. Raised or lowered bed rails. Followed the care plan.
19. Unscreened the person.
20. Completed a safety check of the room.
21. Practiced hand hygiene.
22. Reported and recorded your observations.

	S	U	Comments

Logrolling the Person

Name: _____   Date: _____

Quality of Life	S	U	Comments

Quality of Life

- Knocked before entering the person's room.
- Addressed the person by name.
- Introduced yourself by name and title.
- Explained the procedure before starting and during the procedure.
- Protected the person's rights during the procedure.
- Handled the person gently during the procedure.

Pre-Procedure

1. Followed *Delegation Guidelines:*
   a. *Moving the Person*
   b. *Moving Persons in Bed*
   c. *Turning Persons*
   Saw *Promoting Safety and Comfort:*
   a. *Moving the Person*
   b. *Preventing Work-Related Injuries*
   c. *Turning Persons*
   d. *Logrolling*
2. Asked a co-worker to help you.
3. Obtained the needed assist device.
4. Practiced hand hygiene.
5. Identified the person. Checked the identification (ID) bracelet against the assignment sheet. Used 2 identifiers. Also called the person by name.
6. Provided for privacy.
7. Locked brakes on the bed wheels.
8. Raised the bed for body mechanics. Bed rails were up if used.

Procedure

9. Made sure the bed was flat.
10. Stood on the side opposite to which you turned the person. Your co-worker stood on the other side.
11. Lowered the bed rails if used.
12. Positioned the assist device.
13. Moved the person as a unit to the side of the bed near you. Used the assist device. (If the person had a spinal cord injury or had spinal cord surgery, assisted the nurse as directed.)
14. Placed the person's arms across the chest. Placed a pillow between the knees.
15. Raised the bed rail if used.
16. Went to the other side.
17. Stood near the shoulders and chest. Your co-worker stood near the hips and thighs.
18. Stood with a wide base of support. One foot was in front of the other.
19. Asked the person to hold his or her body rigid.
20. Rolled the person toward you. Or used the assist device. Turned the person as a unit.
21. Removed the slide sheet (if used).

Procedure—cont'd	S	U	Comments

22. Positioned the person in good alignment. Used
    pillows as directed by the nurse and care plan. The
    following are common (unless the spinal cord was involved).
    a. Placed a pillow under the head and neck if allowed.
    b. Adjusted the shoulder. The person was not on an arm.
    c. Placed a small pillow under the upper hand and arm.
    d. Positioned a pillow against the back.
    e. Flexed the upper knee. Positioned the upper leg in
       front of the lower leg.
    f. Supported the upper leg and thigh on pillows.
       Made sure the ankle was supported.

Post-Procedure
23. Provided for comfort.
24. Placed the call light and other needed items within
    reach.
25. Lowered the bed to a safe and comfortable level.
    Followed the care plan.
26. Raised or lowered bed rails. Followed the care plan.
27. Unscreened the person.
28. Completed a safety check of the room.
29. Practiced hand hygiene.
30. Reported and recorded your observations.

Sitting on the Side of the Bed (Dangling)

Name: _____ Date: _____

Quality of Life	S	U	Comments
• Knocked before entering the person's room.	___	___	_____
• Addressed the person by name.	___	___	_____
• Introduced yourself by name and title.	___	___	_____
• Explained the procedure before starting and during the procedure.	___	___	_____
• Protected the person's rights during the procedure.	___	___	_____
• Handled the person gently during the procedure.	___	___	_____

Pre-Procedure

1. Followed *Delegation Guidelines:*
   a. *Moving the Person*
   b. *Dangling*
   Saw *Promoting Safety and Comfort:*
   a. *Moving the Person*
   b. *Preventing Work-Related Injuries*
   c. *Dangling*
2. Asked a co-worker to help you.
3. Practiced hand hygiene.
4. Identified the person. Checked the identification (ID) bracelet against the assignment sheet. Used 2 identifiers. Also called the person by name.
5. Provided for privacy.
6. Decided which side of the bed to use.
7. Moved furniture to provide moving space.
8. Locked brakes on the bed wheels.
9. Raised the bed for body mechanics. Bed rails were up if used.

Procedure

10. Lowered the bed rail if up.
11. Positioned the person in a side-lying position facing you. The person laid on the strong side.
12. Raised the head of the bed to a sitting position.
13. Stood by the person's hips. Faced the foot of the bed.
14. Stood with your feet apart. The foot near the head of the bed was in front of the other foot.
15. Slid 1 arm under the person's neck and shoulders. Grasped the far shoulder. Placed your other hand over the thighs near the knees.
16. Pivoted toward the foot of the bed while moving the person's legs and feet over the side of the bed. As the legs went over the edge of the mattress, the trunk was upright.
17. Had the person hold on to the edge of the mattress. This supported the person in the sitting position. If possible, raised a half-length bed rail (on the person's strong side) for the person to grasp. Had your co-worker support the person at all times.
18. Checked the person's condition.
    a. Asked how the person felt. Asked if the person felt dizzy or light-headed.
    b. Checked the pulse and respirations.
    c. Checked for difficulty breathing.
    d. Noted if the skin was pale or bluish in color.

Procedure—cont'd	**S**	**U**	**Comments**
19. Reversed the procedure to return the person to bed. (Or prepared the person to walk or for a transfer to a chair or wheelchair. Lowered the bed to a safe and comfortable level. The person's feet were flat on the floor.)	_____	_____	_____
20. Lowered the head of the bed after the person returned to bed. Helped him or her move to the center of the bed.	_____	_____	_____
21. Positioned the person in good alignment.	_____	_____	_____

Post-Procedure

	S	**U**	**Comments**
22. Provided for comfort.	_____	_____	_____
23. Placed the call light and other needed items within reach.	_____	_____	_____
24. Lowered the bed to a safe and comfortable level appropriate. Followed the care plan.	_____	_____	_____
25. Raised or lowered bed rails. Followed the care plan.	_____	_____	_____
26. Returned furniture to its proper place.	_____	_____	_____
27. Unscreened the person.	_____	_____	_____
28. Completed a safety check of the room.	_____	_____	_____
29. Practiced hand hygiene.	_____	_____	_____
30. Reported and recorded your observations.	_____	_____	_____

Transferring the Person to a Chair or Wheelchair

Name: _____   Date: _____

Quality of Life	S	U	Comments
• Knocked before entering the person's room.	___	___	_____
• Addressed the person by name.	___	___	_____
• Introduced yourself by name and title.	___	___	_____
• Explained the procedure before starting and during the procedure.	___	___	_____
• Protected the person's rights during the procedure.	___	___	_____
• Handled the person gently during the procedure.	___	___	_____

Pre-Procedure

	S	U	Comments
1. Followed *Delegation Guidelines: Transferring the Person,* Saw *Promoting Safety and Comfort:*	___	___	_____
a. *Transfer/Gait Belts*	___	___	_____
b. *Transferring the Person*	___	___	_____
c. *Stand and Pivot Transfer*	___	___	_____
d. *Bed to Chair or Wheelchair Transfers*	___	___	_____
2. Collected the following:			
• Wheelchair or arm chair	___	___	_____
• Bath blanket	___	___	_____
• Lap blanket (if used)	___	___	_____
• Robe and slip-resistant footwear	___	___	_____
• Paper or sheet	___	___	_____
• Transfer belt (if needed)	___	___	_____
• Seat cushion (if needed)	___	___	_____
3. Practiced hand hygiene.	___	___	_____
4. Identified the person. Checked the identification (ID) bracelet against the assignment sheet. Used 2 identifiers. Also called the person by name.	___	___	_____
5. Provided for privacy.	___	___	_____
6. Decided which side of the bed to use. Moved furniture for a safe transfer.	___	___	_____

Procedure

	S	U	Comments
7. Raised the wheelchair footplates. Removed or swung front rigging out of the way if possible. Positioned the chair or wheelchair near the bed on the person's strong side.	___	___	_____
a. If at the head of the bed, it faced the foot of the bed.	___	___	_____
b. If at the foot of the bed, it faced the head of the bed.	___	___	_____
c. The armrest almost touched the bed.	___	___	_____
8. Placed a folded bath blanket or cushion on the seat (if needed).	___	___	_____
9. Locked (braked) the wheelchair wheels. Made sure that bed wheels were locked.	___	___	_____
10. Fan-folded top linens to the foot of the bed.	___	___	_____
11. Placed the paper or sheet under the person's feet. (This protected linens from footwear.) Put footwear on the person.	___	___	_____
12. Lowered the bed to a safe and comfortable level. Followed the care plan.	___	___	_____
13. Helped the person sit on the side of the bed. Feet were flat on the floor.	___	___	_____
14. Helped the person put on a robe.	___	___	_____
15. Applied the transfer belt if needed. It was applied at the waist over clothing.	___	___	_____

Procedure—cont'd	S	U	Comments

16. *Method 1: Using a transfer belt:*

a. Stood in front of the person.   _____ _____ _____

b. Had the person hold on to the mattress.   _____ _____ _____

c. Made sure the person's feet were flat on the floor.   _____ _____ _____

d. Had the person lean forward.   _____ _____ _____

e. Grasped the transfer belt at each side. Grasped the handles or grasped the belt from underneath. Hands were in an upward position (upward grasp)   _____ _____ _____

f. Prevented the person from sliding or falling. Did one of the following:

  1) Braced your knees against the person's knees. Blocked his or her feet with your feet.   _____ _____ _____

  2) Used the knee and foot of 1 leg to block the person's weak leg or foot. Placed your other foot slightly behind you for balance.   _____ _____ _____

  3) Straddled your legs around the person's weak leg.   _____ _____ _____

g. Explained the following:

  1) You will count "1, 2, 3."   _____ _____ _____

  2) The move will be on "3."   _____ _____ _____

  3) On "3," the person pushes down on the mattress and stands.   _____ _____ _____

h. Asked the person to push down on the mattress and to stand on the "count of 3." Assisted the person to a standing position as you straightened your knees.   _____ _____ _____

17. *Method 2: No transfer belt.* (Note: Used this method only if directed by the nurse and the care plan.)   _____ _____ _____

a. Followed steps 16, a–c.

  1) Stood in front of the person.   _____ _____ _____

  2) Had the person hold on to the mattress.   _____ _____ _____

  3) Made sure the person's feet were flat on the floor.   _____ _____ _____

b. Placed your hands under the person's arms. Your hands were around the shoulder blades.   _____ _____ _____

c. Had the person lean forward.   _____ _____ _____

d. Prevented the person from sliding or falling. Did one of the following:

  1) Braced your knees against the person's knees. Blocked his or her feet with your feet.   _____ _____ _____

  2) Used the knee and foot of 1 leg to block the person's weak leg or foot. Placed your other foot slightly behind you for balance.   _____ _____ _____

  3) Straddled your legs around the person's weak leg.   _____ _____ _____

e. Explained the "count of 3."

  1) You will count "1, 2, 3".   _____ _____ _____

  2) The move will be on "3."   _____ _____ _____

  3) On "3," the person pushes down on the mattress and stands.   _____ _____ _____

f. Asked the person to push down on the mattress and to stand on the "count of 3." Assisted the person up into a standing position as you straightened your knees.   _____ _____ _____

18. Supported the person in the standing position. Held the transfer belt or kept your hands around the person's shoulder blades. Continued to prevent the person from sliding or falling.   _____ _____ _____

19. Helped the person pivot (turn) so he or she could grasp the far arm of the chair or wheelchair. The legs touched the edge of the seat.   _____ _____ _____

Procedure—cont'd

	S	U	Comments
20. Continued to help the person pivot (turn) until the other armrest was grasped.	_____	_____	_____
21. Lowered him or her into the chair or wheelchair as you bent your hips and knees. To assist, the person leaned forward and bent his or her elbows and knees.	_____	_____	_____
22. Made sure the hips were to the back of the seat. Positioned the person in good alignment.	_____	_____	_____
23. Attached the wheelchair front rigging. Positioned the person's feet on the footplates.	_____	_____	_____
24. Covered the person's lap and legs with a lap blanket (if used). Kept the blanket off the floor and the wheels.	_____	_____	_____
25. Removed the transfer belt if used.	_____	_____	_____
26. Positioned the chair as the person preferred. Locked (braked) the wheelchair wheels according to the care plan.	_____	_____	_____

Post-Procedure

	S	U	Comments
27. Provided for comfort.	_____	_____	_____
28. Placed the call light and other needed items within reach.	_____	_____	_____
29. Unscreened the person.	_____	_____	_____
30. Completed a safety check of the room.	_____	_____	_____
31. Practiced hand hygiene.	_____	_____	_____
32. Reported and recorded your observations.	_____	_____	_____
33. Saw procedure: *Transferring the Person From a Chair or Wheelchair to Bed* to return the person to bed.	_____	_____	_____

Transferring the Person From a Chair or Wheelchair to Bed

NATCEP™

Name: _____   Date: _____

Quality of Life	S	U	Comments
• Knocked before entering the person's room.	___	___	_____
• Addressed the person by name.	___	___	_____
• Introduced yourself by name and title.	___	___	_____
• Explained the procedure before starting and during the procedure.	___	___	_____
• Protected the person's rights during the procedure.	___	___	_____
• Handled the person gently during the procedure.	___	___	_____

Pre-Procedure

1. Followed *Delegation Guidelines:*
   a. *Transferring the Person*
   Saw *Promoting Safety and Comfort:*
   a. *Transfer Belts*
   b. *Transferring the Person*
   c. *Stand and Pivot Transfer*
   d. *Bed to Chair or Wheelchair Transfers*
2. Collected a transfer belt if needed.
3. Practiced hand hygiene.
4. Identified the person. Checked the identification (ID) bracelet against the assignment sheet. Used 2 identifiers. Called the person by name.
5. Provided privacy.

Procedure

6. Moved furniture for moving space.
7. Raised the head of the bed to a sitting position. Lowered the bed to a safe and comfortable level for the person. Followed the care plan. When the person transferred to the bed, his or her feet were flat on the floor while sitting on the side of the bed.
8. Moved the call light so it would be to the person's strong side when in bed.
9. Positioned the chair or wheelchair so the person's strong side was next to the bed. Had a co-worker help you if necessary.
10. Locked (braked) the wheelchair and bed wheels.
11. Removed and folded the lap blanket.
12. Removed the person's feet from the footplates. Raised the footplates. Removed or swung front rigging out of the way. Put slip-resistant footwear on the person if not already done.
13. Applied the transfer belt if needed.
14. Made sure the person's feet were flat on the floor.
15. Stood in front of the person.
16. Had the person hold on to the armrests. (If the nurse directed you to do so, placed your arms under the person's arms. Your hands were around the shoulder blades.)
17. Had the person lean forward.
18. Grasped the transfer belt on each side if using it. Grasped underneath the belt. Hands were in an upward position (upward grasp).

Procedure—cont'd

	S	U	Comments
19. Prevented the person from sliding or falling. Did one of the following:			
a. Braced your knees against the person's knees. Blocked his or her feet with your feet.	_____	_____	_____
b. Used the knee and foot of 1 leg to block the person's weak leg or foot. Placed your other foot slightly behind you for balance.	_____	_____	_____
c. Straddled your legs around the person's weak leg.	_____	_____	_____
20. Explained the count of "3."			
a. You will count "1, 2, 3."	_____	_____	_____
b. The move will be on "3."	_____	_____	_____
21. Asked the person to push down on the armrest on the "count of 3." Assisted the person into a standing position as you straightened your knees.	_____	_____	_____
22. Supported the person in the standing position. Held the transfer belt or kept your hands around the person's shoulder blades. Continued to prevent the person from sliding or falling.	_____	_____	_____
23. Helped the person pivot (turn) to reach the edge of the mattress. The legs touched the mattress.	_____	_____	_____
24. Continued to help the person pivot (turn) until he or she reached the mattress with both hands.	_____	_____	_____
25. Lowered him or her onto the bed as you bent your hips and knees. The person leaned forward and bent the elbows and knees.	_____	_____	_____
26. Removed the transfer belt.	_____	_____	_____
27. Removed the robe and footwear.	_____	_____	_____
28. Helped the person lie down.	_____	_____	_____

Post-Procedure

	S	U	Comments
29. Provided for comfort.	_____	_____	_____
30. Placed the call light and other needed items within reach.	_____	_____	_____
31. Raised or lowered bed rails. Followed the care plan.	_____	_____	_____
32. Arranged furniture to meet the person's needs.	_____	_____	_____
33. Unscreened the person.	_____	_____	_____
34. Completed a safety check of the room.	_____	_____	_____
35. Practiced hand hygiene.	_____	_____	_____
36. Reported and recorded your observations.	_____	_____	_____

Transferring the Person To and From the Toilet

Name: _____　Date: _____

	S	U	Comments
Quality of Life			
• Knocked before entering the person's room.	___	___	_____
• Addressed the person by name.	___	___	_____
• Introduced yourself by name and title.	___	___	_____
• Explained the procedure before starting and during the procedure.	___	___	_____
• Protected the person's rights during the procedure.	___	___	_____
• Handled the person gently during the procedure.	___	___	_____

Pre-Procedure

1. Followed *Delegation Guidelines: Transferring the Person,* Saw *Promoting Safety and Comfort:*
   a. *Transfer/Gait Belts*
   b. *Transferring the Person*
   c. *Stand and Pivot Transfer*
   d. *Bed to Chair or Wheelchair Transfers*
   e. *Transferring the Person To and From the Toilet*
2. Practiced hand hygiene.

Procedure

3. Placed slip-resistant footwear on the person.
4. Positioned the wheelchair next to the toilet if there is enough room or positioned the chair at a right angle (90-degree angle) to the toilet. The person's strong side was near the toilet.
5. Locked (braked) the wheelchair wheels.
6. Raised the footplates. Removed or swung front rigging out of the way.
7. Applied the transfer belt.
8. Helped the person unfasten clothing.
9. Used the transfer belt to help the person stand and to pivot (turn) to the toilet. The person used the grab bars to pivot (turn) to the toilet.
10. Supported the person with the transfer belt while he or she lowered clothing. Or had the person hold on to the grab bars for support. Lowered the person's clothing.
11. Used the transfer belt to lower the person onto the toilet seat. Checked for proper positioning on the toilet.
12. Removed the transfer belt.
13. Told the person you would stay nearby. Reminded the person to use the call light or call for you when help was needed. Stayed with the person if required by the care plan.
14. Closed the bathroom door for privacy.
15. Stayed near the bathroom. Completed other tasks in the person's room. Checked on the person every 5 minutes.
16. Knocked on the bathroom door when the person called for you.
17. Helped with wiping, perineal care, flushing, and hand hygiene as needed. Wore gloves and practiced hand hygiene after removing the gloves.
18. Applied the transfer belt.

Procedure—cont'd

	S	U	Comments
19. Used the transfer belt to help the person stand.	_____	_____	_____
20. Helped the person raise and secure clothing.	_____	_____	_____
21. Used the transfer belt to transfer the person to the wheelchair.	_____	_____	_____
22. Made sure the person's buttocks were to the back of the seat. Positioned the person in good alignment.	_____	_____	_____
23. Positioned the feet on the footplates.	_____	_____	_____
24. Removed the transfer belt.	_____	_____	_____
25. Covered the lap and legs with a lap blanket. Kept the blanket off the floor and wheels.	_____	_____	_____
26. Positioned the chair as the person preferred. Locked (braked) the wheelchair wheels according to the care plan.	_____	_____	_____

Post-Procedure

	S	U	Comments
27. Provided for comfort.	_____	_____	_____
28. Placed the call light and other needed items within reach.	_____	_____	_____
29. Unscreened the person.	_____	_____	_____
30. Completed a safety check of the room.	_____	_____	_____
31. Practiced hand hygiene.	_____	_____	_____
32. Reported and recorded your observations.	_____	_____	_____

Moving the Person to a Stretcher

Name: _____   Date: _____

Quality of Life	S	U	Comments
• Knocked before entering the person's room.			
• Addressed the person by name.			
• Introduced yourself by name and title.			
• Explained the procedure before starting and during the procedure.			
• Protected the person's rights during the procedure.			
• Handled the person gently during the procedure.			

Pre-Procedure

1. Followed *Delegation Guidelines: Transferring the Person,* Saw *Promoting Safety and Comfort:*
   a. *Transferring the Person*
   b. *Moving the Person to a Stretcher*
2. Asked 1 or 2 staff members to help you.
3. Collected the following:
   • Stretcher covered with a sheet or bath blanket
   • Bath blanket
   • Pillow(s) if needed
   • Drawsheet, slide sheet, or other lateral transfer device
4. Practiced hand hygiene.
5. Identified the person. Checked the identification (ID) bracelet against the assignment sheet. Used 2 identifiers. Also called the person by name.
6. Provided for privacy.
7. Raised the bed and stretcher for body mechanics.

Procedure

8. Positioned yourself and co-workers.
   a. 1 or 2 workers stood on the side of the bed where the stretcher was.
   b. 1 worker stood on the other side of the bed.
9. Lowered the head of the bed. It was as flat as possible.
10. Lowered the bed rails if used.
11. Covered the person with a bath blanket. Fan-folded top linens to the foot of the bed.
12. Positioned the assist device. Or loosened the drawsheet on each side.
13. Used the assist device to move the person to the side of the bed. This was the side where the stretcher was.
14. Protected the person from falling. Held the far arm and leg.
15. Had your co-workers position the stretcher next to the bed. They stood beside the stretcher.
16. Locked (braked) the bed and stretcher wheels.
17. Grasped the assist device.
18. Transferred the person to the stretcher on the "count of 3." Centered the person on the stretcher.
19. Placed a pillow or pillows under the person's head and shoulder if allowed. Raised the head of the stretcher if allowed.
20. Covered the person. Provided for comfort.
21. Fastened the safety straps. Raised the side rails.
22. Unlocked the stretcher wheels (released the brakes). Transported the person.

Post-Procedure	**S**	**U**	**Comments**
23. Practiced hand hygiene.	_____	_____	_____
24. Reported and recorded:			
• The time of the transport	_____	_____	_____
• Where the person was transported to	_____	_____	_____
• Who went with him or her	_____	_____	_____
• How the transfer was tolerated	_____	_____	_____
25. Reversed the procedure to return the person to bed.	_____	_____	_____

Transferring the Person Using a Stand-Assist Mechanical Lift

Name: _____ Date: _____

Quality of Life

	S	U	Comments
• Knocked before entering the person's room.	___	___	_____
• Addressed the person by name.	___	___	_____
• Introduced yourself by name and title.	___	___	_____
• Explained the procedure before starting and during the procedure.	___	___	_____
• Protected the person's rights during the procedure.	___	___	_____
• Handled the person gently during the procedure.	___	___	_____

Pre-Procedure

1. Followed *Delegation Guidelines: Transferring the Person,* Saw *Promoting Safety and Comfort:*
   a. *Transferring the Person*
   b. *Using a Mechanical Lift*
2. Asked a co-worker to help you (if needed).
3. Collected the following:
   • Stand-assist mechanical lift and sling
   • Arm chair or wheelchair
   • Slip-resistant footwear
   • Bath blanket or cushion
   • Lap blanket (if used)
4. Practiced hand hygiene.
5. Identified the person. Checked the identification (ID) bracelet against the assignment sheet. Used 2 identifiers. Also called the person by name.
6. Provided for privacy.

Procedure

7. Placed the chair (wheelchair) at the head of the bed. It was even with the head-board and about 1 foot away from the bed. Locked (braked) the wheelchair wheels. Placed a folded bath blanket or cushion in the seat if needed.
8. Assisted the person to a seated position on the side of the bed. The person's feet were flat on the floor. Bed wheels were locked.
9. Put footwear on the person.
10. Applied the sling.
    a. Positioned the sling at the lower back.
    b. Brought the straps around to the front of the chest. The straps were positioned under the arms.
    c. Secured the waist belt around the person's waist. Adjusted the belt so it was snug but not tight.
11. Positioned the lift in front of the person.
12. Widened the lift's base.
13. Locked (braked) the lift's wheels.
14. Had the person place the feet on the foot plate and the knees against the knee pad. Assisted as needed. If the lift had a knee strap, secured the strap around the legs. Adjusted the strap so it was snug but not tight.
15. Attached the sling to the sling hooks.
16. Had the person grasp the lift's hand grips.
17. Unlocked the lift's wheels (released the brakes).

Procedure—cont'd   S   U   **Comments**

18. Raised the person slightly off the bed. Checked that the
    sling was secure, the feet were on the foot plate, and the
    knees were against the knee pad. If not, lowered the
    person and corrected the problem before proceeding.   _____   _____   _____

19. Raised the lift until the person was clear of the bed.
    Or raised the person to a standing position. Followed
    the care plan.   _____   _____   _____

20. Adjusted the base's width to move from the bed to the
    chair (wheelchair) if needed. Kept the base in the wide
    or open position as much as possible.   _____   _____   _____

21. Moved the lift to the chair (wheelchair). The person's
    back was toward the seat.   _____   _____   _____

22. Lowered the person into the chair (wheelchair).
    Guided the person into the seat.   _____   _____   _____

23. Locked (braked) the lift's wheels.   _____   _____   _____

24. Unhooked the sling from the sling hooks.   _____   _____   _____

25. Unbuckled the waist belt. Removed the sling.   _____   _____   _____

26. Unlocked the lift's wheels (released the brakes).   _____   _____   _____

27. Had the person lift the feet off of the footplate. Assisted
    as needed. Moved the lift. Positioned the person's feet
    flat on the floor or on the wheelchair footplates.   _____   _____   _____

28. Covered the lap and legs with a lap blanket (if used).
    Kept it off the floor.   _____   _____   _____

Post-Procedure

29. Provided for comfort.   _____   _____   _____

30. Placed the call light and other needed items within reach. _____   _____   _____

31. Unscreened the person.   _____   _____   _____

32. Completed a safety check of the room.   _____   _____   _____

33. Practiced hand hygiene.   _____   _____   _____

34. Reported and recorded your observations.   _____   _____   _____

35. Reversed the procedure to return the person to bed.   _____   _____   _____

Transferring the Person Using a Full-Sling Mechanical Lift

Name: _____   Date: _____

Quality of Life	S	U	Comments

Quality of Life

- Knocked before entering the person's room.
- Addressed the person by name.
- Introduced yourself by name and title.
- Explained the procedure before starting and during the procedure.
- Protected the person's rights during the procedure.
- Handled the person gently during the procedure.

Pre-Procedure

1. Followed *Delegation Guidelines: Transferring the Person,* Saw *Promoting Safety and Comfort:*
   a. *Transferring the Person*
   b. *Using a Mechanical Lift*
2. Asked a co-worker to help you.
3. Collected the following:
   - Full-sling mechanical lift and sling
   - Arm chair or wheelchair
   - Slip-resistant footwear
   - Bath blanket or cushion
   - Lap blanket (if used)
4. Practiced hand hygiene.
5. Identified the person. Checked the identification (ID) bracelet against the assignment sheet. Used 2 identifiers. Also called the person by name.
6. Provided for privacy.
7. Raised the bed for body mechanics. Bed rails were up if used.

Procedure

8. Lowered the head of the bed to a level appropriate for the person. It is as flat as possible.
9. Stood on 1 side of the bed. Your co-worker stood on the other side.
10. Lowered the bed rails if up. Locked (braked) the bed wheels.
11. Centered the sling under the person. To position the sling, turned the person from side to side. Followed the manufacturer's instructions to position the sling.
12. Positioned the person in the semi-Fowler's position.
13. Placed the chair (wheelchair) at the head of the bed. It was even with the head-board and about 1 foot away from the bed. Placed a folded bath blanket or cushion in the seat if needed.
14. Lowered the bed so it was level with the chair.
15. Raised the lift to position it over the person.
16. Positioned the lift over the person.
17. Widened the lift's base. Locked (braked) the lift wheels.
18. Attached the sling to the sling hooks.
19. Raised the head of the bed to a comfortable level for the person.
20. Crossed the person's arms over the chest.
21. Unlocked the lift wheels (released the brakes).

Procedure—cont'd

	S	U	Comments
22. Raised the person slightly from the bed. Checked that the sling was secure. If not, lowered the person and corrected the problem before proceeding.	___	___	_____
23. Raised the lift until the person and sling were free of the bed.	___	___	_____
24. Had your co-worker support the person's legs as you moved the lift and the person away from the bed.	___	___	_____
25. Adjusted the base's width to move from the bed to the chair (wheelchair) if needed. Kept the base in the wide or open position as much as possible.	___	___	_____
26. Positioned the lift so the person's back was toward the chair (wheelchair).	___	___	_____
27. Adjusted the position of the chair (wheelchair) as needed to lower the person into it. Locked (braked) the wheelchair wheels.	___	___	_____
28. Lowered the person into the chair (wheelchair). Guided the person into the seat.	___	___	_____
29. Locked (braked) the lift wheels.	___	___	_____
30. Unhooked the sling. Unlocked the lift's wheels (released the brakes). Moved the lift away from the person. Removed the sling from under the person unless otherwise indicated.	___	___	_____
31. Put footwear on the person. Positioned the feet flat on the floor or on the wheelchair footplates.	___	___	_____
32. Covered the lap and legs with a lap blanket (if used). Kept it off the floor and wheels.	___	___	_____
33. Positioned the chair (wheelchair) as the person preferred. Locked (braked) the wheelchair wheels according to the care plan.	___	___	_____

Post-Procedure

	S	U	Comments
34. Provided for comfort.	___	___	_____
35. Placed the call light and other needed items within reach.	___	___	_____
36. Unscreened the person.	___	___	_____
37. Completed a safety check of the room.	___	___	_____
38. Practiced hand hygiene.	___	___	_____
39. Reported and recorded your observations.	___	___	_____
40. Reversed the procedure to return the person to bed.	___	___	_____

Making a Closed Bed

Name: _____   Date: _____

Quality of Life	S	U	Comments

Quality of Life
- Knocked before entering the person's room.
- Addressed the person by name.
- Introduced yourself by name and title.
- Explained the procedure before starting and during the procedure.
- Protected the person's rights during the procedure.
- Handled the person gently during the procedure.

Pre-Procedure
1. Followed *Delegation Guidelines: Making Beds.* Saw *Promoting Safety and Comfort: Making Beds.*
2. Practiced hand hygiene.
3. Collected clean linens.
   - Mattress pad (if needed)
   - Bottom sheet (flat sheet or fitted sheet)
   - Cotton drawsheet or padded waterproof drawsheet (if needed)
   - Waterproof under-pad (if needed)
   - Top sheet
   - Blanket
   - Bedspread
   - A pillowcase for each pillow
   - Bath towel
   - Hand towel
   - Washcloth
   - Gown or pajamas
   - Bath blanket
   - Gloves
   - Laundry bag
   - Towel, paper towels, or disposable bed protector (as a barrier for clean linens)
4. Placed linens on a clean surface. First placed the barrier between the clean surface and the clean linens if required by agency policy.
5. Raised the bed for body mechanics. Bed rails are down.

Procedure
6. Put on gloves.
7. Removed linens. Rolled each piece away from you. Placed each piece in a laundry bag. (Note: Discarded the incontinence product, disposable bed protector, and disposable drawsheet in the trash. Did not put them in the laundry bag.)
8. Cleaned the bed frame and mattress (if this was your job).
9. Removed and discarded the gloves. Practiced hand hygiene.
10. Moved the mattress to the head of the bed.
11. Put the mattress pad on the mattress. It was even with the top of the mattress.

Procedure—cont'd	**S**	**U**	**Comments**

12. Placed the bottom sheet on the mattress pad. Unfolded it length-wise. Placed the center crease in the middle of the bed. For a flat sheet:
    a. Positioned the lower edge even with the bottom of the mattress. _____ _____ _____
    b. Placed the large hem at the top and the small hem at the bottom. _____ _____ _____
    c. Faced hem-stitching downward, away from the person. _____ _____ _____
13. Opened the sheet. Fan-folded it to the other side of the bed. _____ _____ _____
14. Tucked the corners of a fitted sheet over the mattress at the top and then foot of the bed. For a flat sheet, tucked the top of the sheet under the mattress. The sheet was tight and smooth. _____ _____ _____
15. Made a mitered corner at the top if using a flat sheet. _____ _____ _____
16. Placed the cotton drawsheet or padded waterproof drawsheet on the bed. It was in the middle of the mattress.
    a. Opened and fan-folded the drawsheet to the other side of the bed. _____ _____ _____
    b. Tucked the drawsheet under the mattress. _____ _____ _____
17. Went to the other side of the bed. _____ _____ _____
18. Mitered the top corner of the flat bottom sheet. _____ _____ _____
19. Pulled the bottom sheet tight so there were no wrinkles. Tucked in the sheet. _____ _____ _____
20. Pulled the drawsheets tight so there were no wrinkles. _____ _____ _____
21. *If using a waterproof under-pad*, placed the waterproof under-pad on the bed. It was in the middle of the mattress. _____ _____ _____
22. Went to the other side of the bed. _____ _____ _____
23. Put the top sheet on the bed.
    a. Unfolded it length-wise with the center crease in the middle. _____ _____ _____
    b. Placed the large hem even with the top of the mattress. _____ _____ _____
    c. Opened and fan-folded the sheet to the other side. _____ _____ _____
    d. Faced hem-stitching outward, away from the person. _____ _____ _____
    e. Did not tuck the bottom in yet. _____ _____ _____
    f. Never tucked top linens in on the sides. _____ _____ _____
24. Placed the blanket on the bed.
    a. Unfolded it with the center crease in the middle. _____ _____ _____
    b. Put the upper hem about 6 to 8 inches from the top of the mattress. _____ _____ _____
    c. Opened and fan-folded the blanket to the other side. _____ _____ _____
    d. If steps 30 and 31 were not done, turned the top sheet down over the blanket. Hem-stitching was down, away from the person. _____ _____ _____
25. Placed the bedspread on the bed.
    a. Unfolded it with the center crease in the middle. _____ _____ _____
    b. Placed the upper hem even with the top of the mattress. _____ _____ _____
    c. Opened and fan-folded the bedspread to the other side. _____ _____ _____
    d. Made sure the bedspread facing the door was even. It covered all top linens. _____ _____ _____
26. Tucked in top linens together at the foot of the bed so they were smooth and tight. Made a mitered corner. Left the side of the top linens untucked. _____ _____ _____

Procedure—cont'd

	S	U	Comments
27. Went to the other side.	___	___	_____
28. Straightened all top linens. Worked from the head of the bed to the foot.	___	___	_____
29. Tucked in top linens together at the foot of the bed. Made a mitered corner. Left the top linens untucked.	___	___	_____
30. Turned the top hem of the bedspread under the blanket to form a cuff.	___	___	_____
31. Turned the top sheet down over the bedspread. Hem-stitching was down. (Steps 30 and 31 are not done in some agencies. The bedspread covers the pillow. If so, tucked the bedspread under the pillow.)	___	___	_____
32. Put the pillowcase on the pillow. The zipper, tag, or seam end of the pillow was inserted into the pillowcase first. Folded extra material under the pillow at the open end of the pillowcase.	___	___	_____
33. Placed the pillow on the bed. The open end of the pillowcase was away from the door. The pillowcase seam was toward the head of the bed.	___	___	_____

Post-Procedure

	S	U	Comments
34. Provided for comfort. Note: Omitted this step if the bed was prepared for a new patient or resident.	___	___	_____
35. Attached the call light to the bed. Or placed it within the person's reach.	___	___	_____
36. Lowered the bed to a safe and comfortable level. Followed the care plan. Locked (braked) the bed wheels.	___	___	_____
37. Put the towels, washcloth, gown or pajamas, and bath blanket in the bedside stand.	___	___	_____
38. Completed a safety check of the room.	___	___	_____
39. Followed agency policy for used linens.	___	___	_____
40. Practiced hand hygiene.	___	___	_____

Making an Open Bed

Name: _____ Date: _____

Quality of Life	S	U	Comments

Quality of Life
- Knocked before entering the person's room.
- Addressed the person by name.
- Introduced yourself by name and title.
- Explained the procedure before starting and during the procedure.
- Protected the person's rights during the procedure.
- Handled the person gently during the procedure.

Procedure
1. Followed *Delegation Guidelines: Making Beds*. Saw *Promoting Safety and Comfort: Making Beds*.
2. Practiced hand hygiene.
3. Collected linens for a closed bed.
   - Mattress pad (if needed)
   - Bottom sheet (flat sheet or fitted sheet)
   - Waterproof drawsheet (if needed)
   - Cotton drawsheet (if needed)
   - Waterproof pad
   - Waterproof under-pad (if needed)
   - Top sheet
   - Blanket
   - Bedspread
   - A pillowcase for each pillow
   - Bath towel
   - Hand towel
   - Washcloth
   - Gown or pajamas
   - Bath blanket
   - Gloves
   - Laundry bag
   - Towel, paper towels, or disposable bed protector , (as a barrier for clean linens)
4. Made a closed bed.
   a. Placed linens on a clean surface. First placed the barrier between the clean surface and the clean linens if required by agency policy.
   b. Raised the bed for body mechanics. Bed rails were down.
   c. Put on gloves.
   d. Removed linens. Rolled each piece away from you. Placed each piece in a laundry bag. (Note: Discarded the incontinence product, disposable bed protector, and disposable drawsheet in the trash. Did not put them in the laundry bag.)
   e. Cleaned the bed frame and mattress (if this was your job).
   f. Removed and discarded the gloves. Practiced hand hygiene.
   g. Moved the mattress to the head of the bed.
   h. Put the mattress pad on the mattress. It was even with the top of the mattress.
   i. Placed the bottom sheet on the mattress pad. Unfolded it length-wise. Placed the center crease in the middle of the bed.

Procedure—cont'd	**S**	**U**	**Comments**
For a flat sheet:			
1) Placed the lower edge even with the bottom of the mattress.	___	___	_____
2) Placed the large hem at the top and small hem at the bottom.	___	___	_____
3) Faced hem-stitching downward, away from the person.	___	___	_____
j. Opened the sheet. Fan-folded it to the other side of the bed.	___	___	_____
k. Tucked the corners of a fitted sheet over the mattress at the top and then foot of the bed. For a flat sheet, tucked the top of the sheet under the mattress. The sheet was tight and smooth.	___	___	_____
l. Made a mitered corner at the top if using a flat sheet.	___	___	_____
m. Placed the cotton drawsheet or padded waterproof drawsheet on the bed. It was in the middle of the mattress.	___	___	_____
1) Opened and fan-folded the drawsheet to the other side of the bed.	___	___	_____
2) Tucked the drawsheet under the mattress.	___	___	_____
n. Went to the other side of the bed.	___	___	_____
o. Mitered the top corner of the flat bottom sheet.	___	___	_____
p. Pulled the bottom sheet tight so there were no wrinkles. Tucked in the sheet.	___	___	_____
q. Pulled the drawsheets tight so there were no wrinkles. Tucked both in together or separately.	___	___	_____
r. *If using a waterproof under-pad*, placed the waterproof under-pad on the bed. It was in the middle of the mattress.	___	___	_____
s. Went to the other side of the bed.	___	___	_____
t. Put the top sheet on the bed.			
1) Unfolded it length-wise with the center crease in the middle.	___	___	_____
2) Placed the large hem even with the top of the mattress.	___	___	_____
3) Opened and fan-folded the sheet to the other side.	___	___	_____
4) Faced hem-stitching outward, away from the person.	___	___	_____
5) Did not tuck the bottom in yet.	___	___	_____
6) Never tucked top linens in on the sides.	___	___	_____
u. Placed the blanket on the bed.			
1) Unfolded it with the center crease in the middle.	___	___	_____
2) Put the upper hem about 6 to 8 inches from the top of the mattress.	___	___	_____
3) Opened and fan-folded the blanket to the other side.	___	___	_____
4) If step 4, aa and bb were not done, (not done in some agencies) turned the top sheet down over the blanket. Hem-stitching was down, away from the person.	___	___	_____
v. Placed the bedspread on the bed.			
1) Unfolded it with the center crease in the middle.	___	___	_____
2) Placed the upper hem even with the top of the mattress.	___	___	_____
3) Opened and fan-folded the bedspread to the other side.	___	___	_____
4) Made sure the bedspread facing the door was even. It covered all top linens.			
w. Tucked in top linens together at the foot of the bed so they were smooth and tight. Made a mitered corner. Left the side of the top linens untucked.	___	___	_____

Procedure—cont'd

	S	U	Comments
x. Went to the other side.			
y. Straightened all top linens. Worked from the head of the bed to the foot.			
z. Tucked in top linens together at the foot of the bed. Made a mitered corner. Left the side of top linens untucked.			
aa. Turned the top hem of the bedspread under the blanket to form a cuff.			
bb. Turned the top sheet down over the bedspread. Hem- stitching was down. (Steps aa and bb are not done in some agencies. The bedspread covers the pillow. If so tucked the bedspread under the pillow.)			
cc. Put the pillowcase on the pillow. The zipper, tag, or seam end of the pillow was inserted into the pillowcase first. Folded extra material under the pillow at the open end of the pillowcase.			
dd. Placed the pillow on the bed. The open end of the pillowcase was away from the door. The pillowcase seam was toward the head of the bed.			
5. Fan-folded top linens to the foot of the bed.			

Post-Procedure

	S	U	Comments
6. Placed the call light and other items within reach.			
7. Lowered the bed to a safe and comfortable level. Followed the care plan.			
8. Put the towels, washcloth, gown or pajamas, and bath blanket in the bedside stand.			
9. Provided for comfort.			
10. Completed a safety check of the room.			
11. Followed agency policy for dirty linens.			
12. Practiced hand hygiene.			

Making an Occupied Bed

Name: _____   Date: _____

Quality of Life	S	U	Comments
• Knocked before entering the person's room.	___	___	_____
• Addressed the person by name.	___	___	_____
• Introduced yourself by name and title.	___	___	_____
• Explained the procedure before starting and during the procedure.	___	___	_____
• Protected the person's rights during the procedure.	___	___	_____
• Handled the person gently during the procedure.	___	___	_____

Pre-Procedure

1. Followed *Delegation Guidelines: Making Beds.*
   Saw *Promoting Safety and Comfort:*
   a. *Making Beds*
   b. *The Occupied Bed*
2. Practiced hand hygiene.
3. Collected the following:
   • Gloves
   • Laundry bag
   • Clean linens (same as closed bed)
   • Towel, paper towels, or disposable bed protector (as a barrier for clean linens)
4. Placed linens on a clean surface. First place the barrier between the clean surface and clean linens if required by agency policy.
5. Identified the person. Checked the identification (ID) bracelet against the assignment sheet. Used 2 identifiers. Also called the person by name.
6. Provided for privacy.
7. Removed the call light.
8. Raised the bed for body mechanics. Bed rails were up if used. Bed wheels were locked (braked).
9. Lowered the head of the bed. It was as flat as possible.

Procedure

10. Practiced hand hygiene. Put on gloves.
11. Loosened top linens at the foot of the bed.
12. Lowered the bed rail near you if up.
13. Folded and removed the bedspread. Did the same for the blanket. Placed each over the chair.
14. Covered the person with a bath blanket from the bedside stand.
    a. Unfolded the bath blanket over the top sheet.
    b. Had the person hold the bath blanket. If he or she could not, tucked the top part under the person's shoulders.
    c. Grasped the top sheet under the bath blanket at the shoulders. Brought the sheet down toward the foot of the bed. Removed the sheet from under the blanket.
15. Positioned the person on his or her side facing away from you. Adjusted the pillow for comfort.
16. Loosened bottom linens from the head to the foot of the bed.
17. Fan-folded bottom linens 1 at a time toward the person. Started with the cotton drawsheet. If the mattress pad was re-used, did not fan-fold it.

Procedure—cont'd   S   U   Comments

18. Removed and discarded the gloves. Practiced hand hygiene. Put on clean gloves. _____ _____ _____

19. Placed a clean mattress pad on the bed. Unfolded it length-wise with the center crease in the middle. Fan-folded the top part toward the person. If the mattress pad was re-used, straightened and smoothed any wrinkles. _____ _____ _____

20. Placed the bottom sheet on the mattress pad. Hem-stitching was away from the person. Unfolded the sheet with the crease in the middle. For a flat sheet, the small hem was even with the bottom of the mattress. Fan-folded the top part toward the person. _____ _____ _____

21. Tucked the corners of a fitted sheet over the mattress. For a flat sheet, made a mitered corner at the head of the bed. Tucked the sheet under the mattress from the head to the foot. _____ _____ _____

22. *If using a drawsheet:*
    a. Placed the cotton drawsheet or padded waterproof drawsheet on the bed. It was in the middle of the mattress. _____ _____ _____
    b. Opened the drawsheet. _____ _____ _____
    c. Fan-folded it toward the person. _____ _____ _____
    d. Tucked in excess fabric. _____ _____ _____

23. *If using a waterproof under-pad:*
    a. Placed the waterproof under-pad on the bed. It was in the middle of the mattress. _____ _____ _____
    b. Fan-folded it toward the person. _____ _____ _____

24. Explained to the person that he or she would roll over a "bump." Assured the person that he or she would not fall. _____ _____ _____

25. Helped the person turn to the other side. Adjusted the pillow for comfort. _____ _____ _____

26. Raised the bed rail. Went to the other side and lowered the bed rail. _____ _____ _____

27. Loosened bottom linens. Removed 1 piece at a time. Placed each piece in the laundry bag. (Note: Discarded the disposable bed protector, incontinence product, and disposable drawsheet in the trash. Did not put them in the laundry bag.) _____ _____ _____

28. Removed and discarded the gloves. Practiced hand hygiene. _____ _____ _____

29. Straightened and smoothed the mattress pad. _____ _____ _____

30. Pulled the clean bottom sheet toward you. Tucked fitted sheet corners over the mattress. For a flat sheet, made a mitered corner at the top. Tucked the sheet under the mattress from the head to the foot of the bed. _____ _____ _____

31. Pulled the drawsheets tightly toward you and tucked it in. _____ _____ _____

32. Positioned the person supine in the center of the bed. Adjusted the pillow for comfort. _____ _____ _____

33. Put the top sheet on the bed. Unfolded it length-wise with the crease in the middle. The large hem was even with the top of the mattress. Hem-stitching was on the outside. _____ _____ _____

34. Had the person hold the top sheet so you could remove the bath blanket. Or tucked the top sheet under the person's shoulders. Removed the bath blanket. Placed it in the laundry bag. _____ _____ _____

Procedure—cont'd	S	U	Comments
35. Unfolded the blanket on the bed. The crease was in the middle and it covered the person. The upper hem was 6 to 8 inches from the top of the mattress.	_____	_____	_____
36. Unfolded the bedspread on the bed. The center crease was in the middle and it covered the person. The top hem was even with the mattress top.	_____	_____	_____
37. Turned the top hem of the bedspread under the blanket to make a cuff.	_____	_____	_____
38. Brought the top sheet down over the bedspread to form a cuff.	_____	_____	_____
39. Went to the foot of the bed.	_____	_____	_____
40. Made a 2-inch toe pleat across the foot of the bed. The pleat (fold) was about 6 to 8 inches from the foot of the bed. The pleat prevents pressure on the toes from top linens.	_____	_____	_____
41. Lifted the mattress corner with 1 arm. Tucked all top linens under the bottom of the mattress. Made a mitered corner. Avoided removing the toe pleat. Left the side of the top linens untucked.	_____	_____	_____
42. Raised the bed rail. Went to the other side and lowered the bed rail.	_____	_____	_____
43. Straightened and smoothed top linens.	_____	_____	_____
44. Tucked all top linens under the bottom of the mattress. Made a mitered corner. Left the side of the top linens untucked.	_____	_____	_____
45. Changed the pillowcase(s).	_____	_____	_____

Post-Procedure

	S	U	Comments
46. Provided for comfort.	_____	_____	_____
47. Placed the call light and other needed items within reach.	_____	_____	_____
48. Lowered the bed to a safe and comfortable level. Followed the care plan. The bed wheels were locked (braked).	_____	_____	_____
49. Raised or lowered bed rails. Followed the care plan.	_____	_____	_____
50. Put the clean towels, washcloth, gown or pajamas, and bath blanket in the bedside stand.	_____	_____	_____
51. Unscreened the person.	_____	_____	_____
52. Completed a safety check of the room.	_____	_____	_____
53. Followed agency policy for used linens.	_____	_____	_____
54. Practiced hand hygiene.	_____	_____	_____

Making a Surgical Bed

Name: _____   Date: _____

	S	U	Comments

Pre-Procedure

1. Followed *Delegation Guidelines: Making Beds*.
   Saw *Promoting Safety and Comfort:*
   a. *Making Beds*   _____ _____ _____
   b. *The Surgical Bed*   _____ _____ _____
2. Practiced hand hygiene.   _____ _____ _____
3. Collected the following:
   • Clean linens (same as for closed bed)
   • Gloves   _____ _____ _____
   • Laundry bag   _____ _____ _____
   • Equipment requested by the nurse   _____ _____ _____
   • Towel, paper towels, or disposable bed protector
     (as a barrier for clean linens)   _____ _____ _____
4. Placed linens on a clean surface. First placed the
   barrier between the clean surface and clean linens
   if required by agency policy.   _____ _____ _____
5. Removed the call light.   _____ _____ _____
6. Raised the bed for body mechanics.   _____ _____ _____

Procedure

7. Removed and placed all linens in the laundry bag.
   Wore gloves. Practiced hand hygiene after removing
   and discarding them.   _____ _____ _____
8. Made a closed bed. Did not tuck top linens under the
   mattress.   _____ _____ _____
9. Folded all top linens at the foot of the bed back onto
   the bed. The fold was even with the edge of the mattress. _____ _____ _____
10. Knew on which side of the bed the stretcher would be
    placed. Fan-folded linens length-wise to the other
    side of the bed.   _____ _____ _____
11. Put a pillowcase on each pillow.   _____ _____ _____
12. Placed the pillow(s) on a clean surface.   _____ _____ _____

Post-Procedure

13. Left the bed in its highest position.   _____ _____ _____
14. Left both bed rails down.   _____ _____ _____
15. Put the clean towels, washcloth, gown or pajamas,
    and bath blanket in the bedside stand.   _____ _____ _____
16. Moved furniture away from the bed. Allowed room
    for the stretcher and the staff.   _____ _____ _____
17. Did not attach the call light to the bed.   _____ _____ _____
18. Completed a safety check of the room.   _____ _____ _____
19. Followed agency policy for used linens.   _____ _____ _____
20. Practiced hand hygiene.   _____ _____ _____

Assisting the Person to Brush and Floss the Teeth

Name: _____ Date: _____

Quality of Life	S	U	Comments

- Knocked before entering the person's room.
- Addressed the person by name.
- Introduced yourself by name and title.
- Explained the procedure before starting and during the procedure.
- Protected the person's rights during the procedure.
- Handled the person gently during the procedure.

Pre-Procedure

1. Followed *Delegation Guidelines: Oral Hygiene*. Saw *Promoting Safety and Comfort: Purpose of Oral Hygiene*.
2. Practiced hand hygiene.
3. Collected the following:
   - Toothbrush with soft bristles
   - Toothpaste
   - Mouthwash (or solution noted on care plan)
   - Floss (if used)
   - Water cup with cool water
   - Straw
   - Kidney basin
   - Hand towel
   - Paper towels
   - Gloves
4. Placed the paper towels on the over-bed table. Arranged items on top of them.
5. Identified the person. Checked the ID (identification) bracelet against the assignment sheet. Used 2 identifiers. Also called the person by name.
6. Provided for privacy.
7. Lowered the bed rail near you if up.

Procedure

8. Positioned the person for oral hygiene.
9. Placed the towel over the person's chest. This protected garments and linens from spills.
10. Adjusted the over-bed table in front of the person.
11. Let the person perform oral hygiene. This included brushing the teeth and tongue, rinsing the mouth, flossing, and using mouthwash or other solution.
12. Removed the towel when the person was done.
13. Moved the over-bed table to the side of the bed.

Post-Procedure

14. Assisted with hand hygiene.
15. Provided for comfort.
16. Placed the call light and other needed items within reach.
17. Raised or lowered bed rails. Followed the care plan.

Post-Procedure—cont'd

	S	U	Comments
18. Rinsed the toothbrush. Cleaned, rinsed, and dried equipment. Used clean, dry paper towels for drying. Returned the toothbrush and equipment to their proper place. Wore gloves.	_____	_____	_____
19. Wiped the over-bed table with the paper towels. Discarded the paper towels.	_____	_____	_____
20. Unscreened the person.	_____	_____	_____
21. Completed a safety check of the room.	_____	_____	_____
22. Followed agency policy for dirty linens.	_____	_____	_____
23. Removed and discarded the gloves. Practiced hand hygiene.	_____	_____	_____
24. Reported and recorded your observations.	_____	_____	_____

Brushing and Flossing the Person's Teeth

Name: _____   Date: _____

	S	U	Comments

Quality of Life
- Knocked before entering the person's room.
- Addressed the person by name.
- Introduced yourself by name and title.
- Explained the procedure before starting and during the procedure.
- Protected the person's rights during the procedure.
- Handled the person gently during the procedure.

Pre-Procedure
1. Followed *Delegation Guidelines: Oral Hygiene.* Saw *Promoting Safety and Comfort: Purpose of Oral Hygiene.*
2. Practiced hand hygiene.
3. Collected the following:
   - Toothbrush with soft bristles
   - Toothpaste
   - Mouthwash (or solution noted on care plan)
   - Floss (if used)
   - Water cup with cool water
   - Straw
   - Kidney basin
   - Hand towel
   - Paper towels
   - Gloves
4. Placed the paper towels on the over-bed table. Arranged items on top of them.
5. Identified the person. Checked the ID (identification) bracelet against the assignment sheet. Used 2 identifiers. Also called the person by name.
6. Provided for privacy.
7. Raised the bed for body mechanics. Bed rails were up if used.

Procedure
8. Lowered the bed rail near you if up.
9. Assisted the person to a sitting position or side-lying position near you. (Note: Some state competency tests require that the person be at a 75- to 90-degree angle.)
10. Placed the towel across the person's chest.
11. Adjusted the over-bed table so you could reach it with ease.
12. Practiced hand hygiene. Put on the gloves.
13. Held the toothbrush over the kidney basin. Poured some water over the brush.
14. Applied toothpaste to the toothbrush.
15. Brushed the teeth gently. Brushed the inner, outer, and chewing surfaces of upper and lower teeth.
16. Brushed the tongue gently. Also gently brushed the roof of the mouth, inside of the cheeks, and gums.
17. Allowed the person to rinse the mouth with water. Held the kidney basin under the person's chin. Repeated this step as needed.

Procedure—cont'd	**S**	**U**	**Comments**

18. Flossed the person's teeth (optional).
   a. Broke off an 18-inch piece of dental floss from the dispenser.
   b. Held the floss between the middle fingers of each hand.
   c. Stretched the floss with your thumbs. Held the floss between your thumbs and index fingers.
   d. Started at the upper back tooth on the right side. Worked around to the left side.
   e. Rubbed gently against the side of the tooth. Used up-and-down motions. Did not jerk or snap the floss against the tooth or into the gums.
   f. Curved the floss into a "C" shape against the tooth at the gum line. Rubbed the side of the tooth with the floss from the gum line to the crown. Used gentle up-and-down motions.
   g. Moved to a new section of floss after every second tooth. Remembered to floss the back side of the last tooth.
   h. Flossed the lower teeth. Started on the right side. Worked around to the left side. Remembered to floss the back side of the last tooth.
   i. Discarded the floss.
19. Allowed the person to use mouthwash or other solution. Held the kidney basin under the chin.
20. Wiped the person's mouth. Removed the towel.
21. Removed and discarded the gloves. Practiced hand hygiene.

Post-Procedure

22. Assisted with hand hygiene.
23. Provided for comfort.
24. Placed the call light and other needed items within reach.
25. Lowered the bed to a safe and comfortable level appropriate for the person. Followed the care plan.
26. Raised or lowered bed rails. Followed the care plan.
27. Rinsed the toothbrush. Cleaned, rinsed, and dried equipment. Used clean, dry paper towels for drying. Returned the toothbrush and equipment to their proper place. Wore gloves.
28. Wiped off the over-bed table with the paper towels. Discarded the paper towels.
29. Unscreened the person.
30. Completed a safety check of the room.
31. Followed agency policy for used linens.
32. Removed and discarded the gloves. Practiced hand hygiene.
33. Reported and recorded your observations.

Providing Mouth Care for the Unconscious Person

VIDEO

Name: _____   Date: _____

Quality of Life	S	U	Comments
• Knocked before entering the person's room.			
• Addressed the person by name.			
• Introduced yourself by name and title.			
• Explained the procedure before starting and during the procedure.			
• Protected the person's rights during the procedure.			
• Handled the person gently during the procedure.			

Pre-Procedure

	S	U	Comments
1. Followed *Delegation Guidelines: Purpose of Oral Hygiene.* Saw *Promoting Safety and Comfort:*			
a. *Purpose of Oral Hygiene*			
b. *Mouth Care for the Unconscious Person*			
2. Practiced hand hygiene.			
3. Collected the following:			
• Cleaning agent (checked care plan)			
• Sponge swabs			
• Plastic tongue depressor			
• Water cup with cool water			
• Hand towel			
• Kidney basin			
• Lip lubricant			
• Paper towels			
• Gloves			
4. Placed the paper towels on the over-bed table. Arranged items on top of them.			
5. Identified the person. Checked the ID (identification) bracelet against the assignment sheet. Used 2 identifiers. Also called the person by name.			
6. Provided for privacy.			
7. Raised the bed for body mechanics. Bed rails were up if used.			

Procedure

	S	U	Comments
8. Lowered the bed rail near you.			
9. Positioned the person in a side-lying position near you. Turned the person's head well to the side.			
10. Placed the towel under the person's face and along the chest. This protected the person and the bed.			
11. Put on the gloves.			
12. Placed the kidney basin under the chin.			
13. Separated the upper and lower teeth. Used the plastic tongue depressor. Was gentle. Never used force. If you had problems, asked the nurse for help.			
14. Moistened the sponge swabs moistened with the cleaning agent. Squeezed out excess cleaning agent.			
15. Cleaned the mouth.			
a. Cleaned the chewing and inner surfaces of the teeth.			
b. Cleaned the gums and outer surfaces of the teeth.			
c. Swabbed the roof of the mouth, inside of the cheek, and the lips.			
d. Swabbed the tongue.			
e. Moistened and squeezed out a clean swab. Swabbed the mouth to rinse.			
f. Placed used swabs in the kidney basin.			

Procedure—cont'd	**S**	**U**	**Comments**
16. Removed the kidney basin and supplies.	_____	_____	_____
17. Wiped the person's mouth. Removed the towel.	_____	_____	_____
18. Applied lubricant to the lips.	_____	_____	_____
19. Removed and discarded the gloves. Practiced hand hygiene.	_____	_____	_____

Post-Procedure

	S	**U**	**Comments**
20. Provided for comfort.	_____	_____	_____
21. Placed the call light and other needed items within reach.	_____	_____	_____
22. Lowered the bed to a safe and comfortable level. Followed the care plan.	_____	_____	_____
23. Raised or lowered bed rails. Followed the care plan.	_____	_____	_____
24. Cleaned, rinsed, dried, and returned equipment to its proper place. Used clean, dry paper towels for drying. Discarded disposable items. (Wore gloves.)	_____	_____	_____
25. Wiped off the over-bed table with paper towels. Discarded the paper towels.	_____	_____	_____
26. Unscreened the person.	_____	_____	_____
27. Completed a safety check of the room.	_____	_____	_____
28. Told the person that you were leaving the room. Told the person when you would return.	_____	_____	_____
29. Followed agency policy for dirty linens.	_____	_____	_____
30. Removed and discarded the gloves. Practiced hand hygiene.	_____	_____	_____
31. Reported and recorded your observations.	_____	_____	_____

Providing Denture Care

Name: _____   Date: _____

Quality of Life	S	U	Comments
• Knocked before entering the person's room.	___	___	_____
• Addressed the person by name.	___	___	_____
• Introduced yourself by name and title.	___	___	_____
• Explained the procedure before starting and during the procedure.	___	___	_____
• Protected the person's rights during the procedure.	___	___	_____
• Handled the person gently during the procedure.	___	___	_____

Pre-Procedure

1. Followed *Delegation Guidelines: Purpose of Oral Hygiene.* Saw *Promoting Safety and Comfort:*
   a. *Purpose of Oral Hygiene*
   b. *Denture Care*
2. Practiced hand hygiene.
3. Collected the following:
   • Denture brush or toothbrush (for cleaning dentures)
   • Denture cup and lid labeled with the person's name and room and bed number
   • Denture cleaning agent
   • Denture adhesive as noted in the care plan (if needed)
   • Mouthwash (or other noted solution)
   • Kidney basin
   • 2 hand towels
   • Gauze squares
   • Paper towels
   • Gloves
4. Placed the paper towels on the over-bed table. Arranged items on top of them.
5. Identified the person. Checked the ID (identification) bracelet against the assignment sheet. Used 2 identifiers. Also called the person by name.
6. Provided for privacy.

Procedure

7. Lined the bottom of the sink with a towel. Did not use paper towels. Filled the sink half-way with water.
8. Raised the bed for body mechanics.
9. Lowered the bed rail near you if up.
10. Practiced hand hygiene. Put on gloves.
11. Placed the towel over the person's chest.
12. Asked the person to remove the dentures. Carefully placed them in the kidney basin.
13. Removed the dentures if the person could not do so. Used gauze squares to get a good grip on the slippery dentures.
    a. Grasped the upper denture with your thumb and index finger. Moved it up and down slightly to break the seal. Gently removed the denture. Placed it in the kidney basin.
    b. Grasped and removed the lower denture with your thumb and index finger. Turned it slightly and lifted it out of the person's mouth. Placed it in the kidney basin.
14. Followed the care plan for raising side rails.
15. Took the kidney basin, denture cup, denture brush, and denture cleaning agent to the sink.

Procedure—cont'd	**S**	**U**	**Comments**
16. Rinsed the denture cup and lid.	_____	_____	_____
17. Rinsed each denture under cool or warm running water. Followed center policy for water temperature.	_____	_____	_____
18. Returned dentures to the kidney basin.	_____	_____	_____
19. Applied the denture cleaning agent to the brush.	_____	_____	_____
20. Brushed each denture. Brushed the inner, outer, and chewing surfaces and all surfaces that touched the gums.	_____	_____	_____
21. Rinsed the dentures under running water. Used warm or cool water as directed by the cleaning agent manufacturer.	_____	_____	_____
22. Placed dentures in the denture cup. Covered the dentures with cool or warm water. Followed center policy for water temperature. Closed the lid tightly.	_____	_____	_____
23. Cleaned the kidney basin.	_____	_____	_____
24. Took the denture cup and kidney basin to the over-bed table. Lowered the bed rail if up.	_____	_____	_____
25. Had the person use mouthwash (or noted solution). Held the kidney basin under the chin.	_____	_____	_____
26. Applied denture adhesive if used. Followed the manufacturer's instructions for how to apply and the amount to use.	_____	_____	_____
27. Had the person insert the dentures. Inserted them if the person could not._____			
a. Held the upper denture firmly with your thumb and index finger. Raised the upper lip with the other hand. Inserted the denture. Gently pressed on the denture with your index fingers to make sure it was in place.	_____	_____	_____
b. Held the lower denture with your thumb and index finger. Pulled the lower lip down slightly. Inserted the denture. Gently pressed down on it to make sure it was in place.			
28. Placed the denture cup with the dentures in the top drawer of the bedside stand if the dentures were not worn. The dentures were in water or in a denture soaking solution. Made sure that the lid was on tightly.	_____	_____	_____
29. Wiped the person's mouth. Removed the towel.	_____	_____	_____
30. Removed and discarded the gloves. Practiced hand hygiene.	_____	_____	_____

Post-Procedure

	S	**U**	**Comments**
31. Assisted with hand hygiene.	_____	_____	_____
32. Provided for comfort.	_____	_____	_____
33. Placed the call light and other needed items within reach.	_____	_____	_____
34. Lowered the bed to a safe and comfortable level. Followed the care plan.	_____	_____	_____
35. Raised or lowered bed rails. Followed the care plan.	_____	_____	_____
36. Removed the towel from the sink. Drained the sink.	_____	_____	_____
37. Rinsed the brushes. Emptied and rinsed the denture cup. Cleaned, rinsed, and dried equipment. Used clean, dry paper towels for drying. Returned brushes and equipment to their proper place. Discarded disposable items. Wore gloves for this step.	_____	_____	_____
38. Wiped off the over-bed table with the paper towels. Discarded the paper towels.	_____	_____	_____
39. Unscreened the person.	_____	_____	_____
40. Completed a safety check of the room.	_____	_____	_____
41. Followed center policy for dirty linens.	_____	_____	_____
42. Removed and discarded the gloves. Practiced hand hygiene.	_____	_____	_____
43. Reported and recorded your observations.	_____	_____	_____

Giving a Complete Bed Bath

Name: _____   Date: _____

Quality of Life	S	U	Comments

Quality of Life
- Knocked before entering the person's room.
- Addressed the person by name.
- Introduced yourself by name and title.
- Explained the procedure before starting and during the procedure.
- Protected the person's rights during the procedure.
- Handled the person gently during the procedure.

Pre-Procedure
1. Followed *Delegation Guidelines: Daily Hygiene and Bathing.* Saw *Promoting Safety and Comfort:*
   a. *Daily Hygiene and Bathing*
   b. *Bathing*
2. Practiced hand hygiene.
3. Identified the person. Checked the identification (ID) bracelet against the assignment sheet. Used 2 identifiers. Also called the person by name.
4. Collected clean linens. Placed linens on a clean surface.
5. Collected the following:
   - Wash basin
   - Soap or bodywash
   - Water thermometer
   - Orangewood stick or nail file
   - Washcloth (and at least 4 washcloths for perineal care)
   - 2 bath towels and 2 hand towels
   - Bath blanket
   - Clothing or sleepwear
   - Lotion and powder
   - Deodorant or antiperspirant
   - Brush and comb
   - Other grooming items as requested
   - Paper towels
   - Gloves
6. Covered the over-bed table with paper towels. Arranged items on the over-bed table. Adjusted the height as needed.
7. Provided for privacy.
8. Raised the bed for body mechanics. Bed rails were up if used. Lowered the bed rail near you if up.

Procedure
9. Practiced hand hygiene. Put on gloves.
10. Removed the sleepwear. Did not expose the person. Followed agency policy for used clothing or sleepwear.
11. Covered the person with a bath blanket. Removed top linens.
12. Lowered the head of the bed. It was as flat as possible. The person had at least one pillow.
13. Filled the wash basin 2/3 (two-thirds) full with water. Raised the bed rail before leaving the bedside. Followed the care plan for water temperature. Water temperature was 110°F to 115°F (43.3°C to 46.1°C) for adults. Measured water temperature. Used the water thermometer. Or dipped your elbow or inner wrist into the basin to test the water.

Procedure—cont'd

	S	U	Comments
14. Lowered the bed rail near you if up.	___	___	_____
15. Asked the person to check the water temperature. Adjusted the water temperature as needed. Raised the bed rail before leaving the bedside. Lowered the bed rail when you returned.	___	___	_____
16. Placed the basin on the over-bed table.	___	___	_____
17. Placed a hand towel over the person's chest.	___	___	_____
18. Made a mitt with the washcloth. Used a mitt for the entire bath.	___	___	_____
19. Had the person close his/her eyes. Washed the eyelids and around the eyes with water. Did not use soap.			
a. Cleaned the far eye. Gently wiped from the inner to the outer aspect of the eye with a corner of the mitt.	___	___	_____
b. Cleaned around the eye near you. Used a clean part of the washcloth for each stroke.	___	___	_____
20. Applied soap or body wash to the washcloth if the person prefers for washing the face.	___	___	_____
21. Washed the face and ears. Use soap or the body wash to wash the neck. Rinsed all areas and patted dry with the towel on the chest.	___	___	_____
22. Helped the person move to the side of the bed near you.	___	___	_____
23. Exposed the far arm. Placed a bath towel length-wise under the arm. Applied soap or body wash to the washcloth.	___	___	_____
24. Supported the arm with your palm under the person's elbow. His or her forearm rested on your forearm.	___	___	_____
25. Washed the arm, shoulder, and underarm. Used long, firm strokes. Rinsed and patted dry.	___	___	_____
26. Placed the basin on the towel. Put the person's hand into the water. Washed the hand well with soap. Cleaned under the fingernails with an orangewood stick or nail file.	___	___	_____
27. Had the person exercise the hand and fingers.	___	___	_____
28. Removed the basin. Dried the hand well. Covered the arm with the bath blanket.	___	___	_____
29. Repeated for the near arm.			
a. Placed a bath towel length-wise under the near arm.	___	___	_____
b. Supported the arm with your palm under the person's elbow. His or her forearm rested on your forearm.	___	___	_____
c. Washed the arm, shoulder, and underarm. Used long, firm strokes. Rinsed and patted dry.	___	___	_____
d. Placed the basin on the towel. Put the person's hand into the water. Washed the hand well. Cleaned under the fingernails with an orangewood stick or nail file.	___	___	_____
e. Had the person exercise the hand and fingers.	___	___	_____
f. Removed the basin. Dried the hand well. Covered the arm with the bath blanket.	___	___	_____
30. Placed a bath towel over the chest cross-wise. Held the towel in place. Pulled the bath blanket from under the towel to the waist. Applied soap or body wash to the washcloth.	___	___	_____
31. Lifted the towel slightly and washed the chest. Did not expose the person. Rinsed and patted dry, especially under the breasts.	___	___	_____
32. Moved the towel length-wise over the chest and abdomen. Did not expose the person. Pulled the bath blanket down to the pubic area. Applied soap or body wash to the washcloth.	___	___	_____

Procedure—cont'd   S   U   **Comments**

33. Lifted the towel slightly and washed the abdomen. Rinsed and patted dry.   _____   _____   _____

34. Pulled the bath blanket up to the shoulders. Covered both arms. Removed the towel.   _____   _____   _____

35. Changed soapy or cool water. Measured bath water temperature. Water temperature was 110°F to 115°F (43.3°C to 46.1°C) for adults. Used the water thermometer. Or dipped your elbow or inner wrist into the basin to test the water. If bed rails were used, raised the bed rail near you before leaving the bedside. Lowered it when you returned.   _____   _____   _____

36. Uncovered the far leg. Did not expose the genital area. Placed a towel length-wise under the foot and leg. Applied soap or body wash to the washcloth.   _____   _____   _____

37. Bent the knee and supported the leg with your arm. Washed it with long, firm strokes. Rinsed and patted dry.   _____   _____   _____

38. Placed the basin on the towel near the foot.   _____   _____   _____

39. Lifted the leg slightly. Slid the basin under the foot.   _____   _____   _____

40. Placed the foot in the basin. Used an orangewood stick or nail file to clean under toenails if instructed to do so. If the person could not bend the knees:
    a. Washed the foot with soap or body wash. Carefully separated the toes. Rinsed and patted dry.   _____   _____   _____
    b. Cleaned under the toenails with the orangewood stick or nail file if instructed to do so.   _____   _____   _____

41. Removed the basin. Dried the leg and foot. Applied lotion to the foot if directed by the nurse and care plan. Do not apply lotion between the toes. Covered the leg with the bath blanket. Removed the towel.   _____   _____   _____

42. Repeated for the near leg.
    a. Uncovered the near leg. Did not expose the genital area. Placed a towel length-wise under the foot and leg.   _____   _____   _____
    b. Bent the knee and supported the leg with your arm. Washed it with long, firm strokes. Rinsed and patted dry.   _____   _____   _____
    c. Placed the basin on the towel near the foot.   _____   _____   _____
    d. Lifted the leg slightly. Slid the basin under the foot.   _____   _____   _____
    e. Placed the foot in the basin. Used an orangewood stick or nail file to clean under toenails if instructed to do so. If the person could not bend the knee:
       1) Washed the foot. Carefully separated the toes. Rinsed and patted dry.   _____   _____   _____
       2) Cleaned under the toenails with an orangewood stick or nail file if instructed to do so.   _____   _____   _____
    f. Removed the basin. Dried the leg and foot. Applied lotion to the foot if directed by the nurse and care plan. Covered the leg with the bath blanket. Removed the towel.   _____   _____   _____

43. Changed the water. Measured water temperature. Raised the bed rail near you before leaving the bedside. Lowered it when you returned.   _____   _____   _____

44. Turned the person onto the side away from you. The person was covered with the bath blanket.   _____   _____   _____

45. Uncovered the back and buttocks. Did not expose the person. Placed a towel length-wise on the bed along the back. Applied soap or body wash to the washcloth.   _____   _____   _____

Procedure—cont'd	S	U	Comments

46. Washed the back. Worked from the back of the neck to the lower end of the buttocks. Used long, firm, continuous strokes. Rinsed and dried well.
47. Turned the person onto his or her back.   _____ _____ _____
48. Changed the water for perineal care. Water temperature was 105°F to 109°F (40.5°C to 42.7°C). Followed the care plan for water temperature. Measured water temperature according to agency policy. (Some state competency tests also require changing gloves and hand hygiene completed at this time.) Raised the bed rail near you before leaving the bedside. Lowered it when you returned.   _____ _____ _____
49. Allowed the person to perform perineal care if able. Provided perineal care if the person could not do so. At least 4 washcloths were used. (Practiced hand hygiene and wore gloves for perineal care.)   _____ _____ _____
50. Removed and discarded the gloves. Practiced hand hygiene.   _____ _____ _____
51. Gave a back massage.   _____ _____ _____
52. Applied lotion, powder, deodorant or antiperspirant as requested. Saw *Promoting Safety and Comfort: Bathing.*   _____ _____ _____
53. Put clean garments on the person.   _____ _____ _____
54. Combed and brushed the hair.   _____ _____ _____
55. Made the bed.   _____ _____ _____

Post-Procedure
56. Provided for comfort.   _____ _____ _____
57. Placed the call light and other needed items within reach.   _____ _____ _____
58. Lowered the bed to a safe and comfortable level. Followed the care plan.   _____ _____ _____
59. Raised or lowered bed rails. Followed the care plan.   _____ _____ _____
60. Put on clean gloves.   _____ _____ _____
61. Emptied, cleaned, rinsed, and dried the wash basin. Used clean, dry paper towels for drying. Returned the basin and other supplies to their proper place.   _____ _____ _____
62. Wiped off the over-bed table with paper towels. Discarded the paper towels.   _____ _____ _____
63. Unscreened the person.   _____ _____ _____
64. Completed a safety check of the room.   _____ _____ _____
65. Followed center policy for used linens.   _____ _____ _____
66. Removed and discarded the gloves. Practiced hand hygiene.   _____ _____ _____
67. Reported and recorded your observations.   _____ _____ _____

Assisting With the Partial Bath

Name: _____   Date: _____

	S	U	Comments

Quality of Life

- Knocked before entering the person's room.
- Addressed the person by name.
- Introduced yourself by name and title.
- Explained the procedure before starting and during the procedure.
- Protected the person's rights during the procedure.
- Handled the person gently during the procedure.

Pre-Procedure

1. Followed *Delegation Guidelines: Bathing.* Saw *Promoting Safety and Comfort:*
   a. *Daily Hygiene and Bathing*
   b. *Bathing*
2. Did the following:
   a. Practiced hand hygiene.
   b. Identified the person. Checked the identification (ID) bracelet against the assignment sheet. Used 2 identifiers. Also called the person by name.
   c. Collected clean linens. Placed linens on a clean surface.
   d. Collected the following:
      - Wash basin
      - Soap or bodywash
      - Water thermometer
      - Orangewood stick or nail file
      - Washcloth (and at least 4 washcloths for perineal care).
      - 2 bath towels and 2 hand towels
      - Bath blanket
      - Clothing or sleepwear
      - Lotion and powder
      - Deodorant or antiperspirant
      - Brush and comb
      - Other grooming items as requested
      - Paper towels
      - Gloves
   e. Covered the over-bed table with paper towels. Arranged items on the over-bed table. Adjusted the height as needed.
   f. Provided for privacy.

Procedure

3. Made sure the bed was in the lowest position.
4. Practiced hand hygiene. Put on gloves.
5. Covered the person with a bath blanket. Removed top linens.
6. Filled the wash basin 2/3 (two-thirds) full with water. Water temperature was 110°F to 115°F (43.3°C to 46.1°C) or as directed by the nurse. Measured water temperature with the water thermometer. Or tested bath water by dipping your elbow or inner wrist into the basin.
7. Asked the person to check the water temperature. Adjusted the water temperature as needed.

Procedure—cont'd	S	U	Comments
8. Placed the basin on the over-bed table.	___	___	_____
9. Positioned the person in Fowler's position. Or assisted him or her to sit at the bedside.	___	___	_____
10. Adjusted the over-bed table so the person could reach the basin and supplies.	___	___	_____
11. Helped the person undress. Used the bath blanket for privacy and warmth.	___	___	_____
12. Asked the person to wash easy-to-reach body parts. Explained that you would wash the back and areas the person could not reach.	___	___	_____
13. Placed the call light within reach. Asked him or her to signal when help was needed or bathing was completed.	___	___	_____
14. Removed and discarded the gloves. Practiced hand hygiene. Then left the room.	___	___	_____
15. Returned when the call light was on. Knocked before entering. Practiced hand hygiene.	___	___	_____
16. Changed the bath water. Measured bath water temperature (110°F to 115°F or 43.3°C to 46.1°C or as directed by the nurse). Used the water thermometer. Or tested the water by dipping your elbow or inner wrist into the basin.	___	___	_____
17. Raised the bed for body mechanics. The far bed rail was up if used.	___	___	_____
18. Asked what was washed. Put on gloves. Washed and dried areas the person could not reach. The face, hands, underarms, back, buttocks, and perineal area were washed for the partial bath.	___	___	_____
19. Removed and discarded the gloves. Practiced hand hygiene.	___	___	_____
20. Gave a back massage.	___	___	_____
21. Applied lotion, powder, and deodorant or antiperspirant as requested.	___	___	_____
22. Assisted with clean garments, hair care and other grooming needs.	___	___	_____
23. Made the bed.	___	___	_____

Post-Procedure

	S	U	Comments
24. Provided for comfort.	___	___	_____
25. Placed the call light and other needed items within reach.	___	___	_____
26. Lowered the bed to a safe and comfortable level. Followed the care plan.	___	___	_____
27. Raised or lowered bed rails. Followed the care plan.	___	___	_____
28. Put on clean gloves.	___	___	_____
29. Emptied, cleaned, rinsed, and dried the wash basin. Used clean, dry paper towels for drying. Returned the basin and supplies to their proper place.	___	___	_____
30. Wiped off the over-bed table with the paper towels. Discarded the paper towels.	___	___	_____
31. Unscreened the person.	___	___	_____
32. Completed a safety check of the room.	___	___	_____
33. Followed center policy for used linens.	___	___	_____
34. Removed and discarded the gloves. Practiced hand hygiene.	___	___	_____
35. Reported and recorded your observations.	___	___	_____

Assisting With a Tub Bath or Shower

Name: _____   Date: _____

Quality of Life	S	U	Comments
• Knocked before entering the person's room.	___	___	_____
• Addressed the person by name.	___	___	_____
• Introduced yourself by name and title.	___	___	_____
• Explained the procedure before starting and during the procedure.	___	___	_____
• Protected the person's rights during the procedure.	___	___	_____
• Handled the person gently during the procedure.	___	___	_____

Pre-Procedure

	S	U	Comments
1. Followed *Delegation Guidelines:*			
a. *Bathing*			
b. *Tub Baths and Showers*	___	___	_____
Saw *Promoting Safety and Comfort:*			
a. *Daily Hygiene and Bathing*	___	___	_____
b. *Bathing*	___	___	_____
c. *Tub Baths and Showers*	___	___	_____
2. Reserved the tub or shower room.	___	___	_____
3. Practiced hand hygiene.	___	___	_____
4. Identified the person. Checked the identification (ID) bracelet against the assignment sheet. Used 2 identifiers. Also called the person by name.	___	___	_____
5. Collected the following:			
• Washcloth and 2 bath towels	___	___	_____
• Bath blanket	___	___	_____
• Soap shower gel or bodywash	___	___	_____
• Water thermometer (for tub bath)	___	___	_____
• Clothing or sleepwear	___	___	_____
• Grooming items as requested	___	___	_____
• Robe and slip-resistant footwear	___	___	_____
• Rubber bath mat if needed	___	___	_____
• Disposable bath mat	___	___	_____
• Gloves	___	___	_____
• Wheelchair, shower chair, shower bench, and so on as needed	___	___	_____

Procedure

	S	U	Comments
6. Placed items in the tub or shower room. Used the space provided or a chair.	___	___	_____
7. Cleaned, disinfected, and dried the tub or shower. Also dried the tub or shower room floor. Used clean, dry paper towels for drying. Wore gloves for this step. Practiced hand hygiene after removing and discarding gloves.	___	___	_____
8. Placed a rubber bath mat in the tub or on the shower floor. Did not block the drain.	___	___	_____
9. Placed the disposable bath mat on the floor in front of the tub or shower.	___	___	_____
10. Placed the occupied sign on the door.	___	___	_____
11. Returned to the person's room. Provided for privacy. Practiced hand hygiene.	___	___	_____
12. Helped the person sit on the side of the bed.	___	___	_____
13. Helped the person put on a robe and slip-resistant footwear. Or the person left on clothing.	___	___	_____

Procedure—cont'd	**S**	**U**	**Comments**
14. Assisted or transported the person to the tub or shower room.	_____	_____	_____
15. Had the person sit on a chair if he or she walked to the tub or shower room.	_____	_____	_____
16. Provided for privacy.	_____	_____	_____
17. *For a tub bath:*			
a. Filled the tub halfway with warm water (usually 105°F; 40.5°C). Followed the care plan for water temperature.	_____	_____	_____
b. Measured water temperature. Used the water thermometer or checked the digital display.	_____	_____	_____
c. Asked the person to check the water temperature. Adjusted the water temperature as needed.	_____	_____	_____
18. *For a shower:*			
a. Turned on the shower.	_____	_____	_____
b. Adjusted water temperature and pressure. Checked the digital display. Water temperature is usually 105°F; 40.5°C.	_____	_____	_____
c. Asked the person to check the water temperature. Adjusted the water temperature as needed.	_____	_____	_____
19. Helped the person undress and remove footwear.	_____	_____	_____
20. Helped the person into the tub or shower. Positioned the shower chair and locked (braked) the wheels.	_____	_____	_____
21. Assisted with washing as necessary. Wore gloves.			
a. Washed the face, neck, arms, hands, chest, abdomen, legs, feet, back, and buttocks.	_____	_____	_____
b. Provided perineal care if the person was unable to do it. Wore clean gloves and used clean washcloths. Removed and discarded gloves. Practiced hand hygiene.	_____	_____	_____
c. Followed the care plan and the person's preferences for shampooing hair. Assisted with shampooing as needed.	_____	_____	_____
22. Asked the person to use the call light when done or when help is needed. Reminded the person that a tub bath lasts no longer than 20 minutes.	_____	_____	_____
23. Placed a towel across the chair.	_____	_____	_____
24. Left the room if the person could bathe alone. If not, stayed in the room or nearby. Removed and discarded the gloves and practiced hand hygiene if you left the room.	_____	_____	_____
25. Checked the person at least every 5 minutes.	_____	_____	_____
26. Returned when he or she signaled for you. Knocked before entering. Practiced hand hygiene.	_____	_____	_____
27. Turned off the shower or drained the tub. Covered the person with the bath blanket while the tub drained.	_____	_____	_____
28. Helped the person out of the shower or tub and onto a chair.	_____	_____	_____
29. Helped the person dry off. Patted gently. Dried under the breasts, between skin folds, in the perineal area, and between the toes.	_____	_____	_____
30. Applied lotion, powder, and deodorant or antiperspirant as requested.	_____	_____	_____
31. Helped the person dress and put on footwear.	_____	_____	_____
32. Helped the person return to the room. Provided for privacy.	_____	_____	_____
33. Assisted the person to a chair or into bed.	_____	_____	_____
34. Provided a back massage if the person returned to bed.	_____	_____	_____
35. Assisted with hair care and other grooming needs.	_____	_____	_____

Post-Procedure

	S	U	Comments
36. Provided for comfort.			
37. Placed the call light and other needed items within reach.			
38. Raised or lowered bed rails. Followed the care plan.			
39. Unscreened the person.			
40. Completed a safety check of the room.			
41. Cleaned, disinfected, and dried the tub or shower. Dried the tub or shower room floor. Used clean, dry paper towels for drying. Removed soiled linens. Wore gloves.			
42. Discarded disposable items. Put the unoccupied sign on the door. Returned supplies to their proper place.			
43. Followed center policy for dirty linens.			
44. Removed and discarded the gloves. Practiced hand hygiene.			
45. Reported and recorded your observations.			

Giving Female Perineal Care

Name: _____   Date: _____

Quality of Life	S	U	Comments

Quality of Life
- Knocked before entering the person's room.
- Addressed the person by name.
- Introduced yourself by name and title.
- Explained the procedure before starting and during the procedure.
- Protected the person's rights during the procedure.
- Handled the person gently during the procedure.

Pre-Procedure
1. Followed *Delegation Guidelines: Perineal Care.*
   Saw *Promoting Safety and Comfort:*
   a. *Daily Hygiene and Bathing*
   b. *Perineal Care*
2. Practiced hand hygiene.
3. Collected the following:
   - Soap, bodywash or other cleaning agent as directed
   - At least 4 washcloths
   - Bath towel
   - Bath blanket
   - Water thermometer
   - Wash basin
   - Waterproof under-pad
   - Gloves
   - Laundry bag
   - Paper towels
4. Covered the over-bed table with paper towels. Arranged items on top of them.
5. Identified the person. Checked the identification (ID) bracelet against the assignment sheet. Used 2 identifiers. Also called the person by name.
6. Provided for privacy.
7. Raised the bed for body mechanics. Bed rails were up if used.

Procedure
8. Lowered the bed rail near you if up.
9. Practiced hand hygiene. Put on gloves.
10. Covered the person with a bath blanket. Moved top linens to the foot of the bed.
11. Positioned the person on her back.
12. Draped the person.
13. Raised the bed rail if used.
14. Filled the wash basin. Water temperature was 105°F to 109°F (40.5°C to 42.7°C). Followed the care plan for water temperature. Measured water temperature according to agency policy.
15. Asked the person to check the water temperature. Adjusted the water temperature as needed. Raised the bed rail before leaving the bedside. Lowered it when you returned.
16. Placed the basin on the over-bed table.
17. Lowered the bed rail if up.
18. Helped the person flex her knees and spread her legs. Or helped her spread her legs as much as possible with the knees straight.

Procedure—cont'd

	S	U	Comments
19. Folded the corner of the bath blanket between her legs onto her abdomen.	___	___	_____
20. Placed a waterproof under-pad under her buttocks. Removed any wet or soiled incontinence products.	___	___	_____
21. Removed and discarded the gloves. Practiced hand hygiene. Put on clean gloves.	___	___	_____
22. Wet the washcloths.	___	___	_____
23. Squeezed out water from a washcloth. Made a mitted washcloth. Applied soap, body wash, or other cleansing agent. (Squeezed out excess water every time you changed washcloths. Did not place used washcloths back in the basin. Put used washcloths in the laundry bag.)	___	___	_____
24. Cleaned the perineum. Changed washcloths as needed.			
a. Spread the labia.	___	___	_____
b. Cleaned one side of the labia. Cleaned downward from front to back (top to bottom) with 1 stroke. Used one part of a washcloth.	___	___	_____
c. Cleaned the other side of the labia. Cleaned downward from front to back (top to bottom) with 1 stroke. Used a clean part of a washcloth.	___	___	_____
d. Cleaned the vaginal area. Cleaned downward from front to back (top to bottom) with 1 stroke. Used a clean part of a washcloth.	___	___	_____
25. Rinsed the perineum using a clean washcloth. Changed washcloths as needed.			
a. Separated the labia.	___	___	_____
b. Rinsed one side of the labia. Rinsed downward from front to back (top to bottom) with 1 stroke. Used one part of a washcloth.	___	___	_____
c. Rinsed the other side of the labia. Rinsed downward from front to back (top to bottom) with 1 stroke. Used a clean part of a washcloth.	___	___	_____
d. Rinsed the vaginal area. Rinsed downward front to back (top to bottom) with 1 stroke. Used a clean part of a washcloth.	___	___	_____
26. Patted the perineal area dry with the towel. Dried from front to back.	___	___	_____
27. Folded the blanket back between her legs.	___	___	_____
28. Helped the person lower her legs and turn onto her side away from you.	___	___	_____
29. Applied soap, body wash, or other cleansing agent to a clean mitted washcloth.	___	___	_____
30. Cleaned and rinsed the rectal area.	___	___	_____
a. Cleaned from the vagina to the anus with 1 stroke. Used one part of the washcloth.	___	___	_____
b. Repeated until the area is clean. Used a clean part of the washcloth for each stroke. Changed washcloths as needed.	___	___	_____
c. Rinsed the rectal area with a clean washcloth. Rinsed from the vagina to the anus. Repeated as necessary. Used a clean part of the washcloth for each stroke. Changed washcloths as needed.	___	___	_____
31. Patted the rectal area dry with the towel. Dried from the vagina to the anus.	___	___	_____
32. Removed the waterproof under-pad.	___	___	_____
33. Removed and discarded the gloves. Practiced hand hygiene. Put on clean gloves.	___	___	_____
34. Provided clean and dry linens and incontinence products as needed.			
35. Positioned the person on her back.	___	___	_____

Post-Procedure

	S	U	Comments
36. Covered the person. Removed the bath blanket.	_____	_____	_____
37. Provided for comfort.	_____	_____	_____
38. Placed the call light and other needed items within reach.	_____	_____	_____
39. Lowered the bed to a safe and comfortable level. Followed the care plan.	_____	_____	_____
40. Raised or lowered bed rails. Followed the care plan.	_____	_____	_____
41. Emptied, cleaned, rinsed, and dried the wash basin. Used clean, dry paper towels for drying.	_____	_____	_____
42. Returned the basin and supplies to their proper place.	_____	_____	_____
43. Wiped off the over-bed table with the paper towels. Discarded the paper towels.	_____	_____	_____
44. Unscreened the person.	_____	_____	_____
45. Completed a safety check of the room.	_____	_____	_____
46. Followed agency policy for used linens.	_____	_____	_____
47. Removed and discarded the gloves. Practiced hand hygiene.	_____	_____	_____
48. Reported and recorded your observations.	_____	_____	_____

Giving Male Perineal Care

Name: _____   Date: _____

Quality of Life	S	U	Comments
• Knocked before entering the person's room.			
• Addressed the person by name.			
• Introduced yourself by name and title.			
• Explained the procedure before starting and during the procedure.			
• Protected the person's rights during the procedure.			
• Handled the person gently during the procedure.			

Pre-Procedure

1. Followed *Delegation Guidelines: Perineal Care*. Saw *Promoting Safety and Comfort:*
   a. *Daily Hygiene and Bathing.*
   b. *Perineal Care*
2. Practiced hand hygiene.
3. Collected the following.
   • Soap, bodywash or other cleansing agent as directed
   • At least 4 washcloths
   • Bath towel
   • Bath blanket
   • Water thermometer
   • Wash basin
   • Waterproof under-pad
   • Gloves
   • Laundry bag
   • Paper towels
4. Covered the over-bed table with paper towels. Arranged items on top of them.
5. Identified the person. Checked the identification (ID) bracelet against the assignment sheet. Used 2 identifiers. Also called the person by name.
6. Provided for privacy.
7. Raised the bed for body mechanics. Bed rails were up if used.

Procedure

8. Lowered the bed rail near you if up.
9. Practiced hand hygiene. Put on gloves.
10. Covered the person with a bath blanket. Moved top linens to the foot of the bed.
11. Positioned the person on his back.
12. Draped the person.
13. Raised the bed rail if used.
14. Filled the wash basin. Water temperature was 105°F to 109°F (40.5°C to 42.7°C). Followed the care plan for water temperature. Measured water temperature according to agency policy.
15. Asked the person to check the water temperature. Adjusted the water temperature as needed. Raised the bed rail before leaving the bedside. Lowered it when you returned.
16. Placed the basin on the over-bed table.
17. Lowered the bed rail if up.
18. Folded the corner of the bath blanket between the legs onto his abdomen.

Procedure—cont'd	S	U	Comments
19. Placed a waterproof under-pad under the buttocks. Removed any wet or soiled incontinence products.	___	___	_____
20. Removed and discarded the gloves. Practiced hand hygiene. Put on clean gloves.	___	___	_____
21. Wetted the washcloths.	___	___	_____
22. Squeezed out water from a washcloth. Made a mitted washcloth. Applied soap. (Squeezed out water every time you changed washcloths. Did not place used washcloths back in the basin. Put used washcloths in the laundry bag.)	___	___	_____
23. Retracted the foreskin if the person was uncircumcised.	___	___	_____
24. Grasped the penis.	___	___	_____
25. Cleaned the tip. Used a circular motion. Started at the meatus of the urethra and worked outward. Repeated as needed. Used a clean part of the washcloth each time.	___	___	_____
26. Rinsed the tip with another washcloth. Used the same circular motion.	___	___	_____
27. Returned the foreskin to its natural position immediately after rinsing. After rinsing dried under the foreskin according to agency policy or person preferred.	___	___	_____
28. Cleaned the shaft of the penis. Used firm downward strokes. Used a clean part of a washcloth for each stoke.	___	___	_____
29. Rinsed the shaft. Used firm downward strokes. Used a clean part of a washcloth for each stoke.	___	___	_____
30. Helped the person flex his knees and spread his legs. Or helped him spread his legs as much as possible with his knees straight.	___	___	_____
31. Cleaned the scrotum. Used a clean part of a washcloth.	___	___	_____
32. Rinsed the scrotum. Used a clean part of a washcloth. Observed for redness and irritation of the skin folds.	___	___	_____
33. Patted dry the penis and the scrotum. Used the towel.	___	___	_____
34. Folded the bath blanket back between his legs.	___	___	_____
35. Helped him lower his legs and turn onto his side away from you.	___	___	_____
36. Cleaned the rectal area. Cleaned from scrotum (front or top) to the anus (back or bottom). Rinsed and dried well.	___	___	_____
37. Removed the waterproof under-pad.	___	___	_____
38. Removed and discarded the gloves. Practiced hand hygiene. Put on clean gloves.	___	___	_____
39. Provided clean and dry linens and incontinence products.	___	___	_____
40. Positioned the person for comfort			

Post-Procedure

	S	U	Comments
41. Covered the person. Removed the bath blanket.	___	___	_____
42. Provided for comfort.	___	___	_____
43. Placed the call light and other needed items within reach.	___	___	_____
44. Lowered the bed to a safe and comfortable level. Followed the care plan.	___	___	_____
45. Raised or lowered bed rails. Followed the care plan.	___	___	_____
46. Emptied, cleaned, rinsed, and dried the wash basin. Used clean, dry paper towels for drying.	___	___	_____
47. Returned the basin and supplies to their proper place.	___	___	_____
48. Wiped off the over-bed table with the paper towels. Discarded the paper towels.	___	___	_____
49. Unscreened the person.	___	___	_____
50. Completed a safety check of the room.	___	___	_____
51. Followed agency policy for used linens.	___	___	_____
52. Removed and discarded the gloves. Practiced hand hygiene.	___	___	_____
53. Reported and recorded your observations.	___	___	_____

Brushing and Combing Hair

Name: _____   Date: _____

Quality of Life	S	U	Comments

Quality of Life
- Knocked before entering the person's room.
- Addressed the person by name.
- Introduced yourself by name and title.
- Explained the procedure before starting and during the procedure.
- Protected the person's rights during the procedure.
- Handled the person gently during the procedure.

Pre-Procedure
1. Followed *Delegation Guidelines: Brushing and Combing Hair*. Saw *Promoting Safety and Comfort: Brushing and Combing Hair*.
2. Practiced hand hygiene.
3. Identified the person. Checked the ID (identification) bracelet against the assignment sheet. Used 2 identifiers. Also called the person by name.
4. Asked the person how to style hair.
5. Collected the following:
   - Comb and brush
   - Bath towel
   - Other hair care items as requested
6. Arranged items on the bedside stand.
7. Provided for privacy.

Procedure
8. Lowered the bed rail if up.
9. Positioned the person.
   a. *In a chair*—Helped the person to the chair. The person put on a robe and slip-resistant footwear when up.
   b. *In bed*—Raised the bed for body mechanics. Bed rails were up if used. Lowered the bed rail near you. Assisted the person to a semi-Fowler's position if allowed.
10. Placed a towel across the person's back and shoulders or across the pillow.
11. Had the person remove eyeglasses. Put them in the eyeglass case. Put the case inside the bedside stand.
12. *Hair that was not matted or tangled.*
    a. Used the comb to part the hair.
       1) Parted hair down the middle into 2 sides.
       2) Divided 1 side into 2 smaller sections.
    b. Brushed 1 of the small sections of hair. Started at the scalp and brushed toward the hair ends. Did the same for the other small section of hair. If the person preferred, brushed long hair starting at the hair ends.
    c. Repeated for the other side.
       1) Divided side into 2 smaller sections.
       2) Brushed 1 of the small sections of hair. Started at the scalp and brushed toward the hair ends. Did the same for the other small section of hair. If the person preferred, brushed long hair starting at the hair ends.

Procedure—cont'd | S | U | Comments

13. *Matted or tangled hair.*
   a. Took a small section of hair near the ends.
   b. Combed or brushed through to the hair ends.
   c. Added small sections of hair as you worked up to the scalp.
   d. Combed or brushed through each longer section to the hair ends.
14. Styled the hair as the person preferred.
15. Removed the towel.
16. Allowed the person to put on the eyeglasses.

Post-Procedure

17. Provided for comfort.
18. Placed the call light and other needed items within reach.
19. Lowered the bed to a safe and comfortable level. Followed the care plan.
20. Raised or lowered bed rails. Followed the care plan.
21. Removed hair from the brush or comb. Cleaned, rinsed, dried and returned hair care items to their proper place. Used clean, dry paper towels for drying. Wore gloves for this step. Removed and discarded the gloves. Practiced hand hygiene.
22. Unscreened the person.
23. Completed a safety check of the room.
24. Followed agency policy for used linens.
25. Practiced hand hygiene.

Shampooing the Person's Hair in Bed

Name: _____   Date: _____

Quality of Life	S	U	Comments
• Knocked before entering the person's room.	____	____	_____
• Addressed the person by name.	____	____	_____
• Introduced yourself by name and title.	____	____	_____
• Explained the procedure before starting and during the procedure.	____	____	_____
• Protected the person's rights during the procedure.	____	____	_____
• Handled the person gently during the procedure.	____	____	_____

Pre-Procedure

	S	U	Comments
1. Followed *Delegation Guidelines: Shampooing*. Saw *Promoting Safety and Comfort: Shampooing*.	____	____	_____
2. Practiced hand hygiene.	____	____	_____
3. Collected the following:			
• 2 bath towels	____	____	_____
• Washcloth	____	____	_____
• Shampoo	____	____	_____
• Hair conditioner (if requested)	____	____	_____
• Water thermometer	____	____	_____
• Water Pitcher	____	____	_____
• Shampoo basin	____	____	_____
• Collecting basin	____	____	_____
• Waterproof under-pad	____	____	_____
• Gloves (if needed)	____	____	_____
• Comb and brush	____	____	_____
• Hair dryer	____	____	_____
4. Arranged items nearby. Placed the collecting basin on a chair by the bed.	____	____	_____
5. Identified the person. Checked the ID (identification) bracelet against the assignment sheet. Used 2 identifiers. Also called the person by name.	____	____	_____
6. Provided for privacy.	____	____	_____
7. Raised the bed for body mechanics. Bed rails were up if used.	____	____	_____
8. Practiced hand hygiene.	____	____	_____

Procedure

	S	U	Comments
9. Lowered the bed rail near you if up.	____	____	_____
10. Covered the person's chest with a bath towel.	____	____	_____
11. Brushed and combed the hair to remove snarls and tangles.	____	____	_____
12. Positioned the person for a shampoo in bed .	____	____	_____
a. Lowered the head of the bed and removed the pillow.	____	____	_____
b. Placed the waterproof under-pad and shampoo basin under the head and shoulders.	____	____	_____
c. Supported the head and neck with a folded towel if necessary.	____	____	_____
13. Raised the bed rail if used.	____	____	_____
14. Filled the water pitcher. Water temperature was 105°F (40.5°C). Tested water temperature according to agency policy. Had the person check the water temperature. Adjusted the water temperature as needed. Raised the bed rail before leaving the bedside.	____	____	_____
15. Lowered the bed rail near you if up.	____	____	_____
16. Put on gloves (if needed).	____	____	_____

Procedure—cont'd   S   U   **Comments**

17. Had the person hold a washcloth over the eyes. It did
    not cover the nose and mouth. (Note: A damp washcloth
    is easier to hold. It does not slip. However, your agency
    may require a dry washcloth.)   _____   _____   _____
18. Used the water pitcher to wet the hair. Asked the person
    about the water temperature and adjusted as needed.   _____   _____   _____
19. Applied a small amount of shampoo.   _____   _____   _____
20. Worked up a lather with both hands. Started at the
    hairline. Worked toward the back of the head.   _____   _____   _____
21. Massaged the scalp with your fingertips. Did not
    scratch the scalp with your fingernails.   _____   _____   _____
22. Rinsed the hair until the water ran clear.   _____   _____   _____
23. Repeated the following steps:
    a. Applied a small amount of shampoo.   _____   _____   _____
    b. Worked up a lather with both hands. Started at the
        hairline. Worked toward the back of the head.   _____   _____   _____
    c. Massaged the scalp with your fingertips. Did not
        scratch the scalp with your fingernails.   _____   _____   _____
    d. Rinsed the hair until the water ran clear.   _____   _____   _____
24. Applied conditioner. Followed directions on the container.   _____   _____   _____
25. Squeezed water from the person's hair.   _____   _____   _____
26. Covered the hair with a bath towel.   _____   _____   _____
27. Removed the shampoo basin, collecting basin and
    waterproof under-pad.   _____   _____   _____
28. Dried the person's face with the towel on the chest.   _____   _____   _____
29. Raise the head of the bed.   _____   _____   _____
30. Rubbed the hair and scalp with the towel. Rubbed gently.
    Used the second towel if the first one was wet.   _____   _____   _____
31. Combed the hair to remove snarls and tangles.   _____   _____   _____
32. Dried and styled hair.   _____   _____   _____
33. Removed and discarded the gloves (if used). Practiced
    hand hygiene.   _____   _____   _____

Post-Procedure
34. Provided for comfort.   _____   _____   _____
35. Placed the call light and other needed items within
    reach.   _____   _____   _____
36. Lowered the bed to a safe and comfortable level.
    Followed the care plan.   _____   _____   _____
37. Raised or lowered bed rails. Followed the care plan.   _____   _____   _____
38. Unscreened the person.   _____   _____   _____
39. Completed a safety check of the room.   _____   _____   _____
40. Cleaned the comb and brush. Cleaned, rinsed, dried,
    and returned equipment to its proper place. Used
    clean, dry paper towels for drying. Wore gloves for
    this step. Discarded disposable items. Removed and
    discarded the gloves.   _____   _____   _____
41. Followed agency policy for used linens.   _____   _____   _____
42. Practiced hand hygiene.   _____   _____   _____
43. Reported and recorded your observations.   _____   _____   _____

Shaving the Person's Face With a Safety Razor

Name: _____   Date: _____

Quality of Life	S	U	Comments

Quality of Life
- Knocked before entering the person's room.
- Addressed the person by name.
- Introduced yourself by name and title.
- Explained the procedure before starting and during the procedure.
- Protected the person's rights during the procedure.
- Handled the person gently during the procedure.

Pre-Procedure
1. Followed *Delegation Guidelines: Shaving*. Saw *Promoting Safety and Comfort: Shaving*.
2. Practiced hand hygiene.
3. Collected the following:
   - Wash basin
   - Bath towel
   - Hand towel
   - Washcloth
   - Safety razor
   - Mirror
   - Shaving cream, soap, or lotion
   - Shaving brush
   - After-shave or lotion
   - Tissues or paper towels
   - Gloves
4. Arranged paper towels and supplies on the over-bed table.
5. Identified the person. Checked the ID (identification) bracelet against the assignment sheet. Used 2 identifiers. Also called the person by name.
6. Provided for privacy.
7. Raised the bed for body mechanics. Bed rails are up if used.

Procedure
8. Filled the wash basin with warm water.
9. Placed the basin on the over-bed table.
10. Lowered the bed rail near you if up.
11. Practiced hand hygiene. Put on gloves.
12. Assisted the person to semi-Fowler's position if allowed or the supine position.
13. Adjusted lighting to clearly see the person's face.
14. Placed the towel over the person's chest and shoulders.
15. Adjusted the over-bed table for easy reach.
16. Tightened the razor blade to the shaver if necessary.
17. Washed the person's face. Did not dry.
18. Wet the washcloth or towel. Wrung it out.
19. Applied the washcloth or towel to the face for a few minutes.
20. Applied shaving cream with your hands. (If needed, changed your gloves or wiped excess shaving cream from your gloves using a towel or paper towel.) Or used a shaving brush to apply lather.
21. Held the skin taut with 1 hand.
22. Shaved in the direction of hair growth. Used shorter strokes around the chin and lips.

Procedure—cont'd

	S	U	Comments
23. Rinsed the razor often. Wiped it with tissues or paper towels.			
24. Applied direct pressure to any bleeding areas.	___	___	_____
25. Washed off any remaining shaving cream or soap. Patted dry with a towel.	___	___	_____
26. Applied after-shave or lotion if requested. (If there were nicks or cuts, did not apply after-shave or lotion.)	___	___	_____
27. Removed and discarded the towels and gloves. Practiced hand hygiene.	___	___	_____

Post-Procedure

	S	U	Comments
28. Provided for comfort.	___	___	_____
29. Placed the call light and other needed items within reach.	___	___	_____
30. Lowered the bed to a safe and comfortable level. Followed the care plan.	___	___	_____
31. Raised or lowered bed rails. Followed the care plan.	___	___	_____
32. Cleaned, rinsed, dried, and returned equipment and supplies to their proper place. Used clean, dry paper towels for drying. Discarded the razor blade or disposable razor into the sharps container. Discarded other disposable items. Wore gloves.	___	___	_____
33. Wiped off the over-bed table with clean, dry paper towels. Discarded the paper towels.	___	___	_____
34. Unscreened the person.	___	___	_____
35. Completed a safety check of the room.	___	___	_____
36. Followed agency policy for used linens.	___	___	_____
37. Removed and discarded the gloves. Practiced hand hygiene.	___	___	_____
38. Reported nicks, cuts, irritation, or bleeding to the nurse at once. Also reported and recorded other observations.	___	___	_____

Giving Nail and Foot Care

Name: _____   Date: _____

Quality of Life	S	U	Comments
• Knocked before entering the person's room.	___	___	_____
• Addressed the person by name.	___	___	_____
• Introduced yourself by name and title.	___	___	_____
• Explained the procedure before starting and during the procedure.	___	___	_____
• Protected the person's rights during the procedure.	___	___	_____
• Handled the person gently during the procedure.	___	___	_____

Pre-Procedure

1. Followed *Delegation Guidelines: Nail and Foot Care.* Saw *Promoting Safety and Comfort: Nail and Foot Care.*   ___ ___
2. Practiced hand hygiene.   ___ ___
3. Collected the following:
   - Wash basin or whirlpool foot bath   ___ ___
   - Soap   ___ ___
   - Water thermometer   ___ ___
   - Bath towel   ___ ___
   - Hand towel   ___ ___
   - Washcloth   ___ ___
   - Kidney basin   ___ ___
   - Nail clippers   ___ ___
   - Orangewood stick   ___ ___
   - Emery board or nail file   ___ ___
   - Lotion for the hands   ___ ___
   - Lotion or petroleum jelly for the feet   ___ ___
   - Paper towels   ___ ___
   - Bath mat   ___ ___
   - Gloves   ___ ___
4. Arranged paper towels and other items on the over-bed table.   ___ ___
5. Identified the person. Checked the ID (identification) bracelet against the assignment sheet. Used 2 identifiers. Also called the person by name.   ___ ___
6. Provided for privacy.   ___ ___
7. Assisted the person to the bedside chair. Removed footwear and socks or stockings. Placed the call light and other needed items within reach.   ___ ___

Procedure

8. Placed the bath mat under the feet.   ___ ___
9. Filled the wash basin or whirlpool foot bath 2/3 (two-thirds) full with water. The nurse told you what water temperature to use. (Measured water temperature with a water thermometer. Or tested it by dipping your elbow or inner wrist into the basin. Followed agency policy.) Also asked the person to check the water temperature and adjusted as needed.   ___ ___
10. Placed the basin or foot bath on the bath mat.   ___ ___
11. Put on gloves.   ___ ___
12. Helped the person put his or her bare feet into the basin or foot bath. Both feet were completely covered by water.   ___ ___
13. Adjusted the over-bed table in front of the person.   ___ ___

Procedure—cont'd

	S	U	Comments
14. Filled the kidney basin ⅔ (two-thirds) full with water. The nurse told you what water temperature to use. (Measured water temperature with a water thermometer. Or tested it by dipping your elbow or inner wrist into the basin. Followed agency policy.) Also asked the person to check the water temperature adjusted as needed.			
15. Placed the kidney basin on the over-bed table.	_____	_____	_____
16. Placed the person's fingers into the basin. Positioned the arms for comfort.	_____	_____	_____
17. Allowed the fingers to soak for 5 to 10 minutes. Allowed the feet to soak for 15 to 20 minutes. Re-warmed water as needed.	_____	_____	_____
18. Removed the kidney basin.	_____	_____	_____
19. Dried the hands between the fingers thoroughly.	_____	_____	_____
20. Cleaned under the fingernails with the orangewood stick. Wiped the orangewood stick with a towel after each nail.	_____	_____	_____
21. Pushed cuticles back with the orangewood stick, towel. or a washcloth.	_____	_____	_____
22. Clipped fingernails straight across with nail clippers.	_____	_____	_____
23. Filed and shaped nails with an emery board or nail file. Nails were smooth with no rough edges. Checked each nail for smoothness. Filed as needed.	_____	_____	_____
24. Applied lotion to the hands. Warmed lotion first. To warm lotion, rub some between your hands or hold the bottle under warm water.	_____	_____	_____
25. Moved the over-bed table to the side.	_____	_____	_____
26. Removed and discarded the gloves. Practiced hand hygiene. Put on clean gloves. (Note: Some state competency tests require clean gloves for foot care.)	_____	_____	_____
27. Lifted a foot out of the water. Supported the foot and ankle with 1 hand. With your other hand, washed the foot and between the toes with soap and a washcloth. Returned the foot to the water to rinse the foot and between the toes.	_____	_____	_____
28. Repeated for the other foot. Lifted foot out of the water. Supported the foot and ankle with 1 hand. With your other hand, washed the foot and between the toes with soap and a washcloth. Returned the foot to the water to rinse the foot and between the toes.	_____	_____	_____
29. Removed the feet from the water. Dried thoroughly, especially between the toes. Supported the foot and ankle as needed.	_____	_____	_____
30. Applied lotion or petroleum jelly to the tops, soles, and heels of the feet. Did not apply between the toes. Warmed lotion or petroleum jelly first, by rubbing dome between your hands. Removed excess lotion or petroleum jelly with a towel. Supported the foot and ankle as needed.	_____	_____	_____
31. Removed and discarded the gloves. Practiced hand hygiene.	_____	_____	_____
32. Helped the person put on slip-resistant footwear.	_____	_____	_____

Post-Procedure

	S	U	Comments
33. Provided for comfort.	_____	_____	_____
34. Placed the call light and other needed items within reach.	_____	_____	_____
35. Raised or lowered bed rails. Followed the care plan.	_____	_____	_____
36. Cleaned, rinsed, dried, and returned equipment and supplies to their proper place. Used clean, dry paper towels for drying. Discarded disposable items. Wore gloves.	_____	_____	_____

Post-Procedure—cont'd

	S	U	Comments
37. Unscreened the person.	_____	_____	_____
38. Completed a safety check of the room.	_____	_____	_____
39. Followed agency policy for used linens.	_____	_____	_____
40. Removed and discarded the gloves. Practiced hand hygiene.	_____	_____	_____
41. Reported and recorded your observations.	_____	_____	_____

Undressing the Person

Name: _____   Date: _____

Quality of Life	S	U	Comments
• Knocked before entering the person's room.	____	____	_____
• Addressed the person by name.	____	____	_____
• Introduced yourself by name and title.	____	____	_____
• Explained the procedure before starting and during the procedure.	____	____	_____
• Protected the person's rights during the procedure.	____	____	_____
• Handled the person gently during the procedure.	____	____	_____

Pre-Procedure

1. Followed *Delegation Guidelines: Dressing and Undressing.* Saw *Promoting Safety and Comfort: Dressing and Undressing.*   ____ ____ _____
2. Asked a co-worker to help turn and position the person if needed.   ____ ____ _____
3. Practiced hand hygiene.   ____ ____ _____
4. Collected a bath blanket and clothing as requested by the person.   ____ ____ _____
5. Identified the person. Checked the ID (identification) bracelet against the assignment sheet. Used 2 identifiers. Also called the person by name.   ____ ____ _____
6. Provided for privacy.
7. Raised the bed for body mechanics. Bed rails were up if used.   ____ ____ _____
8. Lowered the bed rail on the person's affected (weak) side.   ____ ____ _____
9. Positioned the person supine.   ____ ____ _____
10. Covered the person with a bath blanket. Fan-folded linens to the foot of the bed.   ____ ____ _____

Procedure

11. Removed garments that opened in the back.
    a. Raised the head and shoulders. Or turned the person onto the side away from you.   ____ ____ _____
    b. Undid buttons, zippers, ties, or snaps.   ____ ____ _____
    c. Brought the sides of the garment to the sides of the person. For a side-lying position, tucked the far side under the person. Folded the near side onto the chest.   ____ ____ _____
    d. Positioned the person supine.   ____ ____ _____
    e. Slid the garment off the shoulder on the unaffected (strong) side. Removed it from the arm.   ____ ____ _____
    f. Removed the garment from the affected (weak) side.   ____ ____ _____
12. Removed garments that opened in the front.
    a. Undid buttons, zippers, ties, or snaps.   ____ ____ _____
    b. Slid the garment off the shoulder and arm on the unaffected (strong) side.   ____ ____ _____
    c. Had the person sit up or raised the head and shoulders. Brought the garment over to the affected (weak) side.   ____ ____ _____
    d. Lowered the head and shoulders. Removed the garment from the affected (weak) side.   ____ ____ _____

Procedure—cont'd	**S**	**U**	**Comments**
e. If you could not raise the head and shoulders:			
1) Turned the person toward you. Tucked the removed part of the garment under the person.	_____	_____	_____
2) Turned the person onto the side away from you.	_____	_____	_____
3) Pulled the side of the garment out from under the person. Made sure the person did not lie on it when supine.	_____	_____	_____
4) Returned the person to the supine position.	_____	_____	_____
5) Removed the garment from the affected (weak) side.	_____	_____	_____
13. Removed pullover garments.			
a. Undid any buttons, zippers, ties, or snaps.	_____	_____	_____
b. Removed the garment from the unaffected (strong) side.	_____	_____	_____
c. Raised the head and shoulders. Or turned the person onto the side away from you. Brought the garment up to the person's neck.	_____	_____	_____
d. Brought the garment over the person's head.	_____	_____	_____
e. Removed the garment from the affected (weak) side.	_____	_____	_____
f. Positioned the person in the supine position.	_____	_____	_____
14. Removed pants or slacks.			
a. Removed footwear and socks.	_____	_____	_____
b. Positioned the person supine.	_____	_____	_____
c. Undid buttons, zippers, ties, snaps, or buckles.	_____	_____	_____
d. Removed the belt.	_____	_____	_____
e. Had the person lift the buttocks off the bed. Slid the pants down over the hips and buttocks. Had the person lower the hips and buttocks.	_____	_____	_____
f. If the person could not raise the hips off the bed:			
1) Turned the person toward you.	_____	_____	_____
2) Slid the pants off the hip and buttocks on the unaffected (strong) side.	_____	_____	_____
3) Turned the person away from you.	_____	_____	_____
4) Slid the pants off the hip and buttocks on the affected (weak) side.	_____	_____	_____
g. Slid the pants down the legs and over the feet.	_____	_____	_____
15. Dressed the person.	_____	_____	_____

Post-Procedure

	S	**U**	**Comments**
16. Provided for comfort.	_____	_____	_____
17. Placed the call light and other needed items within reach.	_____	_____	_____
18. Lowered the bed to a safe and comfortable level. Followed the care plan.	_____	_____	_____
19. Raised or lowered bed rails. Followed the care plan.	_____	_____	_____
20. Unscreened the person.	_____	_____	_____
21. Completed a safety check of the room.	_____	_____	_____
22. Followed agency policy for soiled clothing.	_____	_____	_____
23. Practiced hand hygiene.	_____	_____	_____
24. Reported and recorded your observations.	_____	_____	_____

Dressing the Person

Name: _____   Date: _____

Quality of Life	S	U	Comments

Quality of Life
- Knocked before entering the person's room.
- Addressed the person by name.
- Introduced yourself by name and title.
- Explained the procedure before starting and during the procedure.
- Protected the person's rights during the procedure.
- Handled the person gently during the procedure.

Pre-Procedure
1. Followed *Delegation Guidelines: Dressing and Undressing.* Saw *Promoting Safety and Comfort: Dressing and Undressing.*
2. Asked a co-worker to help turn and position the person if needed.
3. Practiced hand hygiene.
4. Asked the person what he or she would like to wear.
5. Got a bath blanket and clothing requested by the person.
6. Identified the person. Checked the ID (identification) bracelet against the assignment sheet. Used 2 identifiers. Also called the person by name.
7. Provided for privacy.
8. Raised the bed for body mechanics. Bed rails were up if used.
9. Lowered the bed rail (if up) on the person's affected (weak) side.
10. Positioned the person supine.
11. Covered the person with a bath blanket. Fan-folded linens to the foot of the bed.
12. Undressed the person.

Procedure
13. Put on garments that opened in the back.
    a. Slid the garment onto the arm and shoulder of the affected (weak) side.
    b. Slid the garment onto the arm and shoulder of the unaffected (strong) side.
    c. Raised the person's head and shoulders.
    d. Brought the sides to the back.
    e. If you could not raise the person's head and shoulders:
       1) Turned the person toward you.
       2) Brought 1 side of the garment to the person's back.
       3) Turned the person away from you.
       4) Brought the other side to the person's back.
    f. Fastened buttons, zippers, ties, snaps, or other closures.
    g. Positioned the person supine.
14. Put on garments that opened in the front.
    a. Slid the garment onto the arm and shoulder on the affected (weak) side.
    b. Raised the head and shoulders. Brought the side of the garment around to the back. Lowered the person down. Slid the garment onto the arm and shoulder of the unaffected (strong) arm.

Procedure—cont'd	S	U	Comments

Procedure—cont'd

   c. If the person could not raise the head and shoulders:
     1) Turned the person away from you.
     2) Tucked the garment under him or her.
     3) Turned the person toward you.
     4) Pulled the garment out from under him or her.
     5) Turned the person back to the supine position.
     6) Slid the garment over the arm and shoulder of the unaffected (strong) arm.
   d. Fastened buttons, zippers, ties, snaps, or other closures.

15. Put on pullover garments
   a. Slid the arm and shoulder of the garment onto the affected (weak) side.
   b. Raised the person's head and shoulders.
   c. Brought the neck of the garment over the head.
   d. Slid the arm and shoulder of the garment onto the unaffected (strong) side. Brought the garment down.
   e. If the person could not assume a semi-sitting position:
     1) Brought the neck of the garment over the head.
     2) Slid the arm and shoulder of the garment onto the unaffected (strong) side.
     3) Turned the person onto the unaffected (strong) side.
     4) Pulled the garment down on the person's affected (weak) side.
     5) Turned the person onto the affected (weak) side.
     6) Pulled the garment down on the person's unaffected (strong) side.
   f. Positioned the person supine.

16. Put on pants or slacks.
   a. Slid the pants over the feet and up the legs.
   b. Had the person raise the hips and buttocks off the bed.
   c. Brought the pants up over the buttock and hip on the affected (weak) side.
   d. Pulled the pants over the buttock and hip on the unaffected (strong) side.
   e. If the person could not raise the hips and buttocks:
     1) Turned the person onto the unaffected (strong) side.
     2) Pulled the pants over the buttock and hip on the affected (weak) side.
     3) Turned the person onto the affected (weak) side.
     4) Pulled the pants over the buttock and hip on the unaffected (strong) side.
     5) Positioned the person supine.
   f. Fastened buttons, zippers, ties, snaps, a belt buckle, or other closures.

17. Put socks and slip-resistant footwear on the person. Socks were all the way up and smooth

18. Helped the person get out of bed. If the person stayed in bed, covered the person. Removed the bath blanket.

Post-Procedure

19. Provided for comfort.
20. Placed the call light and other needed items within reach.
21. Lowered the bed to a safe and comfortable level. Followed the care plan.
22. Raised or lowered bed rails. Followed the care plan.
23. Unscreened the person.
24. Completed a safety check of the room.
25. Followed agency policy for removed clothing.
26. Practiced hand hygiene.
27. Reported and recorded your observations.

Changing a Standard Patient Gown on a Person With an IV

Name: _____   Date: _____

Quality of Life	S	U	Comments
• Knocked before entering the person's room.	_____	_____	_____
• Addressed the person by name.	_____	_____	_____
• Introduced yourself by name and title.	_____	_____	_____
• Explained the procedure before starting and during the procedure.	_____	_____	_____
• Protected the person's rights during the procedure.	_____	_____	_____
• Handled the person gently during the procedure.	_____	_____	_____

Pre-Procedure

1. Followed *Delegation Guidelines: Changing Patient Gowns.* Saw *Promoting Safety and Comfort: Changing Patient Gowns.*   _____ _____ _____
2. Practiced hand hygiene.   _____ _____ _____
3. Got a clean gown and bath blanket.   _____ _____ _____
4. Identified the person. Checked the ID (identification) bracelet against the assignment sheet. Used 2 identifiers. Also called the person by name.   _____ _____ _____
5. Provided for privacy.   _____ _____ _____
6. Raised the bed for body mechanics. Bed rails were up if used.   _____ _____ _____

Procedure

7. Lowered the bed rail near you (if up).   _____ _____ _____
8. Covered the person with a bath blanket. Fan-folded linens to the foot of the bed.   _____ _____ _____
9. Untied the gown. Freed parts that the person was lying on.   _____ _____ _____
10. Removed the gown from the arm with *no IV*.   _____ _____ _____
11. Gathered up the sleeve of the arm *with the IV*. Slid it over the IV site and tubing. Removed the arm and hand from the sleeve.   _____ _____ _____
12. Kept the sleeve gathered. Slid your arm along the tubing to the bag.   _____ _____ _____
13. Removed the bag from the pole. Slid the bag and tubing through the sleeve. Did not pull on the tubing. Kept the bag above the person.   _____ _____ _____
14. Hung the IV bag on the pole.   _____ _____ _____
15. Gathered the sleeve of the clean gown that went on the arm with the IV infusion.   _____ _____ _____
16. Removed the bag from the pole. Slipped the sleeve over the bag at the shoulder part of the gown. Hung the bag.   _____ _____ _____
17. Slid the gathered sleeve over the tubing, hand, arm, and IV site. Then slid it onto the shoulder.   _____ _____ _____
18. Put the other side of the gown on the person. Fastened the gown.   _____ _____ _____
19. Covered the person. Removed the bath blanket.   _____ _____ _____

Post-Procedure

20. Provided for comfort.   _____ _____ _____
21. Placed the call light and other needed items within reach.   _____ _____ _____
22. Lowered the bed to a safe and comfortable level. Followed the care plan.   _____ _____ _____
23. Raised or lowered bed rails. Followed the care plan.   _____ _____ _____
24. Unscreened the person.   _____ _____ _____
25. Completed a safety check of the room.   _____ _____ _____

Post-Procedure—cont'd

	S	U	Comments
26. Followed agency policy for used linens.	___	___	_____
27. Practiced hand hygiene.	___	___	_____
28. Asked the nurse to check the flow rate.	___	___	_____
29. Reported and recorded your observations.	___	___	_____

Giving the Bedpan

Name: _____   Date: _____

Quality of Life	S	U	Comments

- Knocked before entering the person's room.
- Addressed the person by name.
- Introduced yourself by name and title.
- Explained the procedure before starting and during the procedure.
- Protected the person's rights during the procedure.
- Handled the person gently during the procedure.

Pre-Procedure

1. Followed *Delegation Guidelines:*
   a. *Normal Urination*
   b. *Bedpans.*
   Saw *Promoting Safety and Comfort:*
   a. *Urinary Needs*
   b. *Bedpans*
2. Provided for privacy.
3. Practiced hand hygiene.
4. Put on gloves.
5. Collected the following:
   - Bedpan
   - Bedpan cover (optional)
   - Toilet paper
   - Waterproof under-pad (if required by agency policy)
   - Bath blanket (optional)
6. Arranged equipment on the chair or bed.

Procedure

7. Raised the bed for body mechanics (if the person's needs were not urgent). Lowered the bed rail near you (if up).
8. Lowered the head of the bed. Positioned the person supine. Or raised the head of the bed slightly for comfort.
9. Covered the person with a bath blanket. Folded the top linens and gown out of the way. Kept the lower body covered.
10. Had the person flex the knees and raise the buttocks. He or she did so by pushing against the mattress with the feet.
11. Slid your hand under the lower back. Helped raise the buttocks. If a waterproof under-pad was used, placed it under the buttocks.
12. Slid the bedpan under the person. Made sure the bedpan was centered under the person.
13. If the person could not assist in getting on the bedpan:
    a. Placed the waterproof under-pad under the buttocks (if used).
    b. Turned the person onto the side away from you.
    c. Placed the bedpan firmly against the buttocks.
    d. Held the bedpan securely. Turned the person onto his or her back.
    e. Made sure the bedpan was centered under the person.
14. Covered the person.

Procedure—cont'd	S	U	Comments

15. Raised the head of the bed so the person was in a sitting position (Fowler's position) for a standard bedpan. Or raised the head of the bed to a comfortable level for the person. (Note: Some state competency tests require removing gloves and hand hygiene before you raise the head of the bed.)

16. Made sure the person was correctly positioned on the bedpan.

17. Raised the bed rail if used. Lowered the bed.

18. Placed the toilet paper and call light within reach. (Note: For some state competency tests you ask the person to use hand wipes to clean the hands after wiping with toilet paper.)

19. Asked the person to signal when done or when help was needed. (Stayed with the person if necessary. Was respectful. Provided as much privacy as possible.)

20. Removed and discarded the gloves. Practiced hand hygiene.

21. Left the room and closed the door.

22. Returned when the person signaled. Or checked on the person every 5 minutes. Knocked before entering.

23. Practiced hand hygiene. Put on gloves.

24. Raised the bed for body mechanics. Lowered the bed rail (if used) and lowered the head of the bed.

25. Had the person raise the buttocks. Removed the bedpan. Or held the bedpan and turned the person onto the side away from you.

26. Cleaned the genital area if the person could not do so.
    a. Cleaned from the meatus (front or top) to the anus (back or bottom) with toilet paper. Used fresh toilet paper for each wipe.
    b. Provided perineal care if needed.
    c. Removed and discarded the waterproof under-pad (if used).

27. Covered the bedpan. Took it to the bathroom. Raised the bed rail (if used) before leaving the bedside.

28. Noted the color, amount (output), and character of urine or feces.

29. Emptied the bedpan contents into the toilet and flushed.

30. Rinsed the bedpan. Poured the rinse into the toilet and flushed.

31. Cleaned the bedpan with a disinfectant. Poured disinfectant into the toilet and flushed. Dried the bedpan with clean, dry paper towels.

32. Returned the bedpan to its proper place.

33. Removed and discarded the gloves. Practiced hand hygiene and put on clean gloves.

34. Helped the person with hand hygiene.

35. Removed and discarded the gloves. Practiced hand hygiene.

36. Covered the person with the top linens. Removed the bath blanket (if used).

Post-Procedure

37. Provided for comfort.

38. Placed the call light and other needed items within reach.

39. Lowered the bed to a safe and comfortable level. Followed the care plan.

40. Raised or lowered bed rails. Followed the care plan.

Post-Procedure—cont'd   S   U   **Comments**

41. Unscreened the person.   _____   _____   _____

42. Completed a safety check of the room.   _____   _____   _____

43. Followed agency policy for used linens.   _____   _____   _____

44. Practiced hand hygiene.   _____   _____   _____

45. Reported and recorded your observations. _____   _____   _____

Giving the Urinal

Name: _____   Date: _____

Quality of Life	S	U	Comments
• Knocked before entering the person's room.	___	___	_____
• Addressed the person by name.	___	___	_____
• Introduced yourself by name and title.	___	___	_____
• Explained the procedure before starting and during the procedure.	___	___	_____
• Protected the person's rights during the procedure.	___	___	_____
• Handled the person gently during the procedure.	___	___	_____

Pre-Procedure

	S	U	Comments
1. Followed *Delegation Guidelines:*			
a. *Normal Urination*	___	___	_____
b. *Urinals.*	___	___	_____
Saw *Promoting Safety and Comfort:*			
a. *Urinary Needs*	___	___	_____
b. *Urinals*	___	___	_____
2. Provided for privacy.	___	___	_____
3. Determined if the man would stand, sit, or lie in bed.	___	___	_____
4. Practiced hand hygiene.	___	___	_____
5. Put on gloves.	___	___	_____
6. Collected the following:			
• Urinal	___	___	_____
• Slip-resistant footwear if the man would stand to void	___	___	_____

Procedure

	S	U	Comments
7. *Standing to use the urinal:*			
a. Helped him sit on the side of the bed.	___	___	_____
b. Put slip-resistant footwear on him.	___	___	_____
c. Helped him stand. Provided support if he was unsteady.	___	___	_____
d. Gave him the urinal.			
8. *Using the urinal in bed:*			
a. Gave him the urinal if he was in bed.	___	___	_____
b. Reminded him to tilt the bottom down to prevent spills.	___	___	_____
9. *Positioning the urinal (in bed or standing):*			
a. Helped the person stand if he would stand.	___	___	_____
b. Positioned the urinal.	___	___	_____
c. Placed the penis in the urinal if he could not do so.	___	___	_____
d. Covered him for privacy.	___	___	_____
10. Placed the call light within reach. Asked him to signal when done or when help was needed.	___	___	_____
11. Provided for privacy.	___	___	_____
12. Removed and discarded the gloves. Practiced hand hygiene.	___	___	_____
13. Left the room and closed the door.	___	___	_____
14. Returned when he signaled for you. Or checked on him every 5 minutes. Knocked before entering.	___	___	_____
15. Practiced hand hygiene. Put on gloves.	___	___	_____
16. Closed the cap on the urinal. Took it to the bathroom.	___	___	_____
17. Noted the color, amount (output), and clarity of urine.	___	___	_____
18. Emptied the urinal into the toilet and flushed.	___	___	_____
19. Rinsed the urinal with cold water. Poured rinse into the toilet and flushed.	___	___	_____

Procedure—cont'd	S	U	Comments
20. Cleaned the urinal with a disinfectant. Poured disinfectant into the toilet and flushed. Dried the urinal with clean, dry paper towels.	___	___	_____
21. Returned the urinal to its proper place.	___	___	_____
22. Removed and discarded the soiled gloves. Practiced hand hygiene and put on clean gloves.	___	___	_____
23. Assisted with hand hygiene.	___	___	_____
24. Removed and discarded the gloves. Practiced hand hygiene.	___	___	_____

Post-Procedure

	S	U	Comments
25. Provided for comfort.	___	___	_____
26. Placed the call light and other needed items within reach.	___	___	_____
27. Raised or lowered bed rails. Followed the care plan.	___	___	_____
28. Unscreened him.	___	___	_____
29. Completed a safety check of the room.	___	___	_____
30. Followed agency policy for used linens.	___	___	_____
31. Practiced hand hygiene.	___	___	_____
32. Reported and recorded your observations.	___	___	_____

Helping the Person to the Commode

Name: _____   Date: _____

	S	U	Comments

Quality of Life
- Knocked before entering the person's room.
- Addressed the person by name.
- Introduced yourself by name and title.
- Explained the procedure before starting and during the procedure.
- Protected the person's rights during the procedure.
- Handled the person gently during the procedure.

Pre-Procedure
1. Followed *Delegation Guidelines:*
   a. *Normal Urination*
   b. *Commodes.*
   Saw *Promoting Safety and Comfort:*
   a. *Urinary Needs*
   b. *Commodes*
2. Provided for privacy.
3. Practiced hand hygiene.
4. Put on gloves.
5. Collected the following:
   - Commode
   - Toilet paper
   - Bath blanket
   - Transfer belt
   - Robe and slip-resistant footwear

Procedure
6. Placed the commode next to the bed.
7. Helped the person sit on the side of the bed. Lowered the bed rail if used.
8. Helped the person put on a robe and slip-resistant footwear.
9. Applied the transfer belt.
10. Assisted the person to the commode. Used the transfer belt.
11. Removed the transfer belt. Covered the person with a bath blanket for warmth.
12. Placed the toilet paper and call light within reach.
13. Asked the person to signal when done or when help was needed. (Stayed with the person if necessary. Was respectful. Provided as much privacy as possible.)
14. Removed and discarded the gloves. Practiced hand hygiene.
15. Left the room. Closed the door.
16. Returned when the person signaled. Or checked on the person every 5 minutes. Knocked before entering.
17. Practiced hand hygiene. Put on gloves.
18. Helped the person clean the genital area as needed. Removed and discarded the gloves. Practiced hand hygiene.
19. Applied the transfer belt. Helped the person back to bed; used the transfer belt. Removed the transfer belt, robe, and footwear. Raised the bed rail if used.
20. Put on clean gloves. Removed and covered the commode container. Cleaned the commode.

Procedure—cont'd

	S	U	Comments
21. Took the container to the bathroom.	___	___	_____
22. Observed urine and feces for color, amount (output), and character.	___	___	_____
23. Emptied the container contents into the toilet and flushed.	___	___	_____
24. Rinsed the container. Poured the rinse into the toilet and flushed.	___	___	_____
25. Cleaned and disinfected the container. Poured disinfectant into the toilet and flushed. Dried the container with clean, dry paper towels.	___	___	_____
26. Returned the container to the commode. Closed the lid on the commode. Cleaned other parts of the commode if necessary.	___	___	_____
27. Returned other supplies to their proper place.	___	___	_____
28. Removed and discarded the gloves. Practiced hand hygiene and put on clean gloves.	___	___	_____
29. Assisted with hand hygiene.	___	___	_____
30. Removed and discarded the gloves. Practiced hand hygiene.	___	___	_____

Post-Procedure

	S	U	Comments
31. Provided for comfort.	___	___	_____
32. Placed the call light and other needed items within reach.	___	___	_____
33. Raised or lowered bed rails. Followed the care plan.	___	___	_____
34. Unscreened the person.	___	___	_____
35. Completed a safety check of the room.	___	___	_____
36. Followed center policy for used linens.	___	___	_____
37. Practiced hand hygiene.	___	___	_____
38. Reported and recorded your observations.	___	___	_____

Applying Incontinence Products

Name: _____   Date: _____

Quality of Life	S	U	Comments

Quality of Life
- Knocked before entering the person's room.
- Addressed the person by name.
- Introduced yourself by name and title.
- Explained the procedure before starting and during the procedure.
- Protected the person's rights during the procedure.
- Handled the person gently during the procedure.

Pre-Procedure
1. Followed *Delegation Guidelines: Applying Incontinence Products*. Saw *Promoting Safety and Comfort*:
   a. *Urinary Needs*
   b. *Applying Incontinence Products*
2. Practiced hand hygiene.
3. Collected the following:
   - Incontinence product as directed by the nurse
   - Barrier cream or moisturizer as directed by the nurse
   - Cleaning agent—soap, body wash, or no-rinse incontinence cleanser
   - Items for perineal care
   - Paper towels
   - Trash bags
   - Gloves
   - Slip-resistant footwear if the person stands
4. Covered the over-bed table with paper towels. Arranged items on top of them.
5. Identified the person. Checked the ID (identification) bracelet against the assignment sheet. Used 2 identifiers. Also called the person by name.
6. Marked the date, time, and your initials on the new product. Followed agency policy.
7. Provided for privacy.
8. Filled the wash basin. Water temperature was 105°F to 109°F (40.5°C to 42.7°C). Measured water temperature according to agency policy. Asked the person to check the water temperature. Adjusted water temperature as needed.
9. Raised the bed for body mechanics. Bed rails were up if used. (Omitted this step if the person stood.)

Procedure
10. Lowered the head of the bed. The bed was as flat as possible.
11. Lowered the bed rail near you if up.
12. Practiced hand hygiene. Put on the gloves.
13. Covered the person with a bath blanket. Lowered top linens to the foot of the bed. Lowered the pants or slacks (omitted this step if the person was standing).
14. *To apply an incontinence brief with the person in bed:*
    a. Placed a waterproof under-pad under the buttocks. Asked the person to raise the buttocks off the bed. Or turned the person from side to side.
    b. Loosened the tabs on each side of the used brief.

Procedure—cont'd   S   U   **Comments**

   c. Removed the used brief from front to back
     (top to bottom). Rolled the product up with the
     soiled side inside. Did 1 of the following.
     1) Have the person spread the legs. Roll the front
       of the product toward the back (bottom). Turn
       the person onto the side away from you.
       Removed the brief.
     2) Turned the person onto the side away from you.
       Removed the brief.   _____ _____ _____
   d. Observed the urine as you rolled the product up.
     Estimated the amount of urine: small, moderate,
     large. Observed for urine color and blood.   _____ _____ _____
   e. Placed the used brief in the trash bag. Tied and sealed
     the bag and set the bag aside.   _____ _____ _____
   f. Performed perineal care wearing clean gloves.
     Applied the barrier cream or moisturizer.   _____ _____ _____
   g. Removed and discarded the gloves Practiced hand
     hygiene. Put on clean gloves.
   h. Opened the new brief. Folded it in half length-wise
     along the center.   _____ _____ _____
   i. Inserted the brief between the legs from front to
     back (top to bottom).   _____ _____ _____
   j. Unfolded and spread the back panel.   _____ _____ _____
   k. Centered the brief in the perineal area.   _____ _____ _____
   l. Turned the person onto his or her back.   _____ _____ _____
   m. Unfolded and spread the front panel. Provided a
     "cup" shape in the perineal area. For a man,
     positioned the penis downward.   _____ _____ _____
   n. Made sure the brief was positioned high in the
     groin folds. The brief fit the shape of the body.   _____ _____ _____
   o. Secured the brief.
     1) Pulled the lower tape tab forward on the side near
       you. Attached it at a slightly upward angle. Did
       the same for the other side.   _____ _____ _____
     2) Pulled the upper tape tab forward on the side near
       you. Attached it in a horizontal manner. Did the
       same for the other side.   _____ _____ _____
   p. Smoothed out all wrinkles and folds.   _____ _____ _____
15. *To apply a pad and undergarment with the person in bed:*
   a. Placed a waterproof under-pad under the buttocks.
     Asked the person to raise the buttocks off the bed.
     Or turned the person from side to side.   _____ _____ _____
   b. Turned the person onto the side away from you.   _____ _____ _____
   c. Pulled the undergarment down. The waistband was
     over the knee.   _____ _____ _____
   d. Removed the used pad from the front to back
     (top to bottom). Observed the urine as you rolled the
     product up. Estimated the amount of urine in the used
     product: small, moderate, large. Observed for urine
     color and blood.   _____ _____ _____
   e. Placed the used pad in the trash bag. Tied and sealed
     the bag and set the bag aside.   _____ _____ _____
   f. Performed perineal care wearing clean gloves.
     Applied the barrier cream or moisturizer.   _____ _____ _____
   g. Removed and discarded the gloves Practiced hand
     hygiene. Put on clean gloves.
   h. Folded the new pad in half length-wise along the center.   _____ _____ _____
   i. Inserted the pad between the legs from front to back
     (top to bottom).   _____ _____ _____

Procedure—cont'd   **S**   **U**   **Comments**

    j. Unfolded and spread the back panel.

    k. Centered the pad in the perineal area.

    l. Pulled the garment up at the back.

    m. Turned the person onto his or her back.

    n. Unfolded and spread the front panel. For a man, positioned the penis downward.

    o. Pulled the garment up in front.

    p. Adjusted the pad and under-garment for a good fit.

16. *To apply pull-on underwear with the person standing:*

    a. Helped the person stand. Removed the pants or slacks.

    b. Tore the side seams to remove the used underwear.

    c. Removed the underwear from front to back (top to bottom). Observed the urine as you rolled the underwear up. Estimated the amount of urine in the used product: small, moderate, large. Observed for urine color and blood.

    d. Placed the used underwear in the trash bag. Tied and sealed the bag and set the bag aside.

    e. Performed perineal care wearing clean gloves. Applied barrier cream or moisturizer.

    f. Removed and discarded the gloves Practiced hand hygiene. Put on clean gloves.

    g. Had the person sit on the side of the bed.

    h. Slid the new underwear over the feet to past the knees.

    i. Helped the person stand.

    j. Pulled the underwear up.

    k. Adjusted as needed for a good fit.

17. Asked about comfort. Asked if the product felt too loose or too tight. Checked for wrinkles or creases. Made sure the product did not rub or irritate the groin. Adjusted the product as needed.

18. Removed and discarded the gloves. Practiced hand hygiene.

19. Raised or put on pants or slacks.

Post-Procedure

20. Provided for comfort.

21. Placed the call light and other needed items within reach.

22. Lowered the bed to a safe and comfortable level. Followed the care plan.

23. Raised or lowered bed rails. Followed the care plan.

24. Unscreened the person.

25. Practiced hand hygiene. Put on clean gloves.

26. Cleaned, rinsed, dried, and returned the wash basin and other equipment. Used clean, dry paper towels for drying. Returned items to their proper place.

27. Removed and discarded the gloves. Practiced hand hygiene.

28. Completed a safety check of the room.

29. Followed the agency policy for used linens.

30. Practiced hand hygiene.

31. Reported and recorded your observations.

Giving Catheter Care

Name: _____   Date: _____

Quality of Life	**S**	**U**	**Comments**

- Knocked before entering the person's room.
- Addressed the person by name.
- Introduced yourself by name and title.
- Explained the procedure before starting and during the procedure.
- Protected the person's rights during the procedure.
- Handled the person gently during the procedure.

Pre-Procedure

1. Followed *Delegation Guidelines:*
   a. *Perineal Care*
   b. *Catheter Care*
   Saw *Promoting Safety and Comfort:*
   a. *Perineal Care*
   b. *Urinary Catheters*
   c. *Catheter Care*
2. Practiced hand hygiene.
3. Collected the following:
   - Items for perineal care
   - Gloves
   - Bath blanket
4. Covered the over-bed table with paper towels. Arranged items on top of them.
5. Identified the person. Checked the ID (identification) bracelet against the assignment sheet. Used 2 identifiers. Also called the person by name.
6. Provided for privacy.
7. Filled the wash basin. Water temperature was 105°F to 109°F (40.5°C to 42.7°C). Measured water temperature according to agency policy. Asked the person to check the water temperature. Adjusted water temperature as needed.
8. Raised the bed for body mechanics. Bed rails were up if used.
9. Lowered the bed rail near you if up.

Procedure

10. Practiced hand hygiene. Put on the gloves. (Some state competency tests require gloves be applied after covering the person with the bath blanket.)
11. Covered the person with a bath blanket. Fan-folded top linens to the foot of the bed.
12. Positioned and draped the person for perineal care.
13. Folded back the bath blanket to expose the perineal area.
14. Placed the waterproof under-pad under the buttocks. Had the person flex the knees and raise the buttocks off the bed. Or turned the person from side to side.
15. Checked the drainage tubing. Made sure it was not kinked and that urine could flow freely.
16. Separated the labia (female). In an uncircumcised male, retracted the foreskin. Checked for crusts, abnormal drainage, or secretions.
17. Gave perineal care. Kept the foreskin of the uncircumcised male retracted through step 25.

Procedure—cont'd S U Comments

18. Applied soap, body wash, or other cleansing agent to clean, wet washcloth.
19. Held the catheter at the meatus. Did so for steps 20 through 24.
20. Washed around the catheter at the meatus. Used a circular motion. (Completed this step if required by agency policy or your state competency test.)
21. Cleaned the catheter from the meatus down the catheter at least 4 inches. Cleaned downward, away from the meatus with 1 stroke. Did not tug or pull on the catheter. Repeated as needed with a clean area of the washcloth. Used a clean washcloth if needed.
22. Rinsed around the catheter at the meatus with a clean washcloth. (Completed this step if required by agency policy or your state competency test.)
23. Rinsed the catheter from the meatus down the catheter at least 4 inches. Rinsed downward, away from the meatus with 1 stroke. Did not tug or pull on the catheter. Repeated as needed with a clean area of the washcloth. Used a clean washcloth if needed.
24. Patted dry the areas washed. Dried from the meatus down the catheter at least 4 inches. Did not tug or pull on the catheter.
25. Returned the foreskin (uncircumcised male) to its natural position.
26. Patted dry perineal area. Dried from front to back (top to bottom).
27. Secured the catheter. Positioned the tubing in a straight line or coiled on the bed. Followed the nurse's directions. Secure the tubing to the bottom linens.
28. Removed the waterproof under-pad.
29. Covered the person. Removed the bath blanket.
30. Removed and discarded the gloves. Practiced hand hygiene.

Post-Procedure
31. Provided for comfort.
32. Placed the call light and other needed items within reach.
33. Lowered the bed to a safe and comfortable level. Followed the care plan.
34. Raised or lowered bed rails. Followed the care plan.
35. Cleaned, rinsed, dried, and returned equipment to its proper place. Used clean, dry paper towels for drying. Discarded disposable items. (Wore gloves for this step.)
36. Unscreened the person.
37. Completed a safety check of the room.
38. Followed center policy for used linens.
39. Removed and discarded the gloves. Practiced hand hygiene.
40. Reported and recorded your observations.

Changing a Leg Bag to a Standard Drainage Bag

Name: _____   Date: _____

Quality of Life	S	U	Comments

- Knocked before entering the person's room.
- Addressed the person by name.
- Introduced yourself by name and title.
- Explained the procedure before starting and during the procedure.
- Protected the person's rights during the procedure.
- Handled the person gently during the procedure.

Pre-Procedure

1. Followed *Delegation Guidelines: Urine Drainage Systems.*
   Saw *Promoting Safety and Comfort:*
   a. *Urinary Catheters*
   b. *Urine Drainage Systems*
2. Practiced hand hygiene.
3. Collected the following:
   - Gloves
   - Standard drainage bag and tubing
   - Antiseptic wipes
   - Waterproof under-pad
   - Sterile cap and plug
   - Catheter clamp
   - Paper towels
   - Bedpan
   - Bath blanket
4. Arranged paper towels and equipment on the over-bed table. Placed the bedpan at the foot of the bed.
5. Identified the person. Checked the ID (identification) bracelet against the assignment sheet. Used 2 identifiers. Also called the person by name.
6. Provided for privacy.

Procedure

7. Had the person sit on the side of the bed.
8. Practiced hand hygiene. Put on gloves.
9. Exposed the catheter and leg bag.
10. Emptied the drainage bag.
11. Clamped the catheter. This prevented urine from draining from the catheter into the drainage tubing.
12. Allowed urine to drain from below the clamp into the drainage tubing. This emptied the lower end of the catheter.
13. Helped the person to lie down.
14. Raised the bed rails if used. Raised the bed for body mechanics.
15. Lowered the bed rail near you if up.
16. Covered the person with a bath blanket. Fan-folded top linens to the foot of the bed. Exposed the catheter and leg bag.
17. Placed the waterproof under-pad under the person's leg.
18. Opened the antiseptic wipes. Placed them on paper towels.
19. Opened the package with the sterile cap and plug. Placed the package on the paper towels. Did not let anything touch the sterile cap or plug.

Procedure—cont'd

	S	U	Comments
20. Opened the package with the standard drainage bag and tubing.	___	___	_____
21. Attached the standard drainage bag to the bed frame.	___	___	_____
22. Disconnected the catheter from the drainage tubing. Did not allow anything to touch the ends.	___	___	_____
23. Inserted the sterile plug into the catheter end. Touched only the end of the plug. Did not touch the part that went inside the catheter. (If you contaminated the end of the catheter, wiped the end with an antiseptic wipe. Did so before you inserted the sterile plug.)	___	___	_____
24. Placed the sterile cap on the end of the leg bag drainage tube. (If you contaminated the tubing end, wiped the end with an antiseptic wipe. Did so before you applied the sterile cap.)	___	___	_____
25. Removed the cap from the new standard drainage tubing.	___	___	_____
26. Removed the sterile plug from the catheter.	___	___	_____
27. Inserted the end of the drainage tubing into the catheter.	___	___	_____
28. Removed the clamp from the catheter.	___	___	_____
29. Positioned drainage tubing in a straight line or coiled on the bed. Followed the nurse's directions. Secured the tubing to the bottom linens.	___	___	_____
30. Removed the leg bag. Placed it in the bedpan.	___	___	_____
31. Removed and discarded the waterproof under-pad.	___	___	_____
32. Covered the person. Removed the bath blanket.	___	___	_____
33. Took the bedpan to the bathroom.	___	___	_____
34. Removed and discarded the gloves. Practiced hand hygiene.	___	___	_____

Post-Procedure

	S	U	Comments
35. Provided for comfort.	___	___	_____
36. Placed the call light and other needed items within reach.	___	___	_____
37. Lowered the bed to a safe and comfortable level. Followed the care plan.	___	___	_____
38. Raised or lowered bed rails. Followed the care plan.	___	___	_____
39. Unscreened the person.	___	___	_____
40. Put on clean gloves. Discarded disposable items.	___	___	_____
41. Discarded the drainage tubing and leg bag following center policy. Or cleaned the bag following center policy.	___	___	_____
42. Cleaned and disinfected the bedpan.	___	___	_____
43. Returned the bedpan and other supplies to their proper place.	___	___	_____
44. Removed and discarded the gloves. Practiced hand hygiene.	___	___	_____
45. Completed a safety check of the room.	___	___	_____
46. Followed center policy for used linens.	___	___	_____
47. Practiced hand hygiene.	___	___	_____
48. Reported and recorded your observations.	___	___	_____

Emptying a Urine Drainage Bag

Name: _____   Date: _____

Quality of Life	S	U	Comments
• Knocked before entering the person's room.			
• Addressed the person by name.			
• Introduced yourself by name and title.			
• Explained the procedure before starting and during the procedure.			
• Protected the person's rights during the procedure.			
• Handled the person gently during the procedure.			

Pre-Procedure

1. Followed *Delegation Guidelines: Urine Drainage Systems.* Saw *Promoting Safety and Comfort:*
   a. *Urinary Catheters*
   b. *Urine Drainage Systems*
2. Collected the following:
   • Graduate (measuring container)
   • Gloves
   • Paper towels
   • Antiseptic wipes
3. Practiced hand hygiene.
4. Identified the person. Checked the ID (identification) bracelet against the assignment sheet. Used 2 identifiers. Also called the person by name.
5. Provided for privacy.

Procedure

6. Put on the gloves.
7. Placed paper towel on the floor. Placed graduate on top of it.
8. Positioned the graduate under the drainage bag.
9. Opened the clamp on the drain.
10. Allowed all urine to drain into the graduate. Did not let the drain touch the graduate.
11. Cleaned the end of the drain with an antiseptic wipe.
12. Clamped and positioned the drain in the holder.
13. Measured the urine.
14. Removed and discarded the paper towel.
15. Emptied the contents of the graduate into the toilet and flushed.
16. Rinsed the graduate. Emptied the rinse into the toilet and flushed.
17. Cleaned, disinfected and dried the graduate. Used clean, dry paper towels for drying.
18. Returned the graduate to its proper place.
19. Removed and discarded the gloves. Practiced hand hygiene.
20. Recorded the time and amount of the urine on the intake and output (I&O) record.

Post-Procedure

21. Provided for comfort.
22. Placed the call light and other needed items within reach.
23. Unscreened the person.
24. Completed a safety check of the room.
25. Reported and recorded the amount of urine and other observations.

Removing an Indwelling Catheter

Name: _____ Date: _____

Quality of Life	S	U	Comments
• Knocked before entering the person's room.	___	___	_____
• Addressed the person by name.	___	___	_____
• Introduced yourself by name and title.	___	___	_____
• Explained the procedure before starting and during the procedure.	___	___	_____
• Protected the person's rights during the procedure.	___	___	_____
• Handled the person gently during the procedure.	___	___	_____

Pre-Procedure

1. Followed *Delegation Guidelines: Removing Indwelling Catheters.*
   Saw *Promoting Safety and Comfort:*
   a. *Urinary Catheters*
   b. *Removing Indwelling Catheters*
2. Practiced hand hygiene.
3. Collected the following:
   • Disposable towel
   • Syringe in the size directed by the nurse
   • Disposable bag
   • Gloves
   • Bath blanket
4. Identified the person. Checked the ID (identification) bracelet against the assignment sheet. Used 2 identifiers. Also called the person by name.
5. Provided for privacy.
6. Raised the bed for body mechanics. Bed rails were up if used.

Procedure

7. Lowered the bed rail near you if up.
8. Practiced hand hygiene. Put on gloves.
9. Positioned and draped the person as for perineal care.
10. Covered the person with a bath blanket.
11. Checked the size of the syringe. Knew the amount of water in the balloon. Made sure the syringe was large enough to withdraw all the water from the balloon.
12. Removed the tube holder, leg band, or tape securing the catheter to the person.
13. Positioned the towel.
    a. Female—between her legs
    b. Male—over his thighs
14. Removed all the water from the balloon. (Knew how much water was in the balloon. If the balloon was filled with 10mL of water, you removed 10mL of water.)
    a. Slid the syringe plunger up and down several times. This loosened the plunger.
    b. Pulled the plunger back to the 0.5 (one-half) mL mark.
    c. Attached the syringe to the catheter's balloon port gently. Used only enough force to get the syringe to stay in the port.

Procedure—cont'd   S   U   Comments

    d. Allowed the water to drain into the syringe. Waited
       at least 30 seconds to allow the full amount to drain.
       Did not pull back on the plunger. Pressure in the
       balloon forced the plunger back and filled the syringe.
       If the water was draining slow or not at all, called the
       nurse. Did not remove the catheter if there was water
       in the balloon. The nurse may have had you:
       1. Gently reposition the syringe in the port.   _____   _____   _____
       2. Re-position the person.   _____   _____   _____
       3. Pull back on the syringe gently and slowly.
          Forceful pulling would collapse the catheter. _____   _____   _____

15. Pulled the catheter straight out once all the water was
    removed. Removed the catheter gently.   _____   _____   _____
16. Discarded the catheter into the bag.   _____   _____   _____
17. Dried the perineal area with the towel. Discarded the
    disposable towel in the bag.   _____   _____   _____
18. Removed and discarded the gloves. Practiced hand
    hygiene.   _____   _____   _____
19. Covered the person. Removed the bath blanket.   _____   _____   _____

Post-Procedure

20. Provided for privacy.   _____   _____   _____
21. Placed the call light and other needed items within reach. _____   _____   _____
22. Lowered the bed to a safe and comfortable level.
    Followed the care plan.   _____   _____   _____
23. Raised or lowered bed rails. Followed the care plan. _____   _____   _____
24. Unscreened the person.   _____   _____   _____
25. Put on clean gloves. Discarded disposable items.
    Discarded the syringe according to agency policy. _____   _____   _____
26. Emptied the drainage bag. Noted the amount of urine. _____   _____   _____
27. Discarded the drainage tubing and bag following agency
    policy.   _____   _____   _____
28. Removed and discarded the gloves. Practiced hand
    hygiene.   _____   _____   _____
29. Completed a safety check of the room.   _____   _____   _____
30. Practiced hand hygiene.   _____   _____   _____
31. Reported and recorded your observations.   _____   _____   _____

Applying a Condom Catheter

Name: _____   Date: _____

	S	**U**	**Comments**

Quality of Life
- Knocked before entering the person's room.
- Addressed the person by name.
- Introduced yourself by name and title.
- Explained the procedure before starting and during the procedure.
- Protected the person's rights during the procedure.
- Handled the person gently during the procedure.

Pre-Procedure
1. Followed *Delegation Guidelines:*
   a. *Perineal Care*
   b. *Condom Catheters*
   Saw *Promoting Safety and Comfort:*
   a. *Perineal Care*
   b. *Urinary Catheters*
   c. *Condom Catheters*
2. Practiced hand hygiene.
3. Collected the following:
   - Condom catheter
   - Elastic tape
   - Standard drainage bag or leg bag
   - Cap for the drainage bag
   - Basin of warm water
   - Soap, body wash, or other cleansing agent
   - Towel and washcloths
   - Bath blanket
   - Gloves
   - Waterproof under-pad
   - Paper towels
4. Covered the over-bed table with paper towels. Arranged items on top of them.
5. Identified the person. Checked the ID (identification) bracelet against the assignment sheet. Used 2 identifiers. Also called the person by name.
6. Provided for privacy.
7. Raised the bed for body mechanics. Bed rails were up if used.

Procedure
8. Lowered the bed rail near you if up.
9. Practiced hand hygiene. Put on the gloves.
10. Covered the person with a bath blanket. Lowered top linens to the knees.
11. Asked the person to raise his buttocks off the bed. Or turned him onto his side away from you.
12. Slid the waterproof under-pad under his buttocks.
13. Had the person lower his buttocks. Or turned him onto his back.
14. Secured the standard drainage bag to the bed frame. Or had a leg bag ready. Closed the drain.
15. Exposed the genital area.

Procedure—cont'd   S   U   Comments

16. Removed the condom catheter.
    a. Removed the tape (for the non-adhering type).
       Rolled the sheath off the penis.   _____ _____ _____
    b. Disconnected the drainage tubing from the condom.
       Capped the drainage tube.   _____ _____ _____
    c. Discarded the tape (if used) and condom.   _____ _____ _____
17. Provided perineal care. Observed the penis for reddened
    areas, skin breakdown, and irritations.   _____ _____ _____
18. Removed and discarded the gloves. Practiced hand
    hygiene. Put on clean gloves.   _____ _____ _____
19. Removed the protective backing from the condom.
    This exposed the adhesive strip.   _____ _____ _____
20. Held the penis firmly. Rolled the condom onto the penis.
    Left a 1-inch space between the penis and the end of
    the catheter.   _____ _____ _____
21. Secured the condom.
    a. *Self-adhering condom:* pressed the condom to the penis. _____ _____ _____
    b. *Non-adhering condom secured with elastic tape:* applied
       elastic tape in a spiral. Did not apply tape completely
       around the penis.   _____ _____ _____
22. Made sure the penis tip did not touch the condom.
    Made sure the condom was not twisted.   _____ _____ _____
23. Connected the condom to the drainage tubing.
    Secured excess tubing on the bed. Or attached a
    leg bag.   _____ _____ _____
24. Removed the waterproof under-pad and gloves.
    Discarded them. Practiced hand hygiene.   _____ _____ _____
25. Covered the person. Removed the bath blanket.   _____ _____ _____

Post-Procedure

26. Provided for comfort.   _____ _____ _____
27. Placed the call light and other needed items
    within reach.   _____ _____ _____
28. Lowered the bed to a safe and comfortable level.
    Followed the care plan.   _____ _____ _____
29. Raised or lowered bed rails. Followed the care plan. _____ _____ _____
30. Unscreened the person.   _____ _____ _____
31. Practiced hand hygiene. Put on clean gloves.   _____ _____ _____
32. Measured and recorded the amount of urine in the bag.
    Cleaned or discarded the drainage bag.   _____ _____ _____
33. Cleaned, rinsed, dried, and returned the wash basin
    and other equipment. Used clean, dry paper towels for
    drying. Returned items to their proper place.   _____ _____ _____
34. Removed and discarded the gloves. Practiced hand
    hygiene.   _____ _____ _____
35. Completed a safety check of the room.   _____ _____ _____
36. Reported and recorded your observations.   _____ _____ _____

Checking for and Removing a Fecal Impaction

Name: _____   Date: _____

Quality of Life	S	U	Comments
• Knocked before entering the person's room.			
• Addressed the person by name.			
• Introduced yourself by name and title.			
• Explained the procedure before starting and during the procedure.			
• Protected the person's rights during the procedure.			
• Handled the person gently during the procedure.			

Pre-Procedure

	S	U	Comments
1. Followed *Delegation Guidelines:*			
a. *Bowel Needs*			
b. *Fecal Impaction*			
Saw *Promoting Safety and Comfort:*			
a. *Bowel Needs*			
b. *Fecal Impaction*			
2. Practiced hand hygiene.			
3. Collected the following:			
• Bedpan and cover			
• Bath blanket			
• Toilet paper			
• Gloves			
• Lubricant			
• Waterproof under-pad			
• Basin of warm water			
• Soap or body wash			
• Washcloth			
• Bath towel			
4. Practiced hand hygiene.			
5. Identified the person. Checked the ID (identification) bracelet against the assignment sheet. Used 2 identifiers. Also called the person by name.			
6. Provided for privacy.			
7. Raised the bed for body mechanics. Bed rails were up if used.			

Procedure

	S	U	Comments
8. Lowered the bed rail near you if up.			
9. Covered the person with a bath blanket. Fan-folded top linens to the foot of the bed.			
10. Positioned the person in Sims' position or in a left side-lying position.			
11. Checked the person's pulse. Noted the rate and rhythm.			
12. Practiced hand hygiene. Put on the gloves.			
13. Placed the waterproof under-pad under the buttocks.			
14. Exposed the anal area.			
15. Lubricated your gloved index finger.			
16. Asked the person to take a deep breath through the mouth.			
17. Inserted the gloved finger during the deep breath.			
18. Checked for a fecal mass. Removed your finger and went to step 20 if:			
a. You did not feel a fecal mass.			
b. You felt a fecal mass but did not remove the impaction.			
19. Removed the impaction.			
a. Hooked your index finger around a small piece of feces.			

Procedure—cont'd	S	U	Comments
b. Removed your finger and the feces.	___	___	_____
c. Dropped the stool into the bedpan.	___	___	_____
d. Cleaned your finger with toilet paper. Placed the toilet paper in the bedpan.	___	___	_____
e. Repeated until you no longer felt feces. Reapplied lubricant as needed.			
1) Hooked your index finger around a small piece of feces.	___	___	_____
2) Removed your finger and the feces.	___	___	_____
3) Dropped the stool into the bedpan.	___	___	_____
4) Cleaned your finger with toilet paper. Placed the toilet paper in the bedpan.	___	___	_____
f. *Checked the person's pulse at intervals. Used your clean gloved hand. Noted rate and rhythm. Stopped the procedure if the pulse rate slowed or if the rhythm was irregular. Called for the nurse.*	___	___	_____
20. Wiped the anal area with toilet paper.	___	___	_____
21. Removed and discarded the gloves. Practiced hand hygiene. Put on clean gloves.	___	___	_____
22. Checked the person's pulse. Noted the rate and rhythm.	___	___	_____
23. Helped the person onto the bedpan. Raised the head of the bed and raised the bed rail if used. Or assisted the person to the bathroom or commode. The person wore a robe and slip-resistant footwear when up. The bed was in a low position safe and comfortable for the person.	___	___	_____
24. Placed the call light and toilet paper within reach. Reminded the person not to flush the toilet.	___	___	_____
25. Discarded disposable items.	___	___	_____
26. Removed and discarded the gloves. Practiced hand hygiene.	___	___	_____
27. Left the room if the person could be left alone.	___	___	_____
28. Returned when the person signaled. Or checked on the person every 5 minutes. Knocked before entering.	___	___	_____
29. Practiced hand hygiene and put on gloves. Lowered the bed rail if up.	___	___	_____
30. Observed stools for amount, color, consistency, shape, and odor.	___	___	_____
31. Provided perineal care as needed.	___	___	_____
32. Removed the waterproof under-pad.	___	___	_____
33. Emptied, rinsed, cleaned, and disinfected equipment. If the person had a bowel movement (BM), flushed the toilet after the nurse observed it.	___	___	_____
34. Returned equipment to its proper place.	___	___	_____
35. Removed and discarded the gloves. Practiced hand hygiene after removing and discarding the gloves.	___	___	_____
36. Assisted with hand hygiene. Wore gloves for this step. Practiced hand hygiene after removing and discarding the gloves.	___	___	_____
37. Covered the person. Removed the bath blanket.	___	___	_____

Post-Procedure

	S	U	Comments
38. Provided for comfort.	___	___	_____
39. Placed the call light and other needed items within reach.	___	___	_____
40. Lowered the bed to a safe and comfortable level. Followed the care plan.	___	___	_____
41. Raised or lowered bed rails. Followed the care plan.	___	___	_____
42. Unscreened the person.	___	___	_____
43. Completed a safety check of the room.	___	___	_____
44. Followed agency policy for used linens and used supplies.	___	___	_____
45. Practiced hand hygiene.	___	___	_____
46. Reported and recorded your observations.	___	___	_____

Giving a Cleansing Enema to an Adult

Name: _____   Date: _____

Quality of Life	S	U	Comments
• Knocked before entering the person's room.			
• Addressed the person by name.			
• Introduced yourself by name and title.			
• Explained the procedure before starting and during the procedure.			
• Protected the person's rights during the procedure.			
• Handled the person gently during the procedure.			

Pre-Procedure

1. Followed *Delegation Guidelines:*
   a. *Bowel Needs*
   b. *Enemas*
   Saw *Promoting Safety and Comfort:*
   a. *Bowel Needs*
   b. *Enemas*
2. Practiced hand hygiene.
3. Collected the following before going to the person's room.
   • Disposable enema kit as directed by the nurse (enema bag, tube, clamp, and waterproof under-pad)
   • Water thermometer
   • Waterproof under-pad (if not part of the enema kit)
   • Water-soluble lubricant
   • 3 to 5 mL (1 teaspoon) castile soap or 1 to 2 teaspoons of salt (if needed)
   • IV (intravenous) pole
   • Gloves
4. Arranged items in the person's room and bathroom.
5. Practiced hand hygiene.
6. Identified the person. Checked the ID (identification) bracelet against the assignment sheet. Used 2 identifiers. Also called the person by name.
7. Put on gloves.
8. Collected the following:
   • Commode or bedpan and cover
   • Toilet paper
   • Bath blanket
   • Robe and slip-resistant footwear
   • Paper towels
9. Removed and discarded the gloves. Practiced hand hygiene. Put on clean gloves.
10. Provided for privacy.
11. Raised the bed for body mechanics. Bed rails were up if used.

Procedure

12. Lowered the bed rail near you if up.
13. Covered the person with a bath blanket. Fan-folded top linens to the foot of the bed.
14. Positioned the IV pole so the enema bag was 12 inches above the anus. Or it was at the height directed by the nurse.
15. Raised the bed rail if used.

Procedure—cont'd

	S	U	Comments
16. Prepared the enema.			
a. Closed the clamp on the tube.	_____	_____	_____
b. Adjusted water flow until it was lukewarm.	_____	_____	_____
c. Filled the enema bag for the amount ordered.	_____	_____	_____
d. Measured water temperature with the water thermometer. The nurse told you what water temperature to use.	_____	_____	_____
e. Prepared the solution as directed by the nurse.			
1) *Tap water:* added nothing.	_____	_____	_____
2) *Saline enema:* added salt as directed.	_____	_____	_____
3) *Soapsuds enema (SSE):* added castile soap as directed.	_____	_____	_____
f. Stirred the solution with the water thermometer. Scooped off any suds (SSE).	_____	_____	_____
g. Sealed the bag.	_____	_____	_____
h. Hung the bag on the IV pole.	_____	_____	_____
17. Lowered the bed rail near you if up.	_____	_____	_____
18. Positioned the person in Sims' position or in left side-lying position.	_____	_____	_____
19. Placed a waterproof under-pad under the buttocks.	_____	_____	_____
20. Exposed the anal area.	_____	_____	_____
21. Placed the bedpan behind the person.	_____	_____	_____
22. Positioned the enema tube in the bedpan. Removed the cap from the tubing.	_____	_____	_____
23. Opened the clamp. Allowed solution to flow through the tube to remove air. Clamped the tube.	_____	_____	_____
24. Lubricated the tube 2 to 4 inches from the tip.	_____	_____	_____
25. Separated the buttocks to see the anus.	_____	_____	_____
26. Asked the person to take a deep breath through the mouth.	_____	_____	_____
27. Inserted the tube gently 2 to 4 inches into the adult's rectum. Did this when the person was exhaling. Stopped if the person complained of pain, you felt resistance, or bleeding occurred.	_____	_____	_____
28. Checked the amount of solution in the bag.	_____	_____	_____
29. Unclamped the tube. Gave the solution slowly.	_____	_____	_____
30. Asked the person to take slow, deep breaths. This helped the person relax.	_____	_____	_____
31. Clamped the tube if the person needed to have a bowel movement (BM), had cramping, or started to expel solution. Also clamped the tube if the person was sweating or complained of nausea or weakness. Unclamped when symptoms subsided.	_____	_____	_____
32. Gave the amount of solution ordered. Stopped if the person did not tolerate the procedure.			
33. Clamped the tube before it emptied. This prevented air from entering the bowel.	_____	_____	_____
34. Held toilet paper around the tube and against the anus. Removed the tube.	_____	_____	_____
35. Discarded toilet paper into the bedpan.	_____	_____	_____
36. Wrapped the tubing tip with paper towels. Placed it inside the enema bag.	_____	_____	_____
37. Encouraged retention of the enema for the time ordered.	_____	_____	_____
38. Assisted the person to the bathroom or commode. The person wore a robe and slip-resistant footwear when up. The bed was at a low level that was safe and comfortable for the person. Or helped the person onto the bedpan. Raised the head of the bed. Raised or lowered bed rails according to the care plan.	_____	_____	_____

	S	U	Comments
Procedure—cont'd			
39. Placed the call light and toilet paper within reach. Reminded the person not to flush the toilet.	___	___	_____
40. Discarded disposable items.	___	___	_____
41. Removed and discarded the gloves. Practiced hand hygiene.	___	___	_____
42. Left the room if the person could be left alone.	___	___	_____
43. Returned when the person signaled. Or checked on the person every 5 minutes. Knocked before entering the room or bathroom.	___	___	_____
44. Practiced hand hygiene and put on gloves. Lowered the bed rail if up.	___	___	_____
45. Observed enema results for amount, color, consistency, shape, and odor. Called the nurse to observe results.	___	___	_____
46. Provided perineal care as needed.			
47. Removed the waterproof under-pad.	___	___	_____
48. Emptied, rinsed, cleaned, disinfected and dried equipment. Used clean, dry paper towels for drying. Flushed the toilet after the nurse observed the results.	___	___	_____
49. Returned equipment to its proper place.	___	___	_____
50. Removed and discarded the gloves. Practiced hand hygiene.	___	___	_____
51. Assisted with hand hygiene. Wore gloves for this step. Practiced hand hygiene after removing and discarding the gloves.	___	___	_____
52. Covered the person. Removed the bath blanket.	___	___	_____
Post-Procedure			
53. Provided for comfort.	___	___	_____
54. Placed the call light and other needed items within reach.	___	___	_____
55. Lowered the bed to a safe and comfortable level. Followed the care plan.	___	___	_____
56. Raised or lowered bed rails. Followed the care plan.	___	___	_____
57. Unscreened the person.	___	___	_____
58. Completed a safety check of the room.	___	___	_____
59. Followed center policy for used linens and used supplies.	___	___	_____
60. Practiced hand hygiene.	___	___	_____
61. Reported and recorded your observations.	___	___	_____

Giving a Small-Volume Enema

Name: _____ Date: _____

Quality of Life	S	U	Comments
• Knocked before entering the person's room.	___	___	_____
• Addressed the person by name.	___	___	_____
• Introduced yourself by name and title.	___	___	_____
• Explained the procedure before starting and during the procedure.	___	___	_____
• Protected the person's rights during the procedure.	___	___	_____
• Handled the person gently during the procedure.	___	___	_____

Pre-Procedure

1. Followed *Delegation Guidelines:*
   a. *Bowel Needs* ___ ___ _____
   b. *Enemas* ___ ___ _____
   Saw *Promoting Safety and Comfort:*
   a. *Bowel Needs* ___ ___ _____
   b. *Enemas* ___ ___ _____
2. Practiced hand hygiene. ___ ___ _____
3. Collected the following before going to the person's room.
   • Small-volume enema ___ ___ _____
   • Waterproof under-pad ___ ___ _____
   • Gloves ___ ___ _____
4. Arranged items in the person's room. ___ ___ _____
5. Practiced hand hygiene. ___ ___ _____
6. Identified the person. Checked the ID (identification) bracelet against the assignment sheet. Used 2 identifiers. Also called the person by name. ___ ___ _____
7. Put on gloves. ___ ___ _____
8. Collected the following:
   • Commode or bedpan and cover ___ ___ _____
   • Toilet paper ___ ___ _____
   • Robe and slip-resistant footwear ___ ___ _____
   • Bath blanket ___ ___ _____
9. Removed and discarded the gloves. Practiced hand hygiene. Put on clean gloves. ___ ___ _____
10. Provided for privacy. ___ ___ _____
11. Raised the bed for body mechanics. Bed rails were up if used. ___ ___ _____

Procedure

12. Lowered the bed rail near you if up. ___ ___ _____
13. Covered the person with a bath blanket. Fan-folded top linens to the foot of the bed. ___ ___ _____
14. Positioned the person in Sims' position or in left side-lying position. ___ ___ _____
15. Placed a waterproof under-pad under the buttocks. ___ ___ _____
16. Exposed the anal area. ___ ___ _____
17. Placed the bedpan by the person. ___ ___ _____
18. Removed the cap from the enema tip. ___ ___ _____
19. Separated the buttocks to see the anus. ___ ___ _____
20. Asked the person to take a deep breath through the mouth. ___ ___ _____
21. Inserted the enema tip 2 inches into the adult's rectum. Did this as the person exhaled. Inserted the tip gently. Stopped if the person complained of pain, you felt resistance, or bleeding occurred. ___ ___ _____

Procedure—cont'd	S	U	Comments
22. Squeezed and rolled up the container gently. Released pressure on the bottle after you removed the tip from the rectum.	___	___	_____
23. Put the container into the box, tip first. Discarded the container and box.	___	___	_____
24. Assisted the person to the bathroom or commode when he or she had the urge to have a bowel movement (BM). The person wore a robe and slip-resistant footwear when up. The bed was at a low level that was safe and comfortable. Or helped the person onto the bedpan and raised the head of the bed. Raised or lowered bed rails according to the care plan.	___	___	_____
25. Placed the call light and toilet paper within reach. Reminded the person not to flush the toilet.	___	___	_____
26. Discarded disposable items.	___	___	_____
27. Removed and discarded the gloves. Practiced hand hygiene.	___	___	_____
28. Left the room if the person could be left alone.	___	___	_____
29. Returned when the person signaled. Or checked on the person every 5 minutes. Knocked before entering the room or bathroom.	___	___	_____
30. Practiced hand hygiene. Put on gloves.	___	___	_____
31. Lowered the bed rail if up.	___	___	_____
32. Observed enema results for amount, color, consistency, shape, and odor. Called the nurse to observe results.	___	___	_____
33. Provided perineal care as needed.	___	___	_____
34. Removed the waterproof under-pad.	___	___	_____
35. Emptied, rinsed, cleaned, disinfected and dried equipment. Used clean, dry paper towels for drying. Flushed the toilet after the nurse observed the results.	___	___	_____
36. Returned equipment to its proper place.	___	___	_____
37. Removed and discarded the gloves. Practiced hand hygiene.	___	___	_____
38. Assisted with hand hygiene. Wore gloves for this step. Practiced hand hygiene after removing and discarding the gloves.	___	___	_____
39. Covered the person. Removed the bath blanket.	___	___	_____

Post-Procedure

	S	U	Comments
40. Provided for comfort.	___	___	_____
41. Placed the call light and other needed items within reach.	___	___	_____
42. Lowered the bed to a safe and comfortable level. Followed the care plan.	___	___	_____
43. Raised or lowered bed rails. Followed the care plan.	___	___	_____
44. Unscreened the person.	___	___	_____
45. Completed a safety check of the room.	___	___	_____
46. Followed center policy for used linens and used supplies.	___	___	_____
47. Practiced hand hygiene.	___	___	_____
48. Reported and recorded your observations.	___	___	_____

Giving an Oil-Retention Enema

Name: _____   Date: _____

Quality of Life	S	U	Comments
• Knocked before entering the person's room.	_____	_____	_____
• Addressed the person by name.	_____	_____	_____
• Introduced yourself by name and title.	_____	_____	_____
• Explained the procedure before starting and during the procedure.	_____	_____	_____
• Protected the person's rights during the procedure.	_____	_____	_____
• Handled the person gently during the procedure.	_____	_____	_____

Pre-Procedure

1. Followed *Delegation Guidelines:*
   a. *Bowel Needs*
   b. *Enemas*
   Saw *Promoting Safety and Comfort:*
   a. *Bowel Needs*
   b. *Enemas*
   c. *Oil-Retention Enemas*
2. Practiced hand hygiene.
3. Collected the following before going to the person's room.
   • Oil-retention enema
   • Waterproof under-pads
   • Gloves
   • Bath blanket
4. Arranged items in the person's room.
5. Practiced hand hygiene.
6. Identified the person. Checked the ID (identification) bracelet against the assignment sheet. Used 2 identifiers. Also called the person by name.
7. Provided for privacy.
8. Raised the bed for body mechanics. Bed rails were up if used.

Procedure

9. Put on gloves.
10. Completed the following steps.
    a. Lowered the bed rail near you if up.
    b. Covered the person with a bath blanket. Fan-folded top linens to the foot of the bed.
    c. Positioned the person in Sims' or in left side-lying position.
    d. Placed the waterproof under-pad under the buttocks.
    e. Exposed the anal area.
    f. Positioned the bedpan by the person.
    g. Removed the cap from the enema tip.
    h. Separated the buttocks to see the anus.
    i. Asked the person to take a deep breath through the mouth.
    j. Inserted the enema tip 2 inches into the adult's rectum. Did this as the person exhaled. Inserted the tip gently. Stopped if the person complained of pain, you felt resistance, or bleeding occurred.
    k. Squeezed and rolled up the container gently. Released pressure on the bottle after you removed the tip from the rectum.
    l. Put the container into the box, tip first. Discarded the container and box.

Procedure—cont'd	S	U	Comments
11. Covered the person. Left him or her in the Sims' or left side-lying position.	_____	_____	_____
12. Encouraged retention of the enema until urge to have a bowel movement occurred.	_____	_____	_____
13. Placed more waterproof under-pads on the bed if needed.	_____	_____	_____
14. Removed and discarded the gloves. Practiced hand hygiene.	_____	_____	_____

Post-Procedure

	S	U	Comments
15. Provided for comfort.	_____	_____	_____
16. Placed the call light and other needed items within reach.	_____	_____	_____
17. Lowered the bed to a safe and comfortable level.	_____	_____	_____
18. Raised or lowered bed rails. Followed the care plan.	_____	_____	_____
19. Unscreened the person.	_____	_____	_____
20. Completed a safety check of the room.	_____	_____	_____
21. Followed center policy for used linens and used supplies.	_____	_____	_____
22. Practiced hand hygiene.	_____	_____	_____
23. Reported and recorded your observations.	_____	_____	_____
24. Checked the person often.	_____	_____	_____

Assisting the Person to Empty an Ostomy Pouch

Name: _____   Date: _____

Quality of Life	S	U	Comments

Quality of Life
- Knocked before entering the person's room.
- Addressed the person by name.
- Introduced yourself by name and title.
- Explained the procedure before starting and during the procedure.
- Protected the person's rights during the procedure.
- Handled the person gently during the procedure.

Pre-Procedure

1. *Followed Delegation Guidelines:*
   a *Bowel Needs*
   b *Emptying Ostomy Pouches*
   Saw *Promoting Safety and Comfort:*
   a *Bowel Needs*
   b *Emptying Ostomy Pouches*
2. Practiced hand hygiene.
3. Put on gloves.
4. Arranged the following in the person's bathroom:
   - Toilet paper
   - Pre-moistened wipes
   - Plastic bag (for wipes)
5. Placed a few sheets of toilet paper in the toilet bowl. This helped prevent splashing when the pouch was emptied.
6. Removed and discarded the gloves. Practiced hand hygiene.
7. Identified the person. Checked the ID bracelet against the assignment sheet. Used 2 identifiers (Chapter 13). Also called the person by name.

Procedure

8. Put on gloves.
9. Assisted the person to the bathroom. Closed the bathroom door for privacy.
10. Helped the person sit on the toilet and moved garments out of the way. Made sure the person was comfortable.
11. Had the person spread his or her legs.
12. Positioned the pouch between the legs and over the toilet.
13. Held the pouch outlet over the toilet. Opened the clip or clamp and gently pinched the sides to open the outlet.
14. Allowed the pouch to empty. If necessary, slid your thumb and index finger down the outside of the pouch to push out feces.
15. Cleaned the inside of the outlet with toilet paper or a pre-moistened wipe. Made sure the inside was thoroughly clean. Discarded toilet paper into the toilet. Discarded the wipe into the plastic bag.
16. Cleaned the outside of the pouch outlet and the clip (clamp). Made sure the outside and the clip (clamp) were thoroughly clean. Used toilet paper or a pre-moistened wipe. Discarded toilet paper into the toilet. Discarded the wipe into the plastic bag.
17. Tied or sealed the plastic bag (if used).

Procedure—cont'd	S	U	Comments
18. Closed the pouch outlet with the clip (clamp). Followed the manufacturer's instructions.	_____	_____	_____
19. Observed the color, amount, consistency, and odor of stools. Flushed the toilet.	_____	_____	_____
20. Removed and discarded the gloves. Practiced hand hygiene.	_____	_____	_____
21. Assisted the person with hand-hygiene. Wore gloves for this step.	_____	_____	_____
22. Practiced hand hygiene after removing and discarding gloves.	_____	_____	_____
23. Helped the person back to bed.	_____	_____	_____

Post-Procedure

	S	U	Comments
24. Provided for comfort.	_____	_____	_____
25. Placed the call light and other needed items within reach.	_____	_____	_____
26. Raised or lowered the bed rails. Followed the care plan.	_____	_____	_____
27. Completed a safety check of the room.	_____	_____	_____
28. Followed agency policy for disposal of the plastic bag (if used). Wore gloves for this step.	_____	_____	_____
29. Practice hand hygiene.	_____	_____	_____
30. Reported and recorded your observations.	_____	_____	_____

Preparing the Person for a Meal

Name: _____   Date: _____

Quality of Life	S	U	Comments

Quality of Life
- Knocked before entering the person's room.
- Addressed the person by name.
- Introduced yourself by name and title.
- Explained the procedure before starting and during the procedure.
- Protected the person's rights during the procedure.
- Handled the person gently during the procedure.

Pre-Procedure
1. Followed *Delegation Guidelines: Preparing for Meals*. Saw *Promoting Safety and Comfort: Preparing for Meals*.
2. Practiced hand hygiene.
3. Collected the following:
   - Equipment for oral hygiene
   - Bedpan and cover (optional), urinal, commode, or specimen pan
   - Toilet paper
   - Wash basin
   - Soap
   - Washcloth and towel or handwipes
   - Gloves
4. Provided for privacy.

Procedure
5. Made sure eyeglasses and hearing aids were in place.
6. Assisted with oral hygiene. Made sure dentures were in place. Wore gloves and practiced hand hygiene after removing and discarding gloves.
7. Assisted with elimination. Made sure the incontinent person was clean and dry. Wore gloves and practiced hand hygiene after removing and discarding the gloves.
8. Assisted with hand hygiene. Wore gloves and practiced hand hygiene after removing and discarding them.
9. *Did the following if the person ate in bed.*
   a. Raised the head of the bed to a comfortable position—Fowler's (45 to 60 degrees) or high-Fowler's (60 to 90 degrees). (Note: Some state competency tests require that the person sit upright at least 45 degrees to eat, others require 75 to 90 degrees.)
   b. Removed items from the over-bed table. Cleaned the over-bed table.
   c. Adjusted the over-bed table in front of the person.
10. *Did the following if the person sat in a chair.*
    a. Positioned the person in a chair or wheelchair.
    b. Removed items from the over-bed table. Cleaned the table.
    c. Adjusted the over-bed table in front of the person.
11. For the person who ate in dining area, assisted the person to the dining area.

Post-Procedure

	S	U	Comments
12. Provided for comfort.	_____	_____	_____
13. Placed the call light and other needed items within reach.	_____	_____	_____
14. Emptied, cleaned, rinsed, and disinfected equipment. Used clean, dry paper towels for drying. Returned equipment to its proper place. Wore gloves and practiced hand hygiene after removing and discarding them.	_____	_____	_____
15. Straightened the room. Eliminated unpleasant noise, odors, or equipment.	_____	_____	_____
16. Unscreened the person.	_____	_____	_____
17. Completed a safety check of the room.	_____	_____	_____
18. Practiced hand hygiene.	_____	_____	_____

Serving Meal Trays

Name: _____   Date: _____

Quality of Life	S	U	Comments
• Knocked before entering the person's room.			
• Addressed the person by name.			
• Introduced yourself by name and title.			
• Explained the procedure before starting and during the procedure.			
• Protected the person's rights during the procedure.			
• Handled the person gently during the procedure.			

Pre-Procedure

1. Followed *Delegation Guidelines: Serving Meal Trays*. Saw *Promoting Safety and Comfort: Serving Meal Trays*.
2. Practiced hand hygiene.
3. Prepared the person for a meal if not already done.

Procedure

4. Checked items on the tray with the dietary card. Made sure the tray was complete and had adaptive equipment (assistive devices).
5. Identified the person. Checked the ID (identification) bracelet against the dietary card. Used 2 identifiers. Also called the person by name.
6. Placed the tray within the person's reach. Adjusted the over-bed table as needed.
7. Removed food covers. Opened cartons, cut food into bite-sized pieces, buttered bread, and so on as needed. Seasoned food as the person preferred and the care plan allowed.
8. Placed the napkin, clothes protector, adaptive equipment (assistive devices), and eating utensils within reach. Applied the clothes protector (if needed).
9. Placed the call light within reach.
10. Did the following when the person was done eating.
    a. Measured and recorded fluid intake if ordered.
    b. Noted the amount and type of foods eaten.
    c. Checked for and removed any food in the mouth (pocketing). Wore gloves. Practiced hand hygiene after removing and discarding them.
    d. Removed the tray.
    e. Cleaned spills. Changed used linens and clothing.
    f. Helped the person return to bed if needed.
    g. Assisted with oral hygiene and hand hygiene. Wore gloves. Practiced hand hygiene after removing and discarding the gloves.

Post-Procedure

11. Provided for comfort.
12. Placed the call light and other needed items within reach.
13. Raised or lowered bed rails. Followed the care plan.
14. Completed a safety check of the room.
15. Followed center policy for used linens.
16. Practiced hand hygiene.
17. Reported and recorded your observations.

Feeding the Person

Name: _____   Date: _____

	S	U	Comments

Quality of Life
- Knocked before entering the person's room.
- Addressed the person by name.
- Introduced yourself by name and title.
- Explained the procedure before starting and during the procedure.
- Protected the person's rights during the procedure.
- Handled the person gently during the procedure.

Pre-Procedure
1. Followed *Delegation Guidelines: Feeding the Person.* Saw *Promoting Safety and Comfort:*
   - *Serving Meals*
   - *Feeding the person*
2. Practiced hand hygiene.
3. Positioned the person in a comfortable position for eating—sitting in a chair or in Fowler's (45 to 60 degrees) or high-Fowler's (60 to 90 degrees). (Note: Some state competency tests require at least 45 degrees, others require 75 to 90 degrees.)
4. Got the tray. Placed the tray on the over-bed table or dining table where the person could reach it.

Procedure
5. Checked items on the tray with the dietary card. Made sure the tray was complete.
6. Identified the person. Checked the ID (identification) bracelet with the dietary card. Used 2 identifiers. Also called the person by name.
7. Draped a napkin across the person's chest and underneath the chin. or applied a clothes protector or towel.
8. Cleaned the person's hands. (NOTE: Some state competency tests require soap and water, others allow hand sanitizer or a hand wipe.)
9. Told the person what foods and fluids were on the tray.
10. Prepared food for eating. Cut food into bite-sized pieces. Seasoned foods as the person preferred and as the care plan allowed.
11. Placed a chair where you could sit comfortably. Sat facing the person at eye level.
12. Served foods in the order the person preferred. Identified foods as you served them. Alternated between solid and liquid foods. Used a spoon for safety. Allowed enough time to chew and swallow. Did not rush the person. Also offered water, coffee, tea, or other fluids on the tray.
13. Checked the person's mouth before offering more food or fluids. Made sure the mouth was empty between bites and swallows. Asked if the person was ready for the next bite or drink.
14. Used straws (if allowed) for liquids if the person could not drink out of a glass or cup. Had 1 straw for each liquid. Provided short straws for weak persons. Followed the care plan for using straws.
15. Wiped the person's hands, face, and mouth as needed during the meal. Used a napkin or hand wipe.

Procedure—cont'd   S   U   Comments

16. Followed the care plan if the person had dysphagia.
    (Some persons with dysphagia cannot use a straw.)
    Gave thickened liquids with a spoon.   _____   _____   _____
17. Talked with the person in a pleasant manner.   _____   _____   _____
18. Encouraged the person to eat as much as possible. _____   _____   _____
19. Wiped the person's mouth with a napkin or a hand
    wipe. Discarded the napkin or hand wipe.   _____   _____   _____
20. Noted how much and which foods were eaten.   _____   _____   _____
21. Measured and recorded fluid intake if ordered.   _____   _____   _____
22. Removed the tray.   _____   _____   _____
23. Took the person to his or her room (if in a dining area). _____   _____   _____
24. Assisted with oral hygiene and hand hygiene. Wore
    gloves. Provided for privacy. Practiced hand hygiene
    after removing and discarding the gloves.   _____   _____   _____

Post-Procedure
25. Provided for comfort.   _____   _____   _____
26. Placed the call light and other needed items within reach. _____   _____   _____
27. Raised or lowered bed rails. Followed the care plan. _____   _____   _____
28. Completed a safety check of the room.   _____   _____   _____
29. Returned the food tray to the food cart.   _____   _____   _____
30. Practiced hand hygiene.   _____   _____   _____
31. Reported and recorded your observations.   _____   _____   _____

NATCEP | VIDEO

Measuring Intake and Output

Name: _____ Date: _____

	S	U	Comments

Quality of Life
- Knocked before entering the person's room.
- Addressed the person by name.
- Introduced yourself by name and title.
- Explained the procedure before starting and during the procedure.
- Protected the person's rights during the procedure.
- Handled the person gently during the procedure.

Pre-Procedure
1. Followed *Delegation Guidelines: Intake and Output.* Saw *Promoting Safety and Comfort: Intake and Output.*
2. Practiced hand hygiene.
3. Collected the following:
   - Intake and output (I&O) record
   - 2 Graduates:
   - A graduate for intake
   - A graduate for output
   - Gloves
   - Paper towels

Procedure
4. Put on gloves.
5. Measured intake.
   a. Poured liquid remaining in the container into the graduate used to measure intake. Avoided spills and splashes on the outside of the graduate.
   b. Placed the graduate on a flat surface. Measured the amount at eye level.
   c. Checked the serving amount on the I&O record. Or checked the serving size of each container.
   d. Subtracted the remaining amount from the full serving amount. Noted the amount.
   e. Poured fluid in the graduate back into the container.
   f. Repeated steps for each liquid.
      1) Poured liquid remaining in the container into the graduate used to measure intake. Avoided spills and splashes on the outside of the graduate.
      2) Placed the graduate on a flat surface. Measured the amount at eye level on a flat surface.
      3) Checked the serving amount on the I&O record. Or checked the serving size of each container.
      4) Subtracted the remaining amount from the full serving amount. Noted the amount.
      5) Poured fluid in the graduate back into the container.
   g. Added the amounts from each liquid together.
   h. Recorded the time and amount on the I&O record.
6. Measured output as follows:
   a. Poured fluid into the graduate used to measure output. Avoided spills and splashes on the outside of the graduate.
   b. Placed the device on a paper towel on a flat surface. Measured the amount at eye level.
   c. Disposed of fluid in the toilet. Avoided splashes.

Procedure—cont'd

		S	U	Comments
7.	Cleaned, rinsed, disinfected and dried the graduates. Disposed of rinse in the toilet and flushed. Used clean, dry paper towels for drying. Returned the graduates to their proper place.	_____	_____	_____
8.	Cleaned, rinsed, disinfected and dried the voiding receptacle or drainage container. Disposed of the rinse into the toilet and flushed. Used clean, dry paper towels for drying. Returned item to its proper place.	_____	_____	_____
9.	Removed and discarded the gloves. Practiced hand hygiene.	_____	_____	_____
10.	Recorded the output amount on the person's I&O record.	_____	_____	_____

Post-Procedure

11.	Provided for comfort.	_____	_____	_____
12.	Placed the call light and other items within reach.	_____	_____	_____
13.	Completed a safety check of the room.	_____	_____	_____
14.	Reported and recorded your observations.	_____	_____	_____

NATCEP Providing Drinking Water

Name: _____ Date: _____

Quality of Life	S	U	Comments
• Knocked before entering the person's room.	____	____	_____
• Addressed the person by name.	____	____	_____
• Introduced yourself by name and title.	____	____	_____
• Explained the procedure before starting and during the procedure.	____	____	_____
• Protected the person's rights during the procedure.	____	____	_____
• Handled the person gently during the procedure.	____	____	_____

Pre-Procedure

1. Followed *Delegation Guidelines: Providing Drinking Water*. Saw *Promoting Safety and Comfort: Providing Drinking Water*.   ____ ____ _____
2. Obtained a list of persons who have special fluid orders from the nurse. Or used your assignment sheet.   ____ ____ _____
3. Practiced hand hygiene.   ____ ____ _____
4. Collected the following:
   - Cart   ____ ____ _____
   - Ice chest filled with ice   ____ ____ _____
   - Cover for ice chest   ____ ____ _____
   - Scoop   ____ ____ _____
   - Paper towels   ____ ____ _____
   - Water mugs   ____ ____ _____
   - Water pitcher filled with cold water (optional depending on agency procedure)   ____ ____ _____
   - Towel for the scoop   ____ ____ _____
5. Covered the cart with paper towels. Arranged equipment on top of the paper towels.   ____ ____ _____

Procedure

6. Took the cart to the person's room door. Did not take the cart into the room.   ____ ____ _____
7. Checked the person's fluid orders. Used the list from the nurse.   ____ ____ _____
8. Identified the person. Checked the ID (identification) bracelet against the fluid order sheet or your assignment sheet. Used 2 identifiers. Also called the person by name.   ____ ____ _____
9. Took the mug from the person's over-bed table. Emptied it into the bathroom sink.   ____ ____ _____
10. Determined if a new mug was needed.   ____ ____ _____
11. Used the scoop to fill the mug with ice. Did not let the scoop touch the mug, lid, or straw.   ____ ____ _____
12. Placed the scoop on the towel.   ____ ____ _____
13. Filled the mug with water. Got water from the room sink, or bathroom sink or used the water pitcher on the cart.   ____ ____ _____
14. Placed the mug on the over-bed table.   ____ ____ _____
15. Made sure the mug was within the person's reach.   ____ ____ _____

Post-Procedure   **S**   **U**   **Comments**

16. Provided for comfort.
17. Placed the call light and other needed items within reach.
18. Completed a safety check of the room.
19. Practiced hand hygiene.
20. Repeated for each resident.
    a. Took the cart to the person's room door. Did not take the cart into the room.
    b. Checked the person's fluid orders. Used the list from the nurse.
    c. Identified the person. Checked the ID bracelet against the fluid order sheet or your assignment sheet. Used 2 identifiers. Also called the person by name.
    d. Took the mug from the person's over-bed table. Emptied it into the bathroom sink.
    e. Determined if a new mug was needed.
    f. Used the scoop to fill the mug with ice. Did not let the scoop touch the mug, lid, or straw.
    g. Placed the scoop on the towel.
    h. Filled the mug with water. Got water from the room sink, or the bathroom sink or the water pitcher on the cart.
    i. Placed the mug on the over-bed table.
    j. Made sure the mug was within the person's reach.
    k. Provided for comfort.
    l. Placed the call light and other needed items within reach.
    m. Completed a safety check of the room.
    n. Practiced hand hygiene.

Taking a Temperature With an Electronic Thermometer

Name: _____   Date: _____

Quality of Life	S	U	Comments
• Knocked before entering the person's room.	___	___	_____
• Addressed the person by name.	___	___	_____
• Introduced yourself by name and title.	___	___	_____
• Explained the procedure before starting and during the procedure.	___	___	_____
• Protected the person's rights during the procedure.	___	___	_____
• Handled the person gently during the procedure.	___	___	_____

Pre-Procedure

1. Followed *Delegation Guidelines: Taking Temperatures*. Saw *Promoting Safety and Comfort: Taking Temperatures*.   ___ ___ _____
2. For an oral temperature, asked the person not to eat, drink, smoke, or chew gum for at least 15 to 20 minutes before the measurement or as required by agency policy.   ___ ___ _____
3. Practiced hand hygiene.   ___ ___ _____
4. Collected the following:
   • Thermometer—standard electronic or tympanic membrane, or temporal artery   ___ ___ _____
   • Probe for a standard electronic thermometer (blue–oral or axillary; red– rectal)   ___ ___ _____
   • Probe covers   ___ ___ _____
   • Toilet paper (rectal temperature)   ___ ___ _____
   • Water-soluble lubricant (rectal temperature)   ___ ___ _____
   • Gloves   ___ ___ _____
   • Towel (axillary temperature)   ___ ___ _____
5. Plugged the probe into the thermometer if using a standard electronic thermometer.   ___ ___ _____
6. Practiced hand hygiene.   ___ ___ _____
7. Identified the person. Checked the ID (identification) bracelet against the assignment sheet. Used 2 identifiers. Also called the person by name.   ___ ___ _____

Procedure

8. Provided for privacy. Positioned the person for an oral, rectal, axillary, or tympanic membrane temperature. The Sims' position was used for a rectal temperature.   ___ ___ _____
9. Put on the gloves if contact with blood, body fluids, secretions, or excretions was likely.   ___ ___ _____
10. Inserted the probe into the probe cover.   ___ ___ _____
11. *For an oral temperature:*
    a. Had the person open the mouth and raise the tongue.   ___ ___ _____
    b. Placed the covered probe at the base of the tongue and to 1 side.   ___ ___ _____
    c. Had the person lower the tongue and close the mouth.   ___ ___ _____
    d. Started the thermometer. Held the probe in place until you heard a tone or saw a flashing or steady light.   ___ ___ _____
12. *For a rectal temperature:*
    a. Placed some lubricant on toilet paper.   ___ ___ _____
    b. Lubricated the end of the covered probe.   ___ ___ _____
    c. Exposed the anal area.   ___ ___ _____
    d. Raised the upper buttock.   ___ ___ _____
    e. Inserted the probe ½ inch into the rectum.   ___ ___ _____
    f. Started the thermometer. Held the probe in place until you heard a tone or saw a flashing or steady light.   ___ ___ _____

Quality of Life—cont'd	S	U	Comments

13. *For an axillary temperature:*
    a. Helped the person remove an arm from the gown. Did not expose the person. _____ _____ _____
    b. Dried the axilla with a towel. _____ _____ _____
    c. Placed the covered probe in the center of the axilla. _____ _____ _____
    d. Placed the person's arm over the chest. _____ _____ _____
    e. Started the thermometer. Held the probe in place until you heard tone or saw a flashing or steady light. _____ _____ _____
14. *For a tympanic membrane temperature:*
    a. Asked the person to turn his or her head so the ear was in front of you. _____ _____ _____
    b. Pulled up and back on the adult's ear to straighten the ear canal. If the child was aged 4 years, or less, the nurse may have had you pull the ear down and back. _____ _____ _____
    c. Inserted the covered probe gently. _____ _____ _____
    d. Started the thermometer. Held the probe in place until you heard tone or saw a flashing or steady light. _____ _____ _____
15. *For a temporal artery temperature:*
    a. Placed the device in the center of the forehead. _____ _____ _____
    b. Pressed the scan button. _____ _____ _____
    c. Slid the device right or left across the temporal artery. Used the side of the head that was exposed. Kept the thermometer flat on the forehead and in contact with the skin. _____ _____ _____
    d. Released the scan button when the thermometer reached the hairline. _____ _____ _____
16. Removed the probe from the site. Read the temperature on the display. _____ _____ _____
17. Pressed the eject button to discard the cover. _____ _____ _____
18. Noted the person's name, temperature, and temperature site on your note pad or assignment sheet. _____ _____ _____
19. Returned the probe to the holder. _____ _____ _____
20. Helped the person put the gown back on (axillary temperature). For a rectal temperature:
    a. Wiped the anal area with toilet paper to remove lubricant. _____ _____ _____
    b. Covered the person. _____ _____ _____
    c. Disposed of used toilet paper. _____ _____ _____
    d. Removed and discarded the gloves. Practiced hand hygiene. _____ _____ _____

Post-Procedure
21. Provided for comfort. _____ _____ _____
22. Placed the call light and other needed items within reach. _____ _____ _____
23. Unscreened the person. _____ _____ _____
24. Completed a safety check of the room. _____ _____ _____
25. Returned the thermometer to the charging unit. Follow agency policy for disinfection. _____ _____ _____
26. Practiced hand hygiene. _____ _____ _____
27. Reported and recorded the temperature. Noted the temperature site when reporting and recording. Reported an abnormal temperature at once. _____ _____ _____

Taking a Temperature With a Glass Thermometer

Name: _____   Date: _____

Quality of Life	S	U	Comments

- Knocked before entering the person's room.
- Addressed the person by name.
- Introduced yourself by name and title.
- Explained the procedure before starting and during the procedure.
- Protected the person's rights during the procedure.
- Handled the person gently during the procedure.

Pre-Procedure

1. Followed *Delegation Guidelines: Taking Temperatures.* Saw *Promoting Safety and Comfort:*
   a. *Thermometers Types*
   b. *Taking Temperatures*
2. For an oral temperature, asked the person not to eat, drink, smoke, or chew gum for at least 15 to 20 minutes before the measurement or as required by agency policy.
3. Practiced hand hygiene.
4. Collected the following:
   - Oral or rectal thermometer and holder
   - Tissues
   - Plastic covers if used
   - Gloves
   - Toilet paper (rectal temperature)
   - Water-soluble lubricant (rectal temperature)
   - Towel (axillary temperature)
5. Practiced hand hygiene.
6. Identified the person. Checked the ID (identification) bracelet against the assignment sheet. Used 2 identifiers. Also called the person by name.
7. Provided for privacy.

Procedure

8. Put on the gloves.
9. Rinsed the thermometer under cold running water if it was soaking in disinfectant. Did not use hot water. The substance could expand and break the thermometer. Dried it from the stem to the tip with tissues.
10. Checked for breaks, cracks, or chips. Discarded it following agency policy if it was broken, cracked or chipped.
11. Shook down the thermometer below the lowest number. Held the device by the stem. Stood away from walls, tables, and other hard surfaces. Flexed and snapped your wrist until the substance was below 94 F° or 34 C°.
12. Inserted it into a plastic cover if used.
13. *For an oral temperature:*
    a. Asked the person to moisten the lips.
    b. Placed the bulb end of the thermometer under the tongue and to 1 side.
    c. Asked the person to lower the tongue and close the lips around the thermometer to hold it in place.
    d. Asked the person not to talk or bite down on the thermometer.
    e. Left it in place for 2 to 3 minutes or as required by agency policy.

Procedure—cont'd   S   U   Comments

14. *For a rectal temperature:*
    a. Positioned the person in the Sims' position. _____ _____ _____
    b. Put a small amount of lubricant on toilet paper.
       Lubricant was used for easy insertion and to
       prevent injury. _____ _____ _____
    c. Lubricated the tip of the thermometer. _____ _____ _____
    d. Folded back top linens to expose the anal area. _____ _____ _____
    e. Raised the upper buttock to expose the anus. _____ _____ _____
    f. Inserted the thermometer 1 inch into the rectum.
       Did not force the thermometer. _____ _____ _____
    g. Held the thermometer in place for 2 minutes or as
       required by agency policy. Continued to hold it
       while it was in the rectum. _____ _____ _____
15. *For an axillary temperature:*
    a. Helped the person remove an arm from the gown.
       Did not expose the person. _____ _____ _____
    b. Dried the axilla with the towel. _____ _____ _____
    c. Placed the tip of the thermometer in the center of
       the axilla. _____ _____ _____
    d. Asked the person to place the arm over the chest to
       hold the thermometer in place. Held it and the arm
       in place if he or she could not help. _____ _____ _____
    e. Left the thermometer in place for 5 to 10 minutes or
       as required by agency policy. _____ _____ _____
16. Removed the thermometer. _____ _____ _____
17. *For an oral or axillary temperature:*
    a. Used a tissue to remove the plastic cover. _____ _____ _____
    b. Wiped the thermometer with a tissue if no cover was
       used. Wiped from the stem to the tip. _____ _____ _____
    c. Discarded the tissue and cover (if used). _____ _____ _____
    d. Read the thermometer. _____ _____ _____
    e. Helped the person put the gown back on (axillary
       temperature). _____ _____ _____
18. *For a rectal temperature:*
    a. Used toilet paper to remove the plastic cover. _____ _____ _____
    b. Wiped the thermometer with toilet paper if no cover
       was used. Wiped from the stem to the tip. _____ _____ _____
    c. Placed used toilet paper on several thicknesses of
       clean toilet paper. Discarded the cover (if used). _____ _____ _____
    d. Read the thermometer. _____ _____ _____
    e. Placed the thermometer on clean toilet paper. _____ _____ _____
    f. Wiped the anal area with toilet paper to remove
       lubricant and any feces. Set the used toilet paper
       on several thicknesses of clean toilet paper. _____ _____ _____
    g. Covered the person. _____ _____ _____
    h. Disposed of toilet paper in the toilet. _____ _____ _____
    i. Removed and discarded the glove. Practiced hand
       hygiene. _____ _____ _____
19. Noted the person's name and temperature on your note
    pad or assignment sheet. _____ _____ _____
20. Shook down the thermometer. _____ _____ _____
21. Cleaned the thermometer following agency policy.
    (Wore gloves.) Agency policy may have required that you:
    a. Wiped the thermometer with tissues or toilet paper
       to remove mucus, feces, or sweat. Wiped from the
       stem to the tip.
    b. Rinsed the thermometer under cold running water.
       Did not use hot water. Hot water causes the
       substance to expand and break the thermometer. _____ _____ _____

Procedure—cont'd

	S	U	Comments
22. Stored the thermometer in a holder or a container with a disinfectant solution. Followed agency policy.	_____	_____	_____
23. Removed and discarded the gloves. Practiced hand hygiene.	_____	_____	_____

Post-Procedure

	S	U	Comments
24. Provided for comfort.	_____	_____	_____
25. Placed the call light and other needed items within reach.	_____	_____	_____
26. Unscreened the person.	_____	_____	_____
27. Completed a safety check of the room.	_____	_____	_____
28. Practiced hand hygiene.	_____	_____	_____
29. Reported and recorded the temperature. Noted the temperature site when reporting and recording. Reported an abnormal temperature at once.	_____	_____	_____

Taking a Radial Pulse

Name: _____   Date: _____

Quality of Life	S	U	Comments
• Knocked before entering the person's room.	____	____	_____
• Addressed the person by name.	____	____	_____
• Introduced yourself by name and title.	____	____	_____
• Explained the procedure before starting and during the procedure.	____	____	_____
• Protected the person's rights during the procedure.	____	____	_____
• Handled the person gently during the procedure.	____	____	_____

Pre-Procedure

1. Followed *Delegation Guidelines: Taking Pulses*. Saw *Promoting Safety and Comfort: Taking Pulses*.   ____ ____ _____
2. Practiced hand hygiene.   ____ ____ _____
3. Identified the person. Checked the ID (identification) bracelet against the assignment sheet. Used 2 identifiers. Also called the person by name.   ____ ____ _____
4. Provided for privacy.   ____ ____ _____

Procedure

5. Had the person sit or lie down.   ____ ____ _____
6. Located the radial pulse on the thumb side of the person's wrist. Used your first 2 or 3 middle fingertips.   ____ ____ _____
7. Noted if the pulse was strong or weak, regular or irregular.   ____ ____ _____
8. Counted the pulse for 30 seconds. Multiplied the number of beats by 2 for the number of pulses in 60 seconds (1 minute).   ____ ____ _____
9. Counted the pulse for 1 minute if:
    a. Directed by the nurse and care plan.   ____ ____ _____
    b. Required by agency policy.   ____ ____ _____
    c. The pulse was irregular.   ____ ____ _____
    d. Required for your state competency test.   ____ ____ _____
10. Noted the following on your note pad or assignment sheet.
    a. The person's name   ____ ____ _____
    b. Pulse site   ____ ____ _____
    c. Pulse rate   ____ ____ _____
    d. Pulse strength   ____ ____ _____
    e. If the pulse was regular or irregular   ____ ____ _____

Post-Procedure

11. Provided for comfort.   ____ ____ _____
12. Placed the call light and other needed items within reach.   ____ ____ _____
13. Unscreened the person.   ____ ____ _____
14. Completed a safety check of the room.   ____ ____ _____
15. Practiced hand hygiene.   ____ ____ _____
16. Reported and recorded the pulse rate and your observations. Reported an abnormal pulse at once.   ____ ____ _____

Taking an Apical Pulse and an Apical-Radial Pulse

Name: _____   Date: _____

	S	U	Comments

Quality of Life

- Knocked before entering the person's room.
- Addressed the person by name.
- Introduced yourself by name and title.
- Explained the procedure before starting and during the procedure.
- Protected the person's rights during the procedure.
- Handled the person gently during the procedure.

Pre-Procedure

1. Followed *Delegation Guidelines: Taking Pulses*. Saw *Promoting Safety and Comfort: Using a Stethoscope. Taking Pulses.*
2. Asked a co-worker to help you (for an apical-radial pulse).
3. Practiced hand hygiene.
4. Collected a stethoscope and antiseptic wipes.
5. Practiced hand hygiene.
6. Identified the person. Checked the ID (identification) bracelet against the assignment sheet. Used 2 identifiers. Also called the person by name.
7. Provided for privacy.

Procedure

8. Cleaned the stethoscope ear-pieces and chest-piece with the wipes.
9. For an apical pulse
   a. Had the person sit or lie down.
   b. Exposed the upper part of the left chest. Exposed a woman's breasts only to the extent necessary.
   c. Warmed the diaphragm in your palm.
   d. Placed the stethoscope ear-pieces in your ears. The bends of the tips pointed forward.
   e. Found the apical pulse. Placed the diaphragm 2 to 3 inches to the left of the breastbone.
   f. Counted the pulse for 1 minute. (Counted each lub-dub as 1 beat). Noted if it was regular or irregular.
10. For an apical-radial pulse:
    a. Had the person sit or lie down.
    b. Exposed the upper part of the left chest. Exposed a woman's breasts only to the extent necessary.
    c. Warmed the diaphragm in your palm.
    d. Placed the stethoscope ear-pieces in your ears. The bends of the tips pointed forward.
    e. Found the apical pulse. Placed the diaphragm 2 to 3 inches to the left of the breastbone. Your co-worker found the radial pulse.
    f. Gave the signal to begin counting
    g. Counted the apical pulse for 1 minute. Your co-worker counted the radial pulse for 1 minted.
    h. Gave the signal to stop counting. Asked your co-worker for the radial pulse rate.
11. Covered the person. Removed the stethoscope ear-pieces.

	S	U	Comments

Procedure—cont'd

12. For an apical-radial pulse, subtracted the radial pulse from the apical pulse for the pulse deficit. _____ _____ _____

13. Noted the person's name and pulse site(s), pulse rate(s) and pulse deficit on your note pad or assignment sheet. Noted if the pulse was regular or irregular. _____ _____ _____

Post-Procedure

14. Provided for comfort. _____ _____ _____

15. Placed the call light and other needed items within reach. _____ _____ _____

16. Unscreened the person. _____ _____ _____

17. Completed a safety check of the room. _____ _____ _____

18. Cleaned the stethoscope ear-pieces and chest-piece with the wipes. _____ _____ _____

19. Returned the stethoscope to its proper place. Follow agency policy for disinfection. _____ _____ _____

20. Practiced hand hygiene. _____ _____ _____

21. Reported and recorded your observations. Noted if the pulse was regular or irregular. Recorded the pulse rate with *Ap* for apical. For an apical-radial pulse, recorded the apical and radial pulse rates and the pulse deficit. Reported an abnormal pulse rate at once. _____ _____ _____

Counting Respirations

Name: _____   Date: _____

Procedure	S	U	Comments
1. Followed *Delegation Guidelines: Counting Respirations*.	___	___	_____
2. Kept your fingers or stethoscope over the pulse site.	___	___	_____
3. Did not tell the person you were counting respirations.	___	___	_____
4. Counted chest rises. Each rise and fall of the chest was 1 respiration.	___	___	_____
5. Noted the following:			
a. If respirations were regular	___	___	_____
b. If both sides of the chest rose equally	___	___	_____
c. The depth of the respirations	___	___	_____
d. If the person had any pain or difficulty breathing	___	___	_____
e. An abnormal respiratory pattern	___	___	_____
6. Counted respirations for 30 seconds. Multiplied the number by 2 for the number of respirations in 60 seconds (1 minute).	___	___	_____
7. Counted respirations for 1 minute if:			
a. Directed by the nurse and care plan.	___	___	_____
b. Required by agency policy.	___	___	_____
c. They were abnormal or irregular.	___	___	_____
d. Required for your state competency test.	___	___	_____
8. Noted the person's name, respiratory rate, and other observations on your note pad or assignment sheet.	___	___	_____

Post-Procedure

	S	U	Comments
9. Provided for comfort.			
10. Placed the call light and other needed items within reach.	___	___	_____
11. Unscreened the person.	___	___	_____
12. Completed a safety check of the room.	___	___	_____
13. Practiced hand hygiene.	___	___	_____
14. Reported and recorded the respiratory rate and your observations. Reported abnormal respirations at once.	___	___	_____

Measuring Blood Pressure With an Aneroid Manometer

Name: _____   Date: _____

Quality of Life	S	U	Comments

Quality of Life
- Knocked before entering the person's room.
- Addressed the person by name.
- Introduced yourself by name and title.
- Explained the procedure before starting and during the procedure.
- Protected the person's rights during the procedure.
- Handled the person gently during the procedure.

Pre-Procedure
1. Followed *Delegation Guidelines: Measuring Blood Pressure.* Saw *Promoting Safety and Comfort:*
   a. *Using a Stethoscope*
   b. *Blood Pressure Equipment*
2. Practiced hand hygiene.
3. Collected the following:
   - Aneroid manometer
   - Stethoscope
   - Antiseptic wipes
4. Practiced hand hygiene.
5. Identified the person. Checked the ID (identification) bracelet against the assignment sheet. Used 2 identifiers. Also called the person by name.
6. Provided for privacy.

Procedure
7. Had the person sit or lie down.
8. Positioned the person's arm level with the heart. The palm was up.
9. Wiped the stethoscope ear-pieces and chest-piece with the wipes. Warmed the diaphragm in your palm. Discarded the wipes.
10. Stood no more than 3 feet away from the manometer.
11. Exposed the upper arm.
12. Squeezed the cuff to expel any air. Closed the valve on the bulb.
13. Found the brachial artery at the inner aspect of the elbow. (The brachial artery is on the little finger side of the arm.) Used your fingertips.
14. Located the arrow on the cuff. Aligned the arrow on the cuff over the brachial artery. Wrapped the cuff around the upper arm at least 1 inch above the elbow. It was even and snug.
15. Placed the stethoscope ear-pieces in your ears. Placed the stethoscope's diaphragm over the brachial artery. Did not place it under the cuff.
16. Found the radial pulse for Methods 1 and 2.
17. *Method 1:*
    a. Inflated the cuff until you could no longer feel the pulse. Noted this point.
    b. Inflated the cuff 30 mm Hg beyond the point where you last felt the pulse.

Procedure—cont'd	S	U	Comments

18. *Method 2:*
    a. Inflated the cuff until you no longer felt the pulse. Noted this point.
    b. Inflated the cuff 30 mm Hg beyond the point where you last felt the pulse.
    c. Deflated the cuff slowly. Noted the point where you felt the pulse.
    d. Waited 30 seconds.
    e. Inflated the cuff 30 mm Hg beyond the point where you felt the pulse return.
19. *Method 3:*
    a. Inflated the cuff 160 mm Hg to 180 mm Hg.
    b. Deflated the cuff if you heard a blood pressure (BP) sound. Re-inflated the cuff to 200 mm Hg.
20. Deflated the cuff at an even rate of 2 to 4 millimeters per second. Turned the valve counter-clockwise to deflate the cuff.
21. Noted the point where you heard the first sound. This was the systolic reading. It was near the point where the radial pulse disappeared (Method 1) or returned (Method 2).
22. Continued to deflate the cuff. Noted the point where the sound disappeared (the last sound heard). This was the diastolic reading.
23. Deflated the cuff completely. Removed it from the person's arm. Removed the stethoscope ear-pieces from your ears.
24. Noted the person's name and BP on your note pad or assignment sheet.
25. Returned the cuff to the case or the wall holder.

Post-Procedure
26. Provided for comfort.
27. Placed the call light and other needed items within reach.
28. Unscreened the person.
29. Completed a safety check of the room.
30. Cleaned the ear-pieces and chest-piece with the wipes.
31. Returned the equipment to its proper place. Follow agency policy for disinfection.
32. Practiced hand hygiene.
33. Reported and recorded the BP. Noted which arm was used. Reported an abnormal BP at once.

Measuring Blood Pressure With an Electronic Manometer

Name: _____   Date: _____

Quality of Life	S	U	Comments
• Knocked before entering the person's room.	____	____	_____
• Addressed the person by name.	____	____	_____
• Introduced yourself by name and title.	____	____	_____
• Explained the procedure before starting and during the procedure.	____	____	_____
• Protected the person's rights during the procedure.	____	____	_____
• Handled the person gently during the procedure.	____	____	_____

Pre-Procedure

1. Followed *Delegation Guidelines: Measuring Blood Pressure*.   ____ ____ _____
2. Practiced hand hygiene.   ____ ____ _____
3. Collected the following:
   • Electronic BP monitor   ____ ____ _____
   • BP cuff for use with the device (in the correct size for the person)   ____ ____ _____
4. Practiced hand hygiene.   ____ ____ _____
5. Identified the person. Checked the ID (identification) bracelet against the assignment sheet. Used 2 identifiers. Also called the person by name.   ____ ____ _____
6. Provided for privacy.   ____ ____ _____

Procedure

7. Had the person sit or lie down.
8. Positioned the person's arm level with the heart.   ____ ____ _____
9. Exposed the upper arm. The palm was up.   ____ ____ _____
10. Squeezed the cuff to expel any air.
11. Turned on the electronic BP monitor.
12. Connected the cuff to the monitor's connection tubing.   ____ ____ _____
13. Found the brachial artery at the inner aspect of the elbow. (The brachial artery is on the little finger side of the arm.) Used your fingertips.   ____ ____ _____
14. Located the arrow on the cuff. Aligned the arrow on the cuff over the brachial artery. Wrapped the cuff around the upper arm at least 1 inch above the elbow. It was even and snug.   ____ ____ _____
15. Pressed the start button on the electronic BP monitor. Left the cuff in place while the device measured the BP. Asked the person to be still.   ____ ____ _____
16. Removed the cuff after the BP was measured. The BP was displayed on the monitor.   ____ ____ _____
17. Noted the person's name and BP on your note pad or assignment sheet.   ____ ____ _____
18. Followed the agency policy for where to store the cuff (in the person's room or with the BP monitor).   ____ ____ _____

Post-Procedure   S   U   **Comments**

19. Provided for comfort.
20. Placed the call light and other needed items within reach.   _____   _____   _____
21. Unscreened the person.   _____   _____   _____
22. Completed a safety check of the room.   _____   _____   _____
23. Returned the equipment to its proper place.   _____   _____   _____
24. Practiced hand hygiene.   _____   _____   _____
25. Reported and recorded the BP. Noted which arm was
    used. Reported an abnormal BP at once.   _____   _____   _____

Performing Range-of-Motion Exercises

Name: _____   Date: _____

	S	U	Comments

Quality of Life
- Knocked before entering the person's room.
- Addressed the person by name.
- Introduced yourself by name and title.
- Explained the procedure before starting and during the procedure.
- Protected the person's rights during the procedure.
- Handled the person gently during the procedure.

Pre-Procedure
1. Followed *Delegation Guidelines: Range-of-Motion Exercises.* Saw *Promoting Safety and Comfort: Range-of-Motion Exercises.*
2. Practiced hand hygiene.
3. Identified the person. Checked the ID (identification) bracelet against the assignment sheet. Used 2 identifiers. Also called the person by name.
4. Obtained a bath blanket.
5. Provided for privacy.
6. Raised the bed for body mechanics. Bed rails were up if used.

Procedure
7. Lowered the bed rail near you if up.
8. Positioned the person supine.
9. Covered the person with a bath blanket. Fan-folded top linens to the foot of the bed.
10. Exercised the neck *if allowed by your agency and if the nurse instructed you to do so.*
    a. Placed your hands over the person's ears to support the head. Supported the jaw with your fingers.
    b. Flexion—brought the head forward. The chin touched the chest.
    c. Extension—straightened the head.
    d. Hyperextension—brought the head backward until the chin pointed up.
    e. Rotation—turned the head from side to side.
    f. Lateral flexion—moved the head to the right and to the left.
    g. Repeated flexion, extension, hyperextension, rotation, and lateral flexion 5 times—or the number of times stated on the care plan.

Procedure—cont'd   S   U   **Comments**

11. Exercised the shoulder.
    a. Supported the wrist with 1 hand. Supported the elbow with the other hand.
    b. Flexion—raised the arm straight in front and over the head.
    c. Extension—brought the arm down to the side.
    d. Hyperextension—moved the arm behind the body. (Did this if the person was in a straight-backed chair or was standing.)
    e. Abduction—moved the straight arm away from the side of the body.
    f. Adduction—moved the straight arm to the side of the body.
    g. Internal rotation—bent the elbow. Placed it at the same level as the shoulder. Moved the forearm and hand so the fingers pointed down.
    h. External rotation—moved the forearm and hand so the fingers pointed up.
    i. Repeated flexion, extension, hyperextension, abduction, adduction, and internal and external rotation 5 times—or the number of times stated on the care plan.
12. Exercised the elbow.
    a. Supported the person's wrist with 1 hand. Supported the elbow with your other hand.
    b. Flexion—bent the arm so the same-side shoulder was touched.
    c. Extension—straightened the arm.
    d. Repeated flexion and extension 5 times—or the number of times stated on the care plan.
13. Exercised the forearm.
    a. Continued to support the wrist and elbow.
    b. Pronation—turned the hand so the palm was down.
    c. Supination—turned the hand so the palm was up.
    d. Repeated pronation and supination 5 times—or the number of times stated on the care plan.
14. Exercised the wrist.
    a. Supported the wrist with both of your hands.
    b. Flexion—bent the hand down.
    c. Extension—straightened the hand.
    d. Hyperextension—bent the hand back.
    e. Radial flexion—turned the hand toward the thumb.
    f. Ulnar flexion—turned the hand toward the little finger.
    g. Repeated flexion, extension, hyperextension, and radial and ulnar flexion 5 times—or the number of times stated on the care plan.
15. Exercised the thumb.
    a. Supported the person's hand with 1 hand. Supported the thumb with your other hand.
    b. Abduction—moved the thumb out from the inner part of the index finger.
    c. Adduction—moved the thumb back next to the index finger.
    d. Opposition—touched each fingertip with the thumb.
    e. Flexion—bent the thumb into the hand.
    f. Extension—moved the thumb out to the side of the fingers.
    g. Repeated abduction, adduction, opposition, flexion, and extension 5 times—or the number of times stated on the care plan.

Procedure—cont'd   **S**   **U**   **Comments**

16. Exercised the fingers.
    a. Abduction—spread the fingers and the thumb apart.   _____   _____   _____
    b. Adduction—brought the fingers and thumb together.   _____   _____   _____
    c. Flexion—made a fist.   _____   _____   _____
    d. Extension—straightened the fingers so the fingers, hand, and arm were straight.   _____   _____   _____
    e. Repeated abduction, adduction, flexion, and extension 5 times—or the number of times stated on the care plan.   _____   _____   _____
17. Exercised the hip.
    a. Supported the leg. Placed 1 hand under the knee. Placed your other hand under the ankle.   _____   _____   _____
    b. Flexion—raised the leg.   _____   _____   _____
    c. Extension—straightened the leg.   _____   _____   _____
    d. Hyperextension—moved the leg behind the body. (Did this if the person was standing.)   _____   _____   _____
    e. Abduction—moved the leg away from the body.   _____   _____   _____
    f. Adduction—moved the leg toward the other leg.   _____   _____   _____
    g. Internal rotation—turned the leg inward.   _____   _____   _____
    h. External rotation—turned the leg outward.   _____   _____   _____
    i. Repeated flexion, extension, hyperextension, abduction, adduction, and internal and external rotation 5 times—or the number of times stated on the care plan.   _____   _____   _____
18. Exercised the knee.
    a. Supported the knee. Placed 1 hand under the knee. Placed your other hand under the ankle.   _____   _____   _____
    b. Flexion—bent the knee.   _____   _____   _____
    c. Extension—straightened the knee.   _____   _____   _____
    d. Repeated flexion and extension of the knee 5 times—or the number of times stated on the care plan.   _____   _____   _____
19. Exercised the ankle.
    a. Supported the foot and ankle. Placed 1 hand under the foot. Placed your other hand under the ankle.   _____   _____   _____
    b. Dorsiflexion—pulled the foot upward. Pushed down on the heel at the same time.   _____   _____   _____
    c. Plantar flexion—turned the foot down. Or pointed the toes.   _____   _____   _____
    d. Repeated dorsiflexion and plantar flexion 5 times—or the number of times stated on the care plan.   _____   _____   _____
20. Exercised the foot.
    a. Continued to support the foot and ankle.   _____   _____   _____
    b. Pronation—turned the outside of the foot up and the inside down.   _____   _____   _____
    c. Supination—turned the inside of the foot up and the outside down.   _____   _____   _____
    d. Repeated pronation and supination 5 times—or the number of times stated on the care plan.   _____   _____   _____
21. Exercised the toes.
    a. Flexion—curled the toes.   _____   _____   _____
    b. Extension—straightened the toes.   _____   _____   _____
    c. Abduction—spread the toes apart.   _____   _____   _____
    d. Adduction—pulled the toes together.   _____   _____   _____
    e. Repeated flexion, extension, abduction, and adduction 5 times—or the number of times stated on the care plan.   _____   _____   _____
22. Covered the leg. Raised the bed rail if used.   _____   _____   _____
23. Went to the other side. Lowered the bed rail near you if up.   _____   _____   _____

Procedure—cont'd   S   U   **Comments**

24. Repeated exercises.
    a. Exercised the shoulder.
        1) Supported the wrist with 1 hand. Supported the elbow with the other hand.
        2) Flexion—raised the arm straight in front and over the head.
        3) Extension—brought the arm down to the side.
        4) Hyperextension—moved the arm behind the body. (Did this if the person was in a straight-backed chair or was standing.)
        5) Abduction—moved the straight arm away from the side of the body.
        6) Adduction—Moved the straight arm to the side of the body.
        7) Internal rotation—bent the elbow. Placed it at the same level as the shoulder. Moved the forearm and hand so the fingers pointed down.
        8) External rotation—moved the forearm and hand so the fingers pointed up.
        9) Repeated flexion, extension, hyperextension, abduction, adduction, and internal and external rotation 5 times—or the number of times stated on the care plan.
    b. Exercised the elbow.
        1) Supported the person's wrist with 1 hand. Supported the elbow with your other hand.
        2) Flexion—bent the arm so the same-side shoulder was touched.
        3) Extension—straightened the arm.
        4) Repeated flexion and extension 5 times—or the number of times stated on the care plan.
    c. Exercised the forearm.
        1) Continued to support the wrist and elbow.
        2) Pronation—turned the hand so the palm was down.
        3) Supination—turned the hand so the palm was up.
        4) Repeated pronation and supination 5 times—or the number of times stated on the care plan.
    d. Exercised the wrist.
        1) Supported the wrist with both of your hands.
        2) Flexion—bent the hand down.
        3) Extension—straightened the hand.
        4) Hyperextension—bent the hand back.
        5) Radial flexion—turned the hand toward the thumb.
        6) Ulnar flexion—turned the hand toward the little finger.
        7) Repeated flexion, extension, hyperextension, and radial and ulnar flexion 5 times—or the number of times stated on the care plan.

Procedure—cont'd	**S**	**U**	**Comments**

e. Exercised the thumb.
 1) Supported the person's hand with 1 hand. Supported the thumb with your other hand. ___ ___ _____
 2) Abduction—moved the thumb out from the inner part of the index finger. ___ ___ _____
 3) Adduction—moved the thumb back next to the index finger. ___ ___ _____
 4) Opposition—touched each fingertip with the thumb. ___ ___ _____
 5) Flexion—bent the thumb into the hand. ___ ___ _____
 6) Extension—moved the thumb out to the side of the fingers. ___ ___ _____
 7) Repeated abduction, adduction, opposition, flexion, and extension 5 times—or the number of times stated on the care plan. ___ ___ _____

f. Exercised the fingers.
 1) Abduction—spread the fingers and the thumb apart. ___ ___ _____
 2) Adduction—brought the fingers and the thumb together. ___ ___ _____
 3) Flexion—made a fist. ___ ___ _____
 4) Extension—straightened the fingers so the fingers, hand, and arm were straight. ___ ___ _____
 5) Repeated abduction, adduction, flexion, and extension 5 times—or the number of times stated on the care plan. ___ ___ _____

g. Exercised the hip.
 1) Supported the leg. Placed 1 hand under the knee. Placed your other hand under the ankle. ___ ___ _____
 2) Flexion—raised the leg. ___ ___ _____
 3) Extension—straightened the leg. ___ ___ _____
 4) Hyperextension—moved the leg behind the body. (Did this if the person was standing.) ___ ___ _____
 5) Abduction—moved the leg away from the body. ___ ___ _____
 6) Adduction—moved the leg toward the other leg. ___ ___ _____
 7) Internal rotation—turned the leg inward. ___ ___ _____
 8) External rotation—turned the leg outward. ___ ___ _____
 9) Repeated flexion, extension, hyperextension, abduction, adduction, and internal and external rotation 5 times—or the number of times stated on the care plan. ___ ___ _____

h. Exercised the knee.
 1) Supported the knee. Placed 1 hand under the knee. Placed your other hand under the ankle. ___ ___ _____
 2) Flexion—bent the knee. ___ ___ _____
 3) Extension—straightened the knee. ___ ___ _____
 4) Repeated flexion and extension of the knee 5 times—or the number of times stated on the care plan. ___ ___ _____

i. Exercised the ankle.
 1) Supported the foot and ankle. Placed 1 hand under the foot. Placed your other hand under the ankle. ___ ___ _____
 2) Dorsiflexion—pulled the foot upward. Pushed down on the heel at the same time. ___ ___ _____
 3) Plantar flexion—turned the foot down. Or pointed the toes. ___ ___ _____
 4) Repeated dorsiflexion and plantar flexion 5 times—or the number of times stated on the care plan. ___ ___ _____

	S	U	Comments
Procedure—cont'd			
j. Exercised the foot.			
1) Continued to support the foot and ankle.	_____	_____	_____
2) Pronation—turned the outside of the foot up and the inside down.	_____	_____	_____
3) Supination—turned the inside of the foot up and the outside down.	_____	_____	_____
4) Repeated pronation and supination 5 times—or the number of times stated on the care plan.	_____	_____	_____
k. Exercised the toes.			
1) Flexion—curled the toes.	_____	_____	_____
2) Extension—straightened the toes.	_____	_____	_____
3) Abduction—spread the toes apart.	_____	_____	_____
4) Adduction—put the toes together.	_____	_____	_____
5) Repeated flexion, extension, abduction, and adduction 5 times—or the number of times stated on the care plan.	_____	_____	_____
25. Covered the leg. Raised the bed rail if used.	_____	_____	_____
Post-Procedure			
26. Provided for comfort.	_____	_____	_____
27. Covered the person with the top linens. Removed the bath blanket.	_____	_____	_____
28. Placed the call light and other needed items within reach.	_____	_____	_____
29. Lowered the bed to a safe and comfortable level. Followed the care plan.	_____	_____	_____
30. Raised or lowered bed rails. Followed the care plan.	_____	_____	_____
31. Folded and returned the bath blanket to its proper place. Or followed the agency policy for used linens.	_____	_____	_____
32. Unscreened the person.	_____	_____	_____
33. Completed a safety check of the room.	_____	_____	_____
34. Practiced hand hygiene.	_____	_____	_____
35. Reported and recorded your observations.	_____	_____	_____

Assisting with Ambulation

Name: _____ Date: _____

Quality of Life	S	U	Comments
• Knocked before entering the person's room.	____	____	_____
• Addressed the person by name.	____	____	_____
• Introduced yourself by name and title.	____	____	_____
• Explained the procedure before starting and during the procedure.	____	____	_____
• Protected the person's rights during the procedure.	____	____	_____
• Handled the person gently during the procedure.	____	____	_____

Pre-Procedure

1. Followed *Delegation Guidelines: Assisting with Ambulation.* Saw *Promoting Safety and Comfort: Assisting with Ambulation.* ____ ____ _____
2. Practiced hand hygiene. ____ ____ _____
3. Collected the following:
   • Slip-resistant shoes or footwear ____ ____ _____
   • Paper or towel to protect bottom linens ____ ____ _____
   • Gait (transfer) belt
   • Walker or cane (if needed) ____ ____ _____
4. Identified the person. Checked the ID (identification) bracelet against the assignment sheet. Used 2 identifiers. Also called the person by name. ____ ____ _____
5. Provided for privacy. ____ ____ _____

Procedure

6. Lowered the bed to a safe and comfortable level for the person. Followed the care plan. Locked (braked) the bed wheels. Lowered the bed rail near you if up. ____ ____ _____
7. Fan-folded top linens to the foot of the bed. ____ ____ _____
8. Placed the paper or towel under the person's feet to protect bottom linens. Put the shoes on and fastened. ____ ____ _____
9. Helped the person sit on the side of the bed. ____ ____ _____
10. Made sure the person's feet were flat on the floor. ____ ____ _____
11. Made sure that the person was properly dressed. ____ ____ _____
12. Applied the gait belt at the waist over the clothing. ____ ____ _____
13. Positioned the walker (if used) in front of the person. Or had the person hold the cane (if used) on the strong side. ____ ____ _____
14. Helped the person stand. Grasped the gait belt at each side. ____ ____ _____
15. Stood at the weak side while the person gained balance. Held the belt at the side and back. ____ ____ _____
16. Encouraged the person to stand erect with the head up and back straight. ____ ____ _____
17. *If using a walker or cane:*
    a. Walker—the walker was 6 to 8 inches in front of the person. ____ ____ _____
    b. Cane—the cane was held on the strong side.
       1) The cane tip was 6 to 10 inches to the side of the strong foot.
       2) The cane tip was 6 to 10 inches in front of the strong foot. ____ ____ _____
18. Helped the person walk. Walked to the side and slightly behind the person on the person's weak side. Provided support with the gait belt. Had the person use the hand rail on his or her strong side (unless using a walker or cane). ____ ____ _____

Procedure—cont'd	S	U	Comments

19. *If using a walker or cane:*
    a. Walker—with both hands, the person pushed the walker 6 to 8 inches in front of the feet. ____ ____ _____
    b. Cane:
       1) The cane (on the strong side) was moved forward 6 to 10 inches. ____ ____ _____
       2) The weak leg (opposite the cane) was moved forward even with the cane. ____ ____ _____
       3) The strong leg was moved forward and ahead of the cane and the weak leg. ____ ____ _____
20. Encouraged the person to walk normally. The heel struck the floor first. Discouraged shuffling, sliding, or walking on tip-toes. ____ ____ _____
21. Walked the ordered distance if the person tolerated the activity. Did not rush the person. ____ ____ _____
22. Helped the person return to bed. Removed the gait belt. ____ ____ _____
23. Lowered the head of the bed. Helped the person to the center of the bed. ____ ____ _____
24. Removed the shoes. Removed the paper or towel over the bottom sheet. Discarded the paper or followed agency policy for used linens. ____ ____ _____

Post-Procedure

25. Provided for comfort. ____ ____ _____
26. Placed the call light and other needed items within reach. ____ ____ _____
27. Raised or lowered bed rails. Followed the care plan. ____ ____ _____
28. Returned the robe and shoes to their proper place. ____ ____ _____
29. Unscreened the person. ____ ____ _____
30. Completed a safety check of the room. ____ ____ _____
31. Practiced hand hygiene. ____ ____ _____
32. Reported and recorded your observations. ____ ____ _____

Giving a Back Massage

Name: _____ Date: _____

	S	U	Comments

Quality of Life
- Knocked before entering the person's room.
- Addressed the person by name.
- Introduced yourself by name and title.
- Explained the procedure before starting and during the procedure.
- Protected the person's rights during the procedure.
- Handled the person gently during the procedure.

Pre-Procedure
1. Followed *Delegation Guidelines: The Back Massage.* Saw *Promoting Safety and Comfort: The Back Massage.*
2. Practiced hand hygiene.
3. Identified the person. Checked the ID (identification) bracelet against the assignment sheet. Used 2 identifiers. Also called the person by name.
4. Collected the following:
   - Bath blanket
   - Bath towel
   - Lotion
5. Provided for privacy.
6. Raised the bed for body mechanics. Bed rails were up if used.

Procedure
7. Lowered the bed rail near you if up.
8. Positioned the person in the prone or side-lying position. The back was toward you.
9. Covered the person with a bath blanket. Exposed the back, shoulders, and upper arms.
10. Laid the towel on the bed along the back. Did this if the person was in a side-lying position.
11. Warmed the lotion.
12. Explained that the lotion may feel cool and wet.
13. Applied lotion to the lower back area.
14. Stroked up from the lower back to the shoulders. Then stroked down over the upper arms. Stroked up the upper arms, across the shoulders, and down the back. Used firm strokes. Kept your hands in contact with the person's skin.
15. Repeated stroking up from the lower back to the shoulders. Then stroked down over the upper arms. Stroked up the upper arms, across the shoulders, and down the back. Used firm strokes. Kept your hands in contact with the person's skin. Continued this for at least 3 minutes.
16. Kneaded the back.
    a. Grasped the skin between your thumb and fingers.
    b. Kneaded half of the back. Started at the lower back and moved up to the shoulder. Then kneaded down from the shoulder to the lower back.
    c. Repeated on the other half of the back.

Procedure—cont'd

	S	U	Comments
17. Applied lotion to bony areas. Used circular motions with the tips of your index and middle fingers. *(Did not massage reddened bony areas.)*	___	___	_____
18. Used fast movements to stimulate. Used slow movements to relax the person.	___	___	_____
19. Stroked with long, firm movements to end the massage. Told the person you were finishing.	___	___	_____
20. Straightened and secured clothing or sleepwear.	___	___	_____
21. Covered the person. Removed the towel and bath blanket.	___	___	_____

Post-Procedure

	S	U	Comments
22. Provided for comfort.	___	___	_____
23. Placed the call light and other needed items within reach.	___	___	_____
24. Lowered the bed to a safe and comfortable level. Followed the care plan.	___	___	_____
25. Raised or lowered bed rails. Followed the care plan.	___	___	_____
26. Returned lotion to its proper place.	___	___	_____
27. Unscreened the person.	___	___	_____
28. Completed a safety check of the room.	___	___	_____
29. Followed agency policy for used linens.	___	___	_____
30. Practiced hand hygiene.	___	___	_____
31. Reported and recorded your observations.	___	___	_____

Preparing the Person's Room

Name: _____   Date: _____

Procedure	S	U	Comments
1. Followed *Delegation Guidelines: Admissions, Transfers, and Discharges*.	_____	_____	_____
2. Practiced hand hygiene.	_____	_____	_____
3. Collected the following:			
• Admission kit—wash basin, soap, toothpaste, toothbrush, water mug, and so on.	_____	_____	_____
• Bedpan and urinal (for a man)	_____	_____	_____
• Nursing assistant admission checklist	_____	_____	_____
• Thermometer	_____	_____	_____
• Stethoscope and blood pressure equipment	_____	_____	_____
• Pulse oximeter	_____	_____	_____
• Patient gown or sleepwear (if needed)	_____	_____	_____
• Towels and washcloth	_____	_____	_____
• IV (intravenous) pole (if needed)	_____	_____	_____
• Other items requested by the nurse	_____	_____	_____
4. Placed the following on the over-bed table.			
• Thermometer	_____	_____	_____
• Stethoscope and blood pressure equipment	_____	_____	_____
• Pulse oximeter	_____	_____	_____
• Nursing assistant admission checklist	_____	_____	_____
5. Placed the water mug on the bedside stand or over-bed table.	_____	_____	_____
6. Placed the following in the bedside stand.			
• Admission kit	_____	_____	_____
• Bedpan and urinal	_____	_____	_____
• Patient gown or sleepwear	_____	_____	_____
• Towels and washcloth	_____	_____	_____
7. *If the person arrived by stretcher:*			
a. Made a surgical bed.	_____	_____	_____
b. Raised the bed for a transfer from a stretcher.	_____	_____	_____
8. *If the person was ambulatory or arrived by wheelchair:*			
a. Left the bed closed.	_____	_____	_____
b. Lowered the bed to a safe and comfortable level as directed by the nurse.	_____	_____	_____
9. Attached the call light to the bed linens.	_____	_____	_____
10. Place an IV pole (if needed) next to the head of the bed.	_____	_____	_____
11. Practiced hand hygiene.	_____	_____	_____

Admitting the Person

Name: _____   Date: _____

Quality of Life	S	U	Comments
• Knocked before entering the person's room.	___	___	_____
• Addressed the person by name.	___	___	_____
• Introduced yourself by name and title.	___	___	_____
• Explained the procedure before starting and during the procedure.	___	___	_____
• Protected the person's rights during the procedure.	___	___	_____
• Handled the person gently during the procedure.	___	___	_____

Pre-Procedure

	S	U	Comments
1. Followed *Delegation Guidelines: Admissions, Transfers, and Discharges*. Saw *Promoting Safety and Comfort: Admissions, Transfers, and Discharges*.	___	___	_____
2. Practiced hand hygiene.	___	___	_____
3. Prepared the room.	___	___	_____

Procedure

	S	U	Comments
4. Identified the person. Used 2 identifiers. Checked the information on the admission form and ID (identification) bracelet.	___	___	_____
5. Greeted the person by name. Asked what name he or she preferred.	___	___	_____
6. Introduced yourself to the person and others present. Gave your name and title. Explained that you assist the nurses in giving care.	___	___	_____
7. Introduced the roommate.	___	___	_____
8. Provided for privacy. Asked family or friends to leave the room unless the person preferred that someone stay. Told them how much time you needed and directed them to the waiting area.	___	___	_____
9. Allowed the person to stay dressed if his or her condition permitted. Or helped with changing into a patient gown or sleepwear.	___	___	_____
10. Provided for comfort. The person was in bed or in a chair as directed by the nurse.	___	___	_____
11. Assisted the nurse with assessment.			
a. Measured vital signs.	___	___	_____
b. Measured weight and height.	___	___	_____
c. Collected information for the nursing assistant admission checklist.	___	___	_____

Proceduree—cont'd	S	U	Comments

12. Oriented the person and family to the area.
   a. Gave names of the nurses and nursing assistants.
   b. Explained the purpose of items in the bedside stand.
   c. Explained how to use the over-bed table.
   d. Showed how to use the call light.
   e. Showed the person the bathroom. Explained how to use the call light in the bathroom.
   f. Showed how to use the bed, TV, and light controls.
   g. Explained how to use the agency's phone. Placed the phone within reach.
   h. Explained how to connect to the Internet.
   i. Showed the electrical outlets for charging electronic devices
   j. Explained where to find the nurses' station, lounge, chapel, dining room, and other areas.
   k. Identified staff—housekeeping, dietary, physical therapy, and others. Also identified students in the agency.
   l. Explained when meals and snacks are served.
   m. Explained visiting hours and policies.
13. Filled the water mug if oral fluids were allowed.
14. Placed the call light within reach.
15. Placed other controls and needed items within reach.
16. Provided a denture container if needed. Labeled it with the person's name, room, and bed number.
17. Labeled the person's property and personal care items with his or her name (if not completed by the family). Followed agency policy for labeling items.
18. Completed a clothing and personal belongings list. Followed agency policy for labeling clothing.
19. Helped the person put away clothes and personal items. Used the closet, drawers, and bedside stand. (The family may have helped with this step.)

Post-Procedure

20. Provided for comfort.
21. Lowered the bed to a safe and comfortable level. Followed the nurse's direction.
22. Raised or lowered bed rails as directed by the nurse.
23. Completed a safety check of the room.
24. Practiced hand hygiene.
25. Reported and recorded your observations.

Measuring Weight and Height With a Standing Scale

Name: _____   Date: _____

Quality of Life	S	U	Comments
• Knocked before entering the person's room.			
• Addressed the person by name.			
• Introduced yourself by name and title.			
• Explained the procedure before starting and during the procedure.			
• Protected the person's rights during the procedure.			
• Handled the person gently during the procedure.			

Pre-Procedure

	S	U	Comments
1. Followed *Delegation Guidelines: Weight and Height*.			
2. Asked the person to void.			
3. Practiced hand hygiene.			
4. Brought the standing scale and paper towels to the person's room.			
5. Practiced hand hygiene.			
6. Identified the person. Checked the ID (identification) bracelet against the assignment sheet. Used 2 identifiers. Also called the person by name.			
7. Provided for privacy.			

Procedure

	S	U	Comments
8. Placed the paper towels on the scale platform.			
9. Raised the height rod.			
10. Moved the weights to zero (0). The pointer was in the middle.			
11. Had the person remove the robe and footwear. Assisted as needed. (Note: For some state competency tests, shoes were worn.)			
12. Helped the person stand in the center of the scale. Arms were at the sides. The person did not hold on to anyone or anything.			
13. Moved the lower and upper weights until the balance pointer was in the middle.			
14. Noted the weight on your note pad or assignment sheet.			
15. Asked the person to stand very straight.			
16. Lowered the height rod until it rested on the person's head.			
17. Read the height at the movable part of the height rod. Recorded the height in inches (or in feet and inches) to the nearest ¼ inch.			
18. Noted the height on your note pad or assignment sheet.			
19. Raised the height rod. Helped the person step off of the scale.			
20. Helped the person put on a robe and slip-resistant footwear if he or she would be up. Or helped the person back to bed.			
21. Lowered the height rod. Adjusted the weights to zero (0) if this was your agency policy.			

Post-Procedure

	S	U	Comments
22. Provided for comfort.	_____	_____	_____
23. Placed the call light and other needed items within reach.	_____	_____	_____
24. Raised or lowered bed rails. Followed the care plan.	_____	_____	_____
25. Unscreened the person.	_____	_____	_____
26. Completed a safety check of the room.	_____	_____	_____
27. Discarded the paper towels.	_____	_____	_____
28. Returned the scale to its proper place.	_____	_____	_____
29. Practiced hand hygiene.	_____	_____	_____
30. Reported and recorded the measurements.	_____	_____	_____

Measuring Height—The Person Is in Bed

Name: _____   Date: _____

Quality of Life	S	U	Comments
• Knocked before entering the person's room.	___	___	_____
• Addressed the person by name.	___	___	_____
• Introduced yourself by name and title.	___	___	_____
• Explained the procedure before starting and during the procedure.	___	___	_____
• Protected the person's rights during the procedure.	___	___	_____
• Handled the person gently during the procedure.	___	___	_____

Pre-Procedure

	S	U	Comments
1. Followed *Delegation Guidelines: Weight and Height*.	___	___	_____
2. Practiced hand hygiene.	___	___	_____
3. Asked a co-worker to help you.	___	___	_____
4. Collected a measuring tape and ruler.	___	___	_____
5. Practiced hand hygiene.	___	___	_____
6. Identified the person. Checked the ID (identification) bracelet against the assignment sheet. Used 2 identifiers. Also called the person by name.	___	___	_____
7. Provided for privacy.	___	___	_____
8. Raised the bed for body mechanics. Bed rails were up if used.	___	___	_____

Procedure

	S	U	Comments
9. Lowered the bed rails (if up).	___	___	_____
10. Positioned the person supine if the position was allowed.	___	___	_____
11. Had your co-worker place and hold the beginning of the tape measure at the person's heel.	___	___	_____
12. Pulled the other end of the tape measure along the person's body. Pulled it until it extended past the head.	___	___	_____
13. Placed the ruler flat across the top of the person's head and across the tape measure. Made sure the ruler was level.	___	___	_____
14. Read the height measurement. This was the point where the lower edge of the ruler touched the tape measure.	___	___	_____
15. Noted the height on your note pad or assignment sheet.	___	___	_____

Post-Procedure

	S	U	Comments
16. Provided for comfort.	___	___	_____
17. Placed the call light and other needed items within reach.	___	___	_____
18. Lowered the bed to a safe and comfortable level. Followed the care plan.	___	___	_____
19. Raised or lowered bed rails. Followed the care plan.	___	___	_____
20. Completed a safety check of the room.	___	___	_____
21. Returned equipment to its proper place.	___	___	_____
22. Practiced hand hygiene.	___	___	_____
23. Reported and recorded the height.	___	___	_____

Moving the Person to a New Room

Name: _____ Date: _____

Quality of Life	S	U	Comments
• Knocked before entering the person's room.	_____	_____	_____
• Addressed the person by name.	_____	_____	_____
• Introduced yourself by name and title.	_____	_____	_____
• Explained the procedure before starting and during the procedure.	_____	_____	_____
• Protected the person's rights during the procedure.	_____	_____	_____
• Handled the person gently during the procedure.	_____	_____	_____

Pre-Procedure

	S	U	Comments
1. Followed *Delegation Guidelines: Admissions, Transfers, and Discharges.* Saw *Promoting Safety and Comfort: Admissions, Transfers, and Discharges.*	_____	_____	_____
2. Asked a co-worker to help you.	_____	_____	_____
3. Practiced hand hygiene.	_____	_____	_____
4. Collected the following:			
• Wheelchair or stretcher	_____	_____	_____
• Utility cart	_____	_____	_____
• Bath blanket	_____	_____	_____
5. Practiced hand hygiene.	_____	_____	_____
6. Identified the person. Checked the ID (identification) bracelet against the assignment sheet. Used 2 identifiers. Also called the person by name.	_____	_____	_____
7. Provided for privacy.	_____	_____	_____

Procedure

	S	U	Comments
8. Placed the person's belongings and care equipment on the cart.	_____	_____	_____
9. Transferred the person to a wheelchair or a stretcher. Covered him or her with the bath blanket.	_____	_____	_____
10. Transported the person to the new room. Your co-worker brought the cart.	_____	_____	_____
11. Helped transfer the person to the bed or chair. Helped position the person.	_____	_____	_____
12. Helped arrange the person's belongings and equipment.	_____	_____	_____
13. Reported the following to the receiving nurse.			
a. How the person tolerated the transfer	_____	_____	_____
b. Any observations made during the transfer	_____	_____	_____
c. That the nurse from the previous unit will communicate with him or her	_____	_____	_____

Post-Procedure	**S**	**U**	**Comments**
14. Returned the wheelchair or stretcher and the cart to the storage area.	_____	_____	_____
15. Practiced hand hygiene.	_____	_____	_____
16. Reported and recorded the following:			
• The time of the transfer	_____	_____	_____
• Who helped you with the transfer	_____	_____	_____
• Where the person was taken	_____	_____	_____
• How the person was transferred (bed, wheelchair, or stretcher)	_____	_____	_____
• How the person tolerated the transfer	_____	_____	_____
• Who received the person	_____	_____	_____
• Any other observations	_____	_____	_____
17. Stripped the bed and cleaned the unit. Practiced hand hygiene and put on gloves for this step. (The housekeeping staff may have done this step.)	_____	_____	_____
18. Removed the gloves. Practiced hand hygiene.	_____	_____	_____
19. Followed agency policy for used linens.	_____	_____	_____
20. Made a closed bed.	_____	_____	_____
21. Practiced hand hygiene.	_____	_____	_____

Transferring or Discharging the Person

Name: _____   Date: _____

	S	U	Comments

Quality of Life
- Knocked before entering the person's room.
- Addressed the person by name.
- Introduced yourself by name and title.
- Explained the procedure before starting and during the procedure.
- Protected the person's rights during the procedure.
- Handled the person gently during the procedure.

Pre-Procedure
1. Followed *Delegation Guidelines: Admissions, Transfers, and Discharges.* Saw *Promoting Safety and Comfort: Admissions, Transfers, and Discharges.*
2. Asked a co-worker to help you.
3. Practiced hand hygiene.
4. Identified the person. Checked the ID (identification) bracelet against the assignment sheet. Used 2 identifiers. Also called the person by name.
5. Provided for privacy.

Procedure
6. Helped the person dress as needed.
7. Helped the person pack. Checked the bathroom and all drawers and closets. Made sure all items were collected.
8. Checked off the clothing list and personal belongings. Gave the lists to the nurse.
9. Told the nurse that the person was ready for the final visit. The nurse:
   a. Gave prescriptions written by the doctor.
   b. Provided discharge instructions.
   c. Returned valuables from the safe.
   d. Had the person sign the clothing and personal belongings lists.
10. *If the person left by wheelchair:*
    a. Got a wheelchair and a utility cart for the person's items. Asked a co-worker to help you.
    b. Helped the person into the wheelchair.
    c. Took the person to the exit area.
    d. Locked (braked) the wheelchair wheels.
    e. Helped the person into the vehicle.
    f. Helped put the person's items into the vehicle.
11. *If the person left by ambulance:*
    a. Raised the bed rails.
    b. Placed the call light within reach.
    c. Waited for the ambulance attendants.
    d. Raised the bed for a transfer to the stretcher when the ambulance attendants arrived.

Post-Procedure

	S	U	Comments
12. Returned the wheelchair and cart to the storage area.	___	___	_____
13. Practiced hand hygiene.	___	___	_____
14. Reported and recorded the following:			
• The time of the discharge	___	___	_____
• Who helped you with the procedure	___	___	_____
• How the person was transported	___	___	_____
• Who was with the person	___	___	_____
• The person's destination	___	___	_____
• Any other observations	___	___	_____
15. Stripped the bed and cleaned the unit. Practiced hand hygiene and put on gloves for this step. (The housekeeping staff may have done this step.)	___	___	_____
16. Removed the gloves. Practiced hand hygiene.	___	___	_____
17. Followed agency policy for used linens.	___	___	_____
18. Made a closed bed.	___	___	_____
19. Practiced hand hygiene.	___	___	_____

Preparing the Person for an Examination

Name: _____   Date: _____

Quality of Life	S	U	Comments
• Knocked before entering the person's room.	___	___	_____
• Addressed the person by name.	___	___	_____
• Introduced yourself by name and title.	___	___	_____
• Explained the procedure before starting and during the procedure.	___	___	_____
• Protected the person's rights during the procedure.	___	___	_____
• Handled the person gently during the procedure.	___	___	_____

Pre-Procedure

	S	U	Comments
1. Followed *Delegation Guidelines: Preparing the Person.* Saw *Promoting Safety and Comfort: Preparing the Person.*	___	___	_____
2. Practiced hand hygiene.	___	___	_____
3. Collected the following:			
• Exam form	___	___	_____
• Flashlight	___	___	_____
• Blood pressure equipment	___	___	_____
• Stethoscope	___	___	_____
• Thermometer	___	___	_____
• Pulse oximeter	___	___	_____
• Scale	___	___	_____
• Tongue depressors (blades)	___	___	_____
• Laryngeal mirror	___	___	_____
• Ophthalmoscope	___	___	_____
• Otoscope	___	___	_____
• Nasal speculum	___	___	_____
• Percussion (reflex) hammer	___	___	_____
• Tuning fork	___	___	_____
• Vaginal speculum (for a female)	___	___	_____
• Tape measure	___	___	_____
• Gloves	___	___	_____
• Water-soluble lubricant	___	___	_____
• Cotton-tipped applicators	___	___	_____
• Specimen containers and labels	___	___	_____
• Disposable bag	___	___	_____
• Kidney basin	___	___	_____
• Towel	___	___	_____
• Bath blanket	___	___	_____
• Tissues	___	___	_____
• Drape (sheet, bath blanket, drawsheet, or paper drape)	___	___	_____
• Paper towels	___	___	_____
• Cotton balls	___	___	_____
• Waterproof under-pad	___	___	_____
• Eye chart (Snellen chart)	___	___	_____
• Slides	___	___	_____
• Patient gown	___	___	_____
• Alcohol wipes	___	___	_____
• Wastebasket	___	___	_____
• Container for soiled instruments	___	___	_____
• Marking pencils or pens	___	___	_____
4. Practiced hand hygiene.	___	___	_____
5. Identified the person. Checked the ID (identification) bracelet against the assignment sheet. Used 2 identifiers. Also called the person by name.	___	___	_____
6. Provided for privacy.	___	___	_____

Procedure	S	U	Comments
7. Had the person put on the gown. Told him or her what clothes to remove and where to put them. Assisted as needed.	___	___	_____
8. Asked the person to void. Collected a urine specimen, if needed. Provided for privacy.	___	___	_____
9. Transported the person to the exam room. (Omitted this step when exam was in the person's room.)	___	___	_____
10. Measured weight and height. Recorded the measurements on the exam form.	___	___	_____
11. Helped the person onto the exam table. Provided a step stool if necessary. (Omitted this step for an exam in the person's room.)	___	___	_____
12. Raised the far bed rail (if used). Raised the bed to a safe and comfortable working height. (Omitted this step if an exam table was used.)	___	___	_____
13. Measured vital signs and pulse oximetry. Recorded them on the exam form.	___	___	_____
14. Positioned the person as directed.	___	___	_____
15. Draped the person.	___	___	_____
16. Placed a waterproof under-pad under the buttocks.	___	___	_____
17. Raised the bed rail near you if used.	___	___	_____
18. Provided adequate lighting.	___	___	_____
19. Put the call light on for the examiner. Did not leave the person alone.	___	___	_____

Collecting a Random Urine Specimen

Name: _____   Date: _____

Quality of Life

	S	U	Comments

- Knocked before entering the person's room.
- Addressed the person by name.
- Introduced yourself by name and title.
- Explained the procedure before starting and during the procedure.
- Protected the person's rights during the procedure.
- Handled the person gently during the procedure.

Pre-Procedure

1. Followed *Delegation Guidelines: Urine Specimens.*
   Saw *Promoting Safety and Comfort:*
   a. *Collecting and Testing Specimens*
   b. *Urine Specimens*
2. Practiced hand hygiene.
3. Collected the following before going to the person's room.
   - Laboratory requisition slip
   - Specimen container and lid
   - Voiding device (clean, unused)—bedpan and cover (optional), urinal, or specimen pan
   - Specimen label
   - Disposable bag (if needed)
   - Plastic bag
   - *BIOHAZARD* label (if needed)
   - Gloves
4. Arranged your work area.
5. Practiced hand hygiene.
6. Identified the person. Checked the ID (identification) bracelet against the requisition slip. Compared all information. Also called the person by name. Asked the person to state his or her first and last name and birthdate.
7. Labeled the container in the person's presence.
8. Put on gloves.
9. Collected a commode (if needed) and graduate to measure output.
10. Provided for privacy.

Procedure

11. Placed the specimen pan on the toilet or commode container.
12. Asked the person to urinate into the voiding device. Had the person put toilet paper in the toilet. Or provided a disposable plastic bag and followed agency policy for disposal. Toilet paper was not put in the bedpan or specimen pan.
13. Took the voiding device or commode container to the bathroom.
14. Poured about 120 mL (milliliters) (4 oz [ounces]) into the specimen container.
15. Placed the lid on the specimen container tightly. Put the container in the plastic bag. Did not let the container touch the outside of the bag. Applied a *BIOHAZARD* label.

Procedure—cont'd

	S	U	Comments
16. Measured urine if I&O was ordered. Included the specimen amount.			
17. Emptied, rinsed, cleaned, disinfected, and dried equipment. Used clean, dry paper towels for drying. Returned equipment to its proper place.			
18. Removed and discarded the gloves. Practiced hand hygiene. Put on clean gloves.			
19. Assisted with hand hygiene.			
20. Removed and discarded the gloves. Practiced hand hygiene.			

Post-Procedure

	S	U	Comments
21. Provided for comfort.			
22. Placed the call light and other needed items within reach.			
23. Raised or lowered bed rails. Followed the care plan.			
24. Unscreened the person.			
25. Completed a safety check of the room.			
26. Practiced hand hygiene.			
27. Took the specimen and the requisition slip to the laboratory or storage area. Wore gloves if that was agency policy.			
28. Removed and discarded the gloves. Practiced hand hygiene.			
29. Reported and recorded your observations.			

Collecting a Midstream Specimen

Name: _____   Date: _____

	S	U	Comments
Quality of Life			

Quality of Life
- Knocked before entering the person's room.
- Addressed the person by name.
- Introduced yourself by name and title.
- Explained the procedure before starting and during the procedure.
- Protected the person's rights during the procedure.
- Handled the person gently during the procedure.

Pre-Procedure
1. Followed *Delegation Guidelines: Urine Specimens.* Saw *Promoting Safety and Comfort:*
   a. *Collecting and Testing Specimens*
   b. *Urine Specimens*
   c. *The Midstream Specimen*
2. Practiced hand hygiene.
3. Collected the following before going to the person's room:
   - Laboratory requisition slip
   - Midstream specimen kit—specimen container, label, towelettes, sterile gloves
   - Plastic bag
   - Sterile gloves (if not part of kit and required by agency policy)
   - Disposable gloves
   - BIOHAZARD label (if needed)
4. Arranged your work area.
5. Practiced hand hygiene.
6. Identified the person. Checked the ID (identification) bracelet against the requisition slip. Compared all information. Also called the person by name. Asked the person to state his or her first and last name and birthdate.
7. Put on gloves.
8. Collected the following:
   - Voiding device—bedpan and cover (optional), urinal, commode, or specimen pan if needed
   - Supplies for perineal care
   - Graduate to measure output
   - Paper towel
9. Provided for privacy.

Procedure
10. Provided perineal care. (Wore gloves for this step. Practiced hand hygiene after removing and discarding gloves.)
11. Opened the sterile kit.
12. Put on the gloves. Applied sterile gloves if required by agency policy.
13. Opened the packet of towelettes.
14. Opened the specimen container. Did not touch the inside of the container or the lid. The inside was sterile. Sat the lid down with the inside up.

Procedure—cont'd	S	U	Comments

15. *For a female*—cleaned the perineal area with the towelettes.
     a. Spread the labia with your thumb and index finger. Used your non-dominant hand. (This hand was contaminated and did not touch anything sterile.)
     b. Cleaned down the urethral area from front to back (top to bottom). Used a clean towelette for each stroke.
     c. Kept the labia separated to collect the urine specimen.
         i. Asked the person to void into the device
         ii. Passed the specimen container into the urine stream. (Kept labia separated.)
         iii. Collected about 30 to 60 mL (1 to 2 ounces) of urine.
         iv. Removed the specimen container before the person stopped voiding. Released the labia.
16. *For a male*—cleaned the penis with towelettes.
     a. Held the penis with your non-dominant hand. (This hand was contaminated and did not touch anything sterile.)
     b. Cleaned the penis starting at the meatus. (Retracted the foreskin of the uncircumcised male.) Cleaned in a circular motion. Started at the center and worked outward.
     c. Held the penis (kept the foreskin retracted in the uncircumcised male) until the specimen was collected.
17. Asked the person to void into a device.
18. Passed the specimen container into the urine stream.
19. Collected about 30 to 60 milliliters (1 to 2 ounces) of urine.
20. Removed the specimen container before the person stopped voiding. Released the foreskin of the uncircumcised male. Released the penis.
21. Allowed the person to finish voiding into the device.
22. Put the lid on the specimen container. Touched only the outside of the container and lid. Wiped the outside of the container. Sat the container on a paper towel.
23. Provided toilet paper after the person was done voiding.
24. Took the voiding device to the bathroom.
25. Measured urine if I&O was ordered. Included the specimen amount.
26. Emptied, rinsed, cleaned, disinfected, and dried equipment. Used clean, dry paper towels for drying. Returned equipment to its proper place.
27. Removed and discarded the gloves. Practiced hand hygiene. Put on clean disposable gloves.
28. Labeled the specimen container in the person's presence. Placed the container in the plastic bag. Did not let the container touch the outside of the bag. Applied a *BIOHAZARD* label.
29. Assisted with hand hygiene.
30. Removed and discarded the gloves. Practiced hand hygiene.

Post-Procedure

31. Provided for comfort.
32. Placed the call light and other needed items within reach.
33. Raised or lowered bed rails. Followed the care plan.
34. Unscreened the person.
35. Completed a safety check of the room.
36. Practiced hand hygiene.
37. Took the specimen and the requisition slip to the laboratory or storage area. Wore gloves if that was agency policy.
38. Removed and discarded the gloves. Practiced hand hygiene.
39. Reported and recorded your observations.

Collecting a 24-Hour Urine Specimen

Name: _____ Date: _____

Quality of Life	S	U	Comments

Quality of Life
- Knocked before entering the person's room.
- Addressed the person by name.
- Introduced yourself by name and title.
- Explained the procedure before starting and during the procedure.
- Protected the person's rights during the procedure.
- Handled the person gently during the procedure.

Pre-Procedure
1. Followed *Delegation Guidelines: Urine Specimens*. Saw *Promoting Safety and Comfort*:
   a. *Collecting and Testing Specimens*
   b. *Urine Specimens*
   c. *The 24-Hour Urine Specimen*
2. Practiced hand hygiene.
3. Collected the following before going to the person's room:
   - Laboratory requisition slip
   - Urine container for a 24-hour collection
   - Voiding device (clean, un-used)-bedpan and cover (optional), urinal, or specimen pan
   - Specimen label
   - Preservative if needed
   - Bucket with ice if needed
   - Two 24-hour urine labels
   - Funnel
   - Disposable bag
   - *BIOHAZARD* label
   - Gloves
4. Arranged your work area.
5. Placed one 24-hour urine label in the bathroom. Placed the other near the bed.
6. Practiced hand hygiene.
7. Identified the person. Checked the ID (identification) bracelet against the requisition slip. Compared all information. Also called the person by name. Asked the person to state his or her first and last name and birthdate.
8. Labeled the urine container in the person's presence. Applied the *BIOHAZARD* label. Placed the labeled container in the bathroom.
9. Put on gloves.
10. Collected a commode (if needed) and a graduate to measure output
11. Provided for privacy.

Procedure
12. Asked the person to void. Provided a voiding device. The specimen pan was on the front of the toilet or commode container (if used).
13. Measured and discarded the urine. Noted the time. This started the 24-hour collection period.
14. Marked the time on the urine container.

Procedure—cont'd	S	U	Comments

15. Emptied, rinsed, cleaned, disinfected, and dried equipment. Used clean, dry paper towels for drying. Returned equipment to its proper place. _____ _____ _____

16. Removed and discarded the gloves. Practiced hand hygiene. Put on clean gloves. _____ _____ _____

17. Assisted with hand hygiene. _____ _____ _____

18. Removed and discarded the gloves. Practiced hand hygiene. _____ _____ _____

19. Marked the time the test began and the time it would end on the room and bathroom labels. _____ _____ _____

20. Reminded the person to:
   a. Use the voiding device during the next 24 hours. _____ _____ _____
   b. Not have a BM when voiding. _____ _____ _____
   c. Put toilet paper in the toilet. Or provided a disposable bag. Followed the agency policy for disposal. _____ _____ _____
   d. Put on the call light after voiding. _____ _____ _____

21. Returned to the room when the person signaled for you. Knocked before entering the room. _____ _____ _____

22. Did the following after every voiding.
   a. Practiced hand hygiene. Put on gloves. _____ _____ _____
   b. Measured urine if I&O was ordered. _____ _____ _____
   c. Used the funnel to pour urine into the container. Did not spill any urine. Told the nurse if you spilled or discarded the urine, because the test would have to be restarted. _____ _____ _____
   d. Emptied, rinsed, cleaned, disinfected, and dried equipment. Used clean, dry paper towels for drying. Returned equipment to its proper place. _____ _____ _____
   e. Removed and discarded the gloves. Practiced hand hygiene. Put on clean gloves. _____ _____ _____
   f. Assisted with hand hygiene. _____ _____ _____
   g. Removed and discarded the gloves. Practiced hand hygiene. _____ _____ _____
   h. Did the following:
     1) Provided for comfort. _____ _____ _____
     2) Placed the call light and other needed items within reach. _____ _____ _____
     3) Raised or lowered bed rails. Followed the care plan. _____ _____ _____
     4) Put on gloves. _____ _____ _____
     5) Cleaned, rinsed, dried, and returned equipment to its proper place. Used clean, dry paper towels for drying. Discarded disposable items. _____ _____ _____
     6) Removed and discarded the gloves. Practiced hand hygiene. _____ _____ _____
     7) Unscreened the person. _____ _____ _____
     8) Completed a safety check of the room. _____ _____ _____
     9) Removed and discarded the gloves. Practiced hand hygiene.
     10) Reported and recorded your observations.

Procedure—cont'd   S   U   **Comments**

23. Asked the person to void at the end of the 24-hour
    period.
    a. Practiced hand hygiene. Put on gloves.   _____ _____ _____
    b. Measured urine if I&O was ordered.   _____ _____ _____
    c. Used the funnel to pour urine into the container.
        Did not spill any urine. Told the nurse if you spilled
        or discarded the urine, because the test would have
        to be restarted.   _____ _____ _____
    d. Emptied, rinsed, cleaned, disinfected, and dried
        equipment. Used clean, dry paper towels for drying.
        Returned equipment to its proper place.   _____ _____ _____
    e. Removed and discarded the gloves. Practiced hand
        hygiene. Put on clean gloves.   _____ _____ _____
    f. Assisted with hand hygiene.   _____ _____ _____
    g. Removed and discarded the gloves. Practiced hand
        hygiene.   _____ _____ _____

Post-Procedure

24. Provided for comfort.   _____ _____ _____
25. Placed the call light and other needed items within
    reach.   _____ _____ _____
26. Raised or lowered bed rails. Followed the care plan. _____ _____ _____
27. Put on gloves.   _____ _____ _____
28. Removed the labels from the room and bathroom.   _____ _____ _____
29. Cleaned, rinsed, dried, and returned equipment to its
    proper place. Used clean, dry paper towels for drying.
    Discarded disposable items.   _____ _____ _____
30. Removed and discarded the gloves. Practiced hand
    hygiene.   _____ _____ _____
31. Unscreened the person.   _____ _____ _____
32. Completed a safety check of the room.   _____ _____ _____
33. Took the specimen (labeled urine container) and the
    requisition slip to the laboratory or storage area. Wore
    gloves if that was agency policy.   _____ _____ _____
34. Removed and discarded the gloves. Practiced hand
    hygiene.   _____ _____ _____
35. Reported and recorded your observations.   _____ _____ _____

Collecting a Urine Specimen From an Infant or Child

Name: _____   Date: _____

Quality of Life	S	U	Comments

Quality of Life
- Knocked before entering the child's room.
- Addressed the child by name.
- Introduced yourself by name and title.
- Explained the procedure to the child and parents before starting and during the procedure.
- Protected the child's rights during the procedure.
- Handled the child gently during the procedure.

Pre-Procedure
1. Followed *Delegation Guidelines: Urine Specimens*. Saw *Promoting Safety and Comfort:*
   a. *Collecting and Testing Specimens*
   b. *Urine Specimens*
2. Practiced hand hygiene.
3. Collected the following before going to the child's room.
   - Laboratory requisition slip
   - Collection bag ("wee bag")
   - *BIOHAZARD* label (if needed)
   - Specimen container
   - Plastic bag
   - Scissors
   - Wash basin
   - Bath towel
   - 2 diapers
   - Gloves
4. Arranged your work area.
5. Practiced hand hygiene.
6. Identified the child. Checked the ID (identification) bracelet against the requisition slip. Compared all information. Also called the child by name. Asked the parent to state the child's first and last name and birthdate.
7. Provided for privacy.

Procedure
8. Practiced hand hygiene. Put on gloves.
9. Positioned the child on his or her back.
10. Removed and set aside the diaper.
11. Cleaned the perineal area with cotton balls. Used a new cotton ball for each stroke. Rinsed and dried the area.
12. Removed and discarded the gloves. Practiced hand hygiene.
13. Put on clean gloves.
14. Flexed the child's knees. Spread the legs.
15. Removed the adhesive backing from the collection bag.
16. Applied the bag to the perineum.
17. Cut a slit in the bottom of a new diaper.
18. Diapered the child.
19. Pulled the collection bag through the slit in the diaper.
20. Removed and discarded the gloves. Practiced hand hygiene.
21. Raised the head of the crib if allowed. This helped urine collect in the bottom of the bag.
22. Checked for crib safety. Medical crib rails were raised and locked before leaving the bedside.

Procedure—cont'd	**S**	**U**	**Comments**
23. Unscreened the child.	_____	_____	_____
24. Disposed of the removed diaper. Followed agency policy. Wore gloves for this step.	_____	_____	_____
25. Practiced hand hygiene.	_____	_____	_____
26. Checked the child often.			
a. Checked the bag for urine.	_____	_____	_____
b. Provided for privacy.	_____	_____	_____
c. Wore gloves.	_____	_____	_____
27. Did the following if the child voided.			
a. Provided for privacy.	_____	_____	_____
b. Practiced hand hygiene. Put on clean gloves.	_____	_____	_____
c. Removed the diaper.	_____	_____	_____
d. Removed the collection bag gently.	_____	_____	_____
e. Pressed the adhesive surfaces of the bag together. Made sure the seal was tight and there were no leaks. Or transferred the urine to the specimen container using the drainage tab.	_____	_____	_____
f. Cleaned the perineal area. Rinsed and dried well.	_____	_____	_____
g. Diapered the child.	_____	_____	_____
h. Removed and discarded the gloves. Practiced hand hygiene.	_____	_____	_____
28. Put on clean gloves.	_____	_____	_____
29. Labeled the collection bag or specimen container in the child's presence. Then placed it in the plastic bag. Applied the BIOHAZARD label (if needed).	_____	_____	_____

Post-Procedure

	S	**U**	**Comments**
30. Provided for comfort.	_____	_____	_____
31. Checked for crib safety. Medical crib rails were raised and locked before leaving the bedside.	_____	_____	_____
32. Made sure the call light and other needed items were within reach for the parent.	_____	_____	_____
33. Unscreened the child.	_____	_____	_____
34. Cleaned, rinsed, dried, and returned equipment to its proper place. Used clean, dry paper towels for drying. Discarded disposable items. Wore gloves for this step.	_____	_____	_____
35. Completed a safety check of the room.	_____	_____	_____
36. Removed and discarded the gloves. Practiced hand hygiene.	_____	_____	_____
37. Took the specimen and requisition slip to the laboratory or storage area. Wore gloves if that was agency policy.	_____	_____	_____
38. Removed and discarded the gloves. Practiced hand hygiene.	_____	_____	_____
39. Reported and recorded your observations.	_____	_____	_____

Testing Urine With Reagent Strips

Name: _____   Date: _____

Quality of Life	S	U	Comments
• Knocked before entering the person's room.	___	___	_____
• Addressed the person by name.	___	___	_____
• Introduced yourself by name and title.	___	___	_____
• Explained the procedure before starting and during the procedure.	___	___	_____
• Protected the person's rights during the procedure.	___	___	_____
• Handled the person gently during the procedure.	___	___	_____

Pre-Procedure

1. Followed *Delegation Guidelines: Using Reagent Strips.* Saw *Promoting Safety and Comfort:*
    a. *Collecting and Testing Specimens*   ___ ___ _____
    b. *Using Reagent Strips*   ___ ___ _____
2. Practiced hand hygiene.   ___ ___ _____
3. Collected gloves and the reagent (test) strips ordered.   ___ ___ _____
4. Practiced hand hygiene.   ___ ___ _____
5. Identified the person. Checked the ID (identification) bracelet against the assignment sheet. Used 2 identifiers. Also called the person by name. Asked the person to state his or her first and last name and state his or her birthdate.   ___ ___ _____
6. Put on gloves.   ___ ___ _____
7. Collected equipment for the urine specimen.   ___ ___ _____
8. Provided for privacy.   ___ ___ _____

Procedure

9. Collected the urine specimen.   ___ ___ _____
10. Removed the strip from the bottle. Put the cap tightly on the bottle at once.   ___ ___ _____
11. Dip the test strip areas into the urine.   ___ ___ _____
12. Removed the strip after the correct amount of time. Saw the manufacturer's instructions.   ___ ___ _____
13. Tapped the strip gently against the container. This removed excess urine.   ___ ___ _____
14. Waited the required amount of time. Saw the manufacturer's instructions.   ___ ___ _____
15. Compared the strip with the color chart on the bottle. Read the results.   ___ ___ _____
16. Discarded disposable items and the specimen.   ___ ___ _____
17. Emptied, rinsed, cleaned, disinfected, and dried equipment. Used clean, dry paper towels for drying. Returned equipment to its proper place.   ___ ___ _____
18. Removed and discarded the gloves. Practiced hand hygiene.   ___ ___ _____

Post-Procedure

19. Provided for comfort.   ___ ___ _____
20. Placed the call light and other needed items within reach.   ___ ___ _____
21. Raised or lowered bed rails. Followed the care plan.   ___ ___ _____
22. Unscreened the person.   ___ ___ _____
23. Completed a safety check of the room.   ___ ___ _____
24. Practiced hand hygiene.   ___ ___ _____
25. Reported and recorded the results and any other observations.   ___ ___ _____

Straining Urine

Name: _____   Date: _____

Quality of Life	S	U	Comments

Quality of Life
- Knocked before entering the person's room.
- Addressed the person by name.
- Introduced yourself by name and title.
- Explained the procedure before starting and during the procedure.
- Protected the person's rights during the procedure.
- Handled the person gently during the procedure.

Pre-Procedure
1. Followed *Delegation Guidelines: Urine Specimens.* Saw *Promoting Safety and Comfort:*
   a. *Collecting and Testing Specimens*
   b. *Urine Specimens*
2. Practiced hand hygiene.
3. Collected the following before going to the person's room.
   - Laboratory requisition slip
   - Urine strainer
   - Specimen container
   - Specimen label
   - Voiding device (clean, un-used) -bedpan and cover (optional), urinal or specimen pan
   -
   - 2 STRAIN ALL URINE labels
   - Plastic bag
   - *BIOHAZARD* label (if needed)
   - Gloves
4. Arranged your work area.
5. Placed 1 STRAIN ALL URINE label in the bathroom. Placed the other near the bed.
6. Practiced hand hygiene.
7. Identified the person. Checked the ID (identification) bracelet against the requisition slip. Compared all information. Also called the person by name. Asked the person to state his or her first and last name and birthdate.
8. Labeled the specimen container in the person's presence.
9. Put on gloves.
10. Collected a commode (if needed) and a graduate to measure output.
11. Provided for privacy.

Procedure
12. Asked the person to use the voiding device for urinating. The specimen pan was on the front of the toilet or commode container (if used). Asked the person to put on the call light after voiding.
13. Removed and discarded the gloves. Practiced hand hygiene.
14. Returned to the room when the person signaled for you. Knocked before entering the room.
15. Practiced hand hygiene. Put on clean gloves.
16. Placed the strainer in the graduate.
17. Poured urine into the graduate. Urine passed through the strainer.

Procedure—cont'd	S	U	Comments

18. Placed the strainer in the specimen container if any crystals, stones, or particles appeared. Or transferred them to the specimen container as the nurse directed.   _____ _____ _____
19. Placed the specimen container in the plastic bag. Did not let the container touch the outside of the bag. Applied a *BIOHAZARD* label.   _____ _____ _____
20. Measured urine if I&O was ordered.   _____ _____ _____
21. Emptied, rinsed, cleaned, disinfected, and dried equipment. Used clean, dry paper towels for drying. Returned equipment to its proper place.   _____ _____ _____
22. Removed and discarded the gloves. Practiced hand hygiene. Put on clean gloves.   _____ _____ _____
23. Assisted with hand hygiene.   _____ _____ _____
24. Removed and discarded the gloves. Practiced hand hygiene.   _____ _____ _____

Post-Procedure

25. Provided for comfort.   _____ _____ _____
26. Placed the call light and other needed items within reach.   _____ _____ _____
27. Raised or lowered bed rails. Followed the care plan.   _____ _____ _____
28. Unscreened the person.   _____ _____ _____
29. Completed a safety check of the room.   _____ _____ _____
30. Practiced hand hygiene.   _____ _____ _____
31. Took the specimen container and requisition slip to the laboratory or storage area. Wore gloves if agency policy.   _____ _____ _____
32. Removed and discarded the gloves. Practiced hand hygiene.   _____ _____ _____
33. Reported and recorded your observations.   _____ _____ _____

Collecting and Testing a Stool Specimen

Name: _____   Date: _____

Quality of Life	S	U	Comments
• Knocked before entering the person's room.	____	____	_____
• Addressed the person by name.	____	____	_____
• Introduced yourself by name and title.	____	____	_____
• Explained the procedure before starting and during the procedure.	____	____	_____
• Protected the person's rights during the procedure.	____	____	_____
• Handled the person gently during the procedure.	____	____	_____

Pre-Procedure

1. Followed *Delegation Guidelines: Stool Specimens.* Saw *Promoting Safety and Comfort:*
   a. *Collecting and Testing Specimens*   ____ ____ _____
   b. *Stool Specimens*   ____ ____ _____
2. Practiced hand hygiene.   ____ ____ _____
3. Collected the following before going to the person's room:
   • Laboratory requisition slip   ____ ____ _____
   • Occult blood test kit (if needed)   ____ ____ _____
   • Device to collect the BM (clean, un-used) -bedpan and cover (optional) or specimen pan   ____ ____ _____
   • Specimen container and lid   ____ ____ _____
   • Specimen label   ____ ____ _____
   • Tongue blade (if needed)   ____ ____ _____
   • Disposable bag   ____ ____ _____
   • Plastic bag   ____ ____ _____
   • BIOHAZARD label (if needed)   ____ ____ _____
   • Gloves   ____ ____ _____
4. Arranged your work area.   ____ ____ _____
5. Practiced hand hygiene.   ____ ____ _____
6. Identified the person. Checked the ID bracelet against the requisition slip. Compared all information. Also called the person by name. Asked the person to state his or her first and last name and birthdate.   ____ ____ _____
7. Labeled the specimen container in the person's presence.   ____ ____ _____
8. Put on gloves.   ____ ____ _____
9. Collected the following:
   • Device for voiding—bedpan and cover (optional), urinal, commode, or specimen pan   ____ ____ _____
   • Toilet paper   ____ ____ _____
10. Provided for privacy.   ____ ____ _____

Procedure

11. Asked the person to void. Provided the voiding device if the person did not use the bathroom. Emptied, rinsed, cleaned, disinfected, and dried the device. Used clean, dry paper towels for drying. Returned it to its proper place.   ____ ____ _____
12. Put the specimen pan on the back of the toilet or commode. Or provided a bedpan.   ____ ____ _____
13. Asked the person not to put toilet paper into the bedpan, commode, or specimen pan. Had the person put the toilet paper in the toilet. Or provided a disposable bag and followed agency policy for disposal.   ____ ____ _____

Procedure—cont'd   S   U   Comments

14. Placed the call light and toilet paper within reach. Raised or lowered bed rails. Followed the care plan. _____ _____ _____

15. Removed and discarded the gloves. Practiced hand hygiene. Left the room if the person could be left alone. _____ _____ _____

16. Returned when the person signaled. Or checked on the person every 5 minutes. Knocked before entering. _____ _____ _____

17. Practiced hand hygiene. Put on clean gloves. _____ _____ _____

18. Lowered the bed rail near you if up. Removed the bedpan (if used). Or assisted the person off the toilet or commode (if used). Provided perineal care if needed. _____ _____ _____

19. Noted the color, amount, consistency, and odor of stools. _____ _____ _____

20. Collected the specimen.
    a. Used the spoon attached to the lid to pick up several spoonfuls of stool. Or used a tongue blade to take about 2 tablespoons of stool to the specimen container. Took the sample from:
       1) The middle of a formed stool _____ _____ _____
       2) Areas of pus, mucus, or blood and watery areas _____ _____ _____
       3) The middle and both ends of a hard stool _____ _____ _____
    b. Put the lid on the specimen container tightly. _____ _____ _____
    c. Placed the container in the plastic bag. Did not let the container touch the outside of the bag. Applied a BIOHAZARD label according to agency policy. _____ _____ _____
    d. Wrapped the tongue blade in toilet paper. Discarded it into the disposable bag. _____ _____ _____

21. Removed and discarded the gloves. Practiced hand hygiene. Put on clean gloves. _____ _____ _____

22. Tested the specimen (if needed).
    a. Opened the test kit. _____ _____ _____
    b. Used a tongue blade to obtain a small amount of stool. _____ _____ _____
    c. Applied a thin smear of stool on *box A* on the test paper. _____ _____ _____
    d. Used another tongue blade to obtain stool from another part of the specimen. _____ _____ _____
    e. Applied a thin smear of stool on *box B* on the test paper. _____ _____ _____
    f. Closed the packet. _____ _____ _____
    g. Turned the test packet to the other side. Opened the flap. Applied developer (from the kit) to *boxes A* and *B*. Followed the manufacturer's instructions. _____ _____ _____
    h. Waited 10 to 60 seconds as required by the manufacturer. _____ _____ _____
    i. Noted the color changes on your assignment sheet. _____ _____ _____
    j. Disposed of the test packet. _____ _____ _____
    k. Wrapped the tongue blades with toilet paper. Then discarded them. _____ _____ _____

23. Emptied, rinsed, cleaned, disinfected, and dried equipment. Used clean, dry paper towels for drying. Returned equipment to its proper place. _____ _____ _____

24. Removed and discarded the gloves. Practiced hand hygiene. Put on clean gloves. _____ _____ _____

25. Assisted with hand hygiene. _____ _____ _____

26. Removed and discarded the gloves. Practiced hand hygiene. _____ _____ _____

Post-Procedure   **S**   **U**   **Comments**
27. Provided for comfort.
28. Placed the call light and other needed items within reach.   _____   _____   _____
29. Raised or lowered bed rails. Followed the care plan.   _____   _____   _____
30. Unscreened the person.   _____   _____   _____
31. Completed a safety check of the room.   _____   _____   _____
32. Delivered the specimen and requisition slip to the
    laboratory or storage area. Followed agency policy.
    Wore gloves if that was the agency policy.   _____   _____   _____
33. Removed and discarded the gloves. Practiced hand
    hygiene.   _____   _____   _____
34. Reported and recorded your observations and the test
    results.   _____   _____   _____

Collecting a Sputum Specimen

Name: _____   Date: _____

Quality of Life	S	U	Comments
• Knocked before entering the person's room.	_____	_____	_____
• Addressed the person by name.	_____	_____	_____
• Introduced yourself by name and title.	_____	_____	_____
• Explained the procedure before starting and during the procedure.	_____	_____	_____
• Protected the person's rights during the procedure.	_____	_____	_____
• Handled the person gently during the procedure.	_____	_____	_____

Pre-Procedure

1. Followed *Delegation Guidelines: Sputum Specimens.* Saw *Promoting Safety and Comfort:*
   a. *Collecting and Testing Specimens* _____ _____ _____
   b. *Sputum Specimens* _____ _____ _____
2. Practiced hand hygiene. _____ _____ _____
3. Collected the following before going to the person's room:
   - Laboratory requisition slip _____ _____ _____
   - Sputum specimen container and lid _____ _____ _____
   - Specimen label _____ _____ _____
   - Plastic bag _____ _____ _____
   - *BIOHAZARD* label (if needed) _____ _____ _____
4. Arranged your work area. _____ _____ _____
5. Practiced hand hygiene. _____ _____ _____
6. Identified the person. Checked the ID (identification) bracelet against the assignment sheet. Compared all information. Also called the person by name. Asked the person to state his or her first and last name and birthdate.
7. Labeled the specimen container in the person's presence. _____ _____ _____
8. Collected gloves and tissues. _____ _____ _____
9. Provided for privacy. If able, the person used the bathroom for this procedure. _____ _____ _____

Procedure

10. Put on gloves. _____ _____ _____
11. Asked the person to rinse the mouth out with clear water. _____ _____ _____
12. Had the person hold the container. Only the outside was touched. _____ _____ _____
13. Asked the person to cover the mouth and nose with tissues when coughing. Followed center policy for used tissues. _____ _____ _____
14. Asked the person to take 2 or 3 deep breaths and cough up sputum. _____ _____ _____
15. Had the person expectorate directly into the container. Sputum did not touch the outside of the container. _____ _____ _____
16. Collected 1 to 2 tablespoons of sputum unless told to collect more. _____ _____ _____
17. Put the lid on the container. _____ _____ _____
18. Placed the container in the plastic bag. Did not let the container touch the outside of the bag. Applied a *BIOHAZARD* label according to center policy. _____ _____ _____
19. Removed and discarded the gloves. Practiced hand hygiene. Put on clean gloves. _____ _____ _____

Procedure—cont'd

	S	U	Comments
20. Assisted with hand hygiene.	____	____	_____
21. Removed and discarded the gloves. Practiced hand hygiene.	____	____	_____

Post-Procedure

	S	U	Comments
22. Provided for comfort.	____	____	_____
23. Placed the call light and other needed items within reach.	____	____	_____
24. Raised or lowered bed rails. Followed the care plan.	____	____	_____
25. Unscreened the person.	____	____	_____
26. Completed a safety check of the room.	____	____	_____
27. Practiced hand hygiene.	____	____	_____
28. Delivered the specimen and requisition slip to the laboratory or storage area. Followed center policy. Wore gloves if that was agency policy.	____	____	_____
29. Removed and discarded the gloves. Practiced hand hygiene.	____	____	_____
30. Reported and recorded your observations.	____	____	_____

Measuring Blood Glucose

Name: _____   Date: _____

Quality of Life	S	U	Comments

Quality of Life
- Knocked before entering the person's room.
- Addressed the person by name.
- Introduced yourself by name and title.
- Explained the procedure before starting and during the procedure.
- Protected the person's rights during the procedure.
- Handled the person gently during the procedure.

Pre-Procedure
1. Followed *Delegation Guidelines: Blood Glucose Testing*. Saw *Promoting Safety and Comfort*:
   a. *Collecting and Testing Specimens*
   b. *Blood Glucose Testing*
2. Practiced hand hygiene.
3. Collected the following:
   - Sterile lancet
   - Lancing device (if used)
   - Antiseptic wipes
   - Gloves
   - 2 × 2 gauze squares
   - Glucometer
   - Reagent (test) strips (Used correct ones for the glucometer. Checked expiration date.)
   - Disinfectant
   - Paper towels
   - Warm washcloth
4. Read the manufacturer's instructions for the lancet and glucometer.
5. Disinfected the glucometer. Followed the manufacturer's instructions for the disinfectant.
6. Arranged your work area.
7. Identified the person. Checked the ID (identification) bracelet against the assignment sheet. Used 2 identifiers. Also called the person by name. Asked the person to state his or her first and last name and birthdate.
8. Provided for privacy.
9. Raised the bed for body mechanics. The far bed rail was up if used.

Procedure
10. Helped the person to a comfortable position.
11. Put on gloves.
12. Prepared the supplies.
    a. Opened the antiseptic wipes.
    b. Prepared the lancet. If a lancing device was used, followed the manufacturer's instructions.
    c. Turned on the glucometer.
    d. Followed the prompts. You may have needed to enter a user-ID and the person's ID number. Scanned the bar code on the bottle of test strips if needed. Or compared the code on the bottle of regent strips to the code on the glucometer.
    e. Removed a test strip from the bottle. Closed the cap tightly.
    f. Inserted a test strip into the glucometer.

Procedure—cont'd   S   U   Comments

13. Performed a skin puncture to obtain a drop of blood.
    a. Inspected the person's finger. Selected a puncture site. _____ _____ _____
    b. Did the following to increase blood flow to the puncture side.
       1) Warmed the finger. Rubbed it gently or applied a warm washcloth. _____ _____ _____
       2) Massaged the hand and finger toward the puncture site. _____ _____ _____
       3) Lowered the finger below the person's waist. _____ _____ _____
    c. Held the finger with thumb and index finger. Used your non-dominant hand. Held the finger. _____ _____ _____
    d. Cleaned the site with antiseptic wipe. *Did not touch the site after cleaning.* _____ _____ _____
    e. Allowed the site to dry. _____ _____ _____
    f. Placed the lancet or lancing device against the puncture site. _____ _____ _____
    g. Pushed the button on the lancet to puncture the skin. (Followed the manufacturer's instructions.) _____ _____ _____
    h. Applied gentle pressure below the puncture site. _____ _____ _____
    i. Allowed a large drop of blood to form. _____ _____ _____
14. Collected and tested the specimen. Followed the manufacturer's instructions and agency policy for the glucometer used.
    a. Held the test strip to the drop of blood. The glucometer tested the sample when enough blood was applied. _____ _____ _____
    b. Applied pressure to the puncture site until the bleeding stopped. Used a gauze square. If able, allowed the person to apply pressure to the site. _____ _____ _____
    c. Read the results on the display. Noted the results on your note pad or assignment sheet. Told the person the results. _____ _____ _____
    d. Turned off the glucometer. _____ _____ _____
15. Discarded the lancet into the sharps container. _____ _____ _____
16. Discarded the gauze square and test strip. Followed agency policy. _____ _____ _____
17. Removed and discarded gloves. Practiced hand hygiene. _____ _____ _____

Post-Procedure
18. Provided for comfort. _____ _____ _____
19. Placed the call light and other needed items within reach. _____ _____ _____
20. Lowered the bed to a safe and comfortable level. Followed the care plan. _____ _____ _____
21. Raised or lowered bed rails. Followed the care plan. _____ _____ _____
22. Unscreened the person. _____ _____ _____
23. Discarded used supplies. _____ _____ _____
24. Completed a safety check of the room. _____ _____ _____
25. Followed agency policy for used linens. _____ _____ _____
26. Disinfected the glucometer. Followed the manufacturer's instructions. (Wore gloves. Practiced hand hygiene after removing and discarding the gloves.) _____ _____ _____
27. Returned the glucometer to its proper place. _____ _____ _____
28. Reported and recorded the test results and your observations. _____ _____ _____

Applying Elastic Stockings

Name: _____   Date: _____

Quality of Life	S	U	Comments

Quality of Life
- Knocked before entering the person's room.
- Addressed the person by name.
- Introduced yourself by name and title.
- Explained the procedure before starting and during the procedure.
- Protected the person's rights during the procedure.
- Handled the person gently during the procedure.

Pre-Procedure
1. Followed *Delegation Guidelines: Elastic Stockings.* Saw *Promoting Safety and Comfort: Elastic Stockings.*
2. Practiced hand hygiene.
3. Obtained elastic stockings in the correct size and length. Noted the location of the toe opening.
4. Identified the person. Checked the ID (identification) bracelet against the assignment sheet. Used 2 identifiers. Also called the person by name.
5. Provided for privacy.
6. Raised the bed for body mechanics. Bed rails were up if used.

Procedure
7. Lowered the bed rail near you.
8. Positioned the person supine.
9. Exposed 1 leg. Fan-folded top linens toward the other leg.
10. Gathered or turned the stocking inside out down to the heel.
11. Slipped the foot of the stocking over the toes, foot, and heel. Properly positioned the heel pocket on the heel. The toe opening was over or under the toes. Followed the manufacturer's instructions.
12. Grasped the stocking top. Rolled or pulled the stocking up the leg. It turned right side out as it was rolled or pulled up.
13. Adjusted the stocking as needed. Made sure the stocking did not cause pressure on the toes.
14. Removed twists, creases, or wrinkles. Made sure the stocking was even, snug, smooth, and wrinkle-free.

Procedure—cont'd

	S	U	Comments
15. Covered the leg. Repeated for the other leg.			
a. Exposed the other leg. Fan-folded top linens toward the covered leg.	___	___	_____
b. Gathered or turned the stocking inside out down to the heel.	___	___	_____
c. Slipped the foot of the stocking over the toes, foot, and heel. Properly positioned the heel pocket on the heel. The toe opening was over or under the toes. Followed the manufacturer's instructions.	___	___	_____
d. Grasped the stocking top. Rolled or pulled the stocking up the leg. It turned right side out as it rolled or pulled up.	___	___	_____
e. Adjusted the stocking as needed. Made sure the stocking did not cause pressure on the toes.	___	___	_____
f. Removed twists, creases, or wrinkles. Made sure the stocking was even, snug, smooth, and wrinkle-free.	___	___	_____
16. Covered the person.	___	___	_____

Post-Procedure

	S	U	Comments
17. Provided for comfort.	___	___	_____
18. Placed the call light and other needed items within reach.	___	___	_____
19. Lowered the bed to a safe and comfortable level. Followed the care plan.	___	___	_____
20. Raised or lowered bed rails. Followed the care plan.	___	___	_____
21. Unscreened the person.	___	___	_____
22. Completed a safety check of the room.	___	___	_____
23. Practiced hand hygiene.	___	___	_____
24. Reported and recorded your observations.	___	___	_____

Applying an Elastic Bandage

Name: _____   Date: _____

Quality of Life	S	U	Comments

Quality of Life
- Knocked before entering the person's room.
- Addressed the person by name.
- Introduced yourself by name and title.
- Explained the procedure before starting and during the procedure.
- Protected the person's rights during the procedure.
- Handled the person gently during the procedure.

Pre-Procedure
1. Followed *Delegation Guidelines: Elastic Bandages*. Saw *Promoting Safety and Comfort: Elastic Bandages*.
2. Practiced hand hygiene.
3. Collected an elastic bandage with closures as directed by the nurse
4. Identified the person. Checked the ID bracelet against the assignment sheet. Used 2 identifiers. Also called the person by name.
5. Provided for privacy.
6. Raised the bed for body mechanics. Bed rails were up if used.

Procedure
7. Lowered the bed rail near you if up.
8. Helped the person to a comfortable position in good alignment. Exposed the part to bandage.
9. Made sure the area was clean and dry.
10. Held the bandage with the roll up. The loose end was on the bottom.
11. Applied the bandage to the lower (distal) and smallest part of the wrist, foot, ankle, or knee.
12. Made 2 circular turns around the part.
13. Made over-lapping spiral turns in an upward (proximal) direction. Each turn over-lapped ½ to ¾ of the previous turn. Each over-lap was equal.
14. Applied the bandage smoothly with firm, even pressure. It was not tight.
15. Ended the bandage with 2 circular turns.
16. Secured the bandage in place with the manufacturer's closure. Clips were not under any body part.
17. Checked the fingers or toes for coldness or cyanosis (bluish color). Asked about pain, itching, numbness, or tingling. Removed the bandage if any were noted. Reported your observations.

Post-Procedure
18. Provided for comfort.
19. Placed the call light and other needed items within reach.
20. Lowered the bed to a safe and comfortable level. Followed the care plan.
21. Raised or lowered bed rails. Followed the care plan.
22. Unscreened the person.
23. Completed a safety check of the room.
24. Practiced hand hygiene.
25. Reported and recorded your observations.

Applying a Dry, Non-Sterile Dressing

Name: _____   Date: _____

Quality of Life	S	U	Comments

Quality of Life
- Knocked before entering the person's room.
- Addressed the person by name.
- Introduced yourself by name and title.
- Explained the procedure before starting and during the procedure.
- Protected the person's rights during the procedure.
- Handled the person gently during the procedure.

Pre-Procedure
1. Followed *Delegation Guidelines: Applying Dressings*. Saw *Promoting Safety and Comfort*:
   a. *Wound Care*
   b. *Applying Dressings*
2. Practiced hand hygiene.
3. Collected the following:
   - Gloves
   - PPE (personal protective equipment) as needed
   - Tape or Montgomery ties
   - Dressings as directed by the nurse
   - 4 × 4 gauze
   - Saline solution as directed by the nurse
   - Cleansing solution as directed by the nurse
   - Adhesive remover
   - Dressing set with scissors and forceps
   - Plastic bag
   - Bath blanket
4. Practiced hand hygiene.
5. Identified the person. Checked the ID (identification) bracelet against the assignment sheet. Used 2 identifiers. Also called the person by name.
6. Provided for privacy.
7. Arranged your work area. You did not have to reach over or turn your back on your work area.
8. Raised the bed for body mechanics. Bed rails were up if used.

Procedure
9. Lowered the bed rail near you if up.
10. Helped the person to a comfortable position.
11. Covered the person with a bath blanket. Fan-folded top linens to the foot of the bed.
12. Exposed the affected body part.
13. Made a cuff on the plastic bag. Placed the bag within reach.
14. Practiced hand hygiene.
15. Put on needed PPE. Put on gloves.
16. Removed tape or undid Montgomery ties.
    a. *Tape:* held the skin down. Gently pulled the tape toward the wound.
    b. *Montgomery straps:* undid the straps. Folded the straps away from the wound.
17. Removed any adhesive from the skin. Picked up a gauze square with forceps. Wet a 4 × 4 gauze dressing with adhesive remover. Cleaned away from the wound.

Procedure—cont'd	S	U	Comments

18. Removed dressings with a gloved hand or forceps. Started with the top dressing and removed each layer. Kept the soiled side from the person's sight. Put dressings in the plastic bag. They did not touch the outside of the bag. _____ _____ _____
19. Removed the dressing over the wound very gently. Moistened the dressing with saline if it stuck to the wound. Discarded the dressing by putting it in the plastic bag. It did not touch the outside of the bag. _____ _____ _____
20. Observed the wound, drain site, and wound drainage. _____ _____ _____
21. Removed the gloves and put them in a plastic bag. Practiced hand hygiene. _____ _____ _____
22. Opened the new dressings. _____ _____ _____
23. Put on clean gloves. _____ _____ _____
24. Cleaned the wound with saline as directed by the nurse. _____ _____ _____
25. Applied dressings as directed by the nurse. _____ _____ _____
26. Secured the dressings. Used tape or Montgomery straps. _____ _____ _____
27. Removed the gloves. Put them in the bag. _____ _____ _____
28. Removed and discarded PPE. _____ _____ _____
29. Practiced hand hygiene. _____ _____ _____
30. Covered the person. Removed the bath blanket. _____ _____ _____

Post-Procedure

31. Provided for comfort. _____ _____ _____
32. Placed the call light and other needed items within reach. _____ _____ _____
33. Lowered the bed to a safe and comfortable level. Followed the care plan. _____ _____ _____
34. Raised or lowered bed rails. Followed the care plan. _____ _____ _____
35. Returned equipment and supplies to the proper place. Left extra dressings and tape in the room. _____ _____ _____
36. Discarded used supplies in the bag. Tied the bag closed. Discarded the bag following agency policy. Wore gloves for this step. _____ _____ _____
37. Cleaned your work area. Followed the Bloodborne Pathogen Standard. _____ _____ _____
38. Unscreened the person. _____ _____ _____
39. Completed a safety check of the room. _____ _____ _____
40. Removed and discarded the gloves. Practiced hand hygiene. _____ _____ _____
41. Reported and recorded your observations. _____ _____ _____

Applying Heat and Cold Applications

Name: _____   Date: _____

Quality of Life	S	U	Comments

- Knocked before entering the person's room.
- Addressed the person by name.
- Introduced yourself by name and title.
- Explained the procedure before starting and during the procedure.
- Protected the person's rights during the procedure.
- Handled the person gently during the procedure.

Pre-Procedure

1. Followed *Delegation Guidelines: Hot and Cold Applications; Applying Heat and Cold.* Saw *Promoting Safety and Comfort: Applying Heat and Cold.*
2. Practiced hand hygiene.
3. Collected the following:
   a. *For a hot compress:*
      - Basin
      - Water thermometer
      - Small towel, washcloth, or gauze squares
      - Plastic wrap or aquathermia pad
      - Ties, tape, or rolled gauze
      - Bath towel
      - Waterproof under-pad
   b. *For a hot soak:*
      - Water basin or arm or foot bath
      - Water thermometer
      - Waterproof under-pad
      - Bath blanket
      - Towel
   c. *For a sitz bath:*
      - Disposable sitz bath
      - Water thermometer
      - 2 bath blankets, bath towels, and a clean gown
   d. *For an aquathermia pad:*
      - Aquathermia pad and heating unit
      - Distilled water
      - Flannel cover or other cover as directed
      - Ties, tape, or rolled gauze
   e. *For a hot or cold pack:*
      - Commercial pack
      - Pack cover
      - Ties, tape, or rolled gauze (if needed)
      - Waterproof under-pad
   f. *For an ice bag, ice collar, ice glove,:*
      - Ice bag, collar, glove, or cold pack
      - Crushed ice (except for cold pack)
      - Flannel cover or other cover as directed
      - Paper towels
   g. *For a cold compress:*
      - Large basin with ice
      - Small basin with cold water
      - Gauze squares, washcloths, or small towels
      - Waterproof under-pad
4. Identified the person. Checked the ID (identification) bracelet against the assignment sheet. Used 2 identifiers. Also called the person by name.

Procedure	S	U	Comments
5. Provided for privacy.	___	___	_____
6. Positioned the person for the procedure.	___	___	_____
7. Placed the waterproof under-pad (if needed) under the body part.	___	___	_____
8. *For a hot compress:*			
a. Filled the basin ½ to 2⁄3 (one-half to two-thirds) full with hot water as directed. Measured water temperature.	___	___	_____
b. Placed the compress in the water.	___	___	_____
c. Applied the compress over the area. Noted the time.	___	___	_____
d. Covered the compress as directed. Did 1 of the following:			
1) Applied plastic wrap and then a bath towel. Secured the towel in place with ties, tape, or rolled gauze.	___	___	_____
2) Applied an aquathermia pad.	___	___	_____
9. *For a hot soak:*			
a. Filled a container ½ (one-half) full with hot water. Measured water temperature.	___	___	_____
B. Placed the part into the water. Padded the edge of the container with a towel. Noted the time.	___	___	_____
c. Covered the person with a bath blanket for warmth.	___	___	_____
10. *For a sitz bath:*			
a. Placed the sitz bath on the toilet seat.	___	___	_____
b. Filled the sitz bath 2⁄3 (two-thirds) full with water. Measured water temperature.	___	___	_____
c. Secured the gown above the waist.	___	___	_____
d. Helped the person sit on the sitz bath. Noted the time.	___	___	_____
e. Provided for warmth. Placed a bath blanket around the shoulders. Placed another over the legs.	___	___	_____
f. Stayed with the person if he or she was weak or unsteady.	___	___	_____
11. *For an aquathermia pad:*			
a. Filled the heating unit to the fill line with distilled water.	___	___	_____
b. Removed the bubbles. Placed the pad and tubing below the heating unit. Tilted the heating unit from side to side.	___	___	_____
c. Set the temperature as the nurse directed (usually 105°F [40.5°C]). Removed the key.	___	___	_____
d. Placed the pad in the cover.	___	___	_____
e. Set the heating unit on the bedside stand. Kept the pad and connecting hoses level with the unit.	___	___	_____
f. Plugged in the unit. Allowed water to warm to the desired temperature.	___	___	_____
g. Applied the pad to the part. Noted the time.	___	___	_____
h. Secured the pad in place with ties, tape, or rolled gauze.	___	___	_____
12. *For a hot or cold pack:*			
a. Squeezed, kneaded, or struck the pack as directed by the manufacturer.	___	___	_____
b. Placed the pack in the cover.	___	___	_____
c. Applied the pack. Noted the time.	___	___	_____
d. Secured the pack in place with ties, tape, or rolled gauze. Some packs are secured with Velcro straps.	___	___	_____

Procedure—cont'd	S	U	Comments

13. *For an ice bag, collar, or glove:*
 a. Filled the device with water. Put in the stopper. Turned the device upside down to check for leaks. _____ _____ _____
 b. Emptied the device. _____ _____ _____
 c. Filled the device ½ to 2/3 (one-half to two-thirds) full with crushed ice or ice chips. _____ _____ _____
 d. Removed excess air. Bent, twisted, or squeezed the device. Or pressed it against a firm surface. _____ _____ _____
 e. Placed the cap or stopper on securely. _____ _____ _____
 f. Dried the device with paper towels. _____ _____ _____
 g. Placed the device in the cover. _____ _____ _____
 h. Applied the device. Noted the time. _____ _____ _____
 i. Secured the device in place with ties, tape, or rolled gauze. _____ _____ _____
14. *For a cold compress:*
 a. Placed the small basin with cold water into the large basin with ice. _____ _____ _____
 b. Placed the compress into the cold water. _____ _____ _____
 c. Wrung out the compress. _____ _____ _____
 d. Applied the compress to the part. Noted the time. _____ _____ _____
15. Placed the call light and other needed items within reach. Unscreened the person if appropriate. _____ _____ _____
16. Raised or lowered bed rails. Followed the care plan. _____ _____ _____
17. Did the following every 5 minutes:
 a. Checked the person for signs and symptoms of complications. Removed the application if complications occurred. Told the nurse at once. _____ _____ _____
 b. Checked the application for cooling (hot application) or warming (cold application).
18. Removed the application at the specified time after 15 to 20 minutes. _____ _____ _____

Post-Procedure

19. Provided for comfort. _____ _____ _____
20. Placed the call light and other needed items within reach. _____ _____ _____
21. Raised or lowered bed rails. Followed the care plan. _____ _____ _____
22. Unscreened the person. _____ _____ _____
23. Cleaned, rinsed, dried, (with clean, dry paper towels), and returned re-usable items to the proper place. Followed agency policy for used linens. Wore gloves for this step. _____ _____ _____
24. Completed a safety check of the room. _____ _____ _____
25. Removed and discarded the gloves. Practiced hand hygiene. _____ _____ _____
26. Reported and recorded your observations. _____ _____ _____

Using a Pulse Oximeter

Name: _____   Date: _____

Quality of Life	S	U	Comments
• Knocked before entering the person's room.	___	___	_____
• Addressed the person by name.	___	___	_____
• Introduced yourself by name and title.	___	___	_____
• Explained the procedure before starting and during the procedure.	___	___	_____
• Protected the person's rights during the procedure.	___	___	_____
• Handled the person gently during the procedure.	___	___	_____

Pre-Procedure

1. Followed *Delegation Guidelines: Pulse Oximetry.* Saw *Promoting Safety and Comfort: Pulse Oximetry.*   ___ ___ _____
2. Practiced hand hygiene.   ___ ___ _____
3. Collected the following before going to the person's room:
   - Oximeter
   - Sensor (if not part of the device)
   - Tape (if needed)
   - Alcohol wipe   ___ ___ _____
4. Arranged your work area.   ___ ___ _____
5. Practiced hand hygiene.   ___ ___ _____
6. Identified the person. Checked the ID (identification) bracelet against the assignment sheet. Used 2 identifiers. Also called the person by name.   ___ ___ _____
7. Provided for privacy.   ___ ___ _____

Procedure

8. Provided for comfort.   ___ ___ _____
9. Selected and cleaned the site with an alcohol wipe. If measuring blood pressure, used 1 arm for blood pressure and a site on the other arm for pulse oximetry.   ___ ___ _____
10. Clipped or taped the sensor to the site. If necessary, connected the sensor to the oximeter.   ___ ___ _____
11. Turned on the oximeter.   ___ ___ _____
12. *For continuous monitoring:*
    a. Set the high and low alarm limits for SpO_2 and pulse rate.   ___ ___ _____
    b. Turned on audio and visual alarms.   ___ ___ _____
13. Checked the apical or radial pulse with the pulse on the display. The pulses should have been about the same. Noted both pulses on your assignment sheet.   ___ ___ _____
14. Read the SpO_2 on the display. Noted the value on the flow sheet and your assignment sheet.   ___ ___ _____
15. Left the sensor in place for continuous monitoring. Otherwise, turned off the device and removed the sensor.   ___ ___ _____

Post-Procedure

16. Provided for comfort.   ___ ___ _____
17. Placed the call light and other needed items within reach.   ___ ___ _____
18. Unscreened the person.   ___ ___ _____
19. Completed a safety check of the room.   ___ ___ _____
20. Returned the device to its proper place (unless monitoring was continuous). Followed agency policy for disinfection.   ___ ___ _____
21. Practiced hand hygiene.   ___ ___ _____
22. Reported and recorded the SpO_2, the pulse rate, and your other observations.   ___ ___ _____

Assisting With Deep-Breathing and Coughing Exercises

Name: _____   Date: _____

	S	U	Comments

Quality of Life
- Knocked before entering the person's room.   _____ _____ _____
- Addressed the person by name.   _____ _____ _____
- Introduced yourself by name and title.   _____ _____ _____
- Explained the procedure before starting and during the procedure.   _____ _____ _____
- Protected the person's rights during the procedure.   _____ _____ _____
- Handled the person gently during the procedure.   _____ _____ _____

Pre-Procedure
1. Followed *Delegation Guidelines: Deep Breathing and Coughing.* Saw *Promoting Safety and Comfort: Deep Breathing and Coughing.*   _____ _____ _____
2. Practiced hand hygiene.   _____ _____ _____
3. Identified the person. Checked the ID (identification) bracelet against the assignment sheet. Used 2 identifiers. Also called the person by name.   _____ _____ _____
4. Provided for privacy.   _____ _____ _____

Procedure
5. Lowered the bed rail if up.   _____ _____ _____
6. Helped the person to a comfortable sitting position.
   - Sitting on the side of the bed   _____ _____ _____
   - Semi-Fowler's   _____ _____ _____
   - Fowler's   _____ _____ _____
7. For deep breathing:
   a. Had the person place the hands over the rib cage.   _____ _____ _____
   b. Had the person breathe as deeply as possible. Had the person inhale through the nose.   _____ _____ _____
   c. Asked the person to hold the breath for 2 to 3 seconds.   _____ _____ _____
   d. Asked the person to exhale slowly through pursed lips. Asked the person to exhale until the ribs moved as far down as possible.   _____ _____ _____
   e. Repeated 4 more times. Had the person:
      1) Deep breathe in through the nose.   _____ _____ _____
      2) Hold the breath for 2 to 3 seconds.   _____ _____ _____
      3) Exhale slowly with pursed lips until the ribs moved as far down as possible.   _____ _____ _____
8. For coughing:
   a. *If the person did not have a productive cough:* Had the person place both hands over the chest or abdominal incision. One hand was on top of the other. Or the person held a pillow or folded towel over the chest or abdominal incision.   _____ _____ _____
   b. If the *person had a productive cough:*
      1) Had the person practice cough etiquette.   _____ _____ _____
      2) Splinted the chest or abdominal incision with your hands or a pillow. Wore gloves.   _____ _____ _____
   c. Had the person take in a deep breath.   _____ _____ _____
      i. Deep breathe in through the nose.   _____ _____ _____
      ii. Hold the breath for 2 to 3 seconds.   _____ _____ _____
      iii. Exhale slowly with pursed lips until the ribs moved as far down as possible.   _____ _____ _____
   d. Had the person cough strongly 2 times with the mouth open.   _____ _____ _____
9. Assisted with hand hygiene   _____ _____ _____

Post-Procedure

	S	U	Comments
10. Provided for comfort.	___	___	_____
11. Placed the call light and other needed items within reach.	___	___	_____
12. Raised or lowered bed rails. Followed the care plan.	___	___	_____
13. Unscreened the person.	___	___	_____
14. Completed a safety check of the room.	___	___	_____
15. Practiced hand hygiene.	___	___	_____
16. Reported and recorded your observations.	___	___	_____

Setting Up Oxygen

Name: _____   Date: _____

	S	U	Comments

Quality of Life
- Knocked before entering the person's room.
- Addressed the person by name.
- Introduced yourself by name and title.
- Explained the procedure before starting and during the procedure.
- Protected the person's rights during the procedure.
- Handled the person gently during the procedure.

Pre-Procedure
1. Followed *Delegation Guidelines: Oxygen Set-Up.* Saw *Promoting Safety and Comfort: Oxygen Set-Up.*
2. Practiced hand hygiene.
3. Collected the following before going to the person's room:
   - Oxygen (O_2) device with connecting tubing
   - Flowmeter
   - Humidifier (if ordered)
   - Distilled water (if used humidifier)
4. Arranged your work area.
5. Practiced hand hygiene.
6. Identified the person. Checked the ID (identification) bracelet against the assignment sheet. Used 2 identifiers. Also called the person by name.

Procedure
7. Made sure the flowmeter was in the OFF position.
8. Attached the flowmeter to the wall outlet or to the tank.
9. Filled the humidifier with distilled water.
10. Attached the humidifier to the bottom of the flowmeter.
11. Attached the O_2 device and connecting tubing to the humidifier. *Did not set the flowmeter. Did not apply the O_2 device on the person.*
12. Placed the cap securely on the distilled water. Stored the water according to agency policy.
13. Discarded the packaging from the O_2 device and connecting tubing.

Post-Procedure
14. Provided for comfort.
15. Placed the call light and other needed items within reach.
16. Completed a safety check of the room.
17. Practiced hand hygiene.
18. Told the nurse when you were done. The nurse would then:
    - Turn on the O_2 and set the flow rate.
    - Apply the O_2 device on the person.

Caring for Eyeglasses

Name: _____   Date: _____

	S	U	Comments

Quality of Life
- Knocked before entering the person's room.
- Addressed the person by name.
- Introduced yourself by name and title.
- Explained the procedure before starting and during the procedure.
- Protected the person's rights during the procedure.
- Handled the person gently during the procedure.

Pre-Procedure
1. Followed *Delegation Guidelines: Eyeglasses*. Saw *Promoting Safety and Comfort: Corrective Lenses*.
2. Practiced hand hygiene.
3. Collected the following:
   - Eyeglass case
   - Cleaning solution or warm water
   - Disposable lens cloth or cotton cloth

Procedure
4. Removed the eyeglasses.
   a. Held the frames in front of the ears.
   b. Lifted the frames from the ears. Brought the eyeglasses down away from the face.
5. Cleaned the lenses with cleaning solution or warm water. Cleaned in a circular motion. Dried the lenses with the cloth.
6. *If the person did not wear the glasses:*
   a. Opened the eyeglass case.
   b. Folded the glasses. Put them in the case. Did not touch the clean lenses.
   c. Placed the eyeglass case in the top drawer of the bedside stand.
7. *If the person wore the eyeglasses:*
   a. Held the frames at each side. Placed them over the ears.
   b. Adjusted the eyeglasses so the nose-piece rested on the nose.
   c. Returned the eyeglass case to the top drawer in the bedside stand.

Post-Procedure
8. Provided for comfort.
9. Placed the call light and other needed items within reach.
10. Returned the cleaning solution to its proper place.
11. Discarded the disposable cloth.
12. Completed a safety check of the room.
13. Practiced hand hygiene.
14. Reported and recorded your observations.

Cleaning Baby Bottles

Name: _____   Date: _____

	S	U	Comments

Pre-Procedure

1. See *Promoting Safety and Comfort: Cleaning Baby Bottles.*
2. Practiced hand hygiene.
3. Collected the following:
   - Bottles, nipples, and caps and any other bottle parts (rings, valves, and so on)
   - Wash basin-clean, used only for washing baby-feeding items
   - Bottle brush-clean, used only for washing baby-feeding items
   - Dishwashing soap
   - Other items used to prepare formula
   - Towel

Procedure

4. Practiced hand hygiene.
5. Took apart the bottles. Separated all of the parts—bottles, nipples, caps, and any other parts.
6. Rinsed the bottles, nipples, caps, and other bottle parts in warm or cold running water.
7. Placed the items in the basin.
8. Filled the basin with hot water. Added dishwashing soap.
9. Washed the bottles, nipples, caps, and other bottle parts. Washed any other items used to prepare formula.
10. Cleaned inside baby bottles with the bottle brush.
11. Squeezed hot, soapy water through the nipples. This removed formula.
12. Rinsed all items thoroughly in hot water. Squeezed hot water through the nipples to remove soap.
13. Laid a clean towel on the counter.
14. Stood bottles upside down to drain. Placed nipples, caps, and other items on the towel. Let the items dry.
15. Rinsed the basin and bottle brush well. Let them air-dry after use.

Diapering a Baby

Name: _____   Date: _____

Quality of Life	S	U	Comments
• Knocked before entering the baby's room.	___	___	_____
• Addressed the baby and parents by name.	___	___	_____
• Introduced yourself by name and title.	___	___	_____
• Explained the procedure to the parents before starting and during the procedure.	___	___	_____
• Protected the baby's rights during the procedure.	___	___	_____
• Handled the baby gently during the procedure.	___	___	_____

Pre-Procedure

1. Followed *Delegation Guidelines: Diapering a Baby*. Saw *Promoting Safety and Comfort: Diapering a Baby*.   ___ ___ _____
2. Practiced hand hygiene.   ___ ___ _____
3. Collected the following:
   - Gloves   ___ ___ _____
   - Clean diaper   ___ ___ _____
   - Waterproof changing pad   ___ ___ _____
   - Washcloth   ___ ___ _____
   - Disposable wipes or cotton balls   ___ ___ _____
   - Basin of warm water   ___ ___ _____
   - Baby soap   ___ ___ _____
   - Baby lotion or cream   ___ ___ _____

Procedure

4. Put on the gloves.   ___ ___ _____
5. Placed the changing pad under the baby.   ___ ___ _____
6. Unfastened the dirty diaper. Placed diaper pins out of the baby's reach.   ___ ___ _____
7. Wiped the genital area with the front of the diaper. Wiped from the front to the back (top to bottom).   ___ ___ _____
8. Noted the color and amount of urine and feces. Folded the diaper so urine and feces were inside. Set the diaper aside.   ___ ___ _____
9. Cleaned the genital area from front to back (top to bottom). Used a wet washcloth, disposable wipes, or cotton balls. Washed with mild soap and water for a large amount of feces or if the baby had a rash. Rinsed thoroughly and patted the area dry. Remove and discard the gloves. Practice hand hygiene. Put on clean gloves.   ___ ___ _____
10. Cleaned the circumcision. Follow the nurse's instructions for cord care.   ___ ___ _____
11. Applied cream or lotion to the genital area and buttocks. Did not use too much. Avoided caking lotion.   ___ ___ _____
12. Raised the baby's legs. Slid a clean diaper under the buttocks.   ___ ___ _____
13. Folded a cloth diaper as follows:
    a. *For a boy:* the extra thickness was in the front.   ___ ___ _____
    b. *For a girl:* the extra thickness was in the back.   ___ ___ _____
    c. Brought the diaper between the baby's legs.   ___ ___ _____
14. Made sure the diaper was snug around the hips and abdomen.   ___ ___ _____
    a. It was loose near the penis if the circumcision had not healed.   ___ ___ _____
    b. It was below the umbilicus if the cord stump had not healed.   ___ ___ _____

Procedure—cont'd   S   U   Comments

15. Secured the diaper in place. Used the tape strips or
    Velcro on the disposable diapers. Made sure the tabs
    stuck in place. Used baby pins or Velcro for cloth
    diapers. Pins pointed away from the abdomen.   _____ _____ _____
16. Applied a diaper cover or plastic pants if cloth diapers
    were worn.   _____ _____ _____
17. Placed the baby in the crib, infant seat, or other safe
    place.   _____ _____ _____

Post-Procedure
18. Rinsed feces from the cloth diaper into the toilet and
    flushed.   _____ _____ _____
19. Stored used cloth diapers in a covered pail. Placed a
    disposable diaper in the trash.   _____ _____ _____
20. Removed and discarded the gloves. Practiced hand
    hygiene.   _____ _____ _____
21. Put on clean gloves.   _____ _____ _____
22. Cleaned, rinsed, dried, and returned other items to
    their proper place. Used clean, dry paper towels for
    drying.   _____ _____ _____
23. Removed and discarded the gloves. Practiced hand
    hygiene.   _____ _____ _____
24. Complete a safety check of the room. See the inside of
    the back cover.
25. Reported and recorded your observations.   _____ _____ _____

Giving a Baby a Sponge Bath

Name: _____ Date: _____

Quality of Life	S	U	Comments
• Knocked before entering the baby's room.	___	___	_____
• Addressed the baby and parents by name.	___	___	_____
• Introduced yourself by name and title.	___	___	_____
• Explained the procedure to the parents before starting and during the procedure.	___	___	_____
• Protected the baby's rights during the procedure.	___	___	_____
• Handled the baby gently during the procedure.	___	___	_____

Pre-Procedure

1. Followed *Delegation Guidelines: Bathing an Infant.* Saw *Promoting Safety and Comfort: Bathing an Infant.* ___ ___ _____
2. Practiced hand hygiene. ___ ___ _____
3. Placed the following items in your work area.
   - Baby bathtub ___ ___ _____
   - Water thermometer ___ ___ _____
   - Bath towel ___ ___ _____
   - 2 hand towels ___ ___ _____
   - Receiving blanket ___ ___ _____
   - Washcloth ___ ___ _____
   - Clean diaper ___ ___ _____
   - Clean clothing for the baby ___ ___ _____
   - Cotton balls ___ ___ _____
   - Baby soap (if needed) ___ ___ _____
   - Baby shampoo ___ ___ _____
   - Baby lotion ___ ___ _____
   - Petrolatum gauze or petrolatum jelly (if needed) ___ ___ _____
   - Gloves ___ ___ _____
4. Identified the baby. Checked the ID (identification) bracelet against the assignment sheet. Used 2 identifiers. Followed agency policy. ___ ___ _____
5. Provided for privacy. ___ ___ _____

Procedure

6. Filled the baby bathtub with 2 to 3 inches of warm water. Water temperature was 100°F to 103°F (37.7°C to 40.5°C). Measured water temperature with the water thermometer or used the inside of your wrist. The water felt warm and comfortable. ___ ___ _____
7. Put on gloves. ___ ___ _____
8. Undressed the baby. Left the diaper on. ___ ___ _____
9. Washed the baby's eye lids.
   a. Dipped a cotton ball into the water. ___ ___ _____
   b. Squeezed out excess water. ___ ___ _____
   c. Washed 1 eye lid from the inner part to the outer part. ___ ___ _____
   d. Repeated for the other eye with a new cotton ball. ___ ___ _____
10. Moistened the washcloth and made a mitt. Cleaned the outside of the ear and then behind the ear. Repeated for the other ear. Was gentle. Did not use cotton swabs to clean inside of the ears. ___ ___ _____
11. Rinsed and squeezed out the washcloth. Made a mitt with the washcloth. ___ ___ _____
12. Washed the baby's face. Cleaned inside the nostrils with the washcloth. *Did not use cotton swabs to clean inside the nose.* Patted the face dry. ___ ___ _____

Procedure—cont'd	S	U	Comments

13. Picked up the baby. Held the baby over the baby bathtub basin using the football hold. Supported the baby's head and neck with your wrist and hand.

14. Washed the baby's head.
    a. Squeezed a small amount of water from the washcloth onto the baby's head. Or brought water to the baby's head using a cupped hand.
    b. Applied a small amount of baby shampoo to the head.
    c. Washed the head with circular motions.
    d. Rinsed the head by squeezing water from a washcloth over the baby's head. Or brought water to the baby's head using a cupped hand. Rinsed thoroughly. Did not get soap in the baby's eyes.
    e. Used a small hand towel to dry the head.

15. Laid the baby on the table.

16. Removed the diaper.

17. Washed the front of the body with a washcloth or your hands. Did not get the cord wet. Also washed the arms, hands, fingers, legs, feet, and toes. Washed the genital area and all creases and folds. Rinsed thoroughly. Patted dry.

18. Followed the nurse's instructions for cord care. Cleaned the circumcision.

19. Turned the baby to the prone position. Washed the back and buttocks. Used a washcloth or your hands. Rinsed thoroughly. Patted dry.

20. Applied baby lotion as directed by the nurse.

21. Applied petrolatum gauze or petrolatum jelly to the penis as the nurse directed.

22. Removed and discarded the gloves. Practiced hand hygiene.

23. Put a clean diaper and clean clothes on the baby.

24. Wrapped the baby in the receiving blanket. Put the baby in the crib or other safe area.

Post-Procedure

25. Practiced hand hygiene. Put on gloves.

26. Cleaned, rinsed, dried, and returned equipment and supplies to the proper place. Used clean, dry paper towels for drying. Did this step when the baby was settled.

27. Removed and discarded the gloves. Practiced hand hygiene.

28. Completed a safety check of the room.

29. Reported and recorded your observations.

Giving a Baby a Bath in a Baby Bathtub

Name: _____   Date: _____

Quality of Life	S	U	Comments
• Knocked before entering the baby's room.	___	___	_____
• Addressed the baby and parents by name.	___	___	_____
• Introduced yourself by name and title.	___	___	_____
• Explained the procedure to the parents before starting and during the procedure.	___	___	_____
• Protected the baby's rights during the procedure.	___	___	_____
• Handled the baby gently during the procedure.	___	___	_____

Procedure

1. Did the following:
   a. Followed *Delegation Guidelines: Bathing an Infant*. Saw *Promoting Safety and Comfort: Bathing an Infant*.   ___ ___ _____
   b. Practiced hand hygiene.   ___ ___ _____
   c. Placed the following items in your work area.
      • Baby bathtub   ___ ___ _____
      • Water thermometer   ___ ___ _____
      • Bath towel   ___ ___ _____
      • 2 hand towels   ___ ___ _____
      • Receiving blanket   ___ ___ _____
      • Washcloth   ___ ___ _____
      • Clean diaper   ___ ___ _____
      • Clean clothing for the baby   ___ ___ _____
      • Cotton balls   ___ ___ _____
      • Baby soap (if needed)   ___ ___ _____
      • Baby shampoo   ___ ___ _____
      • Baby lotion   ___ ___ _____
      • Gloves   ___ ___ _____
      • Petrolatum gauze or petrolatum jelly (if needed)   ___ ___ _____
   d. Identified the baby. Checked the ID (identification) bracelet against the assignment sheet. Used 2 identifiers. Followed agency policy.   ___ ___ _____
   e. Provided for privacy.   ___ ___ _____
   f. Filled the baby bathtub with 2 to 3 inches of warm water. Water temperature was 100°F to 103°F (37.7°C to 40.5°C). Measured water temperature with the water thermometer or used the inside of your wrist. The water felt warm and comfortable.   ___ ___ _____
   g. Put on gloves.   ___ ___ _____
   h. Undressed the baby. Left the diaper on.   ___ ___ _____
   i. Washed the baby's eye lids.
      1) Dipped a cotton ball into the water.   ___ ___ _____
      2) Squeezed out excess water.   ___ ___ _____
      3) Washed 1 eye lid from the inner part to the outer part.   ___ ___ _____
      4) Repeated for the other eye with a new cotton ball.   ___ ___ _____
   j. Moistened the washcloth and made a mitt. Cleaned the outside of the ear and then behind the ear. Repeated for the other ear. Was gentle. Did not use cotton swabs to clean inside the ears.   ___ ___ _____
   k. Rinsed and squeezed out the washcloth. Made a mitt with the washcloth.   ___ ___ _____
   l. Washed the baby's face. Cleaned inside the nostrils with the washcloth. *Did not use cotton swabs to clean inside the nose.* Patted the face dry.   ___ ___ _____

Procedure—cont'd

	S	U	Comments
m. Picked up the baby. Held the baby over the baby bathtub basin using the football hold. Supported the baby's head and neck with your wrist and hand.	___	___	___
n. Washed the baby's head.			
1) Squeezed a small amount of water from the washcloth onto the baby's head. Or brought water to the baby's head using a cupped hand.	___	___	___
2) Applied a small amount of baby shampoo to the head.	___	___	___
3) Washed the head with circular motions.	___	___	___
4) Rinsed the head by squeezing water from a washcloth over the baby's head. Or brought water to the baby's head using a cupped hand. Rinsed thoroughly. Did not get soap in the baby's eyes.	___	___	___
5) Used a small hand towel to dry the head.	___	___	___
o. Laid the baby on the table.	___	___	___
p. Removed the diaper.	___	___	___
2. Held the baby.			
a. Placed 1 hand under the baby's shoulders. Your thumb was over the baby's shoulder. Your fingers were under the arm.	___	___	___
b. Supported the buttocks with your other hand. Slid your hand under the thighs. Held the far thigh with your other hand.	___	___	___
3. Lowered the baby into the water feet first.	___	___	___
4. Washed the front of the baby's body. Also washed the arms, hands, fingers, legs, feet, and toes. Washed the genital area and all creases and folds.	___	___	___
5. Reversed your hold. Used your other hand to hold the baby. Kept the baby's face out of the water.	___	___	___
6. Washed the baby's back and buttocks. Rinsed thoroughly.	___	___	___
7. Reversed your hold again. Held the baby with your other hand.	___	___	___
8. Lifted the baby out of the water and onto a towel.	___	___	___
9. Wrapped the baby in the towel. Also covered the baby's head.	___	___	___
10. Patted the baby dry. Dried all folds and creases.	___	___	___
11. Did the following:			
a. Applied baby lotion as directed by the nurse.	___	___	___
b. Removed and discarded the gloves. Practiced hand hygiene.	___	___	___
c. Put a clean diaper and clean clothes on the baby.	___	___	___
d. Wrapped the baby in the receiving blanket. Put the baby in the crib or other safe area.	___	___	___

Post-Procedure

	S	U	Comments
12. Practiced hand hygiene. Put on gloves.	___	___	___
13. Cleaned, rinsed, dried, and returned equipment and supplies to the proper place. Used clean, dry paper towels for drying. Did this when the baby was settled.	___	___	___
14. Removed and discarded the gloves. Practiced hand hygiene.	___	___	___
15. Completed a safety check of the room.	___	___	___
16. Reported and recorded your observations.	___	___	___

Weighing an Infant

Name: _____   Date: _____

Quality of Life	S	U	Comments

Quality of Life
- Knocked before entering the baby's room.
- Addressed the baby and parents by name.
- Introduced yourself by name and title.
- Explained the procedure to the parents before starting and during the procedure.
- Protected the baby's rights during the procedure.
- Handled the baby gently during the procedure.

Pre-Procedure
1. Followed *Delegation Guidelines: Weighing Infants*. Saw *Promoting Safety and Comfort: Weighing Infants*.
2. Practiced hand hygiene.
3. Collected the following:
   - Baby scale
   - Paper for the scale
   - Items for diaper changing
   - Gloves
4. Identified the baby. Checked the ID (identification) bracelet against the assignment sheet. Used 2 identifiers. Followed agency policy.

Procedure
5. Placed the paper on the scale. Adjusted the scale to zero (0).
6. Put on gloves.
7. Undressed the baby and removed the diaper. Cleaned the genital area.
8. Removed and discarded the gloves and practiced hand hygiene. Put on clean gloves.
9. Laid the baby on the scale. Kept 1 hand over the baby to prevent falling.
10. Read the digital display or moved the weights until the scale was balanced.
11. Noted the measurement.
12. Took the baby off of the scale.
13. Diapered and dressed the baby. Laid the baby in the crib.
14. Discarded the paper and soiled diaper.
15. Disinfected the scale; followed agency policy.
16. Removed and discarded the gloves. Practiced hand hygiene.

Post-Procedure
17. Returned the scale to its proper place.
18. Practiced hand hygiene.
19. Complete a safety check of the room. See the inside of the back cover.
20. Reported and recorded your observations.

Assisting With Post-Mortem Care

Name: _____   Date: _____

	S	U	Comments
Pre-Procedure			
1. Followed *Delegation Guidelines: Care of the Body After Death.* Saw *Promoting Safety and Comfort: Care of the Body After Death.*	____	____	_____
2. Practiced hand hygiene.	____	____	_____
3. Collected the following:			
• Post-mortem kit (shroud or body bag, gown, ID [identification] tags, gauze squares, safety pins)	____	____	_____
• Disposable bed protectors	____	____	_____
• Wash basin	____	____	_____
• Bath towel and washcloths	____	____	_____
• Denture cup	____	____	_____
• Items for shaving facial hair	____	____	_____
• Tape	____	____	_____
• Dressings	____	____	_____
• Gloves	____	____	_____
• Cotton balls	____	____	_____
• Valuables envelope	____	____	_____
4. Provided for privacy.	____	____	_____
5. Raised the bed for body mechanics.	____	____	_____
6. Made sure the bed was flat.	____	____	_____
Procedure			
7. Put on gloves.	____	____	_____
8. Positioned the body supine. Arms and legs were straight. A pillow was under the head and shoulders. Or raised the head of the bed 15 to 20 degrees, according to agency policy.	____	____	_____
9. Closed the eyes. Gently pulled the eyelids over the eyes. Applied moist cotton balls gently over the eyelids if the eyes did not stay closed.	____	____	_____
10. Inserted dentures or put them in a labeled denture cup. Followed agency policy.	____	____	_____
11. Closed the mouth. If necessary, placed a rolled towel under the chin to keep the mouth closed.	____	____	_____
12. Removed all jewelry, except for wedding rings if this was agency policy. Listed the jewelry that you removed. Placed the jewelry and the list in a valuables envelope.	____	____	_____
13. Placed cotton balls over the rings. Taped them in place as the nurse directed.	____	____	_____
14. Removed drainage containers.	____	____	_____
15. Removed tubes and catheters with the gauze squares as the nurse directed.	____	____	_____
16. Shaved facial hair if this was agency policy or desired by the family. Some men normally grow facial hair (beard, mustache). If so, do not shave facial hair.	____	____	_____
17. Bathed soiled areas with plain water. Dried thoroughly.	____	____	_____
18. Placed a bed protector under the buttocks.	____	____	_____
19. Removed soiled dressings. Replaced them with clean ones.	____	____	_____
20. Put a clean gown on the body. Positioned the body supine. Arms and legs were straight. A pillow was under the head and shoulders. Or the head of the bed was raised 15 to 20 degrees according to agency policy.	____	____	_____
21. Brushed and combed the hair if necessary.	____	____	_____

Procedure—cont'd	S	U	Comments
22. Covered the body to the shoulders with a sheet if the family viewed the body.	____	____	_____
23. Gathered the person's belongings. Put them in a bag labeled with the person's name. Included eyeglasses, hearing aids, and other valuables.	____	____	_____
24. Removed supplies, equipment, and linens. Straightened the room. Provided soft lighting.	____	____	_____
25. Removed and discarded the gloves. Practiced hand hygiene.	____	____	_____
26. Let the family view the body. Provided for privacy. Returned to the room after they left.	____	____	_____
27. Practiced hand hygiene. Put on gloves.	____	____	_____
28. Filled out the ID tags. Tied 1 to the ankle or to the right big toe.	____	____	_____
29. Placed the body in the body bag or covered it with a sheet. Or applied the shroud.			
a. Positioned the shroud under the body.	____	____	_____
b. Brought the top down over the head.	____	____	_____
c. Folded the bottom up over the feet.	____	____	_____
d. Folded the sides over the body.	____	____	_____
e. Pinned or taped the shroud in place.	____	____	_____
30. Attached the second ID tag to the shroud, sheet, or body bag.	____	____	_____
31. Left the denture cup with the body.	____	____	_____
32. Pulled the privacy curtain around the bed. Or closed the door.	____	____	_____

Post-Procedure

	S	U	Comments
33. Removed and discarded the gloves. Practiced hand hygiene.	____	____	_____
34. Cleaned the unit after the body was removed. Wore gloves.	____	____	_____
35. Removed and discarded the gloves. Practiced hand hygiene.	____	____	_____
36. Reported the following:			
• The time the body was taken by the funeral director	____	____	_____
• What was done with jewelry, other valuables, and personal items	____	____	_____
• What was done with dentures	____	____	_____

Preparing for the Competency Evaluation

After completing your state's training program, you need to pass the competency evaluation. The purpose of the competency evaluation is to make sure you can do your job safely. This section will help you prepare for the test.

Competency Evaluation

The competency evaluation has a written test and a skills test. The number (70+) of questions varies with each state. Each question has 4 answer choices. Although some questions may appear to have more than one possible answer, there is only 1 best answer. You will have about 1 minute to read and answer each question. Some questions take less time to read and answer. Other questions take longer. You should have enough time to take the test without feeling rushed.

The content of the written test varies depending on your state. Content may include:
- Activities of Daily Living—hygiene, dressing and grooming, nutrition and hydration, elimination, rest/sleep/comfort
- Basic Nursing Skills—infection control, safety/emergency, therapeutic/technical procedures (e.g., vital signs, bedmaking), data collection and reporting
- Restorative Skills—prevention, self-care/independence
- Emotional and Mental Health Needs
- Spiritual and Cultural Needs
- The Person's Rights
- Legal and Ethical Behavior
- Being a Member of the Health Care Team
- Communication

The written test is given as a paper and pencil test in most states. Some test sites may use computers. You do not need computer experience to take the test on the computer. If you have difficulty reading English, you may request to take an oral test. Talk with your instructor or employer about details for computer testing or oral testing.

The skills test involves performing 5 nursing skills that you learned in your training program. These skills are chosen randomly. You do not select the skills. You are allowed about 30 minutes to do the skills.

Taking the Competency Evaluation

To register for the test, you need to complete an application. Your instructor or employer tells you when and where the tests are given. There is a fee for the evaluation. If you work in a nursing center, the employer may pay this fee. If you pay the fee, you may need to purchase a money order or certified check. Make sure your name is on the money order or certified check. Cash and personal checks may not be accepted.

Plan to arrive at the test site about 15 to 30 minutes before the evaluation begins. You will not be admitted if you are late. Know the exact location of the test site and room. Drive or take transportation to the test site a few days or a week before the test. Making a "dry run" lets you know how much time you need to travel, park, and get to the test site. It will also help decrease your anxiety level on the test day.

To be admitted to the test, you need two pieces of identification (ID). The first form of ID is a government-issued document such as a driver's license or passport. It must have a current photo and your signature. The name on the ID must be the same as the name on your application form. If your name has changed and you have not been able to have the name changed on your identification documents, ask your instructor or employer what to do. The second form of ID must include your name and signature. Examples include a U.S. state or federal issued ID, student or work ID, or a U.S. financial institution issued ID.

Take several sharpened Number 2 pencils to the test. For the skills test you will need a watch with a second hand.

Taking the written test and skills test may take several hours. You may want to bring snacks or lunch and a beverage to the testing site. Eating and drinking are not allowed during the test. However, you may be told where you can eat while waiting for the test.

You cannot bring textbooks, study notes, or other materials into the testing room. The only exception may be a language translation dictionary that you show to the proctor (a person who monitors the test) before the test begins. Cellphones, laptops, calculators, or other electronic devices are not permitted during testing. Children and pets are not allowed in the testing areas.

Studying for the Competency Evaluation

You began to prepare for the written test and skills test during your training program. You learned the basic nursing content and skills needed to provide safe, quality care. The following suggestions can help you study for the competency evaluation.
- Begin to study at least 2 to 3 weeks before the test. Plan to study for 1 to 2 hours each day.
- Decide on a specific time to study. Choose a study time that is best for you. This may be early in the morning before others are awake. It may be in the evening after others go to sleep. Try to choose a time when you are mentally alert.
- Choose a specific area to study in. This area should be quiet, well lit, and comfortable. You should have enough room to write and to spread out your books, notes, and other study aids. The area does not need to be noise-free. The testing site is not absolutely quiet.

You want to concentrate and not be distracted by the noise around you.

- Collect everything you need before settling down to study. This includes your textbook, notes, paper, highlighters, and pens or pencils.
- Take short breaks when you need them. Take a break when your mind begins to wander or if you feel sleepy.
- Develop a study plan. Write your plan down so you can refer to it. Study one content area before going on to the next. For example, study personal hygiene before going on to vital signs. Do not jump from subject to subject.
- Use a variety of ways to study.
  - Use index cards to help you review abbreviations and terminology. Put the abbreviation or term on the front of the card and place the meaning on the back. Take the cards with you and review them whenever you have a break or are waiting.
  - Record key points. You can listen to the recording while cooking or while riding in the car.
  - Study groups are another way to prepare for a test. Group members can quiz each other.
- To remember what you are learning, try these ideas.
  - Relax when you study. When relaxed, you learn information quickly and recall it with greater ease.
  - Repeat what you are learning. Say it out loud. This helps you remember the idea.
  - Make the information you are learning meaningful. Think about how the information will help you be a good nursing assistant.
  - Write down what you are learning. Writing helps you remember information. Prepare study sheets.
  - Be positive about what you are learning. You remember what you find interesting.
- Suggestions for studying if you have children:
  - When you first come home from work or school, spend time with your children. Then plan study time.
  - Select educational programs on TV that your children can watch as you study.
  - When you take your study breaks, spend time with your children.
  - Ask other adults to take care of the children while you study.
- Take the two practice tests in this section. Each question has the correct answer and the reason why an answer is correct or incorrect. If you practice taking tests, you are more likely to pass them. Take the practice tests under conditions similar to the real test. Work within time limits.
- If your state has a practice test and a candidate handbook, study the content. Some states have practice tests on-line. Information can be obtained at the NCSBN website. https://www.ncsbn.org/nnaap-exam.htm; for additional information go to: www.pearsonvue.com

Managing Anxiety

Almost everyone dreads taking tests. It is common and normal to experience anxiety before taking a test. If used wisely, anxiety can help you do well. When you are anxious, that means you are concerned. You may be concerned about how prepared you are to take the test. Or you may be concerned about how you will feel about yourself if you do not pass the test. Being concerned usually results in some action. To overcome anxiety before the test:

- Study and prepare for the test. That helps increase your confidence as you recall or clarify what you have learned. Anxiety decreases as confidence increases. When you think you know the information, keep studying. This reinforces your learning.
- Develop a positive mental attitude. You can pass this test. You took tests in your training program and passed them. Praise yourself. Talk to yourself in a positive way. If a negative thought enters your mind, stop it at once. Challenge the mental thought and tell yourself you will pass the test.
- Visualize success. Think about how wonderful you will feel when you are notified that you have passed the test.
- Perform breathing exercises. Breathe slowly and deeply.
- Perform regular exercise. Exercise helps you stay physically fit. It also helps keep you calm.
- Good nourishment helps you think clearly. Eat a nourishing meal before the test. Do not skip breakfast. Vitamin C helps fight short-term stress. Protein and calcium help overcome the effects of long-term stress. Complex carbohydrates (pasta, nuts, yogurt) can help settle your nerves. Eat familiar foods the day before and the day of the test. Do not eat foods that could cause stomach or intestinal upset.
- Maintain a normal routine the day before the test.
- Get a good night's sleep before the test. Go to bed early enough so you do not oversleep or are too tired to get up. Set your alarm clock properly. You may want to set two alarm clocks.
- Do not "cram" the evening before or the day of the test. Last-minute cramming increases your anxiety. Do something relaxing with family and friends.
- Avoid drinking large amounts of coffee, colas, water, or other beverages. You do not want to be uncomfortable with a full bladder when you take the test.
- Wear comfortable clothes. Dress in layers so that you are prepared for a cold or warm room.
- If you are a woman, remember that worry and anxiety can affect your menstrual cycle. Wear a panty liner, sanitary napkin, or tampon if you think your period may start. This eliminates worry about soiling your clothing during the test.
- Allow plenty of time for travel, traffic, and parking.
- Arrive early enough to use the restroom before the test begins.
- Do not talk about the test with others. Their panic or anxiety may affect your self-confidence.
- In the unlikely event that you fail the test, do not panic. There are opportunities for you to take it again.

Taking the Test

Follow these guidelines for taking the test.

- Listen carefully and follow the instructions given by the proctor (person administering the test).

- When you receive the test, make certain you have all the test pages.
- Read and follow all directions carefully.
- You are not allowed to ask questions about the content of the test questions.
- Do deep-breathing and muscle-relaxation exercises as needed.
- Cheating of any kind is not allowed. If the proctor sees you giving or receiving any type of assistance, your test booklet is taken and you must leave the testing site.
- If using a computer answer sheet, completely fill in the bubble.
- If you make a mistake, erase the wrong answer completely. Do not make any stray marks on the paper. Not erasing completely or leaving stray marks could cause the computer to misread your answer.
- Do not worry or get anxious if people finish the test before you do. Persons who finish a test early do not necessarily have a better score than those who finish later.
- You cannot take any evaluation materials or notes out of the testing room.

Answering Multiple-Choice Questions

Pace yourself during the test. If you are taking a paper and pencil test, first, answer all the questions that you know. Then go back and answer skipped questions. Sometimes you will remember the answer later. Or another test question may give you a clue to the one you skipped. Spending too much time on a question can cost you valuable time later. To help you answer the questions or statements:

- Always read the questions or statements carefully. Do not scan or glance at questions. Scanning or glancing can cause you to miss important key words. Read each word of the question.
- Before reading the options, decide what the answer is in your own words. Then read all 4 options to the question. Select the 1 best answer.
- Do not read into a question. Take the question as it is asked. Do not add your own thoughts and ideas to the question. Do not assume or suppose "what if." Just respond to the information provided.
- Trust your common sense. If unsure of an answer, select your first choice. Do not change your answer unless you are absolutely sure of the correct answer. Your first reaction is usually correct.

- Look for key words in every question. Sometimes key words are in italics, highlighted, or underlined. Common key words are *always, never, first, except, best, not, correct, incorrect, true,* and *false.*
- Know which words can make a statement correct (e.g., *may, can, usually, most, at least, sometimes*). The word "except" can make a question a false statement.
- Be careful of answers with these key words or phrases: *always, never, every, only, all, none, at all times,* or *at no time.* These words and phrases do not allow for exceptions. In nursing, exceptions are generally present. However, sometimes answers containing these words are correct. For example, which of the following is correct and which are incorrect?
  a. Always use a turning sheet.
  b. Never shake linens.
  c. Soap is used for all baths.
  d. The call light must always be attached to the bed.
  The correct answer is b. Incorrect answers are a, c, and d.
- Omit answers that are obviously wrong. Then choose the best of the remaining answers.
- Go back to the questions you skipped. Answer all questions by eliminating or narrowing your choices. Always mark an answer even if you are not sure.
- Review the test a second time for completeness and accuracy before turning it in.
- Make sure you have answered each question. Also check that you have given only 1 answer for each question.
- Remember, the test is not designed to trick or confuse you. The written competency evaluation tests what you know, not what you do not know. You know more than you are asked.

Computer Testing

The test may be given by computer at the test site. Ask your instructor what computer skills you will need. You usually do not need keyboard or typing skills. You will use a computer mouse to select answers. Also, you will usually receive instruction before the test begins. Computer testing may or may not allow you to return to previous questions. If you plan to take the test by computer, ask your instructor for alternative test-taking strategies.

Note: This review covers selected chapters only based on Competency Evaluation requirements.

CHAPTER 1 INTRODUCTION TO HEALTH CARE AGENCIES

Health Care Agency Purposes

- Health promotion
- Disease prevention
- Detection and treatment of disease
- Rehabilitation and restorative care

Hospitals

- Hospitals provide emergency care, surgery, nursing care, x-ray procedures and treatments, and laboratory testing.
- Hospitals also provide respiratory, physical, occupational, speech, and other therapies.
- Persons cared for in hospitals are called *patients*. Hospital patients have acute, chronic, or terminal illnesses.

Rehabilitation and Sub-Acute Care Agencies

- Medical and nursing care is provided for people who do not need hospital care but are too sick to go home.

Long-Term Care Centers

- Persons who live in long-term care centers are called residents.
- Long-term care is for residents who do not need hospital care but cannot care for themselves at home.
- Centers provide medical and nursing, dietary, recreational, rehabilitative, and social services. Housekeeping and laundry services are also provided.
- Residents are older or disabled.
- Skilled nursing facilities provide more complex care.
- Some residents are recovering from illness, injury, or surgery.
- Some residents return home when well enough. Some residents need nursing care until death.
- Memory care units provide care for residents with Alzheimer disease or other dementias.

Assisted Living Facilities

- Housing, personal care, support services, health care, and social activities are provided in a home-like setting for persons needing help with daily activities.

Other Health Agencies

- Other health agencies include mental health centers, home care, hospice, and health care systems.

The Health Team

- Many health care workers with skills and knowledge contribute to total care.
- The team works together to provide coordinated care to meet each person's needs.
- The team is usually lead by a registered nurse (RN).

The Nursing Team

- The nursing team provides quality care to people.
- Care is coordinated by an RN.

Nursing Assistants

- Nursing assistants report to the licensed nurse supervising their work.
- Delegated tasks are performed under the supervision of a licensed nurse.
- Nursing assistant training and competency evaluation must be successfully completed.

Meeting Standards

Survey Process

- Surveys are done to see if agencies meet standards for licensure, certification, and accreditation.
- A license is issued by the state. A center must have a license to operate and provide care.
- Certification is required to receive Medicare and Medicaid funds.
- Accreditation is voluntary. It signals quality and excellence.

Your Role

- Provide quality care.
- Protect the person's rights.
- Provide for the person's and your own safety.
- Help keep the center clean and safe.
- Conduct yourself in a professional manner.
- Have good work ethics.
- Follow agency policies and procedures.
- Answer questions honestly and completely.

CHAPTER 1 REVIEW QUESTIONS

Circle the BEST answer.

1. Nursing assistants must
   a. Pass a nursing assistant training program and a competency evaluation
   b. Complete a 2, 3, or 4 year program and pass a licensure examination
   c. Obtain advanced skills and certification to assist in the care of hospice patients
   d. Teach people how to make and maintain healthy lifestyle changes

2. Who would the nursing assistant contact if a patient has a question about the medical diagnosis?
   a. Nurse practitioner
   b. RN
   c. Physician's assistant
   d. Physician
3. What is the most important goal of the health team?
   a. Support and respect each other
   b. Treat and cure disease
   c. Provide quality care
   d. Follow the instructions of the RN

Answers to these questions are on p. 537.

CHAPTER 2 THE PERSON'S RIGHTS

- Centers must protect and promote residents' rights. Residents must be free to exercise their rights without interference. If residents are not able to exercise their rights, legal representatives do so for them.

The Omnibus Budget Reconciliation Act of 1987 (OBRA)

- OBRA is a federal law.
- OBRA requires that nursing centers provide care in a manner and in a setting that maintains or improves each person's quality of life, health, and safety.
- OBRA requires nursing assistant training and competency evaluation.
- Resident rights are a major part of OBRA.

Information

- The right to information includes:
  - Access to all records about the person, including medical records, incident reports, contracts, and financial records
  - Information about the person's health condition
  - Information about the person's doctor, including name, specialty, and contact information
- Report any request for information to the nurse.

Refusing Treatment

- The person has the right to refuse treatment.
- A person who does not give consent or refuses treatment cannot be treated against his or her wishes.
- The center must find out what the person is refusing and why.
- Advance directives are part of the right to refuse treatment.
- Report any treatment refusal to the nurse.

Privacy and Confidentiality

- Residents have the right to:
  - Personal privacy. The person's body is not exposed unnecessarily. Only staff directly involved in care and treatments are present. The person must give consent for others to be present. A person has the right to use the bathroom in private. Privacy is maintained for all personal care measures.
  - Visit with others in private—in areas where others cannot see or hear them. This includes phone calls.
  - Send and receive mail without others interfering. No one can open mail the person sends or receives without his or her consent. Unopened mail is given to the person within 24 hours of delivery to the center.
- Information about the person's care, treatment, and condition is kept confidential. So are medical and financial records. Consent is needed to release information to other agencies or persons.

Personal Choice

- Residents have the right to make their own choices. They can:
  - Choose their own doctors.
  - Take part in planning and deciding their care and treatment.
  - Choose activities, schedules, and care based on their preferences.
  - Choose when to get up and go to bed, what to wear, how to spend their time, and what to eat.
  - Choose friends and visitors inside and outside the center.

Grievances

- Residents have the right to voice concerns, questions, and complaints about treatment or care.
- The center must try to correct the matter promptly.
- No one can punish the person in any way for voicing the grievance.

Work

- The person is not required to work or perform services for the center.
- The person has the right to work or perform services if he or she wants to.
- Residents volunteer or are paid for their services.

Taking Part in Resident Groups

- The person has the right to:
  - Form and take part in resident and family groups.
  - Take part in social, cultural, religious, and community events. The resident has the right to help in getting to and from events of their choice.

Personal Items

- The resident has the right to:
  - Keep and use personal items, such as clothing and some furnishings.
  - Have his or her property treated with care and respect. Items are labeled with the person's name.
- Protect yourself and the center from being accused of stealing a person's property. Do not go through a person's closet, drawers, purse, or other space without the person's knowledge and consent. If you have to inspect closets and drawers, follow center policy for reporting and recording the inspection.

Freedom From Abuse, Mistreatment, and Neglect
- Residents have the right to be free from:
  - Verbal, sexual, physical, or mental abuse
  - Involuntary seclusion—separating a person from others against his or her will, confining a person to a certain area, or keeping the person away from his or her room without consent
- No one can abuse, neglect, or mistreat a resident. This includes center staff, volunteers, staff from other agencies or groups, other residents, family members, friends, visitors, and legal representatives.
- Nursing centers must investigate suspected or reported cases of abuse.

Freedom From Restraint
- Residents have the right to not have body movements restricted by restraints or drugs.
- Restraints are used only if required to treat the person's medical symptoms or if necessary to protect the person or others from harm. If a restraint is required, a doctor's order is needed.

Quality of Life
- Residents must be cared for in a manner that promotes dignity and self-esteem. Physical, psychological, and mental well-being must be promoted. Review Box 2-3(p 27), Promoting Dignity and Privacy-OBRA Required Actions in the Textbook.
- Centers must provide activity programs that promote physical, intellectual, social, spiritual, and emotional well-being.
- Residents have the right to a safe, clean, comfortable, and home-like setting. The center must provide a setting and services that meet the person's needs and preferences. The setting and staff must promote the person's independence, dignity, and well-being.

Ombudsman Program
- The Older Americans Act requires a long-term care ombudsman program in every state.
- Ombudsmen are employed by a state agency. They are not nursing center employees. Some are volunteers.
- Ombudsmen protect the health, safety, welfare, and rights of residents. They also may investigate and resolve complaints, provide support to resident and family groups, and help the center manage difficult problems.
- OBRA requires that nursing centers post the names, addresses, and phone numbers of local and state ombudsmen where the residents can easily see it.
- Because a family member or resident may share a concern with you, you must know the state and center policies and procedures for contacting an ombudsman.

CHAPTER 2 REVIEW QUESTIONS

Circle the BEST answer.
1. Which circumstance is a violation of a resident's rights?
   a. Resident refuses a treatment
   b. Resident makes a private telephone call
   c. Resident chooses an activity to attend
   d. Resident is shunned after voicing a grievance
2. What is the primary purpose for the OBRA requirements for nursing assistant training and competency evaluation?
   a. Nursing assistants are trained to provide care that improves or maintains quality of life, health and safety.
   b. Nursing assistants have an easier time getting a job after undergoing the training and competency evaluation.
   c. Nursing care facilities can receive insurance, Medicare and Medicaid funding if nursing assistants are trained.
   d. Nursing care facilities can contain costs by hiring nursing assistants who have completed OBRA approved programs.
3. Which situation best demonstrates that the person is exercising his rights to take part in planning and deciding their care?
   a. Family is told about the benefits and risks of the treatments
   b. Person asks about the expected outcome of the treatment.
   c. Doctor advises the patient that there is no cure for his condition.
   d. Nurse gives the patient and family written information about treatments
4. Which action should be taken if a person volunteers to do some chores around the center?
   a. Tell the person that he can get extra medical supplies in exchange for this work
   b. Ask the family if the person is qualified and able to do the assigned chores
   c. Tell the person that he doesn't need to do any chores because he is paying for services.
   d. Include the volunteer work in the care plan as it fulfills a desire or need to work

Answers to these questions are on p. 537.

CHAPTER 3 THE NURSING ASSISTANT
Federal and State Laws
Nurse Practice Acts
- Each state has a nurse practice act. It regulates nursing practice in that state.

Nursing Assistants
- A state's nurse practice act is used to decide what nursing assistants can do. Some nurse practice acts also regulate nursing assistant roles, functions, education, and certification requirements. Some states have separate laws for nursing assistants.
- Nursing assistants must be able to function with skill and safety. They can have their certification, license, or registration denied, revoked, or suspended.

The Omnibus Budget Reconciliation Act of 1987 (OBRA)
- The purpose of OBRA, a federal law, is to improve the quality of life of nursing center residents.

- OBRA sets minimum training and competency evaluation requirements for nursing assistants. Each state must have a nursing assistant training and competency evaluation program (NATCEP). A nursing assistant must successfully complete a NATCEP to work in a nursing center, hospital, long-term care unit, or home care agency receiving Medicare funds.
- OBRA requires at least 75 hours of instruction. Some states have more hours. At least 16 hours of supervised training in a laboratory or clinical setting are required.
  - The competency evaluation has a written test and a skills test.
  - The written test has multiple-choice questions.
  - The number of questions varies from state to state.
  - The skills test involves performing certain skills learned in the training program.
- OBRA requires a nursing assistant registry in each state. It is an official record that lists persons who have successfully completed the NATCEP.
- Re-training and a new competency evaluation program are required for nursing assistants who have not worked for 24 months. To work in another state, nursing assistants must meet that state's NATCEP.
- Each state's NATCEP must meet OBRA requirements.

Roles and Responsibilities

- Nurse practice acts, OBRA, state laws, and legal and advisory opinions direct what nursing assistants can do.
- The range of functions for nursing assistants varies among states and agencies. Before performing a nursing task make sure that:
  - The state allows nursing assistants to do that task.
  - It is in the job description.
  - You have the necessary education and training.
  - A nurse is available to answer questions and to supervise the task.
- Rules for nursing assistants to follow are in Box 3-2(p 26), Rules for Nursing Assistants, in the Textbook.
  - You are an assistant to the nurse.
  - A nurse assigns and supervises your work.
  - You report observations about the person's physical and mental status to the nurse. Report changes in the person's condition or behavior at once.
  - The nurse decides what should be done for a person. You do not make these decisions.
  - Review directions and the care plan with the nurse before going to the person.
  - Perform only those nursing tasks that you are trained to do.
  - Ask a nurse to supervise you if you are not comfortable performing a nursing task.
  - Perform only the nursing tasks that your state and job description allow.
- State laws and rules limit nursing assistant functions. State laws differ. Know what you can do in the state in which you are working.
- Role limits for nursing assistants are in Box 3-3(p 26), Role Limits, in the Textbook.
  - Never give drugs.
  - Never insert tubes or objects into body openings. Do not remove tubes from the body.

- Never take oral or telephone orders from doctors.
- Never tell the person or family the person's diagnosis or treatment plans.
- Never diagnose or prescribe treatments or drugs for anyone.
- Never supervise others, including other nursing assistants.
- Never ignore an order or request to do something. This includes nursing tasks that you can do, those you cannot do, and those that are beyond your legal limits.

Nursing Assistant Standards

- OBRA defines the basic range of functions for nursing assistants.
- All NATCEPs include those functions. Some states allow other functions.
- Review Box 3-4(p 27), Nursing Assistant Standards, in the Textbook.

Job Description and Job Titles

- Always obtain a written job description when you apply for a job. Do not take a job that requires you to:
  - Act beyond the legal limits of your role.
  - Function beyond your training limits.
  - Perform acts that are against your morals or religion.
- For job purposes, agencies often use other titles for nursing assistants who have completed a NATCEP and are on a state registry. Your job title depends on the setting and your roles and functions in the agency.

CHAPTER 3 REVIEW QUESTIONS

Circle the BEST answer.

1. Which question is a surveyor most likely to ask you about maintaining your clinical competency?
   a. Have you submitted your information to the nursing assistant registry?
   b. Have you ever allowed anyone to use your nursing assistant certificate?
   c. What kind of work did you do before you became a nursing assistant?
   d. How long have you been working for this agency?
2. A resident asks you about his or her medical condition. You
   a. Tell the nurse about the resident's request
   b. Give the resident a copy of the medical record
   c. Ignore the question and quickly change the subject
   d. Tell the resident that you are not allowed to talk about that
3. You answer the telephone. The family starts to give you medical information about the resident. You
   a. Write down the information and promptly give it to the doctor
   b. Politely give your name and title, ask the person to wait and promptly find the nurse
   c. Politely ask the family member to call back later or to call the doctor.
   d. Politely give the nurse's name and tell the family call later and ask for that nurse.

4. When should you refuse a task?
   a. The task is not in your job description.
   b. The task is within the legal limits of your role.
   c. The directions for the task are clear.
   d. A nurse is available for questions and supervision.

Answers to these questions are on p. 537.

CHAPTER 4 DELEGATION
Who Can Delegate
- Registered nurses (RNs) can delegate tasks to nursing assistants. In some states, licensed practical nurses/licensed vocational nurses (LPNs/LVNs) can delegate tasks to nursing assistants.
- An APRN can delegate to RNs, LPNs/LVNs, and nursing assistants.
- A nurse's delegation decisions must protect the person's health and safety. The delegating nurse is legally accountable to the person; accountable for delegation decisions; and accountable for safe and correct task completion.
- Nursing assistants cannot delegate. You cannot delegate any task to other nursing assistants or to any other worker.

The Delegation Process
- Delegation decisions must protect the person's health and safety.
- If you perform a task that places the person at risk, you may face serious legal problems.
- Step 1—Assessment and Planning. The nurse assesses the person's needs and then decides if it is safe to delegate the task.
- Step 2—Communication. The nurse must give clear and complete directions about the task and you must understand the directions to give safe care. After the task, you report and record the care that was given.
- Step 3—Surveillance and Supervision. The nurse observes the care you give and makes sure you complete the task correctly. The nurse must follow up on problems or concerns; e.g., you did not correctly perform the task or the person's condition has changed.
- Step 4—Evaluation and Feedback. The nurse decides if the delegation was successful by observing if the task was done correctly and the outcome and the person's response were as expected. The nurse should provide feedback to the nursing assistant about what was done correctly and what errors should be corrected.

The Five Rights of Delegation
- *The right task.* Is the task in your job description? Does your state allow you to do the task? Were you trained to do the task?
- *The right circumstances.* Do you have experience with the task given the person's condition and needs? Do you understand the purpose of the task? Can you safely perform the task? Do you have the equipment and supplies? Do you know how to use the equipment and supplies?

- *The right person.* Do you have the training and experience to perform the task safely? Do you have concerns about performing the task?
- *The right directions and communication.* Did the nurse give clear directions and instructions. Did the nurse allow questions and help you set priorities? Do you understand what the nurse expects?
- *The right supervision.* Is the nurse available to answer questions. Is the nurse available if the person's condition changes or if problems occur? Did the nurse evaluate the results?

Your Role in Delegation
- When you agree to perform a delegated task on a person, you must protect the person from harm. You are responsible for your own actions. You must complete the task safely. You must ask for help if you have questions or are unsure. Report to the nurse what you did and the observations you made.
- You should refuse to perform a task when:
  o The task is beyond the legal limits of your role.
  o The task is not in your job description.
  o You were not trained to do the task.
  o The task could harm the person.
  o The person's condition has changed.
  o You do not know how to use the supplies or equipment.
  o Directions are not ethical or legal.
  o Directions are against agency policies.
  o Directions are unclear or incomplete.
  o A nurse is not available for supervision.
- Never ignore an order or refuse a task because you do not like it or do not want to do it. Tell the nurse about your concerns.

CHAPTER 4 REVIEW QUESTIONS
Circle the BEST answer.
1. A nurse delegates a task that you did not learn in your training; however, the task is in your job description. Which response is best?
   a. "I must refuse, because I don't know how to do that task."
   b. "I did not learn that task in my training. Can you show me how to do it?"
   c. "I will ask the other nursing assistant to watch me do the task."
   d. "I will ask the other nursing assistant to do the task for me."
2. You are busy with a new resident. It is time for another resident's bath. What should you do first?
   a. Tell the nurse about the delay in the resident's bath
   b. Tell the resident that you will help him bathe later
   c. Delegate the bath to another nursing assistant.
   d. Ask another assistant to help you with the new resident
3. Which task should you refuse to do?
   a. Help another nursing assistant transfer a person
   b. Encourage residents to wake up and eat breakfast
   c. Take vitals signs for another nursing assistant
   d. Bathe a resident who appears to be very ill

Answers to these questions are on p. 537.

CHAPTER 5 ETHICS AND LAWS
Ethical Aspects
- Ethics is the knowledge of what is right conduct and wrong conduct. It also deals with choices or judgments about what should or should not be done. An ethical person does not cause a person harm.
- Ethical behavior involves not being prejudiced or biased. To be prejudiced or biased means to make judgments and have views before knowing the facts. You should not judge a person by your values and standards. Also, do not avoid persons whose standards and values differ from your own.
- Ethical problems involve making choices. You must decide what is the right thing to do.

Codes of Ethics
- Professional groups have codes of ethics. A **code of ethics** has rules, or standards of conduct, for group members to follow.
- Rules of conduct for nursing assistants can be found in Box 5-1(p 40), Code of Conduct for Nursing Assistants, in the Textbook.

Boundaries
- **Professional boundaries** separate helpful actions and behaviors from those that are not helpful.
- A **boundary crossing** is a brief act of over-involvement with the person in order to meet the person's needs, such as giving a crying patient a hug.
- A **boundary violation** is an act or behavior that meets your needs, not the person's. The act or behavior is unethical. Boundary violations include abuse, keeping secrets with a person, or giving a lot of personal information about yourself to another.
- **Professional sexual misconduct** is an act, behavior, or comment that is sexual in nature. It is sexual misconduct even if the person consents or makes the first move.
- To maintain professional boundaries, review Box 5-2(p 41), Professional Boundaries. Be alert to **boundary signs** (acts, behaviors, or thoughts that warn of a boundary crossing or violation).

Legal Aspects
- Ethics is about what you *should or should not do*. Laws tell you what you *can and cannot do*.
- **Negligence** is an unintentional wrong. The negligent person did not act in a reasonable and careful manner and the person or person's property was harmed. The person causing harm did not mean to cause harm.
- **Malpractice** is negligence by a professional person.
- You are legally responsible (liable) for your own actions. The nurse is liable as your supervisor.
- **Defamation** is injuring a person's name and reputation by making false statements to a third person. **Libel** is making false statements in print, writing (including e-mails and texts), or through pictures or drawings. **Slander** is making false statements orally. Never make false statements about a patient, resident, family member, co-worker, or any other person.

- **False imprisonment** is the unlawful restraint or restriction of a person's freedom of movement. It involves threatening to restrain a person, restraining a person, and preventing a person from leaving the agency.
- **Invasion of privacy** is violating a person's right not to have his or her name, photo, or private affairs exposed or made public without giving consent. Review Box 5-3(p 43), Protecting the Right to Privacy, in the Textbook.
- The Health Insurance Portability and Accountability Act (HIPAA) of 1996 protects the privacy and security of a person's health information. **Protected health information** refers to identifying information and information about the person's health care that is maintained or sent in any form (paper, electronic, oral). Direct any questions about the person or the person's care to the nurse.
- **Fraud** is saying or doing something to trick, fool, or deceive a person. The act is fraud if it does or could cause harm to a person or the person's property.
- **Assault** is intentionally attempting or threatening to touch a person's body without the person's consent. The person fears bodily harm.
- **Battery** is touching a person's body without his or her consent. Protect yourself from being accused of assault and battery. Explain to the person what you are going to do and get the person's consent.

Wrongful Use of Electronic Communication
- Electronic communications include e-mail, text messages, faxes, websites, video sites, and social media sites. Video and social media sites include Facebook, Twitter, LinkedIn, YouTube, Instagram, Pinterest, blogs and comments to blog postings, chat rooms, bulletin boards, and so on.
- Wrongful use of electronic communications can result in job loss and loss of your certification (license, registration) for:
  - Defamation
  - Invasion of privacy
  - HIPAA violations
  - Violating the right to confidentiality
  - Patient or resident abuse
  - Unprofessional or unethical conduct

Informed Consent
- A person has the right to decide what will be done to his or her body and who can touch his or her body. Consent is informed when the person clearly understands all aspects of treatment.
- Persons who cannot give consent are persons who are under the legal age or are mentally incompetent. Unconscious, sedated, or confused persons cannot give consent. Informed consent is given by a responsible party—wife, husband, daughter, son, or legal representative.
- You are never responsible for obtaining written consent.

Reporting Abuse

- **Abuse** is
  - The willful infliction of injury, unreasonable confinement, intimidation, or punishment that results in physical harm, pain, or mental anguish. Intimidation means to make afraid with threats of force or violence.
  - Depriving the person (or the person's caregiver) of the goods or services needed to attain or maintain well-being.
- Abuse also includes involuntary seclusion.
- **Vulnerable adults** are persons 18 years old or older who have disabilities or conditions that make them at risk to be wounded, attacked, or damaged. They have problems caring for or protecting themselves due to:
  - A mental, emotional, physical, or developmental disability
  - Brain damage
  - Changes from aging
- All residents are vulnerable. Older persons and children are at risk for abuse.
- **Elder abuse** is any knowing, intentional, or negligent act by a caregiver or another person to an older adult. It may include physical abuse, neglect, verbal abuse, involuntary seclusion, financial exploitation or misappropriation, emotional or mental abuse, sexual abuse, or abandonment. Review Box 5-5(p 48), Signs of Elder Abuse, in the Textbook.
- Federal and state laws require the reporting of elder abuse.
- If you suspect a person is being abused, report your observations to the nurse.
- **Child abuse or neglect** is the intentional harm or mistreatment of a child under 18 years of age. It includes the failure of the parent or caregiver to act which creates immediate risk or results in death, serious physical or emotional harm, sexual abuse or exploitation. Review Box 5-7(p 51), Signs of Child Abuse and Neglect-Signs and Symptoms, in the Textbook.
- **Intimate partner violence is** physical violence, sexual violence, stalking, or psychological aggression by a current or former partner. Review Box 5-8(p 53), Intimate Partner Violence in the Textbook.

CHAPTER 5 REVIEW QUESTIONS

Circle the BEST answer.

1. A resident offers you a gift certificate for being kind to her. You should
   a. Say "thank you for thinking of me" and accept the gift
   b. Ask the nurse what you should do about the gift
   c. Thank the resident and explain that you cannot accept gifts
   d. Accept the gift and ask the resident not to mention it to anyone

2. Which action violates the person's privacy?
   a. Texting about the person's condition to his family member
   b. Discussing the person's treatment with the supervising nurse
   c. Reading the content of the person's mail aloud at his request
   d. Allowing the person to visit with others with the door closed

3. What should you do if you suspect an older person is being abused?
   a. Report the situation to the health department.
   b. Notify the nurse and discuss the observations with him or her.
   c. Notify the doctor about the suspected abuse.
   d. Ask the family why they are abusing the person.

4. A resident needs help going to the bathroom. You do not answer her call light promptly. She gets up without help, falls, and breaks a leg. This is an example of
   a. Negligence
   b. Defamation
   c. False imprisonment
   d. Slander

5. Which member of the health care team has committed defamation?
   a. Nurse implies that a physical therapist uses drugs
   b. Doctor tells the nurse that the patient has a mental illness
   c. Nursing assistant reports seeing a person steal money from a patient
   d. Dietician tells the patient that she needs to lose some weight.

6. Which advice would you give another nursing assistant who tells you that she is a victim of intimate partner violence?
   a. Report the circumstances and violent events to the supervising nurse
   b. Get to a safe place and never speak or interact with the violent partner
   c. Go to a doctor and have injuries checked and documented.
   d. Call the police and report everything that happened including injuries.

7. Which circumstance is false imprisonment?
   a. You gently tell a resident that you will restrain him if he continues to take his roommate's belongings.
   b. You restrain a resident according to the doctor's order and follow the RN's instructions for giving care.
   c. You tell the resident that the bathroom door must be slightly open, so that you can maintain his safety.
   d. You prevent a resident who has dementia and wandering behaviors from going outside by himself.

8. To protect yourself from being accused of assault and battery, what you should you do before touching the person?
   a. Always be polite and consider the other person's needs
   b. Explain to the resident what you plan to do and get consent.
   c. Ask the nurse to verify the goals of care and the tasks to be done
   d. Review the steps of the procedure and then follow through

Answers to these questions are on p. 537.

CHAPTER 6 STUDENT AND WORK ETHICS

- **Professionalism** involves following laws, being ethical, having good work ethics, and having the skills to do your work.
- **Work ethics** deals with behavior in the workplace. Work ethics also applies to students in nursing assistant training and competency evaluation programs (NATCEPs).
- To be a successful student, practice good work ethics in the classroom and clinical setting and in your relationships with instructors and fellow students.

Health, Hygiene, and Appearance

- To give safe and effective care, you must be physically and mentally healthy. You need a balanced diet, sleep and rest, good body mechanics, and exercise on a regular basis. Smoking, drugs, and alcohol can affect performance and safety.
- Personal hygiene needs careful attention. Bathe daily, use deodorant or antiperspirant, and brush your teeth often. Shampoo often. Keep fingernails clean, short, and neatly shaped.
- Review Box 6-1(p 59), Professional Appearance, in the Textbook.

Teamwork

- Practice good work ethics—work when scheduled, be cheerful and friendly, perform delegated tasks, be kind to others, and be available to help others.
- Be ready to work when your shift starts. Arrive on your nursing unit a few minutes early. Stay the entire shift. When it is time to leave, report off duty to the nurse.
- Gossiping is unprofessional and hurtful. To avoid being a part of gossip:
  - Remove yourself from where people are gossiping.
  - Do not make or repeat any comment that can hurt another person or the agency.
  - Do not make or write false statements about another person.
  - Do not talk about residents, family members, patients, visitors, co-workers, or the agency at home or in social settings.
- **Confidentiality** means trusting others with personal and private information. The person's information is shared only among staff involved in his or her care. Agency, family, and co-worker and student information is also confidential.
- Your speech and language must be professional.
  - Do not swear or use foul, vulgar, or abusive language.
  - Do not use slang.
  - Speak softly, gently, and clearly.
  - Do not shout or yell.
  - Do not fight or argue with a person, family member, visitor, or co-worker.
- A courtesy is a polite, considerate, or helpful comment or act.
  - Address others by Miss, Mrs., Ms., Mr., or Doctor. Use the name that the person prefers

  - Say "please" and "thank you." Say "I'm sorry" when you make a mistake or hurt someone.
  - Let residents, families, and visitors enter elevators first.
  - Be thoughtful—compliment others, give praise.
  - Wish the person and family well when they leave the center.
  - Hold doors open for others.
  - Help others willingly when asked.
  - Do not take credit for another person's deeds. Give the person credit for the action.
- Keep personal matters out of the workplace.
  - Make personal phone calls during meals and breaks.
  - Do not let family and friends visit you on the unit.
  - Do not use the agency's computers and other equipment for personal use.
  - Do not take agency supplies for personal use.
  - Do not discuss personal problems at work.
  - Control your emotions.
  - Do not borrow money from or lend money to co-workers.
  - Do not sell things or engage in fund-raising at work.
  - Do not have wireless phones or personal pagers on while at work.
  - Do not text message.
- Leave for and return from breaks and meals on time. Tell the nurse when you leave and return to the unit.
- Protect yourself and others from harm.
  - Understand the roles, functions, and responsibilities in your job description.
  - Follow agency rules, policies, and procedures in the employee handbook or policy and procedure manual.
  - Know what is right and wrong conduct and what you can and cannot do.
  - Follow the nurse's directions and instructions and question unclear directions and things you do not understand. Ask for any training you might need.
  - Help others willingly when asked.
  - Report accurately. This includes measurements, observations, the care given, the person's complaints, and any errors.
  - Accept responsibility for your actions. Admit when you are wrong or make mistakes. Do not blame others. Do not make excuses for your actions. Learn what you did wrong and why. Always try to learn from your mistakes.
  - Handle the person's property carefully and prevent damage.
  - Always follow safety measures.
- Planning your work involves setting priorities. Decide:
  - Which person has the greatest or most life-threatening needs.
  - What task the nurse or person needs done first.
  - What tasks need to be done at a certain time.
  - What tasks need to be done when your shift starts.
  - What tasks need to be done at the end of your shift.
  - How much time it takes to complete a task.
  - How much help you need to complete a task.
  - Who can help you and when.
- Priorities change as the person's needs change.

Managing Stress

- These guidelines can help you reduce or cope with stress.
  - Exercise regularly.
  - Get enough sleep or rest.
  - Eat healthy.
  - Plan personal and quiet time for yourself.
  - Use common sense about what you can do.
  - Do one thing at a time.
  - Do not judge yourself harshly.
  - Give yourself praise.
  - Have a sense of humor.
  - Talk to the nurse if your work or a person is causing too much stress.
- Conflict in the workplace can cause stress and care can be compromised. Resolving conflict involves 6 steps: 1) define the problem, 2) collect information about the problem, 3) identify possible solutions, 4) carry out the best solution, and 6) evaluate the results.
- Communication and good work ethics help prevent and resolve conflicts.
- **Burnout** is a job stress resulting in physical or mental exhaustion and doubts about your abilities or the value of your work. Managing stress can prevent burnout.

Harassment

- **Harassment** means to trouble, torment, offend, or worry a person by one's behavior or comments.
- Harassment is illegal: it can be sexual or it can involve age, race, ethnic background, religion, or disability.
- You must respect others. Do not offend others by your gestures, remarks, or use of touch. Do not offend others with jokes, photos, or other pictures.

CHAPTER 6 REVIEW QUESTIONS

Circle the BEST answer.

1. Which member of the health care team is demonstrating good work ethics?
   a. Nurse works when scheduled, but never works extra shifts.
   b. Nursing assistant is consistently cheerful and friendly.
   c. Nurse declines to assist others to complete their tasks.
   d. Nursing assistant refuses to do tasks that are not assigned

2. A nursing assistant is gossiping about a co-worker. You should
   a. Listen but do not contribute or comment
   b. Discuss the gossipers with a trusted co-worker
   c. Remove yourself from where gossip is occurring
   d. Repeat the comment to trusted co-workers

3. Which health care team member has failed to maintain confidentiality about others?
   a. Nurse talks about a patient's diagnosis with a friend of the patient's family.
   b. Nursing assistant never talks about patients in the elevator, hallway, or dining area.
   c. Physician discusses the diagnosis and treatment with the patient and his wife.
   d. Nursing assistant walks away when encountering people in a private conversation.

4. Which nursing assistant is using professional speech and language?
   a. Nursing Assistant A swears when she accidentally drops a patient's food tray on the floor, "Darn it!"
   b. Nursing Assistant B shouts, "I know you can't hear me, but I am here to help you get out of bed!"
   c. Nursing Assistant C loudly says, "You can't see your mother right now, she didn't sleep well last night."
   d. Nursing Assistant D clearly and softly says, "Mr. Smith, I am going to help you with your bath."

5. Which behavior contributes to your personal health?
   a. Eating a balanced meal before going to the clinical setting
   b. Sleeping and napping whenever you have the time.
   c. Exercising to build strength to independently lift patients
   d. Drinking alcohol and socializing to relax and unwind.

6. Which student is correctly using the phone to attend to personal matters?
   a. Tells instructor that cell phone is on for family emergencies
   b. Makes personal cell phone calls during meal or break time
   c. Turns cell phone on to silent and discretely carries it in a pocket
   d. Uses cell phone only to text and connect to the Internet

Answers to these questions are on p. 537.

CHAPTER 7 COMMUNICATING WITH THE PERSON

Caring for the Person

- The whole person needs to be considered when you provide care—physical, social, psychological, and spiritual parts. These parts are woven together and cannot be separated.
- Follow these rules to address persons with dignity and respect.
  - Call persons by their titles—Mrs. Dennison, Mr. Smith, Miss Turner, or Dr. Gonzalez.
  - Do not call persons by their first names unless they ask you to.
  - Do not call persons by any other name unless they ask you to.
  - Do not call persons Grandma, Papa, Sweetheart, Honey, or other names.

Basic Needs

- A **need** is something necessary or desired for maintaining life and mental well-being.
- According to Maslow, basic needs must be met for a person to survive and function. Needs are arranged in order of importance, lower level to higher level.
  - *Physiological or physical needs*—are required for life. They are oxygen, food, water, elimination, rest, and shelter.
  - *Safety and security needs*—relate to feeling safe from harm, danger, and fear.

o *Love and belonging needs*—relate to love, closeness, affection, and meaningful relationships with others. Family, friends, and the health team can meet love and belonging needs.
o *Self-esteem needs*—relate to thinking well of oneself and to seeing oneself as useful and having value. People often lack self-esteem when ill, injured, older, or disabled.
o *The need for self-actualization*—involves learning, understanding, and creating to the limit of a person's capacity. Rarely, if ever, is it totally met.

Culture and Religion

- **Culture** is the characteristics of a group of people. People come from many cultures, races, and nationalities. Family practices, food choices, hygiene habits, clothing styles, and language are part of their culture. The person's culture also influences health beliefs and practices.
- **Religion** relates to spiritual beliefs, needs, and practices. A person's religion influences health and illness practices. Many may want to pray and observe religious practices. Assist residents to attend religious services as needed. If a person wants to see a spiritual leader or adviser, tell the nurse. Provide privacy during the visit.
- A person may not follow all the beliefs and practices of his or her culture or religion. Some people do not practice a religion.
- Respect and accept the person's culture and religion. Learn about practices and beliefs different from your own. Do not judge a person by your own standards.

Communicating With the Person

- For effective communication between you and the person, you must:
  o Understand and respect the patient or resident as a person.
  o View the person as a physical, psychological, social, and spiritual human being.
  o Appreciate the person's problems and frustrations.
  o Respect the person's rights.
  o Respect the person's religion and culture.
  o Give the person time to understand the information that you give.
  o Repeat information as often as needed.
  o Ask questions to see if the person understood you.
  o Be patient. People with memory problems may ask the same question many times.
  o Include the person in conversations when others are present.

Verbal Communication

- When talking with a person, follow these rules.
  o Face the person. Look directly at the person.
  o Position yourself at the person's eye level.
  o Control the loudness and tone of your voice.
  o Speak clearly, slowly, and distinctly.
  o Do not use slang or vulgar words.

  o Repeat information as needed.
  o Ask one question at a time and wait for an answer.
  o Do not shout, whisper, or mumble.
  o Be kind, courteous, and friendly.
- Use written words if the person cannot speak or hear but can read. Keep written messages brief and concise. Use a black felt pen on white paper and print in large letters.
- Some persons cannot speak or read. Ask questions that have "yes" or "no" answers. A picture board may be helpful.

Nonverbal Communication

- Gestures, facial expressions, posture, body movements, touch, and smell are used to convey messages. Nonverbal messages more accurately reflect a person's feelings than words do. A person may say one thing but act another way. Watch the person's eyes, hand movements, gestures, posture, and other actions.
- Touch conveys comfort, caring, love, affection, interest, trust, concern, and reassurance. Touch should be gentle. Touch means different things to different people. Some people do not like to be touched. To use touch, follow the care plan. Maintain professional boundaries.
- People send messages through their **body language**—facial expressions, gestures, posture, hand and body movements, gait, eye contact, and appearance. Your body language should show interest, enthusiasm, caring, and respect for the person. Often you need to control your body language. Control reactions to odors from body fluids, secretions, or excretions.

Communication Methods

- *Listening* means to focus on verbal and nonverbal communication. You use sight, hearing, touch, and smell. To be a good listener:
  o Face the person.
  o Have good eye contact with the person.
  o Lean toward the person. Do not sit back with your arms crossed.
  o Respond to the person. Nod your head and ask questions.
  o Avoid communication barriers.
- *Paraphrasing* is re-stating the person's message in your own words.
- *Direct questions* focus on certain information. You ask the person something you need to know.
- *Open-ended questions* lead or invite the person to share thoughts, feelings, or ideas. The person chooses what to talk about.
- *Clarifying* lets you make sure that you understand the message. You can ask the person to repeat the message, say you do not understand, or re-state the message.
- *Focusing* deals with a certain topic. It is useful when a person wanders in thought.
- *Silence* is a very powerful way to communicate. Silence gives time to think, organize thoughts, choose words, and gain control. Silence on your part shows caring and respect for the person's situation and feelings.

Communication Barriers

- *Language.* You and the person must use and understand the same language.
- *Cultural differences.* A person from another country may attach different meanings to verbal and nonverbal communication than what you intended.
- *Changing the subject.* Someone changes the subject when the topic is uncomfortable
- *Giving your opinions.* Opinions involve judging values, behaviors, or feelings. Let others express feelings and concerns without adding your opinion. Do not make judgments or jump to conclusions.
- *Talking a lot when others are silent.* Talking too much is usually because of nervousness and discomfort with silence.
- *Failure to listen.* Do not pretend to listen. It shows lack of caring and interest. You may miss complaints of pain, discomfort, or other symptoms that you must report to the nurse.
- *Pat answers.* "Don't worry." "Everything will be okay." These make the person feel that you do not care about his or her concerns, feelings, and fears.
- *Illness and disability.* Speech, hearing, vision, cognitive function, and body movements may be affected. Verbal and nonverbal communication is affected.
- *Age.* Values and communication styles vary among age-groups.

Persons With Special Needs

- Common courtesies and manners apply to any person with a disability. Review Box 7-2(p 81), Disability Etiquette, in the Textbook.
- The person who is comatose is unconscious and cannot respond to others. Often the person can hear and feel touch and pain. Assume that the person hears and understands you. Use touch and give care gently. Practice these measures.
  - Knock before entering the person's room.
  - Tell the person your name, the time, and the place every time you enter the room.
  - Give care on the same schedule every day.
  - Explain what you are going to do.
  - Tell the person when you are finishing care.
  - Use touch to communicate care, concern, and comfort.
  - Tell the person what time you will be back to check on him or her.
  - Tell the person when you are leaving the room.

Family and Friends

- If you need to give care when visitors are there, protect the person's right to privacy. Politely ask the visitors to leave the room when you give care. A partner or family member may help you if the patient or resident consents.
- Treat family and visitors with courtesy and respect.
- Do not discuss the person's condition with family and friends. Refer questions to the nurse. A visitor may upset or tire a person. Report your observations to the nurse.

Behavior Issues

- Many people do not adjust well to illness, injury, and disability. They have some of the following behaviors.
  - *Anger.* Verbal outbursts, shouting, and rapid speech are common. Some people are silent. Others are uncooperative. Nonverbal signs include rapid movements, pacing, clenched fists, and a red face. Glaring and getting close to you when speaking are other signs. Violent behaviors can occur.
  - *Demanding behavior.* Nothing seems to please the person. The person is critical of others.
  - *Self-centered behavior.* The person cares only about his or her own needs. The needs of others are ignored. The person becomes impatient if needs are not met.
  - *Aggressive behavior.* The person may swear, bite, hit, pinch, scratch, or kick. Protect the person, others, and yourself from harm.
  - *Withdrawal.* The person has little or no contact with family, friends, and staff. Some people are generally not social and prefer to be alone.
  - *Inappropriate sexual behavior.* Some people make inappropriate sexual remarks or touch others in the wrong way. These behaviors may be on purpose. Or they are caused by disease, confusion, dementia, or drug side effects.
- You cannot avoid persons with unpleasant behaviors, but you can learn ways to respond. Review Box 7-3(p 83), Dealing With Behavior Issues, in the Textbook.

CHAPTER 7 REVIEW QUESTIONS

Circle the BEST answer.

1. Which circumstance is the best example of providing holistic care?
   a. You cheerfully talk to the resident while helping him with morning hygiene and eating breakfast.
   b. You remind the resident to wear his hearing aid so that he can join others and sing at church service.
   c. You respectfully listen to the resident explain how he needs to prepare for his morning bath.
   d. You assist the resident to go to the chapel and quietly wait for him to finish his morning prays.

2. Which method would you use to address the residents in a long-term care center?
   a. Be friendly, cheerful and polite and use correct pronouns: you, he, she
   b. Use terms of endearment, (Honey, Dear) to show affection
   c. Call everyone by their first name to create a casual atmosphere
   d. Use title and surname, unless the resident prefers something else

3. Based on Maslow's theory of basic needs, which person's needs must be met first?
   a. The person who wants to talk about her grandson
   b. The person who wants to leave the dining room
   c. The person who wants mail sorted and opened
   d. The person who needs assistance to drink more water

4. What is the best strategy when caring for people who have a variety of different cultural backgrounds?
   a. Expect that people from different cultures will follow the doctor's advice.
   b. Give excellent care, because people from all cultures expect good service.
   c. Disregard the person's culture because other care issues are more important.
   d. Learn about other cultures, because culture affects health beliefs and practices.
5. What is your responsibility in relation to a person's religion and spiritual beliefs?
   a. You ask the person how religion influences his health practices.
   b. You assist a person to attend religious services in the nursing center.
   c. You advise the person to find comfort from religion during illness.
   d. You follow and agree with all the beliefs of the person's religion.
6. A person is angry and is shouting at you. What should you do first?
   a. Stay calm and professional
   b. Raise your voice so the person can hear you
   c. Instruct the person to stop yelling
   d. Ask the nurse to deal with the person
7. A person tries to scratch and kick you. You should
   a. Protect yourself from harm
   b. Firmly, but gently hold him down
   c. Leave until the person calms down
   d. Refuse to care for the person
8. Which nursing assistant is using poor communication skills?
   a. Nursing Assistant A positions self at the person's eye level.
   b. Nursing Assistant B speaks slowly, clearly, and distinctly.
   c. Nursing Assistant C speaks as she walks away from person.
   d. Nursing Assistant D asks one question at a time
9. Which nursing assistant is using good listening behavior?
   a. Nursing Assistant A starts talking before the person is finished.
   b. Nursing Assistant B is texting while the person is talking
   c. Nursing Assistant C leans slightly toward the person who is talking.
   d. Nursing Assistant D slouches and crosses arms as the person talks.
10. In which circumstance would you use silence?
    a. You are irritated, because someone has insulted you.
    b. The person wants to share happy news with everyone.
    c. You don't know the answer to the person's question.
    d. The person is upset and needs to gain control.
11. Which nursing assistant needs additional reminders to properly communicate with a person who speaks a foreign language?
    a. Nursing Assistant A says, "Sir, please sit down."
    b. Nursing Assistant B points to a picture of a comb.

c. Nursing Assistant C shouts, "I am here to help you."
   d. Nursing Assistant D repeats the message in a different way
12. When caring for a person who is comatose, which action would you perform?
    a. Talk about normal events that are happening around the unit
    b. Do not say anything, because the person cannot understand
    c. Use touch to communicate care, comfort and concern
    d. Work quickly and quietly to avoid extra stimulation
13. When a person is in a wheelchair, which action would you perform?
    a. Lean on arm rests of the wheelchair while talking to the person
    b. Sit or squat to talk to a person in a wheelchair or chair
    c. Announce obstacles as you push the person in a wheelchair
    d. A friendly pat on the head encourages a person in a wheelchair
14. A person's daughter is visiting and you need to provide care to the person. You
    a. Do any care that doesn't expose the body
    b. Politely ask the daughter to leave the room
    c. Defer the care until the next day
    d. Invite the daughter to help with the care
Answers to these questions are on p. 537.

CHAPTER 8 HEALTH TEAM COMMUNICATIONS
Communication
- For good communication:
  o Use words that mean the same thing to you and the receiver of the message.
  o If you do not know a term, ask what it means
  o Be brief and concise.
  o Give information in a logical and orderly manner.
  o Give facts and be specific.

The Medical Record
- The **medical record, chart, or clinical record** is the permanent, legal account of the person's condition and response to treatment and care. Medical records can be written or stored electronically. The electronic health record (EHR) or electronic medical record (EMR) is the electronic version of the person's medical record. It is a permanent legal document.
- The medical record is a way for the health team to share information about the person. Agencies have policies about medical records and who can see them. Some agencies allow nursing assistants to read and/or record observations in medical records. Follow your agency's policies.
- Medical records can include the person's admission record, advanced directives, health history, graphic

and flow sheets for recording measurements and observations, diagnostic reports and progress reports. See Table 8-1(p 88), Parts of the Medical Record, in the Textbook for additional information.

- The Kardex or care summary is a summary of the person's medical record. The summary can be electronic or on paper as a card file.
- The **nursing process** is the method nurses use to plan and deliver nursing care. It has 5 steps: assessment, nursing diagnosis, planning, implementation, and evaluation.
- **Assessment** involves collecting information about the person. A health history is taken. A registered nurse (RN) assesses the person's body systems and mental systems. Although the nursing assistant does not assess, you play a key role in assessment. You make many observations as you give care and talk to the person.
- **Observation** is using the senses of sight, hearing, touch, and smell to collect information.
- Basic observations are outlined in Box 8-3(p 92), Basic Observations in the Textbook. See Box 8-2(p 91), Observations to Report at Once, in the Textbook):
  - A change in the person's ability to respond
  - A change in the person's mobility
  - Complaints of sudden, severe pain
  - A sore or reddened area on the person's skin
  - Complaints of a sudden change in vision
  - Complaints of pain or difficulty breathing
  - Abnormal respirations
  - Complaints of or signs of difficulty swallowing
  - Vomiting
  - Bleeding
  - Dizziness
  - Vital signs outside the normal ranges
- **Objective data (signs)** are seen, heard, felt, or smelled by an observer. For example, you can feel a pulse.
- **Subjective data (symptoms)** are things a person tells you about that you cannot observe through your senses. For example, you cannot see the person's nausea.
- The nurse uses assessment data to form a **nursing diagnosis,** or a health problem that can be treated by nursing measures.
- The nurse will then conduct **planning** to set priorities and goals for the person's care.
- **Nursing interventions** or **implementations** are the actions taken by the nursing team to help the person reach a goal.
- The nursing diagnoses, goals, and actions for each goal are recorded in the **nursing care plan.** The care plan is a communication tool. Each agency has a care plan tool.
- The RN may conduct a care conference with the health care team to share information and ideas about the person's care.
- The nurse will **evaluate** the planning and implementation based on the person's progress toward the stated goal.
- The nurse may delegate tasks to the nursing assistant via the assignment sheet during any step of the nursing process.

Reporting and Recording

- The health team communicates by reporting and recording.

Reporting

- You report care and observations to the nurse. Report to the nurse:
  - Whenever there is a change from normal or a change in the person's condition. Report these changes at once.
  - When the nurse asks you to do so.
  - When you leave the unit for meals, breaks, or other reasons.
  - Before the end-of-shift report.
- Follow the rules of reporting.
  - Be prompt, thorough, and accurate.
  - Give the person's name and room and bed numbers.
  - Give the time your observations were made or the care was given.
  - Report only what you observed or did yourself.
  - Report care measures that you expect the person to need.
  - Report expected changes in the person's condition.
  - Give reports as often as the person's condition requires or when the nurse asks you to.
  - Report any changes from normal or changes in the person's condition at once.
  - Use your written notes to give a specific, concise, and clear report.

Recording

- When recording or documenting, communicate clearly and thoroughly what you observed, what you did, and the person's response.
- The general rules for recording are:
  - Always use ink. Use the color required by the center.
  - Include the date and time for every recording.
  - Make sure writing is readable and neat.
  - Use only agency-approved abbreviations.
  - Use correct spelling, grammar, and punctuation.
  - Do not use ditto marks.
  - Never erase or use correction fluid. Follow agency procedure for correcting errors.
  - Sign all entries with your name and title as required by agency policy.
  - Do not skip lines.
  - Make sure each form has the person's name and other identifying information.
  - Record only what you observed and did yourself.
  - Never chart a procedure, treatment, or care measure until after it is completed.
  - Be accurate, concise, and factual. Do not record judgments or interpretations.
  - Record in a logical and sequential manner.
  - Be descriptive. Avoid terms with more than one meaning.
  - Use the person's exact words whenever possible. Use quotation marks to show that the statement is a direct quote.
  - Chart any changes from normal or changes in the person's condition. Also chart that you informed the

nurse (include the nurse's name), what you told the nurse, and the time you made the report.
- o Do not omit information.
- o Record safety measures. Example: Reminding a person not to get out of bed.
- Review the 24-hour clock, Figure 8-8(p 96), and Box 8-5(p 96), 24-Hour Clock.
- Review Box 8-6(p 97), Rules for Reporting and Box 8-7(p 99), Rules for Recording

Computers and Other Electronic Devices
- Computers contain vast amounts of information about a person. Therefore the right to privacy must be protected. If allowed access, you must follow the agency's policies.
- Review Box 8-8(p 101), Electronic Devices, in the Textbook.

Phone Communications
- Guidelines for answering phones:
  - o Answer the call after the first ring if possible.
  - o Do not answer the phone in a rushed or hasty manner.
  - o Give a courteous greeting. Identify the nursing unit and your name and title.
  - o When taking a message, write down the caller's name, phone number (with area code and extension), date and time, and who the message is for.
  - o Repeat the message and phone number back to the caller.
  - o Ask the caller to "Please hold" if necessary.
  - o Do not lay the phone down or cover the receiver with your hand when not speaking to the caller. The caller may hear confidential information.
  - o Return to a caller on hold within 30 seconds.
  - o Do not give confidential information to any caller.
  - o Transfer a call if appropriate. Tell the caller you are going to transfer the call. Give the name and phone number in case the call gets disconnected or the line is busy.
  - o End the conversation politely.
  - o Give the message to the appropriate person.

CHAPTER 8 REVIEW QUESTIONS
Circle the BEST answer.
1. Which nursing assistant needs a reminder about the rules of good communication?
   a. Nursing Assistant A uses words with more than one meaning.
   b. Nursing Assistant B use words that are familiar to the person.
   c. Nursing Assistant C gives facts in a brief and concise manner.
   d. Nursing Assistant D gives information in a logical and orderly manner.
2. Which recording reflects application of the rules of recording?
   a. Morning care was provided by another nursing assistant
   b. Resident felt sad and depressed after the visitor left.
   c. Resident had abdomain pane; nurse A was advised
   d. 1200: Resident ate 75% of meal and drank 300 mL of milk

3. Which report to the nurse correctly incorporates the rules for reporting?
   a. Room 102 is asking for pain medication and a sedative
   b. Mr. Smith was having problems breathing about an hour ago.
   c. Mrs. Jones refused to shower, but she washed her face and hands.
   d. Sorry, I forgot to tell you I was going on break; my son called me.
4. Which observations needs to be reported at once?
   a. Person has a bad taste in his mouth.
   b. Person passed a large amount of brown stool.
   c. Person has a reddened area on lower back.
   d. Person independently accomplished his hygiene.
5. Which data is subjective?
   a. The person has pain in his abdomen
   b. The person's pulse is 76
   c. The person's urine is dark amber
   d. The person's breath has an odor

Answers to these questions are on p. 537.

CHAPTER 9 MEDICAL TERMINOLOGY
Medical Terminology and Abbreviations
- Medical terminology and abbreviations are used in health care. Someone may use a word or phrase that you do not understand. If so, ask the nurse to explain its meaning.
- Review Table 9-1(p 105), Word Elements, and Table 9-4(p 110), Common Health Care Terms and Phrases, in the Textbook.
- Use only the abbreviations accepted by the center. If you are not sure that an abbreviation is acceptable, write the term out in full. See the inside back cover of the Textbook for common abbreviations.

CHAPTER 9 REVIEW QUESTIONS
Circle the BEST answer.
1. If a child has a severe sunburn on the posterior surface of the body, you would be extra gentle when you washed the
   a. Face and neck
   b. Back and buttocks
   c. Hands and feet
   d. Top of the head
2. Which term best describes the location of the xiphoid process?
   a. Lateral chest
   b. Proximal to neck
   c. Medial chest
   d. Distal to abdomen
3. You are assigned to care for four patients. Which person is going to require the most time to complete care?
   a. Patient A needs to be NPO after midnight
   b. Patient B requires total assistance with ADLs
   c. Patient C requires VS q 4 hours
   d. Patient D has a UTI and needs I& O

CHAPTER 11 GROWTH AND DEVELOPMENT

- **Growth** is the physical changes that are measured and that occur in a steady and orderly manner.
- **Development** relates to changes in mental, emotional, and social function.
- Growth and development occur in a sequence, order, and pattern. Review the stages of growth and development detailed in the Textbook.
- Middle adulthood (40 to 65 years old). At this stage, developmental tasks are adjusting to physical changes, having grown children, developing leisure-time activities, and adjusting to aging parents.
- Late adulthood (65 years and older). At this stage, developmental tasks are adjusting to decreased strength and loss of health, adjusting to retirement and reduced income, coping with a partner's death, developing new friends and relationships, and preparing for one's own death.

CHAPTER 11 REVIEW QUESTIONS

Circle the BEST answer.

1. Based on the principle of growth and development "simple to complex", which activity would you expect a baby to display first?
   a. Running
   b. Walking
   c. Standing
   d. Sitting
2. During your weekly home visits to an elderly person, you notice that a 3-month old grandchild is alert, but not cooing, smiling or interacting with others. Which action would you take?
   a. Ask the primary caregiver if the baby is ill or tired
   b. Report your observation to the supervising nurse
   c. Do nothing, the baby is not your responsibility
   d. Try smiling, playing and stimulating the baby
3. What is a developmental task of late adulthood?
   a. Accepting changes in appearance
   b. Adjusting to decreased strength
   c. Developing a satisfactory sex life
   d. Performing self-care

Answers to these questions are on p. 537.

CHAPTER 12 THE OLDER PERSON

- Aging is normal. Normal changes occur in body structure and function. Psychological and social changes also occur. The risk for illness or injury increases with aging.

Psychological and Social Changes

- Physical reminders of growing old affect self-esteem and may threaten self-image, self-worth, and independence.
- People adjust to aging in their own way. How they cope depends on their health status, life experiences, finances, education, and social support systems.

- *Retirement.* Many people enjoy retirement. Others are in poor health and have medical bills that can make retirement difficult.
- *Reduced income.* Retirement usually means reduced income. Reduced income may force life-style changes. One example is the person avoids health care or needed drugs.
- *Social relationships.* Social relationships change throughout life. Companionship with people of the same age is important. Hobbies, religious and community events, and new friends provide enjoyment.
- *Children as caregivers.* Some older persons feel more secure when children care for them. Others feel unwanted and useless. Some lose dignity and self-respect. Tensions may occur among the child, parent, and other household members.
- *Death and grieving.* Death of an adult child or a partner can cause immense grief. Emotional needs will be great. The person may be left with few family and friends to provide support.

Physical Changes

- Body processes slow down. Energy level and body efficiency decline.
- *The integumentary system.* The skin loses its elasticity, strength, and fatty tissue layer. Wrinkles appear. Dry skin occurs and may cause itching. The skin is fragile and easily injured. The person is more sensitive to cold. Nails become thick and tough. White or gray hair is common. Hair thins. Facial hair may occur in women. Hair is drier.
- *The musculo-skeletal system.* Muscle and bone strength are lost. Bones become brittle and break easily. Vertebrae shorten. Joints become stiff and painful. Mobility decreases. There is a gradual loss of height.
- *The nervous system.* Confusion and dizziness may occur. Responses are slower. The risk for falls increases. Forgetfulness increases. Memory is shorter. Events from long ago are remembered better than recent ones. Older persons have a harder time falling asleep. Sleep periods are shorter. Older persons wake often during the night and have less deep sleep. Less sleep is needed. They may rest or nap during the day. They may go to bed early and get up early.
- *The senses.* Hearing and vision losses occur. Taste and smell dull. Touch and sensitivity to pain, and pressure are reduced.
- *The circulatory system.* The heart muscle weakens. Arteries narrow and are less elastic.
- Fatigue occurs. Poor circulation occurs in many body parts.
- *The respiratory system.* Respiratory muscles weaken. Lung tissue becomes less elastic. Difficult, or labored breathing may occur with activity. The person may lack strength to cough and clear the airway of secretions.
- *The digestive system.* Less saliva is produced. The person may have difficulty swallowing (dysphagia). Appetite decreases. Indigestion may occur. Loss of teeth and ill-fitting dentures cause chewing problems and digestion problems. Flatulence and constipation can occur.

- *The urinary system.* Bladder muscles weaken. Urinary frequency or urgency may occur. Urinary tract infections are risks. Many older persons have to urinate at night. Urinary incontinence may occur. In men, the prostate gland enlarges. This may cause difficulty urinating or frequent urination.
- *The reproductive system.* In men, testosterone decreases. An erection takes longer. Orgasm is less forceful. Women experience menopause. Female hormones of estrogen and progesterone decrease. The uterus, vagina, and genitalia shrink (atrophy). Vaginal walls thin. There is vaginal dryness. Arousal takes longer. Orgasm is less intense.

Housing Options
- A person's home holds memories and it is a link to neighbors and communities and brings pride and self-esteem.
- Most older people live in their own homes. Others need help from family or community agencies. Review Box 12-2(p 150), In-Home and Community-Based Services, in the Textbook.

Nursing Centers
- The person needing nursing center care may suffer some or all of these losses.
  - Loss of identity as a productive member of a family and community
  - Loss of possessions—home, household items, car, and so on
  - Loss of independence
  - Loss of real-world experiences—shopping, traveling, cooking, driving, hobbies
  - Loss of health and mobility
- The person may feel useless, powerless, and hopeless. The health team helps the person cope with loss and improve quality of life. Treat the person with dignity and respect. Also practice good communication skills. Follow the care plan.

CHAPTER 12 REVIEW QUESTIONS
Circle the BEST answer.
1. Which nursing assistant is verbalizing a myth about aging and older people?
   a. Nursing Assistant A says, "Older people are always so lonely; nobody cares it's sad."
   b. Nursing Assistant B says, "Everybody occasionally forgets something; not just the elderly."
   c. Nursing Assistant C says, "My Grandma is crabby, but she was always unhappy."
   d. Nursing Assistant D says, "A small percentage of the elderly live in nursing centers."
2. In caring for an older person with changes in the integumentary system. Which care measure would you use?
   a. Assist the person to shower daily and use soap to remove body odor
   b. Keep the feet warm by using a heating pad on the lowest setting.

   c. Set the thermostat on a low setting and provide sweaters and socks
   d. Apply lotion and creams to prevent dryness of the skin and itching
3. To assist an older person who has changes of the musculo-skeletal system related to aging, which care measure will you perform?
   a. Assist with range-of-motion exercises as ordered.
   b. Encourage person to use stairs and jog to build muscles
   c. Tell the person to perform own care to maintain mobility
   d. Feed a diet that is high in calories for energy
4. For a person who has age-related changes of the nervous system, which behavior would you expect to observe?
   a. Person's speech is slurred
   b. Person may refuse to eat.
   c. Person may be forgetful.
   d. Person has trouble breathing
5. Which older person needs to have thickened liquids as a care measure for a change in the digestive system?
   a. Person has a decreased appetite
   b. Person has lost several teeth
   c. Person is having flatulence
   d. Person is having trouble swallowing
6. How will age-related changes of the urinary system impact the amount of time you will spend caring for and assisting this person?
   a. Person will have pain, and this will frequently need to be reported to the nurse.
   b. Person will need frequent vital signs that need to be recorded and reported
   c. Person will frequently use the call bell for assistance to go to the bathroom.
   d. Person will desire and need extra amounts of fluid especially in the evening.

Answers to these questions are on p. 537.

CHAPTER 13 SAFETY
Accident Risk Factors
- *Age.* Older persons and children are at risk for injuries.
- *Awareness of surroundings.* Confused or disoriented persons may not understand what is happening to them or around them.
- *Agitated and aggressive behaviors.* Pain, confusion, fear, and decreased awareness of surroundings can cause these behaviors.
- *Vision loss.* Persons can fall or trip over items. Some have problems reading labels on containers.
- *Hearing loss.* Persons may not hear warning signals or fire alarms and will not move to safety.
- *Impaired smell and touch.* Illness and aging affect smell and touch. The person may not detect smoke or gas or may be unaware of injury. Burns are a risk.
- *Impaired mobility.* Some diseases and injuries affect mobility. A person may recognize danger but be unable to move to safety. Some persons are paralyzed. Some persons cannot walk or propel wheelchairs.

- *Drugs*. Drugs have side effects. Reduced awareness, confusion, and disorientation can occur. Report behavior changes and the person's complaints.

Identifying the Person
- You must give the right care to the right person. To identify the person:
  - Compare identifying information on the assignment sheet or treatment card with that on the identification (ID) bracelet.
  - Call the person by name when checking the ID bracelet. Just calling the person by name is not enough to identify him or her. Confused, disoriented, drowsy, hard-of-hearing, or distracted persons may answer to any name.
- Use at least 2 identifiers. Agencies have different requirements. Some may require the person to state and spell his or her name and give a birth date. Others require using the person's ID number. Always follow agency policy.

Preventing Burns
- Smoking, spilled hot liquids, very hot water, and electrical devices are common causes of burns. See Box 13-1(p 161), Preventing Burns, in the Textbook for safety measures to prevent burns.

Preventing Poisoning
- Drugs and household products are common poisons. Poisoning in adults may be from carelessness, confusion, or poor vision when reading labels. To prevent poisoning:
  - Make sure patients and residents cannot reach hazardous materials.
  - Follow agency policy for storing personal care items.
- See Box 13-2(p 162), Preventing Poisoning, in the Textbook for safety measures to prevent poisoning.

Preventing Suffocation
- **Suffocation** is when breathing stops from the lack of oxygen. Death occurs if the person does not start breathing.
- To prevent suffocation, review Box 13-5(p 169), Preventing Suffocation, in the Textbook.

Choking
- Choking or foreign-body airway obstruction occurs when a foreign body (e.g. food or toy) obstructs the airway. Air cannot pass through the air passages into the lungs. The body does not get enough oxygen. This can lead to death.
- Choking often occurs during eating. A large, poorly chewed piece of meat is a common cause. Other common causes include laughing and talking while eating.
- With *mild airway obstruction*, some air moves in and out of the lungs. The person is conscious. Usually the person can speak. Often, forceful coughing can remove the object.
- With *severe airway obstruction*, the conscious person clutches at the throat—the "universal sign of choking." The person has difficulty breathing. Some persons cannot breathe, speak, or cough. The person appears pale and cyanotic (bluish color). Air does not move in and out of the lungs. If the obstruction is not removed, the person will die. Severe airway obstruction is an emergency.
- Use abdominal thrusts to relieve severe choking. Chest thrusts are used for very obese persons and pregnant women.
- Call for help when a person has an obstructed airway. Report and record what happened, what you did, and the person's response.

Preventing Equipment Accidents
- All equipment is unsafe if broken, not used correctly, or not working properly. Inspect all equipment before use. Review Box 13-7(p 175), Preventing Equipment Accidents, in the Textbook.

Hazardous Chemicals
- A hazardous chemical is any chemical in the workplace that can cause harm. Hazardous substances include latex, mercury, disinfectants, and cleaning agents.
- Hazardous substance containers must have a warning label. If a label is removed or damaged, do not use the substance. Take the container to the nurse. Do not leave the container unattended.
- Check the material safety data sheet (MSDS) before using a hazardous substance, cleaning up a leak or spill, or disposing of the substance. Tell the nurse about a leak or spill right away. Do not leave a leak or spill unattended. Review Box 13-8(p 177), Hazardous Chemical Safety Measures, in the Textbook.

Disasters
- A **disaster** is a sudden catastrophic event. The agency has procedures for disasters that could occur in your area. Follow them to keep patients, residents, visitors, staff, and yourself safe.
- Natural disasters include tornadoes, hurricanes, blizzards, earthquakes, volcanic eruptions, floods, and some fires.
- Human-made disasters include auto, bus, train, and airplane accidents. They also include fires, bombings, nuclear power plant accidents, gas or chemical leaks, explosions, and wars.
- Follow agency protocol for a bomb threat or if you find an item that looks or sounds strange.

Fire Safety
- Faulty electrical equipment and wiring, over-loaded electrical circuits, and smoking are major causes of fires.
- Safety measures are needed where oxygen is used and stored.
- Review Box 13-9(p 178), Fire Prevention Measures, in the Textbook.

- Know your center's policies and procedures for fire emergencies. Know where to find fire alarms, fire extinguishers, and emergency exits. Remember the word *RACE*.
  - o **R**—*rescue.* Rescue persons in immediate danger. Move them to a safe place.
  - o **A**—*alarm.* Sound the nearest fire alarm.
  - o **C**—*confine.* Close doors and windows. Turn off oxygen or electrical items.
  - o **E**—*extinguish.* Use a fire extinguisher on a small fire.
- Remember the word *PASS* for using a fire extinguisher.
  - o **P**—*pull* the safety pin.
  - o **A**—*aim* low. Aim at the base of the fire.
  - o **S**—*squeeze* the lever. This starts the stream of water.
  - o **S**—*sweep* back and forth. Sweep side to side at the base of the fire.
- Do not use elevators during a fire.

Elopement

- Elopement is when a resident leaves the agency without staff knowledge. The Centers for Medicare & Medicaid Services (CMS) requires that an agency's emergency prepardness plan address elopement.
- The agency must:
  - o Identify persons at risk for elopement.
  - o Monitor and supervise persons at risk.
  - o Address elopement in the person's care plan.
  - o Have a plan to find a missing patient or resident.

Workplace Violence

- **Workplace violence** is violent acts (including assault or threat of assault) directed toward persons at work or while on duty. Review Box 13-10(p 184), Workplace Violence—Safety Measures, in the Textbook.

CHAPTER 13 REVIEW QUESTIONS
Circle the BEST answer.

1. You see a water spill in the hallway. What will you do?
   a. Notify housekeeping to wipe up the spill.
   b. Wipe up the spill right away.
   c. Report the spill to the nurse.
   d. Ask all residents to walk around the spill.
2. An electrical outlet in a person's room does not work. What will you do?
   a. Tell the administrator about the problem.
   b. Tell the resident to avoid using the outlet.
   c. Put a "do not use" sign over the outlet.
   d. Follow the policy for reporting the problem.
3. Which resident has the greatest risk for accidents?
   a. Resident A walks with a cane
   b. Resident B uses a hearing aid
   c. Resident C is confused and agitated
   d. Resident D uses eyeglasses for reading
4. To prevent burns, which action would you take?
   a. For children, serve hot liquids in sippy cups
   b. Turn cold water on first; turn hot water off first
   c. Turn the heating pad to lowest setting during sleep
   d. Tell older people to stay indoors on sunny days

5. Which nursing assistant has performed an action that puts the person at risk for suffocation?
   a. Nursing Assistant A makes sure the person's dentures fit properly
   b. Nursing Assistant B checks the care plan before giving liquids
   c. Nursing Assistant C leaves the child alone in the bathtub
   d. Nursing Assistant D puts the person in a Fowler's position
6. Which person is showing signs of a severe airway obstruction?
   a. Person A says something is in his throat.
   b. Person B has wheezing and coughing.
   c. Person C is cyanotic and cannot speak.
   d. Person D is forcefully coughing.
7. The "universal sign of choking" is
   a. Clutching at the chest
   b. Clutching at the throat
   c. Not being able to talk
   d. Not being able to breathe
8. Which environment has been safely prepared for a resident who must use supplemental oxygen?
   a. NO SMOKING signs are placed on the resident's door and near the bed.
   b. Candles are arranged in a distant corner of the room.
   c. Wool blankets are used for warmth instead of heaters
   d. Smoking materials are stored with other personal property
9. You discover a fire in the nursing center. What is your first action?
   a. Rescue persons in immediate danger
   b. Sound the nearest fire alarm
   c. Close doors and turn off oxygen
   d. Use a fire extinguisher on a small fire
10. You must use a fire extinguisher to extinguish a small fire. Which action is incorrect?
    a. Pull the safety pin on the fire extinguisher
    b. Aim at the top of the flames
    c. Squeeze the lever to start the stream
    d. Sweep the stream back and forth

Answers to these questions are on p. 537.

CHAPTER 14 PREVENTING FALLS

- Falls are a leading cause of injuries and deaths among older persons. A history of falls increases the risk of falling again.
- Causes for falls are weakness and walking problems, poor lighting, cluttered floors, throw rugs, needing to use the bathroom, out-of-place furniture, wet and slippery floors, bathtubs, and showers. Review Box 14-1(p 192), Fall Risk Factors, in the Textbook.
- Agencies have fall prevention programs. Review Box 14-2(p 193) Preventing Falls, in the Textbook. The person's care plan also lists measures specific for the person.
- Position change alarms alert staff when the person is moving from the bed or chair.

Bed Rails

- A **bed rail** (*side rail*) is a device that serves as a guard or barrier along the side of the bed.
- The nurse and care plan tell you when to raise bed rails. They are needed by persons who are unconscious or sedated with drugs. Some confused and disoriented people need them. When bed rails are needed, always keep them up except when giving bedside nursing care.
- Bed rails present hazards. When bedrails are raised the person cannot get out of bed. He or she can fall when trying to climb over the rails. Or the person can get caught, trapped, entangled, or strangled.
- Bed rails are considered restraints if the person cannot get out of bed or lower them without help.
- Bedrails are only used for the treatment of medical symptoms. The need for bed rails is carefully noted in the person's medical record and the care plan. If a person uses bed rails, check the person often. Record when you checked the person and your observations.
- To prevent falls:
  - Never leave the person alone when the bed is raised.
  - Lower the bed to its lowest position after giving care.
  - If a person does not use bed rails and you need to raise the bed, ask a co-worker to stand on the far side of the bed to protect the person from falling.
  - If you raise the bed to give care, always raise the far bed rail if you are working alone.
  - Be sure the person who uses raised bed rails has access to items on the bedside stand and over-bed table. The call light and personal items should be within the person's reach.

Hand Rails and Grab Bars

- Hand rails give support to persons who are weak or unsteady when walking.
- Grab bars (safety bars) provide support for sitting down or getting up from a toilet. They also are used when standing in the shower and for getting in and out of the shower or tub.

Wheel Locks

- Bed wheels are locked at all times except when moving the bed.
- Wheelchair and stretcher wheels are locked when transferring a person.

Transfer/Gait Belts

- Use a **transfer belt (gait belt)** to support a person who is unsteady or disabled. Always follow the manufacturer's instructions. Apply the belt over clothing and under the breasts. The belt buckle is never positioned over the person's spine. Tighten the belt so it is snug. You should be able to slide your open, flat hand under the belt. Tuck the excess strap under the belt. Remove the belt after the procedure.
- Check with the nurse and care plan before using a transfer/gait belt if the person has:
  - A colostomy, ileostomy, gastrostomy, or urostomy
  - Chronic obstructive pulmonary disease
  - An abdominal wound, incision, or drainage tube
  - A chest wound, incision, or drainage tube
  - Monitoring equipment
  - A hernia
  - Other conditions or care equipment involving the chest or abdomen

The Falling Person

- If a person starts to fall, do not try to prevent the fall. You could injure yourself and the person. Ease the person to the floor and protect the person's head.
- Do not let the person get up before the nurse checks for injuries. An incident report is completed after all falls.

CHAPTER 14 REVIEW QUESTIONS
Circle the BEST answer.

1. You are giving home care to an older person. Which observation should be reported to the nurse as a risk for falls?
   a. Rooms are simply furnished.
   b. Kitchen items are hard to reach.
   c. There is a shower with safety bars.
   d. There is a narrow staircase with handrails
2. If a person needs to be observed as a fall prevention measure, what do you need to clarify with this nurse?
   a. When and where should the person receive meals
   b. How frequently does the person need to be checked.
   c. How long are visitors allowed to stay with person
   d. Is the color-code risk for fall band on the person.
3. A person selects his clothes and dresses himself. Which selection is unsafe?
   a. Slip-resistant footwear is worn.
   b. Long sleeve shirt is buttoned
   c. Pants are too long.
   d. Belt is fastened.
4. In which circumstance would it be correct to raise the bed rails?
   a. The nurse says that medical symptoms warrant the use of bed rails
   b. You hear in report that the person should be restrained as needed for safety.
   c. The person tries to hit you, while you are helping him with morning hygiene.
   d. The family asks you to raise the bed rails because the person might fall out of bed
5. Which nursing assistant is promoting safety and comfort during the use of a transfer/gait belt?
   a. Nursing Assistant A positions the quick release buckle at the person's back
   b. Nursing Assistant B asks the person to stand up to apply the belt around the waist.
   c. Nursing Assistant C applies the belt so that it hangs loosely outside the clothing
   d. Nursing Assistant D lets the excess strap dangle so that the grandchild can hold it
6. A person becomes faint in the hallway and begins to fall. What should you do?
   a. Stand back so that the person will not grab at you as he falls
   b. Catch the person before he falls and call for assistance

c. Take the person back to his room so the nurse can check him
d. Ease the person to the floor and protect the person's head

Answers to these questions are on p. 537.

CHAPTER 15·RESTRAINT ALTERNATIVES AND RESTRAINTS

- The Centers for Medicare & Medicaid Services (CMS), has rules for using restraints. These rules protect the person's right to be free from restraints.
- Restraints may be used for a brief time to treat a medical symptom that would require restraint use or for the immediate physical safety of the person or others. Restraints may be used only when less restrictive measures fail to protect the person or others. They must be discontinued as soon as possible.
- The CMS uses these terms.
  - A **physical restraint** is any manual method or physical or mechanical device, material, or equipment attached to or near the person's body that he or she cannot remove easily and that restricts freedom of movement or normal access to one's body.
  - A **chemical restraint** is a drug that is used for discipline or convenience and not required to treat medical symptoms. The drug or dosage is not a standard treatment for the person's condition.
  - **Freedom of movement** is any change in place or position of the body or any part of the body that the person can control.
  - **Remove easily** is the manual method, device, material, or equipment used to restrain the person that can be removed intentionally by the person in the same manner it was applied by staff.
  - **Convenience** is any action taken to control or manage a person's behavior that requires less effort by the staff; the action is not in the person's best interest.
  - **Discipline** is any action taken by the agency to punish or penalize a patient or resident.
- Federal, state, and accrediting agencies have guidelines about restraint use. They do not forbid restraint use. All other appropriate alternatives must be considered or tried first.
- Every agency has policies and procedures about restraints. They include identifying persons at risk for harm, harmful behaviors, restraint alternatives, and proper restraint use. Staff training is required.

Restraint Alternatives

- Knowing and treating the cause for harmful behaviors can prevent restraint use. There are many alternatives to restraints. See Box 15-1(p 205), Restraint Alternatives.

Safe Restraint Use

- Restraints are used only when necessary to treat a person's medical symptoms—physical, emotional, or behavioral problems. Sometimes restraints are needed to protect the person or others.

Physical and Chemical Restraints

- *Physical restraints* are applied to the chest, waist, elbows, wrists, hands, or ankles. They confine the person to a bed or chair. Or they prevent movement of a body part. Some furniture or barriers prevent free movement.
- Drugs or drug dosages are *chemical restraints* if they:
  - Control behavior or restrict movement.
  - Are not standard treatment for the person's condition.

Risks From Restraints

- Restraints can cause many complications. Injuries occur as the person tries to get free of the restraint. Injuries also occur from using the wrong restraint, applying it wrong, or keeping it on too long. Cuts, bruises, and fractures are common. The most serious risk is death from strangulation. Review Box 15-2(p 207), Risks From Restraint Use, in the Textbook.

Legal Aspects

- *Restraints must protect the person.* A restraint is used only when it is the best safety measure for the person.
- *A doctor's order is required.* The doctor gives the reason for the restraint, what body part to restrain, what to use, and how long to use it.
- *The least restrictive method is used.* It allows the greatest amount of movement or body access possible.
- *Restraints are used only after other measures fail to protect the person.* Box 15-1(p 205), Restraint Alternatives, in the Textbook lists alternatives to restraint use.
- *Unnecessary restraint is false imprisonment.* An unneeded restraint, may lead to false imprisonment charges.
- *Informed consent is required.* The person must understand the reason for the restraint. If the person cannot give consent, his or her legal representative is given the information. The doctor or nurse provides the necessary information and obtains consent.

Safety Guidelines

- Review Box 15-3(p 209), Safety Measures for Using Restraints, in the Textbook.
- *Observe for increased confusion and agitation.* Provide repeated explanations and re-assurance. Spending time with the person has a calming effect.
- *Protect the person's quality of life.* Restraints are used only for a brief time. You must meet the person's physical, emotional, and social needs.
- *Follow the manufacturer's instructions to safely apply and secure the restraints.* The person must be comfortable and able to move the restrained part to a limited and safe extent.
- *Apply restraints with enough help to protect the person and staff from injury.*
- *Observe the person at least every 15 minutes or as often as directed by the nurse and the care plan.* Injuries and deaths can result from improper restraint use and poor observation.

- *Remove or release the restraint, re-position the person, and meet basic needs at least every 2 hours or as often as noted in the care plan.* The restraint is removed for at least 10 minutes. Provide for food, fluid, comfort, safety, hygiene, and elimination needs and give skin care. Perform range-of-motion exercises or help the person walk.

Reporting and Recording

- Report and record the following:
  - Type of restraint applied
  - Body part or parts restrained
  - Safety measures taken
  - Time you applied the restraint
  - Time you removed or released the restraint
  - Care given when restraint was removed
  - Person's vital signs
  - Skin color and condition
  - Condition of the extremities
  - Pulse felt in the restrained part
  - Changes in the person's behavior
- Report these complaints to the nurse at once: complaints of discomfort; a tight restraint; difficulty breathing; or pain, numbness, or tingling in the restrained part.

CHAPTER 15 REVIEW QUESTIONS

Circle the BEST answer.

1. Which care measure would be considered an alternative to restraints?
   a. Tucking the sheets tightly, so that the person does not fall out of bed
   b. Raising the bedrails to prevent getting up without calling for assistance
   c. Putting the bed close to the wall so that the person will not fall out.
   d. Having a companion or family member sit at the person's bedside

2. Which nursing assistant has used a restraint as a convenience?
   a. Nursing Assistant A puts the person in a chair with a lap-top tray for meals
   b. Nursing Assistant B raises a bedrail so that the person can use it to move in bed
   c. Nursing Assistant C puts the person in a belt restraint during shift change
   d. Nursing Assistant D places a mitt restraint according to the care plan.

3. You walk into a room and see that a person is being strangled by the restraint. What is the first thing you should do?
   a. Run to the nurses' station to get the nurse
   b. Release the restraint or cut it with scissors
   c. Call the Rapid Response Team or the doctor
   d. Start cardiopulmonary resuscitation and rescue breathing

4. The person with a restraint should be observed at least every
   a. 15 minutes
   b. 30 minutes

   c. Hour
   d. 2 hours

5. Restraints need to be removed at least every
   a. Hour
   b. 2 hours
   c. 3 hours
   d. 4 hours

6. Which documentation related to restraints is correct?
   a. Person was restrained for bad behavior until he calmed down.
   b. Restraints were in place for the entire shift, with no problems.
   c. Restraints removed for 10 minutes and fluids offered at 1400.
   d. Vital signs were deferred, because both arms were restrained

Answers to these questions are on p. 537.

CHAPTER 16 PREVENTING INFECTION

- An **infection** is a disease state resulting from the invasion and growth of microbes in the body. Infection is a major safety hazard.
- Following certain practices and procedures prevents the spread of infection (**infection control**).

Microorganisms

- A **microorganism (microbe)** is a small (*micro*) living plant or animal (*organism*).
- Some microbes are harmful and can cause infections (**pathogens**). Others do not usually cause infection (**non-pathogens**).

Multidrug-Resistant Organisms

- *Multidrug-resistant organisms (MDROs)* can resist the effects of antibiotics. Such organisms are able to change their structures to survive in the presence of antibiotics. The infections they cause are harder to treat.
- MDROs are caused by prescribing antibiotics when they are not needed (over-prescribing). Not taking antibiotics for the prescribed days is also a cause.
- Two common types of MDROs are resistant to many antibiotics.
  - *Methicillin-resistant Staphylococcus aureus (MRSA)*
  - *Vancomycin-resistant Enterococcus (VRE)*

Infection

- **A local infection** is in a body part.
- **A systemic infection** involves the whole body.
- Older persons may not show the normal signs and symptoms of infection. The person may have only a slight fever or no fever at all. Redness and swelling may be very slight. The person may not complain of pain. Confusion and delirium may occur.
- Infections can become life-threatening before the older person has obvious signs and symptoms. Be alert to minor changes in the person's behavior or condition.
- Report any concerns to the nurse at once. Review Box 16-1(p 223), Infection-Signs and Symptoms, in the Textbook.

Healthcare-Associated Infection

- A **healthcare-associated infection (HAI)** is an infection that develops in a person who has received health care in any setting where health care is given. Hospitals, nursing centers, clinics, and home care settings are examples. Review Box 16-2(p 224), Healthcare-Associated Infections—Examples in the Textbook.
- The health team must prevent the spread of HAIs by:
  - Medical asepsis. This includes hand hygiene.
  - Surgical asepsis.
  - Standard Precautions
  - Transmission-Based Precautions
  - Bloodborne Pathogen Standard.

Medical Asepsis

- **Asepsis** is the absence of disease-producing microbes.
- **Medical asepsis (clean technique)** refers to the practices used to:
  - Reduce the number of microbes
  - Prevent microbes from spreading from 1 person or place to another person or place.

Common Aseptic Practices

- To prevent the spread of microbes, wash your hands:
  - After elimination.
  - After changing tampons or sanitary pads.
  - After contact with your own or another person's blood, body fluids, secretions, or excretions. This includes saliva, vomitus, urine, feces, vaginal discharge, mucus, semen, wound drainage, pus, and respiratory secretions.
  - After coughing, sneezing, or blowing your nose.
  - Before and after handling, preparing, or eating food.
  - After smoking.
- Also do the following:
  - Provide all persons with their own linens and personal care items.
  - Cover your nose and mouth when coughing, sneezing, or blowing your nose.
  - If without tissues, cough or sneeze into your upper arm. Do not cough or sneeze into your hands.
  - Bathe, wash hair, and brush your teeth regularly.
  - Wash fruits and raw vegetables before eating or serving them.
  - Wash cooking and eating utensils with soap and water after use.

Hand Hygiene

- *Hand hygiene is the easiest and most important way to prevent the spread of infection.* Practice hand hygiene before and after giving care. Review Box 16-3(p 227), Rules of Hand Hygiene, in the Textbook.

Supplies and Equipment

- Most health care equipment is disposable. Bedpans, urinals, wash basins, water pitchers, and drinking cups are multi-use items and should be labeled with the person's name, room number and bed number. Do not "borrow" these items for another person.
- Non-disposable items are cleaned and then disinfected. Then they are sterilized.

Other Aseptic Measures

- Review Box 16-4 (p 231), Aseptic Measures, in the Textbook.

Bloodborne Pathogen Standard

- The health team is at risk for exposure to human immunodeficiency virus (HIV) and the hepatitis B virus (HBV). HIV and HBV are bloodborne pathogens found in the blood.
- The Bloodborne Pathogen Standard is intended to protect you from exposure.
- Staff at risk for exposure to HIV and HBV receive free training.
- *Hepatitis B vaccination.* You can receive the hepatitis B vaccination within 10 working days of being hired. The agency pays for it. If you refuse the vaccination, you must sign a statement. You can have the vaccination at a later date.

Laundry

- OSHA requires these measures for contaminated laundry.
  - Handle it as little as possible.
  - Wear gloves or other needed PPE.
  - Bag contaminated laundry where it is used.
  - Mark laundry bags or containers with the BIOHAZARD symbol for laundry sent off-site.
  - Place wet, contaminated laundry in leak-proof containers before transport. The containers are color-coded in red or have the BIOHAZARD symbol.

Equipment

- Contaminated equipment and work surfaces are cleaned and decontaminated with a proper disinfectant:
  - Upon completing tasks
  - At once when there is obvious contamination
  - At the end of the work shift if the surfaces have been contaminated since the last cleaning

Exposure Incidents

- An **exposure incident** is any eye, mouth, other mucous membrane, non-intact skin, or parenteral contact with blood or OPIM (other potentially infectious materials).
- Report exposure incidents at once. Medical evaluation, follow-up, and required tests are free. Your blood is tested for HIV and HBV. Confidentiality is important.

Personal Protective Equipment (PPE)

- OSHA requires these measures for PPE: gloves, goggles, face shields, masks, laboratory coats, gowns, shoe covers, and surgical caps.
  - Remove PPE before leaving the work area.
  - Remove PPE when a garment becomes contaminated.
  - Place used PPE in marked areas or containers when being stored, washed, decontaminated, or discarded.
  - Wear gloves when you expect contact with blood or OPIM.
  - Wear gloves when handling or touching contaminated items or surfaces.
  - Replace worn, punctured, or contaminated gloves.
  - Do not wash or decontaminate disposable gloves for re-use.

o Discard utility gloves that show signs of cracking, peeling, tearing, or puncturing. Utility gloves are decontaminated for re-use if the process will not ruin them.

Work Practice Controls

- *Work practice controls* reduce employee exposure in the workplace. All tasks involving blood or other potentially infectious materials (OPIM) are done in ways to limit splatters, splashes, and sprays.
  - o Do not eat, drink, smoke, apply cosmetics or lip balm, or handle contact lenses in areas of occupational exposure.
  - o Do not store food or drinks where blood or OPIM are kept.
  - o Practice hand hygiene after removing gloves.
  - o Wash hands as soon as possible after skin contact with blood or OPIM.
  - o Do not re-cap, bend, or remove needles by hand.
  - o Do not shear or break needles.
  - o Discard needles and sharp instruments (razors) in containers that are closable, puncture-resistant, and leak-proof. Containers are color-coded in red and have the BIOHAZARD symbol.

Surgical asepsis

- o **Surgical asepsis (sterile technique)** are the practices used to remove all microbes.
- o Surgical asepsis is required any time the skin or sterile tissues are entered. Review Box 16-6(p 237), Surgical Asepsis—Principles and Practices

CHAPTER 16 REVIEW QUESTIONS

Circle the BEST answer.

1. Which action would you take to prevent healthcare-associated infections?
   a. Wear sterile gloves when caring for people with infections
   b. Perform hand hygiene before and after giving care
   c. Get the hepatitis B vaccination series
   d. Immediately report an exposure incident
2. In which circumstance would the use of an alcohol-based hand sanitizer be acceptable?
   a. Before eating your lunch
   b. After removing gloves
   c. After cleaning up diarrheal feces
   d. After known exposure to *Clostridium difficile*
3. Which nursing assistant is correctly following the procedure for hand-washing?
   a. Nursing Assistant A stands away from the sink and clothes do not touch the sink
   b. Nursing Assistant B raises hands above elbows towards the faucet
   c. Nursing Assistant C quickly washes hands by rubbing palms several times
   d. Nursing Assistant D dries hands with a paper towel; then uses towel to turn off faucet
4. Which person has a healthcare-associated infection?
   a. Nursing assistant develops a cold after her son gets a cold at school.
   b. Person develops a urinary infection because catheter care was not performed.
   c. Nursing assistant gets hepatitis after getting stuck with a dirty needle
   d. Person becomes HIV positive after unprotected sex with several partners.
5. Which member of the health care team is following work practice controls to prevent bloodborne pathogen exposure?
   a. Nurse recaps needle before putting it in the sharps box
   b. Nursing assistant throws a disposable razor in the trash can
   c. Doctor performs hand hygiene after removing gloves
   d. Nursing assistant applies lip balm in a procedure area

Answers to these questions are on p. 537.

CHAPTER 17 ISOLATION PRECAUTIONS

- Isolation precautions prevent the spread of **communicable diseases (contagious diseases).** They are diseases caused by pathogens that spread easily.
- The Centers for Disease and Control and Prevention's (CDC's) isolation precautions guideline has 2 tiers of precautions.
  - o Standard Precautions
  - o Transmission-Based Precautions

Standard Precautions

- Standard Precautions reduce the risk of spreading pathogens and known and unknown infections. Standard Precautions are used for all persons whenever care is given. They prevent the spread of infection from:
  - o Blood.
  - o All body fluids, secretions, and excretions even if blood is not visible. Sweat is not known to spread infections.
  - o Non-intact skin (skin with open breaks).
  - o Mucous membranes.
- Review Box 17-1(p 242), Standard Precautions, in the Textbook.

Transmission-Based Precautions

- Some infections require Transmission-Based Precautions. Review Box 17-2(p 243), Transmission-Based Precautions, in the Textbook.
- Agency policies may differ from those in the Textbook. The rules in Box 17-3(p 244), Rules for Transmission-Based Precautions, in the Textbook are a guide for giving safe care.

Gloves

- Wear gloves whenever contact with blood, body fluids, secretions, excretions, mucous membranes, and non-intact skin is likely. Wearing gloves is the most common protective measure used with Standard Precautions and Transmission-Based Precautions. Remember the following when using gloves.
  - o Outer surface of gloves is considered contaminated.
  - o Gloves are easier to put on when your hands are dry.

o Do not tear gloves when putting them on.

o Remove and discard torn, cut, or punctured gloves at once. Practice hand hygiene. Then put on a new pair.

o Apply a new pair for every person.

o Wear gloves once. Discard them after use.

o Put on clean gloves just before touching mucous membranes or non-intact skin.

o Put on new gloves whenever gloves become contaminated with blood, body fluids, secretions, or excretions. A task may require more than 1 pair of gloves.

o Change gloves whenever moving from a contaminated body site to a clean body site.

o Change gloves if interacting with the person involves touching portable computer keyboards or other mobile equipment that is transported from room to room.

o Put on gloves last when worn with other PPE.

o Make sure gloves cover your wrists. If you wear a gown, gloves cover the cuffs.

o Remove gloves so the inside part is on the outside. The inside is clean.

o Practice hand hygiene after removing gloves.

- Latex allergies are common and can cause skin rashes. Difficulty breathing and shock are more serious problems. Report skin rashes and breathing problems at once. If you or a resident has a latex allergy, wear latex-free gloves.

Personal Protective Equipment (PPE)

- The PPE needed —gloves, a gown, a mask, and goggles or a face shield—depends on the task, the procedures, care measures, and the type of Transmission-Based Precautions used. The nurse will tell you what equipment is needed.

- Gowns must completely cover you from your neck to mid-thigh or below. The gown front and sleeves are considered contaminated. A wet gown is contaminated. Gowns are used once. When removing a gown, roll it inside out into a bundle.

- Masks are disposable. A wet or moist mask is contaminated. When removing a mask, touch only the ties or elastic bands. The front of the mask is contaminated.

- The front of goggles or a face shield is contaminated. Use the device's ties, headband, or ear-pieces to remove the device.

Donning and Removing PPE

- According to the CDC, PPE is donned in the following order.
  o Gown
  o Mask or respirator
  o Eyewear (goggles or face shield)
  o Gloves

- Removing PPE (removed at the doorway before leaving the person's room):
  o *Method 1*
    1. Gloves
    2. Eyewear (goggles or face shield)
    3. Gown

    4. Mask or respirator (respirator is removed after leaving the person's room and closing the door)
    5. Wash hands or use an alcohol-based hand sanitizer immediately after removing all PPE
  o *Method 2*
    1. Gown and gloves
    2. Eyewear (goggles or face shield)
    3. Mask or respirator (respirator is removed after leaving the person's room and closing the door)
    4. Wash hands or use an alcohol-based hand sanitizer immediately after removing all PPE

- Review Figure 17-4 (pp 247, 248, 249), Donning and Removing PPE, in the Textbook.

- Practice hand hygiene after removing PPE. Practice hand hygiene between steps if your hands become contaminated. Then practice hand hygiene again after removing all PPE.

- NOTE: Some state competency tests require hand hygiene after removing each PPE item. And some states use a different order for donning and removing PPE. Follow the procedures used in your state and agency.

- Some very severe and deadly infections require additional PPE and special training.

Bagging Items

- Contaminated items, linens, and trash are bagged to remove them from the person's room. Leak-proof plastic bags are used. They have the BIOHAZARD symbol. Double-bagging is not needed unless the outside of the bag is wet, soiled, or may be contaminated.

Collecting Specimens

- Follow agency procedures to collect, store, and transport specimens (e. g., blood, body fluids, secretions, and excretions) when a person is on Transmission-Based Precautions. Specimens are transported to the laboratory in biohazard specimen bags.

CHAPTER 17 REVIEW QUESTIONS

Circle the BEST answer.

1. What is the most common measure that would be used in caring for any person who needs Standard or Transmission-Based Precautions?
   a. Respiratory hygiene
   b. Using shoe covers
   c. Donning gloves
   d. Wearing a mask

2. When would you perform hand hygiene?
   a. After donning a gown
   b. When the mask is contaminated.
   c. When the gown is contaminated
   d. After removing PPE

3. Which nursing assistant is using PPE correctly?
   a. Nursing Assistant A removes PPE when it becomes contaminated.
   b. Nursing Assistant B wears gloves during all encounters with patients
   c. Nursing Assistant C removes contaminated gloves in the nurses' station
   d. Nursing Assistant D wears PPE for warmth, because the unit is cold.

4. When do you need to change gloves?
   a. You take the dirty linen off the bed; then you put it in the laundry hamper
   b. You empty the bedpan; then you need to flush and clean the toilet
   c. You give perineal care; then the person asks you to clean her feet
   d. You help a person brush her teeth; then she needs to rinse and spit
5. In which circumstance would you anticipate the need to don a mask?
   a. You must transport a person on droplet precautions to the x-ray department
   b. You enter the room of a person on droplet precautions to assist with hygiene
   c. You enter the room of a person on contact precautions to deliver a meal tray
   d. You take vital signs on a person who needs standard precautions

CHAPTER 18 BODY MECHANICS
Principles of Body Mechanics
- The strongest and largest muscles are in the shoulders, upper arms, hips, and thighs. Use these muscles to lift and move persons and heavy objects.
- For good body mechanics:
  - Bend your knees and squat to lift a heavy object. Do not bend from your waist.
  - Hold items close to your body and base of support.
- Review Box 18-1(p 258), Rules for Body Mechanics, in the Textbook.

Work-Related Injuries
- **Musculo-skeletal disorders (MSDs)** are injuries and disorders of the muscles, tendons, ligaments, joints, and cartilage.
- The Occupational Safety and Health Administration (OSHA) identifies MSD risk factors as:
  - Force: the amount of physical effort needed to perform a task.
  - Repeating action: doing the same motions or series of motions continually or frequently.
  - Awkward postures: assuming positions that place stress on the body.
  - Heavy lifting: manually lifting people who cannot lift themselves.
- According to the U.S. Department of Labor, nursing assistants are at the greatest risk for MSDs.
- Always report a work-related injury as soon as possible. Early attention can help prevent the problem from becoming worse. Review Box 18-3(p 260), Preventing Work-Related Injuries, in the Textbook.

Positioning the Person
- The person must be positioned correctly at all times. Regular position changes and good alignment promote comfort and well-being. Breathing is easier. Circulation is promoted. Pressure injuries and contractures are prevented.

- Whether in bed or in a chair, the person is re-positioned at least every 2 hours. To safely position a person:
  - Use good body mechanics.
  - Ask a co-worker to help you if needed.
  - Explain the procedure to the person.
  - Be gentle when moving the person.
  - Provide for privacy.
  - Use pillows as directed by the nurse for support and alignment.
  - Provide for comfort after positioning.
  - Place the call light within reach after positioning.
  - Complete a safety check before leaving the room.
- **Fowler's position** is a semi-sitting position. In **semi-Fowler's** position, the head of the bed is raised 30 degrees but some agencies define semi-Fowler's position as raising the head of the bed 30 degrees and the knee portion 15 degrees. In **high-Fowler's** position, the head of the bed is raised between 60 and 90 degrees.
- The **supine position (dorsal recumbent position)** is the back-lying position.
- In the **prone position**, the person lies on the abdomen with the head turned to one side.
- A person in the **lateral position (side-lying position)** lies on one side or the other.
- The **Sims' position (semi-prone side position)** is a left side-lying position. The upper (right) leg is sharply flexed so it is not on the lower (left) leg. The lower (left) arm is behind the person.
- Persons who sit in chairs must hold their upper bodies and heads erect. For good alignment:
  - The person's back and buttocks are against the back of the chair.
  - Feet are flat on the floor or wheelchair footplates. Never leave feet unsupported.
  - Backs of the knees and calves are slightly away from the edge of the seat.

CHAPTER 18 REVIEW QUESTIONS
Circle the BEST answer.
1. To lift and move residents and heavy objects you should
   a. Use the muscles in your lower arms, hands and fingers
   b. Use the muscles in your lower legs and upper back
   c. Use the muscles in your shoulders, upper arms, hips, and thighs
   d. Use the muscles in your chest, abdomen and lower back
2. Which nursing assistant is not using good body mechanics?
   a. Nursing Assistant A bends his knees and squats to lift a heavy object
   b. Nursing Assistant B bends over at her waist to lift a heavy object
   c. Nursing Assistant C holds items close to her body and base of support
   d. Nursing Assistant D bends his legs and does not bend his back

3. Which person is most likely to benefit from being placed in the Fowler's position?
   a. A person with a respiratory disorder who has difficulty breathing
   b. A person who is comatose and has a contracture of the right forearm.
   c. A person who has fragile skin and is at risk for a pressure injury.
   d. A person who has a work- related musculo-skeletal back injury.
4. In high-Fowler's position
   a. The head of the bed is raised to 30 degrees
   b. The head of the bed is raised between 30 and 45 degrees
   c. The head of the bed is raised between 45 and 60 degrees
   d. The head of the bed is raised between 60 and 90 degrees

Answers to these questions are on p. 537.

CHAPTER 19 MOVING THE PERSON
Preventing Work-Related Injuries
- Good body mechanics alone will not prevent injury. The Occupational Safety and Health Administration (OSHA) recommends
  o Minimizing manual lifting in all cases.
  o Eliminating manual lifting whenever possible.
- Careful planning is needed to move the person safely. You must know the person's physical abilities, the number of staff needed, what procedure to use, and the equipment needed.

Protecting the Skin
- Protect the person's skin from friction and shearing. Both cause infection and pressure injuries. To reduce friction and shearing:
  o Roll the person.
  o Use friction-reducing devices such as a lift sheet (turning sheet), turning pads, and slide sheets.

Moving Persons in Bed
- Know how much help and what equipment or friction-reducing devices are needed.
- Review Box 19-1(p 270), Moving Persons in Bed- Guidelines, in the Textbook.

Raising the Person's Head and Shoulders
- You can raise the person's head and shoulders easily and safely by locking arms with the person (do not pull on the person's arm or shoulder).
- Have help with older persons and with those who are heavy or hard to move.

Moving the Person Up in Bed
- You may be able to independently move light-weight adults up in bed if they can assist using a trapeze.
- Two or more staff members are needed to move heavy, weak, and very old persons up in bed. Always protect the person and yourself from injury.

Moving the Person Up in Bed With an Assist Device
- Assist devices are used to reduce shearing and friction. Such assist devices include a drawsheet (lift sheet), flat sheet folded in half, turning pad, slide sheet, and large re-usable waterproof underpads.
- Assist devices are used to move most patients and residents and at least 2 staff members are needed to position and use the assist device.
- Moving the person to the side of the bed can be done alone if the person is small enough. You move the person in segments by placing your hands and arms underneath the person. Move the upper body first (while supporting the person's neck), then the lower body, and finally the legs and feet.

Turning Persons
- Turning persons onto their sides helps prevent complications from bed rest. Procedures and care measures often require the side-lying position. After the person is turned, position him or her in good alignment. Use pillows as directed to support the person in the side-lying position.
- **Logrolling** is turning the person as a unit, in alignment, with 1 motion. The spine is kept straight.

Sitting on the Side of the Bed (Dangling)
- Many persons become dizzy or faint when getting out of bed too fast. They may need to sit on the side of the bed for 1 to 5 minutes before walking or transferring. Some persons increase activity in stages—bed rest, to dangling, to sitting in a chair, to walking.
- While dangling, the person coughs and deep breathes. He or she moves the legs in circles to stimulate circulation.
- If dizziness or faintness occurs, lay the person down. Report this to the nurse.

Re-Positioning in a Chair or Wheelchair
- The person can slide down into the chair. For good alignment and safety, the person's back and buttocks must be against the back of the chair.
- Follow the nurse's directions and the care plan for the best way to re-position a person in a chair or wheelchair. Do not pull the person from behind the chair or wheelchair.
- If the chair reclines, have a co-worker assist, recline the chair, put an assist device under the person, and use the assist device to move the person up.
- If the person is in a wheelchair and has strength to assist, lock the wheels of the wheelchair and move the foot rests to the sides. Position a transfer belt around the person, stand in front of the person, block the person's knees with your knees and grasp the transfer belt with both hands. Ask the person to push with his or her feet and arms on the count of 3 and move the person back into the wheelchair while the person pushes with his or her feet and arms.

CHAPTER 19 REVIEW QUESTIONS

Circle the BEST answer.

1. Which care measure is the best to reduce friction and shearing while moving the person in bed?
   a. Use the bed controls to move the bed
   b. Ask the person to slide himself
   c. Link arms with person and pull him across
   d. Use a slide board or slide sheet
2. The number of staff required to safely move a person depends on
   a. The person's height, weight, cognitive function, and physical abilities.
   b. The person's age, health status and desire for independence
   c. The person's strength in the extremities and ability to balance
   d. The person's medical diagnosis and willingness to co-operate
3. In which circumstance would you logroll the person?
   a. Person gets dizzy when he first sits up to dangle.
   b. Person is recovering from spinal surgery.
   c. Person can reach across grasp the siderail with coaching.
   d. Person needs limited assistance according to the care plan.

Answers to these questions are on p. 537.

CHAPTER 20 SAFELY TRANSFERRING THE PERSON

- A transfer is how a person safely moves to and from a surface.
- The amount of help needed and the method used vary with the person's ability.

Wheelchair and Stretcher Safety

- Wheelchairs are used for persons who cannot walk or who have severe problems walking. Stretchers are used to transfer persons who are seriously ill, cannot sit up, or must stay in a lying position.
- Review Box 20-1(p 289), Wheelchair and Stretcher Safety, in the Textbook.

Stand and Pivot Transfers

- Some persons can stand and pivot (to turn one's body from a set standing position). Use this transfer if the person's legs are strong enough to bear weight and the person is cooperative and can follow directions and assist in the transfer.
- Transfer belts (gait belts) are used to support persons during transfers and to re-position persons in chairs and wheelchairs.

Chair or Wheelchair Transfers

- Arrange the room so there is enough space for a safe transfer. Correct placement of the chair, wheelchair, or other device also is needed for a safe transfer.
- Have the person wear slip-resistant footwear for transfers.
- Lock the wheels of the bed, wheelchair, stretcher, or other assist device.
- The person must not put his or her arms around your neck when assisting the person to stand.
- After the transfer, position the person in good alignment.
- For bed to chair or wheelchair transfers, the strong side moves first. Help the person out of bed on his or her strong side. When transferring the person from the chair or wheelchair back to bed, the same rules apply. Help the person from the wheelchair to the bed on his or her strong side. If the person is weak on 1 side, position the chair or wheelchair so that the person's strong side is nearest the bed. The strong side moves first.

Transferring To and From the Toilet

- Transferring the person to and from the toilet is often hard because bathrooms are small. If the wheelchair can fit in the bathroom, place it at a 90-degree angle to the toilet and use a sliding board or the stand and pivot transfer from the wheelchair to the toilet.

Lateral Transfers

- A lateral transfer moves a person between 2 horizontal surfaces, such as from a bed to a stretcher. The person slides from 1 surface to the other.
- Use friction-reducing devices to protect the skin from friction and shearing during lateral transfers.
- When moving a person from a bed to a stretcher, use a friction-reducing device and at least 2 or 3 staff members to assist. If the person weighs more than 200 pounds, a lateral transfer device, or a mechanical ceiling lift is used.
- Persons who cannot help themselves are transferred with mechanical lifts. So are persons who are too heavy for the staff to transfer.
- Before using a mechanical lift, you must be trained in its use. The sling, straps, hooks, and chains must be in good repair. The person's weight must not exceed the lift's capacity. At least 2 staff members are needed. Always follow the manufacturer's instructions for using the lift.
- Falling from the lift is a common fear. To promote the person's mental comfort, always explain the procedure before you begin. Also show the person how the lift works.

CHAPTER 20 REVIEW QUESTIONS

Circle the BEST answer.

1. Which action would you use to transfer a person from the bed to a wheelchair?
   a. Help the person put on slip-resistant footwear after he/she is sitting in the wheelchair.
   b. Encourage the person to put his/her arms around your neck to rise to a standing position.
   c. Apply a belt restraint and check it for a snug fit before helping the person to stand.
   d. Ensure that the wheels are locked on the bed and wheelchair before transferring the person.

2. A person has a weak left side and a strong right side. Which action is correct for transferring the person from the bed to the wheelchair?
   a. Place the wheelchair on the left side of bed before transfer
   b. Lower the weak side into the wheelchair first.
   c. Get the person out of bed on the strong side.
   d. Use the weak side for balance and the strong side for strength
3. When using a mechanical lift, what is an important safety feature to remember?
   a. The wheels of the lift should always locked.
   b. Persons who are very thin are at risk to slip through the straps
   c. In a narrow space, the lift is stable in a narrow position.
   d. The lift is most stable with the base in the open position.

Answers to these questions are on p. 537.

CHAPTER 21 THE PERSON'S UNIT

- A person's unit is the space, furniture, and equipment used by the person in the agency. CMS requires that resident units be as personal and home-like as possible.
- Keep the person's room clean, neat, safe, and comfortable. Follow the rules in Box 21-1(p 309), Maintaining the Person's Unit, and Box 21-2(p 309), and CMS Requirements for Resident Rooms, in the Textbook.

Comfort

- Age, illness, and activity affect comfort.
- Temperature, ventilation, noise, odors, and lighting are factors that are controlled to meet the person's needs.

Temperature and Ventilation

- Older persons and those who are ill may need higher temperatures for comfort. Ventilation systems provide fresh air and move air within the room.
- To protect older and ill persons from drafts, make sure the person wears enough clothing, offer a lap cover when sitting in a chair and cover the legs, use a bath blanket when providing care, and move the person from drafty areas.

Odors

- To reduce odors in nursing centers:
  - Empty, clean, and disinfect bedpans, urinals, commodes, and kidney basins promptly.
  - Check to make sure toilets are flushed.
  - Check incontinent people often.
  - Clean persons who are wet or soiled from urine, feces, vomitus, or wound drainage.
  - Change wet or soiled linens and clothing promptly.
  - Keep laundry containers closed.
  - Follow agency policy for wet or soiled linens and clothing.
  - Dispose of incontinence and ostomy products promptly.
  - Provide good hygiene to prevent body and breath odors.
  - Use room deodorizers as needed and as allowed by agency policy.
- If you smoke, practice hand-washing after handling smoking materials and before giving care. Pay attention to your uniforms, hair, and breath because of smoke odors.

Noise

- To decrease noise:
  - Control your voice.
  - Handle equipment carefully.
  - Keep equipment in good working order.
  - Answer phones, call lights, and intercoms promptly.

Lighting

- Adjust lighting to meet the person's needs. Glares, shadows, and dull lighting can cause falls, headaches, and eyestrain. A bright room is cheerful. Dim light is better for relaxing and rest. Persons with poor vision need bright light. Always keep light controls within the person's reach.

Room Furniture and Equipment

- Rooms are furnished and equipped for safety and to meet basic needs.

The Bed

- Beds are raised to give care. This reduces bending and reaching.
- Bed wheels are locked at all times except when moving the bed.
- Use bed rails as the nurse and care plan direct.
- Basic bed positions:
  - *Flat*—the usual sleeping position.
  - *Fowler's position*—a semi-sitting position. The head of the bed is raised between 45 and 60 degrees.
  - *High-Fowler's position*—a semi-sitting position. The head of the bed is raised 60 to 90 degrees.
  - *Semi-Fowler's position*—the head of the bed is raised 30 degrees. Some agencies define semi-Fowler's position as when the head of the bed is raised 30 degrees and the knee portion is raised 15 degrees. Know the definition used by your agency.
  - *Trendelenburg's position*—the head of the bed is lowered and the foot of the bed is raised. A doctor orders the position.
  - *Reverse Trendelenburg's position*—the head of the bed is raised and the foot of the bed is lowered. A doctor orders the position.

Bed Safety

- *Entrapment* means getting caught, trapped, or entangled in spaces created by bed rails, the mattress, the bed frame, or the head-board and foot-board. Head, neck, or chest entrapment can cause serious injuries and deaths. Always check for entrapment. If a person is caught, trapped, or entangled, try to release the person. Call for the nurse at once.

The Over-Bed Table

- Only clean and sterile items are placed on the table. Never place bedpans, urinals, or soiled linens on the over-bed table or on top of the bedside stand.

- Clean the table and bedside stand after using them for a work surface and before serving meal trays.

Privacy Curtains
- Always pull the curtain completely around the bed before giving care. Privacy curtains do not block sound or conversations.

The Call System
- Always keep the call light within the person's reach—in the room, bathroom, and shower or tub room. You must:
  - Place the call light on the person's strong side.
  - Remind the person to signal when help is needed.
  - Answer call lights promptly.
  - Answer bathroom and shower or tub room call lights at once.
- Persons with limited hand mobility may need special communication measures.
- Be careful when using the intercom. Remember confidentiality. Persons nearby can hear what you and the person say.

The Bathroom
- Grab bars are by the toilet so persons can use them to get on and off the toilet.
- Some toilet seats are raised to make transfers easier and for persons with joint problems.
- A call light or button is within reach of the toilet if the person needs assistance.
- Towel racks, toilet paper, soap, paper towels and a wastebasket should be within reach.

Closet and Drawer Space
- The person must have free access to the closet and its contents. You must have the person's permission to open or search closets or drawers.
- Agency staff can inspect a person's closet or drawers if hoarding is suspected. The person is informed of the inspection and is present when it takes place. Have a co-worker present when you inspect a person's closet.

CHAPTER 21 REVIEW QUESTIONS
Circle the BEST answer.
1. Which person and situation create the greatest risk for entrapment?
   a. An older person is sitting in a wheelchair and visiting with family
   b. An obese person is learning to use the trapeze over the bariatric bed.
   c. A small, frail older person is confused and very restless in bed.
   d. A frail older person is sitting in the dining room and refuses to eat.
2. Which bed position, would most people prefer for sleeping?
   a. Semi-Fowler's
   b. Flat
   c. Trendelenburg
   d. High-Fowler's

3. Which task is a nursing assistant responsibility?
   a. You should clean the bedside stand if you use it for a work surface.
   b. You should routinely check closets and drawers for unsafe items.
   c. You should encourage independent residents not to use call lights
   d. You should clean upholstered furniture and rugs every day.
4. Which person needs additional measures to be protected from drafts?
   a. Person is wearing a sleeveless t-shirt and a short skirt
   b. Person is sitting in a wheelchair with a lab robe over legs
   c. Person is covered with a bath blanket during morning hygiene
   d. Person is provided an extra blanket while taking a nap
5. Which action would you perform to reduce odors?
   a. Empty and clean commodes at the end of the shift
   b. Keep laundry containers open in well-ventilated areas
   c. Use circulating fans to move air and disperse odors
   d. Clean persons who are wet or soiled from urine or feces
6. Which nursing assistant needs to be counseled about the call lights?
   a. Nursing Assistant A ensures that the call light is within the person's reach.
   b. Nursing Assistant B places the call light on the person's strong side.
   c. Nursing Assistant C only answers the call lights of assigned residents.
   d. Nursing Assistant D promptly answers a bathroom call light.
7. You suspect a resident is hoarding food in her closet. Before you inspect the closet, what do you do?
   a. Tell the resident that hoarding violates agency policy.
   b. Inspect the closet when the resident is not in the room.
   c. Tell the family to check the closet for unwanted items.
   d. Ask the resident if you can inspect the closet.

Answers to these questions are on p. 537.

CHAPTER 22 BEDMAKING
- Clean, dry, and wrinkle-free linens promote comfort and help to prevent skin breakdown and pressure injuries.
- To keep beds neat and clean:
  - Change linens whenever they become wet, soiled, or damp.
  - Straighten linens whenever loose or wrinkled and at bedtime.
  - Check for and remove food and crumbs after meals and snacks.
  - Check linens for dentures, eyeglasses, hearing aids, sharp objects, and other items.
  - Follow Standard Precautions and the Bloodborne Pathogen Standard.

Types of Beds
- Beds are made in these ways.
  - A closed bed is not in use or the bed is ready for a new resident. Top linens are not folded back.
  - An open bed is in use. Top linens are fan-folded back so the person can get into bed. A closed bed becomes an open bed by fan-folding back the top linens.
  - An occupied bed is made with the person in it.
  - A surgical bed is made to transfer a person from a stretcher. This bed is also made for persons who arrive by ambulance.

Linens
- When handling linens and making beds:
  - Practice medical asepsis.
  - Always hold linens away from your body and uniform. Your uniform is considered dirty.
  - Never shake linens.
  - Place clean linens on a clean surface.
  - Never put clean or used linens on the floor.
- Collect enough linens. Do not bring unneeded linens to the person's room. Once in the room, extra linens are considered contaminated. They cannot be used for another person.
- Roll each piece of used linens away from you. The side that touched the person is inside the roll and away from you.

Making Beds
- When making beds, safety and medical asepsis are important. Use good body mechanics. Follow the rules for safe resident handling, moving, and transfers. Practice hand hygiene before handling clean linens and after handling used linens. To save time and energy, make beds with a co-worker.
- Review Box 22-1(p 327), Rules for Bedmaking, in the Textbook.
- Closed beds are made for nursing center residents who are up and away from the bed for all or most of the day. Change linens as needed. For beds awaiting new residents or patients, the entire bed requires clean linens after the bed system has been cleaned and disinfected.
- The closed bed becomes an open bed by fan-folding back the top linens so the person can get into bed with ease.
- An occupied bed is made while the person stays in bed. Keep the person in good alignment. Follow restrictions or limits in the person's movement or position. Explain each procedure step to the person before it is done. This is important even if the person cannot respond to you.

CHAPTER 22 REVIEW QUESTIONS
Circle the BEST answer.
1. Which aspect of bedmaking is most likely to be of interest to a surveyor who is observing at your facility?
   a. How you make a mitered corner
   b. How you transport linens
   c. How you position the pillow on the bed
   d. How you center bed linen

2. Which item do you obtain first when you are collecting a stack of linen to change a soiled bed?
   a. Bottom sheet
   b. Top sheet
   c. Pillowcase
   d. Mattress pad
3. Which action would you use when changing a soiled bed?
   a. Wear gloves when removing soiled linens from the bed.
   b. Reach across bed and roll soiled linens towards you
   c. Gather soiled linens in a tight ball in the middle of the bed
   d. Pull soiled linens from bed directly into a laundry bag
4. Which action would you take to keep beds neat and clean?
   a. Encourage residents to leave their rooms after the beds are made
   b. Check for and remove food and crumbs after meals
   c. Ask the nurse if you should use the closed or open bed method
   d. Change linens whenever the residents want you to change them
5. Which nursing assistant needs to be reminded about the rules for bedmaking?
   a. Nursing Assistant A practices medical asepsis when handling linens.
   b. Nursing Assistant B holds linens away from her body and uniform.
   c. Nursing Assistant C shakes linens to remove crumbs and food
   d. Nursing Assistant D put soiled linens in the used laundry bin.

Answers to these questions are on p. 537.

CHAPTER 23 ORAL HYGIENE
Oral Hygiene
- Oral hygiene keeps the mouth and teeth clean. It prevents mouth odors and infections, increases comfort, and makes food taste better. Mouth care also reduces the risk for cavities and periodontal disease.
- Ask the person about his/her preferences for when and how often oral hygiene is performed. Follow the care plan.
- Follow Standard Precautions and the Bloodborne Pathogen Standard.

Brushing and Flossing Teeth
- Flossing removes plaque and tartar from the teeth as well as food from between the teeth.
- Flossing is recommended at least once a day and can be done when the person desires.
- You need to floss for persons who cannot do so themselves.
- Some persons need help gathering and setting up equipment for oral hygiene. Perform oral care for persons who are weak, cannot move their arms, or are too confused to brush their teeth.

Mouth Care for the Unconscious Person

- Unconscious persons have dry mouths and crusting on the tongue and mucous membranes. Oral hygiene keeps the mouth clean and moist. It also helps prevent infection.
- Use sponge swabs to apply the cleaning agent. To prevent cracking of the lips, apply a lubricant to the lips. Follow the care plan.
- To prevent aspiration on the unconscious person:
  - Position the person on his/her side with the head turned well to the side.
  - Use only a small amount of fluid to clean the mouth.
  - Do not insert dentures. Dentures are not worn when the person is unconscious.
- When giving oral hygiene, keep the person's mouth open with a plastic tongue depressor.
- Mouth care is given at least every 2 hours. Follow the care plan.

Denture Care

- Mouth care is given and dentures are cleaned as often as natural teeth. Dentures are usually removed at bedtime. Some persons remove dentures at meal time. Remind people not to wrap dentures in tissues or napkins at meal time, as they could be discarded accidentally.
- Dentures are slippery when wet. Hold them firmly. During cleaning, hold them over a sink that is half-filled with water and lined with a towel. Use a cleaning agent and follow the manufacturer's instructions.
- Hot water causes dentures to lose their shape. If dentures are not worn after cleaning, store them in a container with cool water or a denture soaking solution.
- Label the denture cup with the person's name, room number, and bed number. Report lost or damaged dentures to the nurse at once. Losing or damaging dentures is negligent conduct.
- Many people do not like being seen without their dentures. Privacy is important. If you clean dentures, return them to the person as quickly as possible.
- Persons with partial dentures have some natural teeth. They need to brush and floss the natural teeth.

Reporting and Recording

- Dry, cracked, swollen, or blistered lips
- Mouth or breath odor
- Redness, swelling, irritation, sores, or white patches in the mouth or on the tongue
- Bleeding, swelling, or redness of the gums
- Loose teeth
- Rough, sharp, or chipped areas on dentures
- Loose fitting dentures

CHAPTER 23 REVIEW QUESTIONS

Circle the BEST answer.

1. The person lacks appetite and you notice that he is eating less than he did before. What is the logical time to offer to help him with oral hygiene?
   a. At night, just before he goes to bed
   b. Before he goes to the dining room for meals
   c. In the morning as soon as he gets up
   d. After he has finished eating meals or snacks
2. When giving oral hygiene, what should you report and record?
   a. Dry, cracked, swollen, or blistered lips
   b. Position and angle of the toothbrush
   c. Amount of time to accomplish hygiene
   d. The number of fillings a person has
3. Which nursing assistant needs a reminder about how to do mouth care for a person who is unconscious?
   a. Nursing Assistant A uses a small amount of fluid to clean the mouth
   b. Nursing Assistant B uses her fingers to keep the person's mouth open
   c. Nursing Assistant C explains each step of care before proceeding
   d. Nursing Assistant D gives mouth care at least every 2 hours
4. What is the rationale for cleaning dentures over a sink half-filled with water and lined with a towel?
   a. This action prevents breakage if you accidentally drop them
   b. Dentures fit more comfortably into the mouth if they are wet
   c. Food particles, mucous and plaque must be scrubbed and rinsed off
   d. Dentures will warp or loose shape if they are too dry

Answers to these questions are on p. 537.

CHAPTER 24 DAILY HYGIENE AND BATHING

- Besides cleansing, good hygiene prevents body and breath odors. It is relaxing and increases circulation.
- Many factors affect daily hygiene needs—perspiration (sweating), elimination, vomiting, drainage from wounds or body openings, bedrest, and activity.

Daily Care

- Most people have hygiene routines and habits. Hygiene measures are often done before and after meals and at bedtime. You assist with hygiene whenever it is needed. Protect the person's right to privacy and to personal choice.

Bathing

- Bathing cleans the skin. The mucous membranes of the genital and anal areas are cleaned as well. A bath is refreshing and relaxing. Circulation is stimulated and body parts exercised. Talk to the person while assisting with hygiene and make observations.
- Review Box 24-2(p 354), Rules for Bathing, in the Textbook.
- Review Promoting Safety and Comfort: Bathing (p 356), in the Textbook
- Soap dries the skin. Therefore older persons usually need a complete bath or shower twice a week. Partial baths are taken the other days. Some bathe daily but not with soap. Thorough rinsing is needed when using soap. Lotions and oils keep the skin soft.

- Water temperature for complete bed baths and partial bed baths is between 110°F and 115°F. Older persons have fragile skin and need lower water temperatures. Measure water temperature according to agency policy.
- Report and record:
  - The color of the skin, lips, nail beds, and sclera (whites of the eyes)
  - If the skin appears pale, gray-ish, yellow (jaundice), or bluish (cyanotic)
  - The location and description of rashes
  - Skin texture—smooth, rough, scaly, flaky, dry, moist
  - Diaphoresis—profuse (excessive) sweating
  - Bruises or open areas
  - Pale or reddened areas, particularly over bony parts
  - Drainage or bleeding from wounds or body openings
  - Swelling of the feet and legs
  - Corns or calluses on the feet
  - Skin temperature
  - Complaints of pain or discomfort

The Complete Bed Bath

- The complete bed bath involves washing the person's entire body in bed. Wash around the person's eyes with water. Do not use soap. Gently wipe from the inner to the outer aspect of the eye. Use a clean part of the washcloth for each stroke. Ask the person if you should use soap to wash the face. Let the person wash the genital area if he or she is able.
- Give a back massage after the bath. Apply deodorant or antiperspirant, lotion, and powder as requested. Comb and brush the hair. Empty and clean the wash basin.

The Partial Bath

- The partial bath involves bathing the face, hands, axillae (underarms), back, buttocks, and perineal area. You assist the person as needed. Most need help washing the back.

Tub Baths and Showers

- Falls, burns, and chilling from water are risks. Review Box 24-2(p 354), Rules for Bathing, and Promoting Safety and Comfort: Tub Baths and Showers (p 364), in the Textbook.
- A tub bath can cause a person to feel faint, weak, or tired. The person may need a bathing lift, a tub with a side entry door, or a mechanical lift to get in and out of the tub.
- Some people can use a regular shower. Have the person use the grab bars for support during the shower. Use a bath math if the shower does not have slip resistant surfaces. Never let weak or unsteady persons stand in the shower. They may need to use shower chairs, shower stalls or cabinets, or shower trolleys. Some shower rooms have 2 or more stations. Protect the person's privacy. Properly screen and cover the person.
- Water temperature for tub baths and showers is usually 105°F/ 40. 5° C
- Report and record dizziness and light-headedness.
- Clean and disinfect the tub or shower before and after use.

Perineal Care

- Perineal care involves cleaning the genital and anal areas. It is done daily during the bath and whenever

the area is soiled with urine or feces. The person does perineal care if able.

- *Perineal* and *perineum* are not common terms. Most people understand *privates, private parts, crotch, genitals,* or *the area between the legs*. Use terms the person understands.
- Standard Precautions, medical asepsis, and the Bloodborne Pathogen Standard are followed.
- Work from clean to the dirty—commonly called cleaning from "front to back." On a woman, clean from the urethra (cleanest) to the anal (dirtiest) area. On a male, start at the meatus of the urethra and work outward.
- Use warm water. Use washcloths, towelettes, cotton balls, or swabs according to agency policy. Rinse thoroughly. Pat dry. Water temperature is usually 105°F to 109°F.
- Report and record:
  - Bleeding, redness, swelling, irritation, discharge
  - Complaints of pain, burning, or other discomfort
  - Signs of urinary or fecal incontinence
  - Signs of skin breakdown
  - Odors

CHAPTER 24 REVIEW QUESTIONS

Circle the BEST answer.

1. In hospitals, what is the most common time for bathing?
   a. After breakfast
   b. Before going to bed
   c. After procedures
   d. Before being discharged

2. The water temperature for a complete bed bath is
   a. 102°F to 108°F
   b. 110°F to 115°F
   c. 115°F to 120°F
   d. 120°F to 125°F

3. You are assisting a person who has a respiratory disorder. If you are not careful when applying powder after a bath or shower, what could happen to the person?
   a. Respiratory disease causes dry skin and powder will worsen the dryness
   b. Respiratory disorders cause a person to sweat and powder will cake
   c. Powder could cause a skin rash with severe itching
   d. Inhaled powder could irritate the lungs and the airways

4. When washing a person's eyes, what would you do?
   a. Have the person rinse the eyes with cool water
   b. Avoid the eye area unless given specific instructions
   c. Gently wipe from the outer to the inner aspect of the eye
   d. Use a clean part of the washcloth for each stroke

5. When giving female perineal care, you should.
   a. Cleanse the anal area first with a paper towel
   b. Cleanse from the urethra to the anal area
   c. Have the person soak in tub of warm water
   d. Coach the person as she performs self-care

6. When giving male perineal care,
   a. Use the bag bath method
   b. Ask the person to retract the foreskin
   c. Start at the meatus and work outward
   d. Clean the scrotum first; it is cleaner than the penis

CHAPTER 25 GROOMING

- Hair care, shaving, nail and foot care prevent infection and promote comfort.

Hair Care

- You assist patients and residents with brushing and combing hair and with shampooing as needed and according to the care plan.

Brushing and Combing Hair

- Encourage residents to brush and comb their own hair but assist as needed.
- Daily brushing and combing prevent tangled and matted hair.
- When brushing and combing hair, start at the scalp and brush or comb to the hair ends.
- Never cut hair for any reason.
- Special measures are needed for curly, coarse, and dry hair. Check the care plan.
- When giving hair care, place a towel across the person's back and shoulders to protect garments from falling hair. If the person is in bed, give hair care before changing the linens and pillowcase.

Shampooing

- Shampooing frequency depends on the person's needs and preferences.
- Keep shampoo away from and out of eyes. Have the person hold a washcloth over the eyes.
- Wear gloves if the person has scalp sores, nits, lice or other hair or scalp problems.
- Follow Standard Precautions and the Bloodborne Pathogen Standard.
- Water temperature is usually 105°F.
- Hair is dried and styled as soon as possible after the shampooing.
- During shampooing, report and record:
  - Scalp sores
  - Flaking
  - Itching
  - Presence of nits or lice
  - Hair falling out in patches; patches of hair loss
  - Very dry or very oily hair
  - Matted or tangled hair
  - How the person tolerated the procedure

Shaving

- Shaving is common for facial hair, underarms and legs.
- Electric shaver or safety razors are used. Some persons have their own shavers. Do not use safety razors on persons with healing problems or persons taking anticoagulant drugs. Older persons with wrinkled skin are at risk for nicks and cuts. Safety razors are not used to shave them or persons with dementia.
- Wash and comb mustaches and beards daily and as needed. Ask the person how to groom his mustache or beard. Never shave or trim a mustache or a beard.
- Many women shave their legs and underarms. This practice varies among cultures. Legs and underarms are shaved after bathing when the skin is soft.
- Review Box 25-1(p 383), Rules for Shaving, in the Textbook.

Nail and Foot Care

- Nail and foot care prevent infection, injury, and odors.
- Nails are easier to trim and clean right after soaking or bathing.
- Use nail clippers to cut fingernails. Never use scissors. Use extreme caution to prevent damage to nearby tissues.
- Some agencies do not let nursing assistants cut or trim toenails. Follow agency policy.
- Follow Standard Precautions and the Bloodborne Pathogen Standard.
- Report and record:
  - Dry, reddened, irritated, or callused areas
  - Breaks in the skin
  - Corns on top of and between the toes
  - Blisters
  - Very thick nails
  - Loose nails
- You do not cut or trim toenails if a person has diabetes or poor circulation to the legs and feet or takes drugs that affect blood clotting. Also, do not cut or trim toenails if the person has nail fungus, very thick nails or ingrown toenails. The nurse or podiatrist cuts toenails and provides foot care for these persons.
- When doing foot care, check between the toes for cracks and sores. If left untreated, a serious infection could occur.
- The feet of persons with decreased sensation or circulatory problems may easily burn because they do not feel hot temperatures.
- After soaking, apply lotion to the feet. Because the lotion can cause slippery feet, help the person put on slip-resistant footwear before you transfer the person or let the person walk.

CHAPTER 25 REVIEW QUESTIONS

Circle the BEST answer.

1. Which aspect of grooming is a surveyor most likely to observe for?
   a. Personal grooming supplies are stored in the bathroom
   b. Female residents are wearing nail polish
   c. Shared items, such as nail clippers are stored in the proper place
   d. Residents have their hair combed and styled
2. A person's hair is matted and tangled. What should you do?
   a. Shampoo the hair first and then use a wide-tooth comb
   b. Get the nurse's permission to cut the hair at the tangled area

c. Brush through the matting and tangling from the hair ends to the scalp.

d. Wet the hair, apply conditioner and wait for the hair shaft to soften

3. While combing the resident's hair you observe small white oval shapes and tan colored insects that are about the size of a sesame seed. You report this to the nurse. Which instruction is the nurse most likely to give you?

a. Wash the person's hair twice and use generous amounts of shampoo.

b. Always wear gloves whenever you perform any care for the person

c. Report to the employee health clinic for exposure to infection

d. Wash linens from the bed and person's clothing in hot water

4. When should you wear gloves for shampooing a person's hair?

a. The person has oily hair

b. The person has sores on the scalp

c. The person likes a long scalp massage

d. The person has very thin hair

5. Which adverse outcome could occur, when a new and inexperienced nursing assistant uses a blade razor to shave a person who is taking an anticoagulant medication?

a. The hair is brittle and breaks under the razor blade

b. The skin is fragile and easily torn during shaving

c. Shaving will be uncomfortable, because the hair is coarse

d. A nick or a cut could cause serious bleeding

6. Which action would you perform before you begin to shave facial hair?

a. Brush out the whiskers and hair

b. Gently rub the face with a towel

c. Apply lotion or after-shave

d. Apply a warm moist towel

7. Which nursing assistant needs a reminder about the rules and guidelines for grooming?

a. Nursing Assistant A uses scissors to trim the fingernails and toenails

b. Nursing Assistant B brushes out tangles before shampooing the hair

c. Nursing Assistant C stores the person's eyeglasses before combing hair

d. Nursing Assistant D reports to the nurse that the person has corn on the toe

8. What is included in the daily care of mustaches and beards?

a. Clipping

b. Combing

c. Trimming

d. Shaving

9. For a person who has diabetes, which aspect of grooming is not part of your duties?

a. Trimming the toenails

b. Shampooing the hair

c. Assisting with shaving

d. Styling the hair

10. Fingernails are cut with

a. Scissors

b. Nail clippers

c. An emery board

d. A nail file

CHAPTER 26 DRESSING AND UNDRESSSING

Changing Garments

- Garments are changed after the bath and whenever wet or soiled or on admission or discharge

- To assist with dressing and undressing, you need this information from the nurse and the care plan.
  - How much help the person needs
  - Which side is the person's unaffected side (strong side)
  - If certain garments are needed

- What observations to report and record:
  - How much help was given
  - How the person tolerated the procedure
  - Complaints by the person
  - Changes in the person's behavior
  - When to report observations
  - What patient or resident concerns to report at once

- When changing clothing:
  - Provide for privacy. Do not expose the person.
  - Encourage the person to do as much as possible.
  - Let the person choose what to wear. Make sure the right under-garments are chosen.
  - Make sure garments and footwear are the correct size.
  - Remove clothing from the strong (unaffected) side first.
  - Put clothing on the weak (affected) side first.
  - Support the arm or leg when removing or putting on a garment.
  - Move or handle the body gently. Do not force a joint beyond its range of motion or to the point of pain.

- When changing gowns, remove the gown from the strong arm first while supporting the weak arm. Put a clean gown on the weak arm first and then the strong arm.

- To change the gown of a person with an intravenous (IV) bag, gather the sleeve of the arm with the IV bag and slide it over the IV site and tubing. Remove the IV bag, draw it through the sleeve, and re-hang the IV bag. Gather the sleeve of the clean gown, remove the IV bag, slide the sleeve over the IV bag, then re-hang the bag. Slide the sleeve over the tubing, hand, arm, and IV site. Do not pull on the tubing.

- Have the nurse check the flow rate after changing the gown of a person with an IV. If the person is on an IV pump, do not change the gown; ask the nurse for instructions.

CHAPTER 26 REVIEW QUESTIONS
Circle the BEST answer.

1. Which nursing assistant needs a reminder about assisting residents to dress and undress?

a. Nursing Assistant A provides privacy when residents are changing clothes.

b. Nursing Assistant B helps residents to don street clothes for the day.

c. Nursing Assistant C encourages the residents to choose what to wear.

d. Nursing Assistant D stretches the residents' clothes so they are easier to put on

2. Which action would be the best to use in assisting a person with Alzheimer's to get dressed?
   a. Assist him to dress at the same time everyday
   b. Ask him what he would like to wear
   c. Assist him to find his long johns
   d. Give him a button hook dressing aid

3. What is the primary purpose of labeling residents' clothing and shoes on the inside?
   a. To ensure that residents are wearing their own clothes
   b. To help confused residents recognize their items
   c. To respect and preserve dignity of residents
   d. To prevent theft of residents' personal items

4. You are assisting a person who is lying in bed to remove his pants. You instruct him to lift his hips and buttocks, but he is unable. What would you do?
   a. Ask a co-worker to lift him up
   b. Tug on his pants one side at a time
   c. Assist him to stand up
   d. Turn him towards you

5. Which nursing assistant has performed the correct acting while changing the gown of a person who has an IV?
   a. Nursing Assistant A turns the IV pump off in order to thread the tubing through the sleeve
   b. Nursing Assistant B places the IV bag on the bed while assisting the patient with the gown
   c. Nursing Assistant C asks the nurse to check the IV flow rate after the gown is changed
   d. Nursing Assistant D cuts off the standard gown and obtains a clean gown with snap fasteners

Answers to these questions are on p. 537.

CHAPTER 27 URINARY NEEDS
Normal Urination
- The healthy adult produces about 1500 milliliters (mL) of urine a day.
- The frequency of urination is affected by amount of fluid intake, habits, availability of toilet facilities, activity, work, and illness. People usually void at bedtime, after sleep, and before meals. Some people void every 2 to 3 hours. The need to void at night disturbs sleep. Some persons need help getting to the bathroom and others use bedpans, urinals, or commodes. Review Box 27-1(p 402), Rules for Normal Urination, in the Textbook.

Observations
- Observe urine for color, clarity, odor, amount, particles, and blood. Normal urine is pale yellow, straw-colored, or amber. It is clear with no particles. A faint odor is normal.
- Some foods and drugs affect urine color. Ask the nurse to observe urine that looks or smells abnormal.

- Report the following urinary problems.
  o **Dysuria**—painful or difficult urination
  o **Enuresis**—involuntary loss or leakage of urine during sleep: bedwetting
  o **Hematuria**—blood in the urine
  o **Nocturia**—frequent urination at night
  o **Oliguria**—scant amount of urine; less than 500 mL in 24 hours
  o **Polyuria**—abnormally large amounts of urine
  o **Urinary frequency**—voiding at frequent intervals
  o **Urinary retention**—not being able to completely empty the bladder
  o **Urinary incontinence**—involuntary loss or leakage of urine
  o **Urinary urgency**—the need to void at once

Assisting with a Bedpan, Urinal or Commode
- Follow Standard Precautions and the Bloodborne Pathogen Standard when handling bedpans, urinals, commodes, and their contents.
- Bedpans are used when the person cannot be out of bed.
- Urinals for men or women can be used standing, sitting, or lying down (supine or lateral position). Female urinals are shaped to fit snugly under the urethra. See Delegation Guidelines: Urinals (p 406), in the Textbook. Remind people not to place urinals on over-bed tables and bedside stands.
- Commodes are chairs or wheelchairs with an opening for a container. Persons unable to walk to the bathroom often use commodes. See Delegation Guidelines: Commodes (p 408), in the Textbook.
- Thoroughly clean and disinfect bedpans, urinals, and commodes after use.

Urinary Incontinence
- **Urinary incontinence** is the involuntary loss or leakage of urine.
- If urinary incontinence is a new problem, tell the nurse at once.
- Incontinence is embarrassing. Garments are wet and odors develop. Skin irritation, infection, and pressure injuries are risks. The person's pride, dignity, and self-esteem are affected. Social isolation, loss of independence, and depression are common.
- Good skin care and dry garments and clean linens are essential. Promoting normal urinary elimination prevents incontinence in some people. Other people may need bladder training.
- Review Box 27-3(p 411), Urinary Incontinence-Nursing Measures, in the Textbook.
- Caring for persons with incontinence is stressful. Remember, the person does not choose to be incontinent. If you find yourself becoming short-tempered and impatient, talk to the nurse at once. Kindness, empathy, understanding, and patience are needed.

Applying Incontinence Products
- Incontinence products are used to keep the person dry. Most are disposable and only used once.

- Incontinence products include a complete incontinence brief, a pad and under-garment, pull-on underwear, or a belted under-garment. Follow the manufacturer's instructions for applying incontinence products.
- Observations to report and record:
  - Complaints of pain, burning, irritation, or the need to void
  - Signs and symptoms of skin breakdown, including redness, irritation, blisters, and complaints of pain, burning, itching, or tingling
  - The amount of urine and urine color
  - Blood in the urine
  - Leakage or a poor product fit
- Review Box 27-4(p 413), Applying Incontinence Products, in the Textbook.

Bladder Training

- Bladder training helps some persons with urinary incontinence. Control of urination is the goal. Bladder control promotes comfort and quality of life. It also increases self-esteem.
- You assist with bladder training as directed by the nurse and the care plan. The care plan may include one of the following: bladder rehabilitation, prompted voiding, habit training/scheduled voiding, or catheter clamping.

CHAPTER 27 REVIEW QUESTIONS

Circle the BEST answer.

1. Which observation is abnormal and needs to be reported to the nurse?
   a. Urine is straw-colored.
   b. Urine is a pale-yellow color
   c. Urine is an amber color
   d. Urine is a bright red color
2. Which observation needs to be promptly reported to the nurse?
   a. Person is having new onset of urinary urgency
   b. Person has been assisted to the commode 3 times
   c. Person needs a larger size of incontinence underwear
   d. Person voided a large amount of yellow urine after lunch
3. Which liquid may contribute to bladder irritation and temporary incontinence?
   a. Water
   b. Low-fat milk
   c. Coffee
   d. Apple juice
4. Which person is demonstrating functional incontinence?
   a. Confused person can't find the bathroom
   b. Older woman passes urine when she sneezes
   c. Older man has dribbling and a weak stream
   d. Person is being treated for a urinary tract infection
5. The goal of bladder training is to
   a. Allow the person to use the toilet
   b. Improve perineal hygiene
   c. Gain control of urination
   d. Decrease dependence on staff

Answers to these questions are on p. 537.

CHAPTER 28 URINARY CATHETERS

- A catheter is a tube used to drain or inject fluid through a body opening. A urinary catheter is inserted through the urethra into the bladder and is used to drain urine.
- The types of catheters are a **straight catheter,** which is used to drain the urine and then removed, and an **indwelling catheter (retention or Foley catheter),** which is left in the bladder and drains urine constantly into a drainage bag. A **supra-pubic catheter** is surgically inserted into the bladder through an incision above (supra) the pubis bone (pubic).

Catheter Care

- The risk of a urinary tract infection (UTI) is high. Review Box 28-1(p 422), Indwelling Catheter Care, in the Textbook.
- The catheter must not pull at the insertion site. Hold the catheter securely during catheter care. Then properly secure the catheter. Also make sure the tubing is not under the person. Besides obstructing urine flow, lying on the tubing is uncomfortable. It can also cause skin breakdown.
- Follow Standard Precautions and the Bloodborne Pathogen Standard.
- Report and record:
  - Complaints of pain, burning, irritation, or the need to void (report at once)
  - Crusting, abnormal drainage, or secretions
  - The color, clarity, and odor of urine
  - Particles in the urine
  - Blood in the urine
  - Cloudy urine
  - Urine leaking at the insertion site
  - Drainage system leaks

Urine Drainage Systems

- A closed urinary drainage system is used for indwelling catheters. Infections can occur if microbes enter the drainage system. The two types of drainage bags are standard drainage bags and leg bags.
- The standard drainage bag hangs from the bed frame, chair, or wheelchair. It must not touch the floor. The bag is always kept lower than the person's bladder. Do not hang the drainage bag on a bed rail.
- If the drainage system is disconnected accidentally, tell the nurse at once. Do not touch the ends of the catheter or tubing. Do the following:
  - Practice hand hygiene. Put on gloves.
  - Wipe the end of the drainage tube with an antiseptic wipe.
  - Wipe the end of the catheter with another antiseptic wipe.
  - Do not put the ends down. Do not touch the ends after you clean them.
  - Connect the drainage tubing to the catheter.
  - Discard the wipes into a biohazard bag.
  - Remove the gloves. Practice hand hygiene.
- Check with the nurse and care plan about when to empty and measure the urine in the drainage bag.

Follow Standard Precautions and the Bloodborne Pathogen Standard.
- A leg bag is a drainage system that attaches to the thigh or calf. Empty and measure a leg bag when it is half full.
- Report and record:
  o The amount of urine measured
  o The color, clarity, and odor of urine
  o Particles in the urine
  o Blood in the urine
  o Cloudy urine
  o Complaints of pain, burning, irritation, or the need to urinate
  o Drainage system leaks

Removing Indwelling Catheters
- Before removing an indwelling catheter, be sure that your state allows you to perform this procedure, the procedure is in your job description, you know how to use the supplies and equipment, and you review the procedure with the nurse.
- The balloon of an indwelling catheter is inflated with water injected with a syringe. A syringe is also used to remove the water. Before removing the indwelling catheter, learn the size of the balloon before deflating it. If the balloon is 5 mL in size, you must withdraw 5 mL of water with the syringe. Do not remove the catheter if water remains in the balloon. Call the nurse.
- Report and record the following observations.
  o The amount of urine in the drainage bag
  o The color, clarity, and odor of urine
  o Particles in the urine
  o Blood in the urine
  o How the person tolerated the procedure
  o Complaints of pain, burning, irritation, or the need to void

Condom Catheters
- Condom catheters are often used for incontinent men. They are also called external catheters, Texas catheters, and urinary sheaths.
- These catheters are changed daily after perineal care.
- To apply a condom catheter, follow the manufacturer's instructions. Thoroughly wash and dry the penis before applying the catheter.
- Some condom catheters are self-adhering. Other catheters are secured in place with elastic tape in a spiral manner. Never use adhesive tape to secure catheters. It does not expand. Blood flow to the penis is cut off, injuring the penis.
- When removing or applying a condom catheter, report and record the following observations.
  o Reddened or open areas on the penis
  o Swelling of the penis
  o Color, clarity, and odor of urine
  o Particles in the urine
  o Blood in the urine
  o Cloudy urine

- Do not apply a condom catheter if the penis is red, is irritated, or shows signs of skin breakdown. Report your observations to the nurse at once.

CHAPTER 28 REVIEW QUESTIONS
Circle the BEST answer.
1. Which statement is correct?
   a. The urine drainage system is placed on the floor under the person's bed
   b. The urine drainage system is placed on the bed during stretcher transfers
   c. The urine drainage system is placed on the person's lap if he/she is in a wheelchair
   d. The urine drainage system must be kept lower than the person's bladder.
2. If the drainage system becomes accidentally disconnected, you need to
   a. Call the nurse right away
   b. Use antiseptic wipes to clean the ends of the tubing
   c. Put on gloves and clamp the tubing
   d. Put the ends of the tubing on paper towels
3. Before removing an indwelling catheter, what do you do first?
   a. Gently tug to see if it will come out.
   b. Wipe the meatus with an antiseptic wipe.
   c. Drain the balloon with a syringe.
   d. Check the balloon size.
4. How often are condom catheters changed?
   a. Condom catheters are changed daily.
   b. Condom catheters are changed at the end of each shift.
   c. Whenever the tape becomes loose
   d. When the penis is sore or red

Answers to these questions are on p. 537.

CHAPTER 29 BOWEL NEEDS
Normal Bowel Elimination
- Bowel movements (BMs) vary from person to person—daily, 2 to 3 times a day, every 2 to 3 days. Time of day also varies.
- Carefully observe stools before disposing of them. Observe and report the color, amount, consistency, odor, and shape of stools. Also observe and report the presence of blood or mucus, the time the person had the bowel movement (BM), the frequency of BMs, and any complaints of pain or discomfort.

Factors Affecting Bowel Elimination
- *Privacy.* Bowel elimination is a private act.
- *Habits.* Many people have a BM after breakfast. Some read. Defecation is easier when a person is relaxed.
- *Diet—high-fiber foods.* Fiber helps prevent constipation.
- *Diet—other foods.* Some foods cause constipation. Other foods cause frequent stools or diarrhea.
- *Fluids.* Drinking 6 to 8 glasses of water daily promotes normal bowel elimination. Warm fluids—coffee, tea, hot cider, warm water—increase peristalsis.
- *Activity.* Exercise and activity maintain muscle tone and stimulate peristalsis.

- *Drugs*. Drugs can prevent constipation or control diarrhea. Some have diarrhea or constipation as side effects.
- *Disability*. Some people cannot control BMs. A bowel training program is needed.
- *Aging*. Older persons are at risk for constipation. Some older persons lose bowel control and have fecal incontinence.
- To provide comfort and safety during bowel elimination, review Box 29-1(p 440), Safety and Comfort—Bowel Needs, in the Textbook. Follow Standard Precautions and the Bloodborne Pathogen Standard.

Common Problems

- Common problems include constipation, fecal impaction, diarrhea, fecal incontinence, and flatulence.
- **Constipation** is the passage of a hard, dry stool.
- Common causes of constipation are a low-fiber diet and ignoring the urge to defecate. Other causes include decreased fluid intake, inactivity, drugs, aging, and certain diseases.
- Dietary changes, fluids, and activity prevent or relieve constipation. So do stool softeners, laxatives, suppositories, and enemas.
- A **fecal impaction** is the prolonged retention and buildup of feces in the rectum.
- Fecal impaction results if constipation is not relieved. The person cannot defecate. Liquid feces pass around the hardened fecal mass in the rectum. The liquid feces seep from the anus.
- Signs and symptoms of fecal impaction include: abdominal discomfort, abdominal distention, nausea, cramping, and rectal pain. Older persons have poor appetite or confusion. Some persons have a fever. Report these signs and symptoms to the nurse.
- Checking for and removing a fecal impaction can be dangerous, because the vagus nerve can be stimulated, resulting in a slowing of the heart rate. Check with your state and agency policies to determine if you may perform this procedure.
- **Diarrhea** is the frequent passage of liquid stools.
- The need to have a BM is urgent. Some people cannot get to a bathroom in time. Abdominal cramping, nausea, and vomiting may occur.
- Assist with elimination needs promptly, dispose of stools promptly, and give good skin care. Liquid stools irritate the skin. So does frequent wiping with toilet paper. Skin breakdown and pressure injuries are risks.
- Follow Standard Precautions and the Bloodborne Pathogen Standard when in contact with stools.
- Report signs of diarrhea at once. Ask the nurse to observe the stool.
- **Fecal incontinence** is the inability to control the passage of feces and gas through the anus.
- Fecal incontinence affects the person emotionally. Frustration, embarrassment, anger, and humiliation are common. The person may need:
  - Bowel training
  - Help with elimination after meals and every 2 to 3 hours

- Incontinence products to keep garments and linens clean
- Good skin care
- **Flatulence** is the excessive formation of gas or air in the stomach and intestines.
- Causes include swallowing air while eating and drinking and bacterial action in the intestines. Other causes may be gas-forming foods, constipation, bowel and abdominal surgeries, and drugs that decrease peristalsis.
- If flatus is not expelled, the intestines distend (swell or enlarge from the pressure of gases). Abdominal cramping or pain, shortness of breath, and a swollen abdomen occur. "Bloating" is a common complaint. Exercise, walking, moving in bed, and the left side-lying position often produce flatus. Enemas and drugs may be ordered.

Bowel Training

- Bowel training has 2 goals.
  - To gain control of BMs.
  - To develop a regular pattern of elimination. Fecal impactions, constipation, and fecal incontinence are prevented.
- Factors that promote elimination are part of the care plan and bowel training program.

Suppositories

- A suppository is a cone-shaped, solid drug that is inserted into a body opening. A rectal suppository is inserted into the rectum. Suppositories melt at body temperature.
- A BM occurs about 30 minutes after inserting a suppository.
- Check with your state and agency policies to determine if you can insert a suppository.

Enemas

- An **enema** is the introduction of fluid into the rectum and lower colon.
- Doctors order enemas to:
  - Remove feces.
  - Relieve constipation, fecal impaction, or flatulence.
  - Clean the bowel of feces before certain surgeries and diagnostic procedures.
- Review Box 29-2(p 445), Giving Enemas, in the Textbook.
- The preferred position for an enema is the Sims' or left side-lying position.
- A cleansing enema is used to clean the bowel of feces and flatus and to relieve constipation and fecal impaction. Cleansing enemas take effect in 10 to 20 minutes.
- A small-volume enema irritates the bowel and distends the rectum, causing a BM. The person should retain the enema solution until he or she needs to have a BM, which usually takes 1-5 minutes or as long as 10 minutes.
- An oil-retention enema relieves constipation and fecal impaction by softening the feces and lubricating the

rectum so the feces can pass. The oil is retained for 30 minutes to 1 to 3 hours.

The Person With an Ostomy

- Sometimes part of the intestines is removed surgically. An ostomy is sometimes necessary. An **ostomy** is a surgically created opening for the elimination of body wastes. The opening is called a **stoma.** The person wears an ostomy pouch over the stoma to collect stools and flatus.
- Stools irritate the skin. Skin care prevents skin breakdown around the stoma. The skin is washed and dried. Then a skin barrier is applied around the stoma. It prevents stools from having contact with the skin. The skin barrier is part of the ostomy pouch or a separate device.
- The pouch has an adhesive backing that is applied to the skin. Sometimes pouches are secured to ostomy belts.
- The pouch is changed every 3 to 7 days and when it leaks. Frequent pouch changes can damage the skin.
- An ostomy pouch is emptied when it is about one-third (1/3) to one-half (1/2) full with feces or gas. Depending on the person, ostomy type, and ostomy location, pouches are usually emptied 2 to 6 times a day. Many pouches have a drain at the bottom that closes with a clip, clamp, or wire closure. The drain is opened to empty the pouch. The drain is wiped with toilet tissue before it is closed.
- Observations to report and record include signs of skin breakdown, color, amount, consistency, and odor of stools, and complaints of pain or discomfort.

CHAPTER 29 REVIEW QUESTIONS

Circle the BEST answer.

1. Which habit is most likely to contribute to constipation?
   a. Eats whole grain cereal and fruit for breakfast
   b. Spends most of the day sitting in a chair
   c. Drinking 6 to 8 glasses of water daily.
   d. Having 2 cups of coffee in the morning
2. Which food is gas-forming and will therefore stimulate peristalsis?
   a. Biscuit
   b. Cottage cheese
   c. Chocolate
   d. Cabbage
3. A person has fecal incontinence. How often should you assist him to go to the bathroom?
   a. Whenever you have extra time
   b. After meals and every 2 to 3 hours
   c. In the morning and at bedtime
   d. Every 30 minutes while awake
4. The preferred position for an enema is the
   a. Sims' position or the left side-lying position
   b. Prone position
   c. Supine position
   d. Trendelenburg's position

Answers to these questions are on p. 537.

CHAPTER 30 NUTRITION NEEDS

- A poor diet and poor eating habits:
  - Increase the risk for disease and infection.
  - Cause chronic illnesses to become worse.
  - Cause healing problems.
  - Increase the risk of accidents and injuries.

Basic Nutrition

- **Nutrition** is the process involved in the ingestion, digestion, absorption, and use of foods and fluids by the body. Good nutrition is needed for growth, healing, and body functions.
- A *nutrient* is a substance that is ingested, digested, absorbed, and used by the body.
- A *calorie* is the fuel or energy value of food.

Dietary Guidelines for Americans

- The Dietary Guidelines help people attain and maintain a healthy weight, reduce the risk of chronic disease, and promote overall health. The Dietary Guidelines focus on consuming fewer calories, making informed food choices, and being physically active.

MyPlate

- The MyPlate symbol, issued by the United States Department of Agriculture (USDA), helps you make wise food choices by balancing calories, increasing certain foods like fruits and vegetables, and reducing certain foods with excess salt and sugar.

Nutrients

- A well-balanced diet ensures an adequate intake of essential nutrients.
- *Protein*—is needed for tissue growth and repair. Sources include meat, fish, poultry, eggs, milk and milk products, cereals, beans, peas, and nuts.
- *Carbohydrates*—provide energy and fiber for bowel elimination. They are found in fruits, vegetables, breads, cereals, and sugar.
- *Fats*—provide energy, add flavor to food, and help the body use certain vitamins. Sources of healthy fats include salmon, avocados, and olive oil. Unhealthy fats usually come from animal sources (meats and dairy foods).
- *Vitamins*—are needed for certain body functions. The body stores vitamins A, D, E, and K. The vitamin C and the B complex vitamins are not stored and must be ingested daily.
- *Minerals*—are needed for bone and tooth formation, nerve and muscle function, fluid balance, and other body processes.
- *Water*—is needed for all body processes.
- Review Tables 30-2(p 462), Common Vitamins, and 30-3(p 463), Common Minerals, in the Textbook

Centers for Medicare & Medicaid Services Dietary Requirements

- CMS has requirements for food served in nursing centers.
  - Each person's nutritional and dietary needs are met.
  - Each person's religious and cultural needs and preferences are met.

○ The person's diet is well-balanced. It is nourishing and tastes good. Food is well-seasoned.
○ Food is appetizing. It has an appealing aroma and is attractive.
○ Hot food is served hot. Cold food is served cold.
○ Food is served promptly.
○ Food is prepared to meet each person's needs. Some people need food cut, ground, or chopped. Others have special diets.
○ Other foods are offered if the person refused the food served. Substituted food must have a similar nutritional value to the first foods served.
○ Each person receives at least 3 meals a day. A bedtime snack is offered.
○ The center provides needed adaptive equipment and utensils.

Factors Affecting Eating and Nutrition

- *Culture.* Culture influences dietary practices, food choices, and food preparation.
- *Religion.* Selecting, preparing, and eating food often involve religious practices. A person may follow all, some, or none of the dietary practices of his or her faith.
- *Finances.* People with limited incomes often buy the cheaper carbohydrate foods. Their diets often lack protein and certain vitamins and minerals.
- *Appetite.* Illness, drugs, anxiety, pain, and depression can cause loss of appetite. Unpleasant sights, thoughts, and smells are other causes.
- *Personal choice.* Food likes and dislikes are influenced by foods served in the home. Usually food likes expand with age and social experiences.
- *Body reactions.* People usually avoid foods that cause allergic reactions. They also avoid foods that cause nausea, vomiting, diarrhea, indigestion, gas, or headaches.
- *Illness.* Appetite usually decreases during illness and recovery from injuries. However, nutritional needs are increased.
- *Drugs.* Drugs can cause loss of appetite, confusion, nausea, constipation, impaired taste, or changes in gastro-intestinal (GI) function. They can cause inflammation of the mouth, throat, esophagus, and stomach.
- *Chewing problems.* Mouth, teeth, and gum problems can affect chewing. Examples include oral pain, dry or sore mouth, gum disease, and dentures that fit poorly. Broken, decayed, or missing teeth also affect chewing, especially the meat group.
- *Swallowing problems.* Stroke, pain, confusion, dry mouth, and diseases of the mouth, throat, and esophagus can affect swallowing.
- *Disability.* Disease or injury can affect the hands, wrists, and arms. Adaptive equipment lets the person eat independently.
- *Impaired cognitive function.* Impaired cognitive function may affect the person's ability to use eating utensils. And it may affect eating, chewing, and swallowing.
- *Age.* Many GI changes occur with aging.

Special Diets
The Sodium-Controlled Diet

- A sodium-controlled diet decreases the amount of sodium in the body. The diet involves:
○ Omitting high-sodium foods. Review Box 30-2 (p 467), High-Sodium Foods, in the Textbook.
○ Not adding salt when eating.
○ Limiting the amount of salt used in cooking.
○ Diet planning.

Diabetes Meal Planning

- Diabetes meal planning is for people with diabetes. It involves the person's food preferences and calories needed. It also involves eating meals and snacks at regular times.
- Serve the person's meals and snacks on time to maintain a certain blood sugar level.
- Always check the tray to see what was eaten. Tell the nurse what the person did and did not eat. If not all the food was eaten, a between-meal nourishment is needed. The nurse tells you what to give. Tell the nurse about changes in the person's eating habits.

The Dysphagia Diet

- **Dysphagia** means difficulty swallowing. Food thickness is changed to meet the person's needs. Review Box 30-3(p 468), Dysphagia, in the Textbook.
- You may need to feed a person with dysphagia. To promote the person's comfort:
○ Know the signs and symptoms of dysphagia. Review Box 30-3(p 468), Dysphagia-Signs and Symptoms, in the Textbook.
○ Feed the person according to the care plan.
○ Follow the ordered diet; fluid thickeners are used to meet the person's needs.
○ Follow aspiration precautions (see Box 30-3(p 468), Aspiration Precautions, in the Textbook) and the care plan.
○ Report changes in how the person eats.
○ Report choking, coughing, or difficulty breathing during or after meals. Also report abnormal breathing or respiratory sounds. Report these observations at once.

Food Intake

- Food intake is measured in different ways. Follow agency policy for the method use.
- *Percentage of food eaten.* Some agencies measure the percent of the whole meal tray. Other agencies measure the percent of each food item eaten.
- *Calorie counts.* Note what the person ate and how much. A nurse or dietitian converts the portion amounts into calories.

Preparing the Person for Meals

- Preparing residents for meals promotes their comfort.
○ Assist with elimination needs.
○ Provide oral hygiene. Make sure dentures are in place.
○ Make sure eyeglasses and hearing aids are in place.
○ Make sure incontinent persons are clean and dry.
○ Position the person in a comfortable position.

○ Reduce or remove unpleasant odors, sights and sounds.
○ Follow the care plan for pain relief measures
○ Assist the person with hand-hygiene.
- Food is served in containers that keep foods at the correct temperature. Hot food is kept hot. Cold food is kept cold.
- Prompt serving keeps food at the correct temperature.

Feeding the Person
- Serve food and fluid in the order the person prefers. Offer fluids during the meal.
- Use teaspoons to feed the person.
- Persons who need to be fed are often angry, humiliated, and embarrassed. Some are depressed or refuse to eat. Let them do as much as possible. If strong enough, let them hold milk or juice glasses. Never let them hold hot drinks.
- Tell the visually impaired person what is on the tray. Describe what you are offering. For persons who feed themselves, use the numbers on the clock for the location of foods.
- Many people pray before eating. Allow time and privacy for prayer.
- Meals provide social contact with others. Engage the person in pleasant conversations. Sit facing the person. Allow time to chew and swallow. The person will eat better if not rushed. Wipe the person's hands, face, and mouth as needed during the meal.
- Report and record:
  ○ The amount and kind of food eaten
  ○ Complaints of nausea or dysphagia
  ○ Signs and symptoms of dysphagia
  ○ Signs and symptoms of aspiration
- Many special diets involve between-meal snacks. These snacks are served upon arrival on the nursing unit. Follow the same considerations and procedures for serving meal trays and feeding persons.

CHAPTER 30 REVIEW QUESTIONS
Circle the BEST answer.
1. A person is on a sodium-controlled diet. Which snack would be best for this person?
   a. Apple slices and plain almonds
   b. Biscuit and peanut butter
   c. Pretzels and tomato juice
   d. Cheese and crackers
2. You are checking dietary cards and you see that the person is supposed to be on a clear liquid diet. Which item needs to be taken off the tray?
   a. Gelatin
   b. Iced-tea
   c. Broth
   d. Milk
3. Which person needs to have thickened liquids?
   a. Has dysphagia and frequently chokes and coughs during a meal
   b. Has diabetes and needs consistent calories throughout the day
   c. Has heart problems and blood pressure is higher than normal

d. Has constipation, is inactive and prefers low fiber foods
4. When feeding a person, what would you do?
   a. Feed all of the protein foods first
   b. Offer fluids at the end of the meal
   c. Hand the person a spoon and check on him frequently
   d. Wipe the person's hands, face and mouth as needed.
5. A person is visually impaired. What would you do?
   a. Draw a map of how the food is arranged on the plate
   b. Use the numbers on a clock to indicate the location of food
   c. Talk about your favorite foods and share recipes
   d. Let the person smell the food as you offer each bite

Answers to these questions are on p. 537.

CHAPTER 31 FLUID NEEDS
Fluid Balance
- Fluid balance is needed for health. The amount of fluid taken in (**intake**) and the amount of fluid lost (**output**) must be approximately equal. If fluid intake exceeds fluid output, body tissues swell with water (**edema**).
- **Dehydration** is a decrease in the amount of water in body tissues. Fluid output exceeds intake. Review Box 31-1(p 481), Dehydration, in the Textbook.

Normal Fluid Requirements
- An adult needs 1500 milliliters (mL) of water daily to survive. About 2000 to 2500 mL of fluid per day is needed for normal fluid balance. Water requirements increase with hot weather, exercise, fever, illness, and excess fluid loss.
- Older persons may have a decreased sense of thirst. Their bodies need water but they may not feel thirsty. Offer fluids according to the care plan.

Electrolytes
- Sodium, potassium, calcium, and magnesium are some electrolytes. Electrolytes are needed for:
  ○ Fluid balance
  ○ Acid-base (pH) balance (Chapter 10)
  ○ Movement of nutrients into the cells and wastes out of the cells
  ○ Nerve, muscle, heart, and brain function

Special Fluid Orders
- The doctor may order the amount of fluid a person can have in 24 hours. Intake and output (I&O) measurements may be ordered by the doctor or nurse.
- *Encourage fluids.* The person drinks an increased amount of fluid.
- *Restrict fluids.* Fluids are limited to a certain amount.
- *Nothing by mouth (NPO).* The person cannot eat or drink.
- *Thickened liquids.* All liquids are thickened, including water.

Intake and Output

- All fluids taken by mouth are measured and recorded—such as, water and milk. So are foods that melt at room temperature—ice cream, sherbet, custard, pudding, gelatin, and Popsicles.
- Output includes urine, vomitus, diarrhea, and wound drainage.

Measuring Intake and Output (I&O)

- To measure I&O, you need to know:
  - 1 cubic centimeter (cc) equals 1 mL.
  - 1 teaspoon equals 5 mL.
  - 1 ounce (oz) equals 30 mL.
  - 1 cup equals 240 mL
  - A pint is about 500 mL.
  - A quart is about 1000 mL.
  - 1 liter equals 1000mL.
  - The serving sizes of bowls, dishes, cups, pitchers, glasses, and other containers.
- An I&O record is kept at the bedside. Record I&O measurements in the correct column. Amounts are totaled at the end of the shift. The totals are recorded in the person's chart. They are also shared during the end-of-shift report.
- The urinal, commode, bedpan, or specimen pan is used for voiding. Remind the person not to void in the toilet. Also remind the person not to put toilet paper into the receptacle.

Providing Drinking Water

- Patients and residents need fresh drinking water each shift. Follow the agency's procedure for providing fresh water.
- Water mugs and pitchers can spread microbes. To prevent the spread of microbes:
  - Label the water mug with the person's name and room and bed number.
  - Do not touch the rim or inside of the mug or lid.
  - Do not let the ice scoop touch the mug, lid, or straw.
  - Place the ice scoop in the holder or on a towel, not in the ice container or dispenser.
  - Keep ice chest closed when not in use.
  - Make sure the person's water mug is clean and free of cracks and chips. Provide a new mug as needed.

CHAPTER 31 REVIEW QUESTIONS

Circle the BEST answer.

1. Which person has a sign or symptom of dehydration?
   a. Person A has a swollen leg
   b. Person B has dark amber urine
   c. Person C has trouble swallowing
   d. Person D has an intake of 2000mL
2. A person is on intake and output. Which item is recorded as intake?
   a. Ice cream
   b. Apple slices
   c. Toast
   d. Strawberry jam

3. A person drank a pint of milk at lunch. You record this as
   a. 250 mL of milk
   b. 350 mL of milk
   c. 500 mL of milk
   d. 750 mL of milk
4. The soup bowl holds 6 ounces. A person ate all of the soup. You record his intake as
   a. 50 mL
   b. 120 mL
   c. 180 mL
   d. 200 mL
5. Which person is most likely to need frequent oral hygiene?
   a. Person A is on "encourage fluids"
   b. Person B needs "restricted fluids"
   c. Person C needs "thickened fluids"
   d. Person D is on "regular fluids"

Answers to these questions are on p. 537.

CHAPTER 33 VITAL SIGNS

Vital Signs

- The vital signs of body function are temperature, pulse, respirations, blood pressure, and, in some agencies, pain or pulse oximetry.
- Accuracy is essential when you measure, record, and report vital signs. If unsure of your measurements, promptly ask the nurse to take them again.
- Report the following at once.
  - Any vital sign that is changed from a prior measurement
  - Vital signs above or below the normal range

Body Temperature

- Thermometers are used to measure temperature. It is measured using the Fahrenheit (F) and centigrade or Celsius (C) scales.
- Temperature sites are the mouth, rectum, axilla (underarm), tympanic membrane (ear), and temporal artery (forehead).
- Review Box 33-2(p 505), Temperature Sites, in the Textbook.
- Normal range for body temperatures depends on the site.
  - Oral: 97.6°F to 99.6°F (36.5°C to 37.5°C)
  - Rectal: 98.6°F to 100.6°F (37.0°C to 38.1°C)
  - Axillary: 96.6°F to 98.6°F (35.9°C to 37.0°C)
  - Tympanic membrane: 98.6°F (37°C)
  - Temporal artery: 99.6°F (37.5°C)
- Older persons have lower body temperatures than younger persons.

Thermometers

- Electronic thermometers include:
  - Standard electronic thermometers with a blue probe for oral and axillary temperatures and red probes for rectal temperatures. A disposable cover protects the probe.
  - Tympanic membrane thermometer, which measures body temperature at the tympanic membrane in the ear.

- ○ Temporal artery thermometer, which measures body temperature at the temporal artery in the forehead.
  - ○ Digital thermometers, which measure body temperature at the oral, axillary, or rectal sites.
- Other thermometers include disposable thermometers which are used for oral temperatures and glass thermometers. Glass thermometers are less common but may be used in home settings. When using glass thermometers, rectal temperatures require 2 minutes; oral requires 2- 3 minutes and axillary requires 5-10 minutes.

Taking Temperatures

- *The oral site.* Place the thermometer under the person's tongue and to the side.
- *The rectal site.* Lubricate the tip end of the rectal thermometer. Privacy is important.
- *The axillary site.* The axilla must be dry. Place the probe in the center of the axilla and place the person's arm over the chest to hold the probe in place.
- Tympanic membrane thermometers are inserted gently into the ear. Pull the adult ear up and back to straighten the ear canal.
- Temporal thermometers. Use the exposed side of the head. Do not use the side that was on a pillow.

Pulse

- The adult pulse rate is between 60 and 100 beats per minute. Report these abnormal rates to the nurse at once.
  - ○ *Tachycardia*—the heart rate is more than 100 beats per minute.
  - ○ *Bradycardia*—the heart rate is less than 60 beats per minute.
- The rhythm of the pulse should be regular. Report and record an irregular pulse rhythm.
- Report and record if the pulse force is strong, full, bounding, weak, thready, or feeble.

Taking Pulses

- The radial pulse is used for routine vital signs. Place the first 2 or 3 fingers against the radial pulse. Do not use your thumb to take a pulse. Count the pulse for 30 seconds and multiply by 2 if the agency policy permits. If the pulse is irregular, count it for 1 minute. Report and record if the pulse is regular or irregular, strong or weak.
- The apical pulse is located 2-3 inches to the left of the sternum. A stethoscope is used to measure the apical or the apical-radial pulse. Count the apical pulse for 1 minute.

Respirations

- The healthy adult has 12 to 20 respirations per minute. Respirations are normally quiet, effortless, and regular. Both sides of the chest rise and fall equally.
- Count respirations when the person is at rest. Count respirations right after taking a pulse.
- Count respirations for 30 seconds and multiply the number by 2 if the agency policy permits.

If an abnormal pattern is noted, count the respirations for 1 minute.
- Report and record:
  - ○ The respiratory rate
  - ○ Equality and depth of respirations
  - ○ If the respirations were regular or irregular
  - ○ If the person has pain or difficulty breathing
  - ○ Any respiratory noises
  - ○ An abnormal respiratory pattern

Blood Pressure

Normal and Abnormal Blood Pressures

- Blood pressure has normal ranges.
  - ○ *Systolic pressure* (upper number)—90 mm Hg and higher but lower than 120 mm Hg
  - ○ *Diastolic pressure* (lower number)—60 mm Hg and higher but lower than 80 mm Hg
- **Hypertension**—blood pressure measurements that remain above a systolic pressure of 140 mm Hg or a diastolic pressure of 90 mm Hg. Report any systolic measurement above 120 mm Hg. Also report a diastolic pressure above 80 mm Hg.
- **Hypotension**—when the systolic blood pressure is below 90 mm Hg and the diastolic pressure is below 60 mm Hg. Report a systolic pressure below 90 mm Hg. Also report a diastolic pressure below 60 mm Hg.
- Review Box 33-5(p 525), Measuring Blood Pressure—Guidelines, in the Textbook.

CHAPTER 33 REVIEW QUESTIONS
Circle the BEST answer.

1. The nurse ask you to take the temperature of a confused older person. Which method would you use?
   a. Oral electronic probe thermometer
   b. Axillary glass thermometer
   c. Temporal artery thermometer
   d. Rectal glass thermometer
2. Which pulse rate should you report at once?
   a. A pulse rate of 52 beats per minute
   b. A pulse rate of 60 beats per minute
   c. A pulse rate of 76 beats per minute
   d. A pulse rate of 100 beats per minute
3. Which nursing assistant needs a reminder about how to take a pulse?
   a. Nursing Assistant counts an irregular pulse for 1 minute.
   b. Nursing Assistant B uses her thumb to check the radial pulse rate.
   c. Nursing Assistant C locates the radial pulse to count the rate.
   d. Nursing Assistant D uses a stethoscope to take an apical pulse
4. Which blood pressure should you report?
   a. 120/80 mm Hg
   b. 88/62 mm Hg
   c. 110/70 mm Hg
   d. 92/68 mm Hg

Answers to these questions are on p. 538.

CHAPTER 34 EXERCISE AND ACTIVITY

Bed rest

- Bed rest means restricting the person to bed for health reasons.
- Bed rest is ordered to:
  - Reduce oxygen needs.
  - Reduce pain.
  - Reduce swelling.
  - Promote healing.

Complications From Bed rest

- Pressure injuries, constipation, and fecal impactions can result. Urinary tract infections and renal calculi (kidney stones) can occur. So can blood clots and pneumonia.
- The musculo-skeletal system is affected by lack of exercise and activity. These complications must be prevented to maintain normal movement.
  - A **contracture** is caused by abnormal shortening of a muscle; this results in decreased motion and joint stiffness. Common sites are the fingers, wrists, elbows, toes, ankles, knees, and hips. The site is deformed and disabled.
  - **Atrophy** is the decrease in size or the wasting away of tissue. Tissues shrink in size.
- **Orthostatic hypotension (postural hypotension)** is abnormally low blood pressure when the person stands up suddenly. The person can experience dizziness, weakness, or see spots before the eyes. Fainting can occur. To prevent orthostatic hypotension, have the person change slowly from a lying or sitting position to a standing position.

Positioning

- Supportive devices are often used to support and maintain the person in a certain position.
  - *Bed-boards*—are placed under the mattress to prevent the mattress from sagging.
  - *Foot-boards*—are placed at the foot of mattresses to prevent plantar flexion that can lead to footdrop.
  - *Trochanter rolls*—prevent the hips and legs from turning outward (external rotation).
  - *Hip abduction wedges*—keep the hips abducted (apart).
  - *Hand rolls or hand grips*—prevent contractures of the thumb, fingers, and wrist.
  - *Splints*—keep the elbows, wrists, thumbs, fingers, ankles, and knees in normal position.
  - *Bed cradles*—keep the weight of top linens off the feet and toes.

Range-of-Motion Exercises

- **Range-of-motion (ROM)** exercises involve moving the joints through their complete range of motion without causing pain. They are usually done at least 2 times a day.
  - *Active ROM*—exercises are done by the person.
  - *Passive ROM*—you move the joints through their range of motion.
  - *Active-assistive ROM*—the person does the exercises with some help.

- Review Box 34-1(p 535), Range-of-Motion Exercises, in the Textbook.
- ROM exercises can cause injury if not done properly. Practice these rules.
  - Exercise only the joints the nurse tells you to exercise.
  - Expose only the body part being exercised.
  - Use good body mechanics.
  - Support the part being exercised at all times
  - Move the joint slowly, smoothly, and gently.
  - Do not force a joint beyond its present range of motion or to the point of pain.
  - Ask the person if he or she has pain or discomfort.
  - Stop if you meet resistance or suspect pain. Tell the nurse
  - Perform ROM exercises to the neck only if allowed by your agency and if the nurse instructs you to do so.

Ambulation

- **Ambulation** is the act of walking.
- Follow the care plan when helping a person walk. Use a gait (transfer) belt if the person is weak or unsteady. The person uses hand rails along the wall. Always check the person for orthostatic hypotension.
- When you help the person walk, walk to the side and slightly behind the person on the person's weak side. Encourage the person to use the hand rail on his or her strong side.

Walking Aids

- A cane is held on the strong side of the body. The cane tip is about 6 to 10 inches to the side of the foot. It is about 6 to 10 inches in front of the foot on the strong side. The grip is level with the hip. To walk:
  - Step A: The cane is moved forward 6 to 10 inches.
  - Step B: The weak leg (opposite the cane) is moved forward even with the cane.
  - Step C: The strong leg is moved forward and ahead of the cane and the weak leg.
- A walker gives more support than a cane. Wheeled walkers are common. They have wheels on the front legs and rubber tips on the back legs. The person pushes the walker about 6 to 8 inches in front of his or her feet.
- Crutches are used when the person cannot use 1 leg or when 1 or both legs need to gain strength. Tips are checked. Bolts are tightened. Person should wear slip-resistant shoes. Crutches should be placed within the person's reach.
- Braces support weak body parts, prevent or correct deformities, or prevent joint movement. A brace is applied over the ankle, knee, or back. Skin and bony points under braces are kept clean and dry. Report redness or signs of skin breakdown at once. Also report complaints of pain or discomfort. The care plan tells you when to apply and remove a brace.

CHAPTER 34 REVIEW QUESTIONS
Circle the BEST answer.

1. To prevent orthostatic hypotension, you should
   a. Move the person from the supine position to the standing position
   b. Check the person's vital signs after you help him or her to stand up
   c. Move a person slowly from the lying or sitting position to a standing position
   d. Keep the person in bed if he or she usually feels dizzy when getting up

2. You are reviewing the assignment sheet to plan your work. Which person is likely to need the most help throughout the day?
   a. Person A is on strict bed rest
   b. Person B is on bed rest
   c. Person C is on bed rest with commode privileges
   d. Person D is on bed rest with bathroom privileges

3. The nurse tells you to use a trochanter roll to help maintain a person's body alignment. Which piece of equipment would you obtain?
   a. Rubber ball
   b. Splint
   c. Bath blanket
   d. Bed cradle

4. A person's left leg is weaker than his right.
   a. The person holds the cane on his right side.
   b. The person holds the cane on his left side.
   c. The person holds the cane in his dominant hand
   d. The person holds the cane in his non-dominant hand

Answers to these questions are on p. 538.

CHAPTER 35 COMFORT, REST, AND SLEEP
- Comfort is a state of well-being. Person has no physical or emotional pain.
- Pain or discomfort means to ache, hurt, or be sore. Pain is subjective. You must rely on what the person says.
- Pain is often considered a vital sign. Report the person's complaints of pain and your observations to the nurse.

Factors Affecting Pain
- *Past experience.* The severity of pain, its cause, how long it lasted, and if relief occurred all affect the person's current response to pain.
- *Anxiety.* Pain and anxiety are related. Pain can cause anxiety. Anxiety increases how much pain the person feels. Reducing anxiety helps lessen pain.
- *Rest and sleep.* Pain seems worse when a person is tired or restless. Pain often seems worse at night.
- *Attention.* The more a person thinks about pain, the worse it seems.
- *Personal and family duties.* Often pain is ignored because of responsibilities related to job, school, children, partner or parents. Some deny pain if a serious illness is feared.
- *The value or meaning of pain.* To some people, pain is a sign of weakness. Or it may signal the need for tests or treatment. For some persons, pain means avoiding work, daily routines, and certain people. Some people like attention and pampering by others.
- *Support from others.* Dealing with pain is often easier when family and friends offer comfort and support. Facing pain alone is hard for persons.
- *Culture.* Culture affects pain responses. Non–English-speaking persons may have problems describing pain.
- *Illness.* Some diseases cause decreased pain sensations.
- *Age.* Older persons may have chronic pain that masks new pain. They may deny or ignore new pain, thinking it is related to a known problem. Or they may deny or ignore pain because they are afraid of what it may mean. For persons who cannot tell you about pain, changes in usual behavior may signal pain. Loss of appetite also signals pain. Report any changes in a person's usual behavior to the nurse.

Signs and Symptoms
- Rely on what the person tells you. Promptly report any information you collect about pain. Use the person's exact words when reporting and recording pain.
- The nurse needs the following information.
  - *Location.* Where is the pain?
  - *Onset and duration.* When did the pain start? How long has it lasted?
  - *Intensity.* Ask the person to rate the pain. Use a pain scale.
  - *Description.* Ask the person to describe the pain.
  - *Factors causing pain.* Ask what the person was doing before the pain started and when it started.
  - *Factors affecting pain.* Ask what makes the pain better and what makes it worse.
  - *Vital signs.* Increases often occur with acute pain. They may be normal with chronic pain.
  - *Other signs and symptoms.* Dizziness, nausea, vomiting, weakness, numbness, and tingling.
- Review Box 35-3(p 551), Pain-Signs and Symptoms, and Box 35-4(p 552), Comfort and Pain-Relief Measures, in the Textbook.

The Back Massage
- The back massage can promote comfort and relieve pain. It relaxes muscles and stimulates circulation.
- A good time to give a massage is after baths and showers and with evening care. Massages last 3 to 5 minutes.
- Observe the skin for breaks, bruises, reddened areas, and other signs of skin breakdown.
- Lotion reduces friction during the massage. It is warmed before applying.
- Use firm strokes. Keep your hands in contact with the person's skin.
- After the massage, apply some lotion to the elbows, knees, and heels.
- Back massages are dangerous for persons with certain heart diseases, back injuries, back and other surgeries, skin diseases, and some lung disorders. Check with the nurse and the care plan before giving back massages to persons with these conditions.

- Do not massage reddened bony areas. Reddened areas signal skin breakdown and pressure injuries. Massage can lead to more tissue damage.
- Wear gloves if the person's skin is not intact. Always follow Standard Precautions and the Bloodborne Pathogen Standard.
- Report and record skin breakdown, redness, bruising, and breaks in the skin.

Rest

- *Rest* means to be calm, at ease, and relaxed with no anxiety or stress. Rest may involve inactivity. Or the person does things that are calming and relaxing.
- Promote rest by meeting physical, safety, and security needs.
  - Thirst, hunger, pain or discomfort, and elimination needs can affect rest. A comfortable position and good alignment are important. A quiet setting promotes rest.
  - The person must feel safe from falling or other injuries. The person is secure with the call light within reach. Understanding the reasons for care and knowing how care is given also help the person feel safe.
- Many persons have rituals or routines before resting. Follow them whenever possible.
- Love and belonging are important for rest. Visits or calls from family and friends may relax the person. Reading cards and letters may also help.
- Meet self-esteem needs.
- Some persons are refreshed after a 15- or 20-minute rest. Others need more time.
- Ill or injured persons need to rest more often. Do not push the person beyond his or her limits.

Sleep

- Sleep is a basic need. Tissue healing and repair occur during sleep. Sleep lowers stress, tension, and anxiety. It refreshes and renews the person. The person regains energy and mental alertness. The person thinks and functions better after sleep.

Factors Affecting Sleep

- *Illness.* Illness increases the need for sleep.
- *Nutrition.* Sleep needs increase with weight gain. Foods with caffeine prevent sleep.
- *Exercise.* Exercise can help people to sleep better.
- *Usual sleep settings.* Changes in usual sleep settings (e.g., bed, pillow, lighting) can interfere with sleep.
- *Drugs and other substances.* Sleeping pills promote sleep. Drugs for anxiety, depression, and pain can induce sleep. Some drugs may cause nightmares or interfere with normal sleep patterns. Caffeine can prevent sleep.
- *Life-style changes.* Changes in daily routines may affect sleep.
- *Emotional problems.* Fear, worry, depression, and anxiety affect sleep.
- *Age.* The amount of sleep needed decreases with age.

Sleep Disorders

- **Insomnia** is a chronic condition in which the person cannot sleep or stay asleep all night.
- **Sleep deprivation** means that the amount and quality of sleep are inadequate. Function and alertness are decreased.
- **Sleepwalking** is when the person leaves the bed and walks about. If a person is sleepwalking, protect the person from injury. Guide sleepwalkers back to bed. They startle easily. Awaken them gently.

Promoting Sleep

- To promote sleep, allow a flexible bedtime, provide a comfortable room temperature, and have the person void before going to bed. Review Box 35-7(p 557), Promoting Sleep, in the Textbook for other measures.

CHAPTER 35 REVIEW QUESTIONS

Circle the BEST answer.

1. A person complains of pain. Which question would you ask?
   a. Where is the pain?
   b. Has this pain happened before?
   c. When did you take the last pain pill?
   d. Why does it hurt?
2. Which of the following should be investigated as a possible non-verbal signal of pain?
   a. Illness
   b. Mental alertness
   c. Loss of appetite
   d. Hyperactivity
3. Which nursing assistant needs a reminder about the procedure for giving a back massage?
   a. Nursing Assistant A uses long firm strokes to stimulate circulation.
   b. Nursing Assistant B gives the massage after the bath.
   c. Nursing Assistant C observes the skin before beginning the massage.
   d. Nursing Assistant D uses cold lotion for the massage.
4. You are assigned to care for a person who occasionally sleepwalks. What is the priority concern?
   a. Risk for falls
   b. Startles easily
   c. Fatigue
   d. Memory loss
5. Which action would promote sleep for a person?
   a. Offer the person coffee and cookies
   b. Accompany the person on a walk
   c. Encourage usual bedtime rituals
   d. Tell the person to go to bed

Answers to these questions are on p. 538.

CHAPTER 36 ADMISSIONS, TRANSFERS, AND DISCHARGES

- Admission is the official entry of a person into a health care setting. It can cause anxiety and fear in patients, residents, and families.

- Transfer is moving the person to another health care setting or moving the person to a new room within the agency.
- Discharge is the official departure of a person from a health care setting.
- During the admission process:
  - Identifying information is obtained from the person or family.
  - The person is given an identification (ID) number and bracelet.
  - The person signs admitting papers and a general consent form.
- You prepare the person's room before the person arrives.

Admitting the Person

- Admission is your first chance to make a good impression. You must:
  - Greet the person by name and title. Use the admission records to find out the person's name.
  - Introduce yourself by name and title to the person, family, and friends.
  - Make roommate introductions.
  - Act in a professional manner.
  - Treat the person with dignity and respect.
- During the admission procedure the nurse may ask you to:
  - Collect some information for the nursing assistant admission checklist.
  - Measure the person's weight and height.
  - Measure the person's vital signs.
  - Obtain a urine specimen (if needed).
  - Complete a clothing and personal belongings list.
  - Orient the person to the room, nursing unit, and agency.

Weight and Height

- When weighing a person, follow the manufacturer's instructions and center procedures for using the scales. Follow these guidelines when measuring weight and height.
  - The person wears only a gown or sleepwear. No footwear is worn.
  - The person voids before being weighed and a dry incontinence product is worn if needed.
  - Weigh the person at the same time of day. Before breakfast is the best time.
  - Use the same scale for daily, weekly, and monthly weights.
  - Balance the scale at zero before weighing the person.

Moving the Person to a New Room

- Sometimes a person is moved to a new room because of a change in condition or care needs, the person requests a room change, or roommates do not get along. Support and reassure the person moving to a new room.
- The person is transported by wheelchair, stretcher, or the bed.

Transfers and Discharges

- When transferred or discharged, the person leaves the agency. He or she goes home or to another health care setting.
- Transfers and discharges are usually planned in advance by the health team.
- For discharges, the health team teaches the person and family about diet, exercise, and drugs. They also teach them about procedures and treatments and arrange for home care, equipment, and therapies as needed.
- The nurse tells you when to start the transfer or discharge procedure. Usually a wheelchair is used. If leaving by ambulance, a stretcher is used.
- If a person wants to leave the agency without the doctor's permission, tell the nurse at once. The nurse or social worker handles the matter.

CHAPTER 36 REVIEW QUESTIONS
Circle the BEST answer.

1. You are preparing a person to transfer to another long-term facility that will be closer to the person's family. You observe that the person seems tearful. What is the best response?
   a. "You should be cheerful; you will get to see your family."
   b. "Don't cry; everything is going to be just fine."
   c. "You seem sad; is there anything that I can do for you?"
   d. "I am sure that the new facility will be much nicer than this one."
2. When a person is admitted, what would you do?
   a. Greet the person by name and title
   b. Go get a co-worker if the person is obese
   c. Ask the family to take responsibility for valuables
   d. Ask the nurse how much time to spend on the admission process
3. When weighing the person, which action is correct?
   a. Have the person void before being weighed.
   b. Tell the person not to eat until after being weighed
   c. Balance the scale at zero after weighing every person
   d. Have the person wear shoes when being weighed.
4. A person wants to leave the hospital without the doctor's permission. What would you do?
   a. Persuade the person to stay
   b. Tell the nurse at once
   c. Call hospital security
   d. Stay with the person and close the door

Answers to these questions are on p. 538.

CHAPTER 38 COLLECTING AND TESTING SPECIMENS

Collecting Specimens

- When collecting specimens:
  - Follow the rules for medical asepsis.
  - Follow Standard Precautions and the Bloodborne Pathogen Standard.
  - Use a clean container for each specimen.
  - Use the correct container.
  - Do not touch the inside of the container or the inside of the lid.

o Identify the person.
o Label the container in the person's presence.
o Collect the specimen at the correct time.

Urine specimens
- There are different types of urine specimens: random, midstream, 24-hour, catheter or urine from an infant or child. The purpose of the specimen and the collection process will vary. When you are asked to obtain a urine specimen you need to know:
  o Type of voiding device—bedpan, urinal, commode, or toilet with specimen pan
  o The type of specimen needed
  o What time to collect the specimen
  o What special measures are needed
  o If you need to test the specimen
  o If measuring intake and output (I&O) is ordered
  o Straining urine is done when stones (calculi) are present or suspected.
  o Urine can be tested with a reagent strip to detect: urine pH, blood (hematuria), glucose (glucosuria), ketones, infection and protein.

Stool Specimens
- Stools are studied for fat, microbes, worms, blood, and other abnormal contents.
- Stool specimens should not be contaminated with urine or toilet paper.
  o Take the sample from:
  o The middle of a formed stool
  o Areas of pus, mucus, or blood and watery areas
  o The middle and both ends of a hard stool
  o To detect occult blood, a thin smear of stool is applied to the test kit. Developer is added and color changes are noted.

Sputum Specimens
- Sputum is collected in the morning. Have the person rinse the mouth with water first. If tuberculosis is known or suspected, wear a respirator mask for your protection.

Blood Glucose Testing
- Blood glucose testing is used for persons with diabetes.
- If you are delegated to perform glucose testing, first know if your state and agency allow you to perform the procedure.
- Information that you need from the nurse includes:
  o What sites to avoid for a skin puncture
  o When to collect and test the specimen—usually before meals and at bedtime
  o If the person receives drugs that affect blood clotting

CHAPTER 38 REVIEW QUESTIONS
Circle the BEST answer.
1. The nurse asks you to test a person's urine for glucose and ketones. Which equipment do you need to obtain?
   a. Glucometer
   b. Bottle of reagent strips
   c. Occult blood kit
   d. Syringe
2. Which person needs to drink 8 to 12 glasses of water per day?
   a. Child who is wearing a urine collection bag ("wee bag")
   b. Person who is collecting urine for a 24-hour urine specimen
   c. Person who is having all urine strained for stones
   d. Older adult who needs to produce a midstream urine specimen
3. Which type of specimen may require suctioning?
   a. Urine
   b. Stool
   c. Blood
   d. Sputum
4. You are asked to perform blood glucose testing on a person who takes a medication that affects blood clotting. What would you do?
   a. Decline to do the procedure
   b. Apply firm pressure until bleeding stops
   c. Puncture the middle fleshy part of the finger
   d. Perform the procedure very quickly

Answers to these questions are on p. 538.

CHAPTER 39 THE PERSON HAVING SURGERY
- Surgery may be in-patient, requiring a hospital stay, or same-day surgery, also called out-patient, 1-day, or ambulatory surgery. The person is prepared for what happens before, during, and after surgery.

Pre-Operative Care
- The person may have special tests such as chest x-ray or electrocardiogram (ECG). Nutrition and fluids may be restricted 6 to 8 hours before surgery.
- Personal care before surgery includes:
  o A complete bath, shower, or tub bath and shampoo. A special soap or shampoo may be ordered to reduce the number of microbes and the risk of infection.
  o Make-up, nail polish, and fake nails are removed.
  o Hair accessories, wigs, and hairpieces are removed and a surgical cap keeps the hair out of the face and the operative site.
- Being NPO causes thirst and a dry mouth. The person must not swallow any water during oral hygiene.
- Dentures, eyeglasses, contact lenses, hearing aids, and other prostheses are removed.
- Often elastic stockings and sequential compression devices are put on before transport to the OR.

Post-Operative Care
- The person's room must be ready. Make a surgical bed, place supplies in the room, and move furniture out of the way for a stretcher.
- Your role in post-operative care depends on the person's condition. Vital signs, including and pulse oximetry are taken. The nurse tells you how often to check the person. Review Box 39-2(p 608), Post-Op Complications and Observations, in the Textbook.

- The person is re-positioned every 1 to 2 hours to prevent respiratory and circulatory complications. Turning may be painful. Provide support and use smooth, gentle motions.
- Coughing and deep-breathing exercises help prevent respiratory complications.
- Circulation must be stimulated for blood flow in the legs. If blood flow is sluggish, blood clots may form.
- Report the following at once.
  o Swollen area of a leg.
  o Pain or tenderness in a leg. This may occur only when standing or walking.
  o Warmth in the part of the leg that is swollen or painful.
  o Red or discolored skin.

Leg Exercises

- Leg exercises promote venous blood flow and help prevent thrombi. They are usually done 5 times, at least every 1 or 2 hours, while the person is awake.
  o Make circles with the toes. This rotates the ankles.
  o Dorsiflex and plantar flex the feet.
  o Flex and extend 1 knee and then the other.
  o Raise and lower the leg off the bed. Repeat with the other leg.

Elastic Stockings

- Elastic stockings exert pressure on the veins. The pressure promotes venous blood return to the heart. The stockings help prevent blood clots in the leg veins.
- Elastic stockings are also called AE (anti-embolism or anti-embolic) stockings or TED (thrombo-embolic disease) hose.
- The nurse measures the person for the correct size of elastic stockings. Most stockings have an opening near the toes that is used to check circulation, skin color, and skin temperature.
- The person usually has 2 pairs of stockings. One pair is washed; the other pair is worn.
- Stockings should not have twists, creases, or wrinkles after you apply them. Twists can affect circulation. Creases and wrinkles can cause skin breakdown.
- Loose stockings do not promote venous blood return to the heart. Stockings that are too tight can affect circulation. Tell the nurse if the stockings are too loose or too tight.

CHAPTER 39 REVIEW QUESTIONS
Circle the BEST answer.
1. You report a swollen calf that is red, warm to the touch and painful because these are possible signs and symptoms of
   a. Hypovolemia
   b. Thrombus
   c. Dehiscence
   d. Pneumonia
2. What is the purpose of the toe opening on the elastic stockings?
   a. The toe opening is used to determine the correct size of the elastic stockings

   b. The toe opening allows the person to move toes and gives access for hygiene for feet
   c. The toe opening allows access to smooth creases or wrinkles after application
   d. The toe opening is used to check circulation, skin color, and temperature in the toes
3. The nurse tells you that a person will soon arrive from PACU. Which task is the nurse most likely to ask you to do?
   a. Take vital signs with pulse oximeter reading every 5 minutes
   b. Position the person in high Fowler's to improve breathing
   c. Stay with the person because he will not be able to call for help
   d. Make a surgical bed, raise the bed, and lower the side rails

Answers to these questions are on p. 538.

CHAPTER 40 WOUND CARE
- A **wound** is a break in the skin or mucous membrane.
- The wound is a portal of entry for microbes. Infection is a major threat. Wound care involves preventing infection and further injury to the wound and nearby tissues.

Skin Tears
- A **skin tear** is a break or rip in the skin.
- Skin tears are caused by friction, shearing, pulling, or pressure on the skin. Bumping a hand, arm, or leg on any hard surface can cause a skin tear. Beds, bed rails, chairs, wheelchair footplates, and tables are dangers. So is holding the person's arm or leg too tight, removing tape or adhesives, bathing, dressing, and other tasks. Buttons, zippers, jewelry, or long or jagged finger or toenails can also cause skin tears.
- Skin tears are painful. They are portals of entry for microbes. Wound complications can develop. Tell the nurse at once if you cause or find a skin tear.
- Review Box 40-1(p 619), Preventing Skin Tears, in the Textbook.

Circulatory Ulcers
- *Circulatory ulcers (vascular ulcers)* are open sores on the lower legs or feet. They are caused by decreased blood flow through the arteries or veins.
- Review Box 40-2(p 620), Preventing Circulatory Ulcers, in the Textbook.
- *Venous ulcers (stasis ulcers)* are open sores on the lower legs or feet. They are caused by poor blood flow through the veins. The heels and inner aspect of the ankles are common sites for venous ulcers.
- *Arterial ulcers* are open wounds on the lower legs or feet caused by poor arterial blood flow. They are found between the toes, on top of the toes, and on the outer side of the ankle.
- A *diabetic foot ulcer* is an open wound on the foot caused by complications from diabetes.

- With nerve damage, the person can lose sensation in a foot or leg. The person may not feel pain, heat, or cold. Therefore the person may not feel a cut, blister, burn, or other trauma to the foot. Infection and a large sore can develop. Blood flow to the foot decreases; tissues and cells do not get oxygen and nutrients. A sore does not heal properly. Tissue death (gangrene) can occur. Review Box 40-3(p 621), Diabetes Foot Care, in the Textbook.

Prevention and Treatment

- Check the person's feet and legs every day. Report any sign of a problem to the nurse at once. Follow the care plan to prevent and treat circulatory ulcers.
- Complications of wounds include hemorrhage and infection
- Report wound observations. Review Box 40-4(p 624), Wound Observations in the Textbook.
- Some agencies let you apply simple, dry, non-sterile dressings to simple wounds. Follow the rules in Box 40-5 (p 627), Applying Dressings, in the Textbook.

CHAPTER 40 REVIEW QUESTIONS

Circle the BEST answer.

1. Which action could you perform to prevent skin tears?
   a. Use an assist device to move and turn the person in bed.
   b. Firmly hold a confused person to prevent sudden movements
   c. Instruct the person not to wear rings, watches, bracelets
   d. Tell a confused person to cooperate with care
2. A person is diabetic. How often would you inspect the feet for problems?
   a. Every 4 hours
   b. Every day
   c. Once a week
   d. Once a month
3. Elastic stockings are used to prevent
   a. Circulatory ulcers
   b. Skin tears
   c. Excoriation
   d. Wound infection

Answers to these questions are on p. 538.

CHAPTER 41 PRESSURE INJURIES

- A **pressure injury** is defined by the National Pressure Ulcer Advisory Panel as localized damage to the skin and/or underlying soft tissue.
- Pressure injuries usually occur over a bony prominence— e.g., shoulder blades, elbows, hips, spine, sacrum, knees, ankles, heels, and toes.
- Pressure, shearing, and friction are common causes of skin breakdown and pressure injuries. Risk factors include breaks in the skin, poor circulation to an area, moisture, dry skin, and irritation by urine and feces. Review Box 41-1(p 635), Pressure Injury Risk Factors in the Textbook.

Persons at Risk

- Persons at risk for pressure injuries are those who:
  o Are confined to a bed or chair.
  o Need some or total help in moving.
  o Are agitated or have involuntary muscle movements.
  o Have loss of bowel or bladder control.
  o Are exposed to moisture.
  o Have poor nutrition or poor fluid balance.
  o Have limited awareness.
  o Have problems sensing pain or pressure.
  o Have circulatory problems.
  o Are obese or very thin.
  o Have a medical device.
  o Have a healed pressure injury.

Pressure injury Stages

- Pressure injuries range from reddened intact skin to tissue loss with bone exposure. See Box 41-2(p 636), Pressure Injury Stages.
- Figures 41-6 to 4-12(pp 637, 638, 639), in the Textbook shows the stages of pressure injuries.

Prevention and Treatment

- Good nursing care, cleanliness, and skin care are essential. Managing moisture, good nutrition and fluid balance, and relieving pressure also are key measures.
- Preventing pressure injuries is much easier than trying to heal them. Review Box 41-3(p 641), Preventing Pressure Injuries, in the Textbook.
- The person at risk for pressure injuries may be placed on a foam, air, alternating air, gel, or water mattress.
- Protective devices are often used to prevent and treat pressure injuries and skin breakdown. Protective devices include:
  o Bed cradle
  o Heel and elbow protectors
  o Heel and foot elevators
  o Gel or fluid-filled pads and cushions
  o Special beds
  o Other equipment—pillows, trochanter rolls, and foot-boards

CHAPTER 41 REVIEW QUESTIONS

Circle the BEST answer.

1. Which medical device could cause a pressure injury?
   a. Trochanter roll
   b. Oxygen tubing
   c. Foot elevator
   d. Fluid-filled pad
2. Which device would be the best to use to prevent shearing?
   a. Alternating air mattress
   b. Bed cradle
   c. Draw sheet
   d. Pillow
3. Which action would help to prevent a mucosal membrane injury?
   a. Frequently checking on a person who is placed on a bedpan

b. Reporting redness and irritation at the urinary meatus
c. Reminding person who is sitting to shift position every 15 minutes
d. Keeping the head of the bed at 30° or less according to care plan

4. A person likes to sit in a wheelchair in the dayroom. Which action will help to prevent shearing?
   a. Encouraging the person to recline back in the chair
   b. Locking the wheels after person is positioned
   c. Positioning the person's feet on the footrests
   d. Making sure that the armrests are well padded

Answers to these questions are on p. 538.

CHAPTER 42 HEAT AND COLD APPLICATIONS
Heat Applications
- Heat relieves pain, relaxes muscles, promotes healing, reduces tissue swelling, and decreases joint stiffness.

Complications
- High temperatures can cause burns. Report pain, excessive redness, and blisters at once. Also observe for pale skin.
- Metal implants pose risks. Pacemakers and joint replacements are made of metal. Do not apply heat to an implant area.
- Heat is not applied to a pregnant woman's abdomen. The heat can affect fetal growth.

Moist and Dry Heat Applications
- In moist heat applications, water is in contact with the skin. Moist heat applications include hot compresses, hot soaks, sitz baths, and hot packs.
- Dry heat applications do not use water, allowing the application to stay at the desired temperature longer. Aquathermia pads, some hot packs and warming therapy pads are dry heat applications.

Cold Applications
- Cold applications reduce pain, prevent swelling, and decrease circulation and bleeding. Cold is useful right after an injury.
- Complications include pain, burns, blisters, and poor circulation. Burns and blisters occur from intense cold. They also occur when dry cold is in direct contact with the skin.

Applying Heat and Cold
- Protect the person from injury during heat and cold applications. Review Box 42-1(p 650), Applying Heat and Cold, in the Textbook.

CHAPTER 42 REVIEW QUESTIONS
Circle the BEST answer.

1. Heat applications are most likely to be used for
   a. Abdominal pain
   b. Wound infections
   c. Musculo-skeletal injuries
   d. Post-surgical pain

2. When heat is applied to an area, which of these is an expected response?
   a. The skin is red and warm.
   b. The skin is pale, white, or gray.
   c. The person begins to shiver.
   d. The area is excessively red.

Answers to these questions are on p. 538.

CHAPTER 43 OXYGEN NEEDS
Altered Respiratory Function
- Hypoxia means that cells do not have enough oxygen.
- Restlessness, dizziness, and disorientation are early signs of hypoxia.
- Report signs and symptoms of hypoxia to the nurse at once. Hypoxia is life-threatening.
- Review Box 43-1(p 657), Altered Respiratory Function, in the Textbook.

Abnormal Respirations
- Adults normally have 12 to 20 respirations per minute. They are quiet, effortless, and regular. Both sides of the chest rise and fall equally.
- Abnormal patterns are listed below. Report these observations at once.
  - **Tachypnea**—rapid breathing. Respirations are 20 or more per minute.
  - **Bradypnea**—slow breathing. Respirations are fewer than 12 per minute.
  - **Apnea**—lack or absence of breathing.
  - **Hypoventilation**—respirations are slow, shallow, and sometimes irregular.
  - **Hyperventilation**—respirations are rapid and deeper than normal.
  - **Dyspnea**—difficult, labored, painful breathing.
  - **Cheyne-Stokes respirations**—respirations gradually increase in rate and depth. Then they become shallow and slow. Breathing may stop for 10 to 20 seconds.
  - **Orthopnea**—breathing deeply and comfortably only when sitting.
  - **Biot's respirations**—rapid and deep respirations followed by 10 to 30 seconds of apnea.
  - **Kussmaul respirations**—very deep and rapid respirations.

Pulse Oximetry
- Pulse oximetry measures the oxygen concentration in arterial blood.
- A sensor attaches to a finger, toe, earlobe, nose, or forehead.
- Avoid swollen sites and sites with skin breaks. Bright light, poor blood flow to the fingers, fake nails, nail polish and movements can affect the measurements.

Promoting Oxygenation
- Breathing is usually easier in semi-Fowler's and Fowler's positions. Persons with difficulty breathing often prefer the **orthopneic position** (sitting up and leaning over a table to breathe).

- Deep breathing moves air into most parts of the lungs. Coughing removes mucus. Deep breathing and coughing are usually done every 1 to 2 hours while the person is awake. They help prevent pneumonia and atelectasis (the collapse of a portion of the lung).
  - The incentive spirometer is a machine used to improve lung function and prevent complications. Your role may be to assist or remind the person to use the spirometer. See Delegation Guidelines: Incentive Spirometry (p 663), in the Textbook.

Oxygen Devices

- A nasal cannula allows eating and drinking. Tight prongs can irritate the nose. Pressure on the ears and cheekbones is possible.
- There are different kinds of face masks that cover the nose and mouth. Talking and eating are hard to do with a mask. Listen carefully. Moisture can build up under the mask. Keep the face clean and dry. Masks are removed for eating. Usually oxygen is given by cannula during meals.

Oxygen Flow Rates

- When giving care and checking the person, always check the flow rate. Tell the nurse at once if it is too high or too low. A nurse or respiratory therapist will adjust the flow rate.

Oxygen Safety

- You do not give oxygen. You assist the nurse in providing safe care.
- Always check the oxygen level when you are with or near persons using oxygen systems that contain a limited amount of oxygen. Oxygen tanks and liquid oxygen systems are examples. Report a low oxygen level to the nurse at once.
- Follow the rules for fire and the use of oxygen in Chapter 13 (p 180), in the Textbook.
- Never remove the oxygen device. However, turn off the oxygen flow if there is a fire.
- Make sure the oxygen device is secure but not tight.
- Check for signs of irritation from the oxygen device—behind the ears, under the nose, around the face, and on the cheekbones.
- Keep the face clean and dry when a mask is used.
- Never shut off the oxygen flow.
- Do not adjust the flow rate unless allowed by your state and agency.
- Tell the nurse at once if the flow rate is too high or too low.
- Tell the nurse at once if the humidifier is not bubbling.
- Secure tubing to the person's garment. Follow agency policy.
- Make sure there are no kinks in the tubing.
- Make sure the person does not lie on any part of the tubing.
- Report signs of hypoxia, respiratory distress, or abnormal breathing to the nurse at once.
- Give oral hygiene as directed. Follow the care plan.

- Make sure the oxygen device is clean and free of mucus.
- Make sure the oxygen tank is secure in its holder.

CHAPTER 43 REVIEW QUESTIONS
Circle the BEST answer.

1. Which piece of equipment will the nurse ask you to obtain for a person who has orthopnea?
   a. Oxygen face mask
   b. Over-the-bed table
   c. Box of tissues
   d. Incentive spirometer
2. Adults normally have
   a. 8 to 10 respirations per minute
   b. 12 to 20 respirations per minute
   c. 10 to 12 respirations per minute
   d. 20 to 24 respirations per minute
3. What is the best description of dyspnea?
   a. Breathing appears difficult, labored, or painful
   b. Breathing is slow with 12 or fewer respirations per minute
   c. Breathing is rapid with 24 or more respirations per minute
   d. Breathing seems absent or barely measurable
4. You are helping a new nursing assistant who is performing a pulse oximeter reading on a person. For which action would you intervene?
   a. Tells the person that the sensor clips on snugly, but pain is not expected
   b. Places the blood pressure cuff and the pulse oximeter on the same arm
   c. Checks the fingers and toes for swelling, skin breaks or nail polish
   d. Checks the SpO2 and pulse rate and records information on the flow sheet
5. The nurse tells you to play with the child and use a pinwheel and to help her blow bubbles. What is the purpose of the play activities?
   a. Encourages and promotes deep breathing
   b. Distracts the child from the oxygen therapy
   c. Prevents hyperventilation
   d. Strengths chest muscles

Answers to these questions are on p. 538.

CHAPTER 45 REHABILITATION AND RESTORATIVE NURSING CARE

- A **disability** is any lost, absent, or impaired physical or mental function.
- **Rehabilitation** is the process of restoring the person to his or her highest possible level of physical, psychological, social, and economic function. The focus is on improving abilities. This promotes function at the highest level of independence.
- **Restorative nursing care** is care that helps persons regain health and strength for safe and independent living. Restorative nursing measures promote healing, self-care, elimination, positioning, mobility, communication and cognitive function

Rehabilitation and the Whole Person
- Rehabilitation takes longer in older persons. Changes from aging affect healing, mobility, vision, hearing, and other functions. Chronic health problems can slow recovery.

Physical Aspects
- Rehabilitation starts when the person first seeks health care. Complications, such as contractures and pressure injuries, are prevented.
- *Elimination.* Bowel or bladder training may be needed. Fecal impaction, constipation, and fecal incontinence are prevented.
- *Self-care.* Self-care for activities of daily living (ADL) is a major goal. Self-help devices are often needed.
- *Mobility.* The person may need to learn how to move in bed and how to perform transfers. Crutches, a walker, a cane, a brace, or a wheelchair may be needed.
- *Nutrition.* The person may need a dysphagia diet or enteral nutrition.
- *Communication.* Speech therapy and communication devices may be helpful.

Psychological and Social Aspects
- A disability can affect function and appearance. Self-esteem and relationships may suffer. The person may feel less than whole, useless, unattractive, unclean, or undesirable. The person may deny the disability. The person may expect therapy to correct the problem. He or she may be depressed, angry, and hostile.
- Successful rehabilitation depends on the person's attitude. The person must accept his or her limits and be motivated. The focus is on abilities and strengths. Despair and frustration are common. Progress may be slow.
- Remind persons of their progress. They need help accepting disabilities and limits. Give support, re-assurance, and encouragement. Spiritual support helps some people. Psychological and social needs are part of the care plan.

The Rehabilitation Team
- Rehabilitation is a team effort. The person is the key member. The health team and family help the person set goals and plan care. The focus is to help the person regain function and independence.

Your Role
- Every part of your job focuses on promoting the person's independence. Preventing decline in function also is a goal. Review Box 45-2(p 684), Assisting With Rehabilitation Needs, in the Textbook.

Quality of Life
- To promote quality of life:
  - Protect the right to privacy.
  - Protect the right to be free from abuse and mistreatment.
  - Learn to deal with your anger and frustration.
  - Encourage activities.
  - Provide a safe setting.
  - Show patience, understanding, and sensitivity.

CHAPTER 45 REVIEW QUESTIONS
Circle the BEST answer.
1. If you are a restorative aide, it means you have
   a. Special training in restorative nursing and rehabilitation skills
   b. Cared for people that have rehabilitation needs
   c. Read material on how to perform rehabilitation duties
   d. Seniority at a rehabilitation facility
2. What would you do if a person with a disability expressed angry or hostility when you encouraged him to wash his own face?
   a. Take over and perform the hygienic care for him
   b. Tell him you will come back after he has calmed down
   c. Be patient and talk to the nurse if the behavior continues
   d. Firmly tell him that you are just trying to do your job
3. A person attempts to tie his shoe, but the knot doesn't hold, and the shoelace comes untied. Which response is best?
   a. "Tying your shoelaces is not that hard; try again."
   b. "Here, let me do it for you. I'm sorry that it's so hard for you."
   c. "You used the wrong kind of knot, try to remember what to do."
   d. "That was a good try and you had a nice hold on the laces."
4. You see a family member hit and scream at a person. What should you do?
   a. Check the person to see if there are any serious injuries
   b. Call the police and report the abusive behavior
   c. Talk to the nurse and describe what you saw and heard
   d. Tell the family member to leave at once and don't come back
5. A person has a weak left arm. You will
   a. Place the call light on his left side
   b. Place the call light on his right side
   c. Give him sympathy and pity
   d. Tell him to call out loudly when he needs help
Answers to these questions are on p. 538.

CHAPTER 46 HEARING, SPEECH, AND VISION PROBLEMS
Hearing Loss
- Hearing loss is not being able to hear the normal range of sounds associated with normal hearing. Deafness is hearing loss in which it is impossible for the person to understand speech through hearing alone.

- Obvious signs and symptoms of hearing loss include:
  - Speaking too loudly
  - Leaning forward to hear
  - Turning and cupping the better ear toward the speaker
  - Straining to understand a conversation
  - Answering questions or responding inappropriately
  - Asking others to repeat themselves, speak louder or to speak more slowly and clearly
  - Having trouble hearing over the phone
  - Finding it hard to follow conversations when 2 or more people are talking
  - Turning up the TV, radio, or music volume so loud that others complain
- Persons with hearing loss may wear hearing aids or lip-read (speech-read). They watch facial expressions, gestures, and body language. Some people learn American Sign Language (ASL). Others may have hearing assistance dogs.
- Review Box 46-3(p 691), Measures to Promote Hearing, in the Textbook.
- Hearing aids are battery-operated. If they do not seem to work properly:
  - Check if the hearing aid is on. It has an on and off switch.
  - Check the battery position.
  - Insert a new battery if needed.
  - Clean the hearing aid. Follow the nurse's direction and the manufacturer's instructions.
- Hearing aids are turned off when not in use. The battery is removed.
- Handle and care for hearing aids properly. If lost or damaged, report it to the nurse at once.
- Review Box 46-4(p 692), Hearing Aids-Care Measures in the Textbook

Speech Disorders
Aphasia
- **Aphasia** is the total or partial loss of the ability to use or understand language.
- *Expressive aphasia* relates to difficulty expressing or sending out thoughts. Thinking is clear. The person knows what to say but has difficulty or cannot speak the words.
- *Receptive aphasia* relates to difficulty understanding language. The person has trouble understanding what is said or read. People and common objects are not recognized.
- *Global aphasia* is a difficulty in speaking and understanding language.

Eye Disorders
- *Cataract.* Cataract is a clouding of the lens in the eye. Signs and symptoms include cloudy, blurry, or dimmed vision. Persons may also be sensitive to light and glares or see halos around lights. Poor vision at night and double vision in one eye are other symptoms. Surgery is the only treatment.
- *Age-related macular degeneration (AMD).* AMD blurs central vision needed for reading, sewing, driving, and seeing faces and fine detail. Treatment may stop or slow the disease progress.
- *Diabetic retinopathy.* Diabetic retinopathy causes blood vessels in the retina to become damaged. Usually both eyes are affected. It is a leading cause of blindness. Control of diabetes, blood pressure, and cholesterol can help to decrease risk or worsening of diabetic retinopathy.
- *Glaucoma.* Glaucoma results when fluid builds up in the eye and causes pressure on the optic nerve. The optic nerve is damaged. Vision loss with eventual blindness occurs. Drugs and surgery can control glaucoma and prevent further damage to the optic nerve. Prior damage cannot be reversed.
- See Box 46-6(p 695), Vision Problems- Signs and Symptoms in the Textbook

Impaired Vision and Blindness
- Blindness is absence of sight. The legally blind person sees at 20 feet what a person with normal vision sees at 200 feet.
- Review Box 46-7(p 698), Caring for Blind and Visually Impaired Persons, in the Textbook.

Corrective Lenses
- Clean eyeglasses daily and as needed.
- Protect eyeglasses from loss or damage. When not worn, put them in their case.
- Contact lenses are cleaned, removed, and stored according to the manufacturer's instructions.

CHAPTER 46 REVIEW QUESTIONS
Circle the BEST answer.

1. Which nursing assistant needs a reminder about measures that promote hearing?
   a. Nursing Assistant A pauses slightly between sentences
   b. Nursing Assistant B speaks clearly, distinctly, and slowly
   c. Nursing Assistant C uses facial expressions and gestures to give clues
   d. Nursing Assistant D chats with the person while making the bed
2. A person who uses a hearing aid is preparing to go to bed. Which action would you perform?
   a. Turn the hearing aid off, then put it in the ear canal
   b. Discard the battery and store the hearing aid
   c. Place the hearing aid in the storage case
   d. Clean the hearing aid and assist with re-positioning
3. Which nursing assistant needs a reminder about caring for a person who is blind?
   a. Nursing Assistant A identifies self when entering the room
   b. Nursing Assistant B cleans up and stores personal items in the closet
   c. Nursing Assistant C describes people, places, and things thoroughly
   d. Nursing Assistant D asks how much the person can see

4. Fluid buildup in the eye that causes pressure on the optic nerve is
   a. Cataract
   b. Cerumen
   c. Glaucoma
   d. Tinnitus

Answers to these questions are on p. 538.

CHAPTER 47 CANCER, IMMUNE SYSTEM, AND SKIN DISORDERS

Cancer

- Cancer is the second leading cause of death in the United States. Risk factors include: age, tobacco, radiation, infections, immunosuppressive drugs, alcohol, hormones, diet and obesity, and environment.
- Review Box 47-1(p 706), Cancer-Signs and Symptoms, in the Textbook.
- Treatments include: surgery, radiation therapy, chemotherapy, hormone therapy, immune therapy, targeted therapy, stem cell transplants and complementary and alternative medicine.
- Persons with cancer have many needs. They include:
  o Pain relief or control
  o Rest and exercise
  o Fluids and nutrition
  o Preventing skin breakdown
  o Preventing bowel problems (constipation, diarrhea)
  o Dealing with treatment side effects
  o Psychological and social needs
  o Spiritual needs
  o Sexual needs
- Anger, fear, and depression are common. Some surgeries are disfiguring. The person may feel unwhole, unattractive, or unclean.
- Talk to the person. Do not avoid the person because you are uncomfortable. Use touch and listening to show that you care.

Immune System Disorders

- The immune system protects the body from microbes, cancer cells, and other harmful substances. It defends against threats inside and outside the body.

HIV/AIDS

- Acquired immunodeficiency syndrome (AIDS) is caused by the human immunodeficiency virus (HIV). The virus is spread through body fluids—blood, semen, vaginal secretions, rectal fluids, and breast-milk. HIV is not spread by air, saliva, tears, sweat, sneezing, coughing, insects, casual contact, closed mouth or social kissing, or toilet seats.
- Persons with AIDS are at risk for pneumonia, tuberculosis, Kaposi's sarcoma (a cancer), nervous system disorders, mental health disorders, and dementia.
- To protect yourself and others from HIV, follow Standard Precautions and the Bloodborne Pathogen Standard.
- Review Box 47-4(p713), Caring for the Person With AIDS, in the Textbook.

- Older persons also get AIDS. They get and spread HIV through sexual contact and intravenous (IV) drug use. Aging and some diseases can mask the signs and symptoms of AIDS. Older persons are less likely to be tested for HIV/AIDS.

Skin Disorders—Shingles

- Shingles is caused by the same virus that causes chicken pox. A rash or blisters can occur. Pain is mild to intense and itching is a common complaint.
- Shingles is most common in persons over 50 years of age. Persons at risk are those who have had chicken pox as children and who have weakened immune systems. Shingles lesions are infectious until they crust over.
- Treatments include anti-viral and pain-relief drugs. A vaccine is available to prevent shingles.

CHAPTER 47 REVIEW QUESTIONS

Circle the BEST answer.

1. Which personal protective equipment is the most important to maintain safety when caring for a person who is receiving chemotherapy?
   a. Shoe covers
   b. Gown
   c. Mask
   d. Gloves
2. Benign tumors
   a. Do not spread to other body parts
   b. Invade healthy tissue
   c. Are always very small
   d. Divide in a rapidly uncontrolled way
3. Which body fluid is most likely to be a source of HIV?
   a. Breast milk
   b. Tears
   c. Saliva
   d. Sweat
4. Which nursing assistant should inform the nurse about a personal condition that would affect care assignment to a person who has shingles in the infectious stage?
   a. Nursing Assistant A has a child who the chicken pox vaccination.
   b. Nursing Assistant B is taking antibiotics for a respiratory infection
   c. Nursing Assistant C recently found out that she is pregnant
   d. Nursing Assistant D has an elderly parent who had the shingles vaccination

Answers to these questions are on p. 538.

CHAPTER 48 NERVOUS SYSTEM AND MUSCULO-SKELETAL DISORDERS

Nervous System Disorders

Stroke

- Stroke is also called a brain attack or cerebrovascular accident (CVA). Stroke is caused by bleeding in the brain (cerebral hemorrhage) or by a blood clot in the brain.

- Review Box 48-1(p 719), Stroke: Warning Signs, in the Textbook.
- The effects of stroke include:
  - Loss of face, hand, arm, leg, or body control
  - **Hemiplegia**—paralysis on one side of the body
  - Changing emotions (crying easily or mood swings, sometimes for no reason)
  - Difficulty swallowing (dysphagia)
  - Aphasia or slowed or slurred speech
  - Changes in sight, touch, movement, and thought
  - Impaired memory
  - Urinary frequency, urgency, or incontinence
  - Loss of bowel control or constipation
  - Depression and frustration
  - Behavior changes
- The health team helps the person regain the highest possible level of function. Review Box 48-2(p 720), Stroke Care Measures, in the Textbook.

Parkinson's Disease

- Parkinson's disease is a slow, progressive disorder with no cure. Persons over the age of 60 are at risk. Signs and symptoms become worse over time. They include:
  - *Tremors*—often start in one finger and spread to the whole arm. Pill-rolling movements—rubbing the thumb and index finger—may occur. The person may have trembling in the hands, arms, legs, jaw, and face.
  - *Rigid, stiff muscles*—in the arms, legs, neck, and trunk.
  - *Slow movements*—the person has a slow, shuffling gait.
  - *Stooped posture and impaired balance*—it is hard to walk. Falls are a risk.
  - *Mask-like expression*—the person cannot blink and smile. A fixed stare is common.
  - *Speech changes*— the person may have slurred, monotone, and soft speech.
- Other signs and symptoms that develop over time include swallowing and chewing problems, constipation, and bladder problems. Sleep problems, depression, emotional changes (fear, insecurity), memory loss and slow thinking can occur.
- Drugs are ordered to treat and control the disease. Exercise and physical therapy improve strength, posture, balance, and mobility. Therapy is needed for speech and swallowing problems. The person may need help with eating and self-care. Safety measures are needed to prevent falls and injury.

Multiple Sclerosis

- Multiple sclerosis (MS) is a chronic disease. The myelin (which covers nerve fibers) in the brain and spinal cord is destroyed. Nerve impulses are not sent to and from the brain in a normal manner. Functions are impaired or lost. There is no cure.
- Symptoms usually start between the ages of 15 and 60. Signs and symptoms may include vision problems, muscle weakness that usually starts on one side of the body, and balance and coordination problems. Tingling, prickling, or numb sensations may occur. Partial or complete paralysis and pain may occur. Other problems include; fatigue; hearing loss; tremors; dizziness; depression; bladder function; sexual function; and changes in speech, concentration, attention, memory, and judgment.
- Persons with MS are kept active and independent as long as possible. Skin care, hygiene, and range-of-motion (ROM) exercises are important. So are turning, positioning, and deep breathing and coughing. Bowel and bladder elimination are promoted. Injuries and complications from bed rest are prevented.

Amyotrophic lateral sclerosis (ALS)

- Memory and intellect are usually unaffected; but affected nerve cells in the brain and spinal cord stop sending messages to the voluntary muscles. The muscles weaken, waste away (atrophy), and twitch. The person cannot move the arms, legs, and body. Muscles for speaking, chewing and swallowing, and breathing also are affected. Eventually respiratory muscles fail.
- The person is kept active and independent to the extent possible.

Head Injuries

- Traumatic brain injury (TBI) occurs from violent injury to the brain. Common causes include falls, traffic accidents, violence, sports, explosive blasts, and combat injuries. Review Box 48-3(p 722), Traumatic Brain Injury-Signs and Symptoms, in the Textbook.
- Disabilities from TBI include cognitive problems, sensory problems, communications problems, and emotional problems.

Spinal Cord Injury

- Spinal cord injuries can permanently damage the nervous system. Common causes are motor vehicle crashes, falls, violence, sports injuries, alcohol use, and cancer and other diseases.
- The higher the level of injury, the more functions lost.
  - Lumbar injuries—sensory and muscle functions in the legs are lost. The person has **paraplegia**—paralysis and loss of sensory function in the legs and lower trunk.
  - Thoracic injuries—sensory and muscle function below the chest is lost. The person has paraplegia.
  - Cervical injuries—sensory and muscle functions of the arms, legs, and trunk are lost. Paralysis in the arms, legs, and trunk is called **quadriplegia** or **tetraplegia**.
- Review Box 48-4(p 724), Paralysis-Care Measures, in the Textbook.

Musculo-Skeletal Disorders

Arthritis

- Arthritis means joint inflammation.
- *Osteoarthritis (degenerative joint disease)*. The fingers, spine (neck and lower back), and weight-bearing joints (hips, knees, and feet) are often affected.
- *Rheumatoid arthritis*. Rheumatoid arthritis (RA) causes joint pain, swelling, stiffness, and loss of function. Fatigue and fever may occur.
- Treatments for osteoarthritis and RA are similar.
  - Pain control.

o Heat and cold.
o Exercise.
o Rest and joint care.
o Assistive (adaptive) devices.
o Weight control.
o Healthy life-style.
o Safety.
o Joint replacement surgery.

Fractures

- A fracture is a broken bone. Falls, accidents, sports injuries, bone tumors, and osteoporosis are some causes.
- Signs and symptoms of a fracture include:
  o Severe pain
  o Swelling and tenderness
  o Problems moving the part
  o Deformity (the part looks out of place)
  o Bruising and skin color changes at the fracture site
  o Bleeding (internal or external)
  o Numbness and tingling
- Review Box 48-7(p 729), Cast Care, Box 48-8(p 731), Traction Care, Box 48-9(p 731), Hip Fracture Care in the Textbook.

CHAPTER 48 REVIEW QUESTIONS

Circle the BEST answer.

1. The person had a stroke. Which action would you perform?
   a. Keep the side rails up at all times
   b. Re-position the person every 2 hours
   c. Assist the person to a supine position
   d. Place personal items on the affected side
2. The person with hemiplegia
   a. Is paralyzed on one side of the body
   b. Is paralyzed in both arms
   c. Has paralysis in both legs
   d. Has paralysis in all extremities
3. The leading cause of disability in the United States is
   a. Head injuries
   b. Arthritis
   c. Stroke
   d. Spinal cord injuries
4. The person has paralysis in the legs and lower trunk. This is called
   a. Quadriplegia
   b. Paraplegia
   c. Hemiplegia
   d. Tetraplegia
5. You observe that a person who has a cast on her wrist is wearing her wedding ring. What should you do?
   a. Tell her to remove the ring and store it in a safe place
   b. Check to see if there is swelling or discoloration near the ring
   c. Do nothing; people have a right to wear personal jewelry
   d. Inform the nurse about your observation

Answers to these questions are on p. 538.

CHAPTER 49 CARDIOVASCULAR, RESPIRATORY, AND LYMPHATIC DISORDERS

Cardiovascular Disorders

- *Hypertension.* Hypertension (high blood pressure) occurs when the systolic pressure is 140 mm Hg or higher or the diastolic pressure is 90 mm Hg or higher. Narrowed blood vessels are a common cause. Review Box 49-1(p 739), Cardiovascular Disorders-Risk Factors, in the Textbook.
- *Coronary artery disease (CAD).* In CAD, the coronary arteries become hardened and narrow and the heart muscle gets less blood and oxygen. The most common cause is atherosclerosis, or plaque buildup on artery walls. Complications of CAD are angina, heart attack, heart failure, irregular heartbeats, and sudden death. CAD complications may require cardiac rehabilitation, which consists of exercise training and education, counseling, and training for life-style changes.
- *Angina.* Angina is chest pain. It is caused by reduced blood flow to part of the heart muscle. Chest pain is described as tightness, pressure, squeezing, or burning in the chest. Pain can occur in the shoulders, arms, neck, jaw, or back. The person may be pale, feel faint, and perspire. Dyspnea, nausea, fatigue, and weakness may occur. Some persons complain of "gas" or indigestion. Chest pain lasting longer than a few minutes and not relieved by rest and nitroglycerin may signal heart attack. The person needs emergency care.
- *Myocardial infarction (MI).* MI is also called *heart attack, acute myocardial infarction (AMI),* and *acute coronary syndrome (ACS).* Blood flow to the heart muscle is suddenly blocked. Part of the heart muscle dies. MI is an emergency. Sudden cardiac death *(sudden cardiac arrest)* can occur. Review Box 49-2(p 741), Myocardial Infarction-Signs and Symptoms, in the Textbook.
- *Heart failure.* Heart failure or congestive heart failure (CHF) occurs when the heart is weakened and cannot pump normally. Blood backs up. Tissue congestion occurs. Drugs are given to strengthen the heart. They also reduce the amount of fluid in the body. A sodium-controlled diet is ordered. Oxygen is given. Semi-Fowler's position is preferred for breathing. Intake and output (I&O), daily weight, elastic stockings, and range-of-motion (ROM) exercises are part of the care plan.
- *Dysrhythmias.* Dysrhythmias are abnormal heart rhythms. Rhythms may be too fast, too slow, or irregular. Dysrhythmias are caused by changes in the heart's electrical system. Some abnormal rhythms are treated with a pacemaker.

Respiratory Disorders

Chronic Obstructive Pulmonary Disease

- Chronic bronchitis and emphysema are two types of *chronic obstructive pulmonary disease (COPD).* These disorders obstruct airflow. Lung function is gradually lost.

- *Chronic bronchitis*. Bronchitis means inflammation of the bronchi. Chronic bronchitis occurs after repeated episodes of bronchitis. Smoking is the major cause. Smoker's cough is the main symptom of chronic bronchitis. Over time, the cough becomes more frequent. The person has difficulty breathing and tires easily. The person must stop smoking. Oxygen therapy and breathing exercises are often ordered. If a respiratory tract infection occurs, the person needs prompt treatment.
- *Emphysema*. In emphysema, the alveoli enlarge and become less elastic. They do not expand and shrink normally when breathing in and out. Air becomes trapped when exhaling. Smoking is the most common cause. The person has shortness of breath and a cough. Fatigue is common. The person works hard to breathe in and out. Breathing is easier when the person sits upright and slightly forward. The person must stop smoking. Respiratory therapy, breathing exercises, oxygen, and drug therapy are ordered.

Asthma
- In asthma, the airway becomes inflamed and narrow. Extra mucus is produced. Dyspnea results. Wheezing, coughing, pain and tightening in the chest are common. Asthma usually is triggered by allergies. Other triggers include air pollutants and irritants, smoking and second-hand smoke, respiratory tract infections, and exertion. Asthma is treated with drugs. Severe attacks may require emergency care.

Sleep Apnea
- Pauses in breathing last a few seconds to over a minute and can occur many times during sleep.
- The most common cause is blockage of the airway.
- During sleep, the person may use: Continuous positive airway pressure (CPAP) or Bilevel positive airway pressure (BiPAP).
- In these therapies a mask is attached to a pump. Air pressure is forced through the mask. The air keeps the airway open.

Pneumonia
- Pneumonia is an inflammation and infection of lung tissue. Bacteria, viruses, and other microbes are causes.
- High fever, chills, painful cough, chest pain on breathing, and rapid pulse occur. Shortness of breath and rapid breathing also occur. Cyanosis may be present.
- Drugs are ordered for infection and pain. Fluid intake is increased. Intravenous (IV) therapy and oxygen may be needed. The semi-Fowler's position eases breathing. Rest is important. Standard Precautions are followed. Isolation precautions are used depending on the cause.

Tuberculosis
- Tuberculosis (TB) is a bacterial infection in the lungs. TB is spread by airborne droplets with coughing, sneezing, speaking, singing, or laughing. Those who have close, frequent contact with an infected person are at risk. TB is more likely to occur in close, crowded areas. Age (very young or very old), poor nutrition, and human immunodeficiency virus (HIV) infection are other risk factors.
- Signs and symptoms are tiredness, loss of appetite, weight loss, fever, and night sweats. Cough and sputum production increase over time. Sputum may contain blood. Chest pain occurs.
- Drugs for TB are given. Standard Precautions and airborne precautions are needed. The person must cover the mouth and nose with tissues when sneezing, coughing, or producing sputum. Tissues are discarded in a no-touch waste container. Hand-washing after contact with sputum is essential.

Lymphatic Disorders
Lymphedema
- Lymphedema usually occurs in an arm or a leg because of a blockage or damage to the lymph system. Treatment may include careful exercise, good skin care, massage therapy and pressure garments (compression sleeves, lymphedema sleeves or stockings). It is important to avoid putting pressure on the affected limb (e.g., no blood pressure cuff). See Box 49-5(p 748), Lymphedema-Care Measures in the Textbook.

CHAPTER 49 REVIEW QUESTIONS
Circle the BEST answer.
1. What is the most important information to remember when caring for a person who has angina?
   a. You should know the person's typical pain and symptom pattern and how drugs and rest usually affect the symptoms
   b. The person should stop all activities, rest, and have nitroglycerin tablets available before angina occurs
   c. Systolic pressure that is 140 mm Hg or higher or diastolic pressure that is 90 or higher should be immediately reported.
   d. Pain that is severe, lasts longer than a few minutes, or is not relieved by rest or drugs may signal a heart attack.
2. For a person has heart failure. Which task would you perform?
   a. Measure intake and output
   b. Measure weight every week
   c. Promote a diet that is high in salt
   d. Encourage fluids for hydration
3. Which position is usually best for the person with pneumonia?
   a. Semi-Fowler's
   b. Prone
   c. Supine
   d. Trendelenburg's
4. In which situation would you expect to use airborne precautions?
   a. Person is being treated for an acute asthma attack
   b. Person has chronic bronchitis and continues to smoke
   c. Person has signs and symptoms of tuberculosis
   d. Person has emphysema and is coughing up sputum

Answers to these questions are on p. 538.

CHAPTER 50 DIGESTIVE AND ENDOCRINE DISORDERS

Digestive Disorders

Gastro-Esophageal Reflux Disease (GERD)

- GERD occurs when stomach contents flow back up into the esophagus. Drugs to prevent stomach acid production or to promote stomach emptying may be ordered. Life-style changes include limiting smoking and alcohol, losing weight, eating small meals, wearing loose belts and clothing, sitting upright for 3 hours after meals, and raising the head of the bed 6 to 9 inches so that head and shoulders are higher than the stomach.

Vomiting

- These measures are needed.
  - Follow Standard Precautions and the Bloodborne Pathogen Standard.
  - Turn the person's head well to the side. This prevents aspiration.
  - Place a kidney basin under the person's chin.
  - Move vomitus away from the person.
  - Provide oral hygiene.
  - Observe vomitus for color, odor, and undigested food. If it looks like coffee grounds, it contains undigested blood. This signals bleeding. Report your observations.
  - Measure, report, and record the amount of vomitus. Also record the amount on the intake and output (I&O) record.
  - Save a specimen for laboratory study.
  - Dispose of vomitus after the nurse observes it.
  - Eliminate odors.
  - Provide for comfort.

Hepatitis

- Hepatitis is an inflammation of the liver. It can be mild or cause death. Signs and symptoms are listed in Table 50-1(p 756), Hepatitis, in the Textbook. Some people do not have symptoms.
- Protect yourself and others. Follow Standard Precautions and the Bloodborne Pathogen Standard. Isolation precautions are ordered as necessary. Assist the person with hygiene and hand-washing as needed.

Endocrine Disorders

Diabetes

- In this disorder the body cannot produce or use insulin properly. Insulin is needed for glucose to move from the blood into the cells. Sugar builds up in the blood. Cells do not have enough sugar for energy and cannot function.
- Diabetes must be controlled to prevent complications. Complications include eye problems, renal failure, nerve damage, stroke, heart attack, and slow healing. Foot and leg wounds can lead to infection and amputation.
- Blood glucose is monitored for:
  - *Hypoglycemia*—low sugar in the blood.
  - *Hyperglycemia*—high sugar in the blood.
- Review Table 50-2(p 760), Hypoglycemia and Hyperglycemia in the Textbook. Either condition can lead to death if not corrected. You must call for the nurse at once.

CHAPTER 50 REVIEW QUESTIONS
Circle the BEST answer.

1. You walk into a person's room; the person is in a supine position and vomiting. What should you should do first?
   a. Obtain a kidney basin
   b. Notify the nurse immediately
   c. Turn the person's head to one side
   d. Observe emesis for blood, color and odor

2. Which task is part of your responsibility in helping a person with GERD successfully achieve the lifestyle modifications for this disorder?
   a. Encourage him to maintain the eating habits he is used to
   b. Tell him that he is not allowed to lie down for 3 hours after eating
   c. Assist him to select and don a loose-fitting belt and loose clothes
   d. Place him a in supine position to rest after dinner

3. Which symptom is the person most likely to report during a "gallbladder attack"?
   a. Pain in the right upper abdomen
   b. Constipation and pain with straining
   c. Rectal bleeding and bloody stools
   d. Severe itching and hot dry skin

4. You are caring for a person who has hepatitis A. What is the most important measure for infection control?
   a. Isolating the person
   b. Good hand hygiene
   c. Vaccination
   d. Cough etiquette

5. A person with diabetes is trembling, sweating, and feels hungry and faint. You
   a. Get the person a cool cloth and a fan
   b. Get the person something to eat
   c. Place him in a supine position with feet up
   d. Tell the nurse immediately

Answers to these questions are on p. 538.

CHAPTER 51 URINARY AND REPRODUCTIVE DISORDERS

Urinary System Disorders

Urinary Tract Infections (UTIs)

- UTIs are common. Urologic exams, intercourse, poor perineal hygiene, immobility, and poor fluid intake are common causes. Urinary catheters create a high risk; UTIs is a common health care associated infection.

Prostate Enlargement

- The prostate grows larger as a man grows older. This is called benign prostatic hyperplasia (BPH). The enlarged prostate presses against the urethra. This obstructs urine flow through the urethra.

Urinary Diversion

- A urinary diversion is a surgically created pathway for urine to leave the body.
- Often an ostomy is involved. Good skin care is needed to prevent skin breakdown. Observe and report skin

changes around the stoma. See "The Person With an Ostomy" in Chapter 29 (p 450).

Kidney Stones
- Kidney stones (calculi) can cause severe pain and changes in urination: pain, frequency, urgency, hematuria (blood in urine), and cloudy foul-smelling urine.
- Urine is strained for stones. Fluids help to flush the stone; 2000 to 3000mL/day is encouraged.

Kidney Failure
- In kidney failure (renal failure) the kidneys do not function or are severely impaired. Waste products are not removed from the blood. Fluid is retained.
- Acute kidney failure is sudden. Blood flow to the kidneys is severely decreased.
- With chronic kidney failure the kidneys cannot meet the body's needs. Hypertension and diabetes are common causes. Review Box 51-2(p 766), Chronic Kidney Disease-Signs and Symptoms, and Box 51-3(p 767), Kidney Failure-Care Measures in the Textbook.

Reproductive Disorders
Sexually Transmitted Diseases
- A sexually transmitted disease (STD), also known as sexually transmitted infection (STI), is spread by oral, vaginal, or anal sex. Some people do not have signs and symptoms or are not aware of an infection. Standard Precautions and the Bloodborne Pathogen Standard are followed. Review Box 51-4(p 768), Sexually Transmitted Diseases/Sexually Transmitted Infections in the Textbook.

CHAPTER 51 REVIEW QUESTIONS
Circle the BEST answer.

1. An older man has benign prostatic hyperplasia. Which symptom is he most likely to report?
   a. Hiccups
   b. Fever and chills
   c. Flank pain
   d. Dribbling after voiding
2. In caring for a person with acute renal failure, what important role do you have that helps the doctor and the nurse to monitor the kidney function?
   a. Performing perineal care
   b. Measuring intake and output
   c. Adhering to Standard Precautions
   d. Straining the urine
3. You are assisting an elderly person with perineal care and you notice a sore on the shaft of his penis. Which action would you take before reporting your observation to the nurse?
   a. Gently cleanse the sore with mild soap and apply an antiseptic cream
   b. Initiate contact and wound precautions with gloving and gowning
   c. Use Standard Precautions and the Bloodborne Pathogen Standard
   d. Ask the person how long the sore has been there and if it is painful

Answers to these questions are on p. 538.

CHAPTER 52 MENTAL HEALTH DISORDERS
- **Mental health** involves a person's emotional, psychological, and social well-being.
- **Mental health disorders** are serious illnesses that can affect a person's thinking, mood, behavior, function, and ability to relate to others. Review Box 52-1(p 771), Mental Health Disorders in the Textbook for warning signs and risk factors.
- **Stress** is the response or change in the body caused by any emotional, psychological, physical, social, or economic factor.

Anxiety Disorders
- **Anxiety** is feeling of worry, nervousness, or fear about an event or situation. Anxiety is a normal reaction to stress and helps a person to stay alert and focused and to cope.
- Coping and defense mechanisms are used to relieve anxiety. Review Box 52-3(p 772), Defense Mechanisms, in the Textbook.
- Some common anxiety disorders are generalized anxiety disorder, panic disorder, obsessive-compulsive disorder, phobias, and post-traumatic stress disorder.
- *Generalized anxiety disorder.* **Generalized anxiety disorder** is characterized by extreme anxiety, fear, or worry that occurs most days for at least 6 months. The person has worry and concern about many things.
- *Panic disorder.* **Panic** is an intense and sudden feeling of fear, anxiety, or dread. Onset is sudden with no obvious reason. The person cannot function. Review Box 52-2 (p 771), Anxiety-Signs and Symptoms, in the Textbook.
- *Obsessive-compulsive disorder (OCD).* An **obsession** is frequent, upsetting and unwanted thoughts, ideas, or images. **Compulsion** is an overwhelming urge to repeat certain rituals, acts or behaviors.
- *Phobias.* **Phobia** means an intense fear. The person has an intense fear of an object, situation, or activity that has little or no actual danger. The person avoids what is feared. When faced with the fear, the person has high anxiety and cannot function.
- *Post-traumatic stress disorder (PTSD).* PTSD occurs in some people after a terrifying, traumatic, scary or dangerous event that involved physical harm or threat of physical harm. Review Box 52-4(p 773), Post-Traumatic Stress Disorder: Signs and Symptoms, in the Textbook. Flashbacks are common. A **flashback** is reliving the trauma in thoughts during the day and in nightmares during sleep. The traumatic event can seem like it is happening all over again. Some people recover within 6 months, for others the condition is chronic.

Psychotic Disorders
- **Schizophrenia** is a serious brain illness affecting how a person thinks feels and behaves. Symptoms include:
  - *Psychosis*—a state of severe mental impairment. The person does not view the real or unreal correctly.
  - *Hallucinations*—seeing, hearing, smelling, or feeling something that is not real.
  - *Delusion*—a false belief.

- Delusion of grandeur—an exaggerated belief about one's importance, wealth, power, or talents.
- Delusion of persecution—the false belief that one is being mistreated, abused, or harassed.
- Thought disorders—trouble organizing thoughts or connecting thoughts logically.
- Movement disorders—include agitated body movements; repeating motions over and over; and sitting for hours without moving, speaking, or responding.
- Emotional and behavioral problems—normal functions are impaired or absent, including losing motivation or interest in daily activities, being unable to plan, lacking emotions, neglecting personal hygiene, and withdrawing socially.
- Cognitive problems—trouble paying attention, understanding, or remembering information.

- The person with schizophrenia has problems relating to others. He or she may be paranoid. The person may have difficulty organizing thoughts. Responses are inappropriate. Communication is disturbed. The person may withdraw. Some people regress to an earlier time or condition. Some persons with schizophrenia attempt suicide.

Mood Disorders
Bipolar Disorder
- The person with bipolar disorder has severe extremes in mood, energy, and ability to function. There are emotional lows (depression) and emotional highs (mania). This disorder must be managed throughout life. Review Box 52-5(p 774), Bipolar Disorder-Signs and Symptoms, in the Textbook. Bipolar disorder can damage relationships and affect school or work performance. Some people are suicidal.

Depression
- Depression causes distressing symptoms that affect feeling, thinking, and daily activities. Review Box 52-5(p 774), Bipolar Disorder-Signs and Symptoms; Depressive Episode in the Textbook.
- Depression is common in older persons. There are many losses—death of family and friends, loss of health, loss of body functions, and loss of independence. Loneliness and the side effects of some drugs also are causes. Review Box 52-6(p 775), Depression in Older Persons-Signs and Symptoms, in the Textbook. Depression in older persons is often overlooked or a wrong diagnosis is made.

Substance Abuse Disorder
- Addiction is a chronic disease involving substance seeking behaviors and use that is compulsive and hard to control despite the harmful effects. The person must have the substance. Persons addicted to drugs or alcohol cannot stop taking the substance without treatment.
- Alcoholism—alcohol dependence involves:
  - Craving—a strong need to drink

- Loss of control—not being able to stop drinking once started
- Physical dependence—withdrawal symptoms
- Tolerance—the need for more alcohol for the same effect
- **Withdrawal syndrome** is the physical and mental response after stopping or severely reducing use of a substance that was used regularly. The body responds with anxiety, restlessness, insomnia, irritability, poor attention, and physical illness.

Suicide
- **Suicide** means to end one's life on purpose.
- Suicide is most often linked to depression, alcohol or substance abuse, or stressful events. Review Box 52-8(p 778), Suicide, in the Textbook.
- If a person mentions or talks about suicide, take the person seriously. Call for the nurse at once. Do not leave the person alone.

Care and Treatment
- Treatment of mental health disorders involves having the person explore his or her thoughts and feelings. Often drugs are ordered.
- The care plan reflects the person's needs. The physical, safety and security, and emotional needs of the person must be met.
- Communication is important. Be alert to nonverbal communication.
- Protect yourself. Call for help. Do not try to handle the situation on your own.
- Keep a safe distance between you and the person.
- Be aware of your setting. Do not let the person block your exit.

CHAPTER 52 REVIEW QUESTIONS
Circle the BEST answer.
1. You are caring for a person with mysophobia. Which action would you perform?
   a. Carefully clean the over-the-bed table before bringing the meal tray
   b. Make sure that the room always has light; at night turn on a nightlight
   c. Reassure the person that the activity is conducted in a small private room
   d. Allow the person to choose a shower, tub bath, or a small basin of water
2. Notify the nurse, because the physical symptoms of a panic attack could mimic
   a. A seizure
   b. A heart attack
   c. An opioid overdose
   d. A urinary tract infection
3. Which behavior is characteristic of bulimia nervosa and needs to be reported to the nurse?
   a. Eats only a small amount of certain foods
   b. Goes to the bathroom and induces vomiting
   c. Eats a large amount of food and asks for more
   d. Plays with food by pushing it around the plate

4. A person says, "Everyone would be better off without me." What would you do?
   a. Convince the person that he is valued
   b. Give the person privacy to consider his thoughts
   c. Help the person focus on the reality of his life
   d. Take the person seriously; notify the nurse
5. Which person has the greatest risk for suicide contagion?
   a. Grandmother whose grandson has suicidal thoughts
   b. Teenager whose best friend committed suicide
   c. Nursing assistant knows a patient who committed suicide
   d. Nursing instructor who teaches students about suicide prevention
6. As you enter a room to assist a person with bipolar disorder, manic phase, she throws a shoe at you and shouts profanities. What would you do first?
   a. Tell her to quiet down and stop throwing things
   b. Quickly close the door and immediately get the nurse
   c. Stand in the open doorway and calmly call for assistance
   d. Cautiously approach her and use a friendly caring tone of voice

Answers to these questions are on p. 538.

CHAPTER 53 CONFUSION AND DEMENTIA

- Changes in the brain and nervous system occur with certain diseases and aging. Review Box 53-1(p 783), Nervous System Changes from Aging, in the Textbook.
- **Cognitive function** involves memory, thinking, reasoning, ability to understand, judgment, and behavior.

Confusion

- Confusion is a state of being disoriented to person, time, place, situation, or identity. Diseases, brain injury, infections, fever, alcohol or drug use and drug side effects are some of the causes.
- The care of the confused person includes treatment that is aimed at the cause. Some measures help to improve function and basic needs must be met. Review Box 53-2(p 783), Confusion-Care Measures in the Textbook.

Delirium

- **Delirium** is a state of sudden, severe confusion and rapid changes in brain function. Usually temporary and reversible, it occurs with physical or mental illness. Delirium is an emergency. Be alert for signs and symptoms and notify the nurse. Review Box 53-3(p 783), Delirium-Signs and Symptoms in the Textbook.

Dementia

- **Dementia** is the loss of cognitive function that interferes with routine personal, social, and occupational activities.
- Dementia is not a normal part of aging; however, risk does increase with age.

- Some early warning signs include problems with language, dressing, cooking, personality changes, poor or decreased judgment, and driving as well as getting lost in familiar places and misplacing items.
- Alzheimer's disease is the most common type of permanent dementia.

Alzheimer's Disease

- Alzheimer's disease (AD) is a brain disease. Memory, thinking, reasoning, judgment, language, behavior, mood, and personality are affected. Onset is gradual.

Signs of AD

- Warning signs include:
  o Gradual loss of short-term memory.
  o Asking the same questions over and over again.
  o Repeating the same story—word for word, again and again.
  o Forgetting activities that were once done regularly with ease.
  o Losing the ability to pay bills or balance a checkbook.
  o Getting lost in familiar places. Or misplacing household objects.
  o Neglecting to bathe or wearing the same clothes over and over again. Meanwhile, the person insists that a bath was taken or that clothes were changed.
  o Relying on someone else to make decisions or answer questions that the person would have handled.
- Review Box 53-5(p 785), Signs of Alzheimer's Disease-Early Signs and Symptoms, in the Textbook for other signs of AD.

Behaviors

- The following behaviors are common with AD.
  o *Wandering.* Persons with AD are not oriented to person, place, and time. They may wander away from home and not find their way back. The person cannot tell what is safe or dangerous.
  o *Sundowning.* With sundowning, signs, symptoms, and behaviors of AD increase during hours of darkness. As daylight ends, confusion, restlessness, anxiety, agitation, and other symptoms increase.
  o *Hallucinations.* The person with AD may see, hear, or feel things that are not real.
  o *Delusions.* People with AD may think they are some other person. A person may believe that the caregiver is someone else.
  o *Paranoia.* The person has false beliefs and suspicion about a person or situation.
  o *Catastrophic reactions.* The person reacts as if there is a disaster or tragedy.
  o *Agitation and aggression.* The person may pace, hit, or yell.
  o *Communication changes.* The person has trouble expressing thoughts and emotions.
  o *Screaming.* Persons with AD may scream to communicate.
  o *Repetitive behaviors.* Persons with AD repeat the same motions over and over again.

o *Rummaging and hiding things*. The person may search for things by moving things around, turning things over, or looking through something such as a drawer or closet. The person may hide things, throw things away, or lose something.

o *Changes in intimacy and sexuality*. The person with AD may depend on and cling to his or her partner or may not remember life with or feelings for his or her partner. Sexual behaviors may involve the wrong person, the wrong time, and the wrong place. Persons with AD cannot control behavior.

Care of Persons With AD and Other Dementias

- People with AD do not choose to be forgetful, incontinent, agitated, or rude. Nor do they choose to have other behaviors, signs, and symptoms of the disease. The disease causes the behaviors.
- Safety, hygiene, nutrition and fluids, elimination, comfort, sleep, and activity needs must be met. Review Box 53-9(p 791), Care of Persons With AD and Other Dementias, in the Textbook.
- The person can have other health problems and injuries. However, the person may not recognize pain, fever, constipation, incontinence, or other signs and symptoms. Carefully observe the person. Report any change in the person's usual behavior to the nurse.
- Infection is a risk. Provide good skin care, oral hygiene, and perineal care after bowel and bladder elimination.
- Supervised activities meet the person's needs and cognitive abilities.
- Impaired communication is a common problem. Avoid giving orders, expecting the truth, or correcting the person's errors.
- Always look for dangers in the person's room and in the hallways, lounges, dining areas, and other areas on the nursing unit. Remove the danger if you can.
- Every staff member must be alert to persons who wander. Such persons are allowed to wander in safe areas.

The Family

- The family may have physical, emotional, social, and financial stresses. The family often feels hopeless. No matter what is done, the person only gets worse. Anger and resentment may result. Guilt feelings are common.
- The family is an important part of the health team. They may help plan the person's care. For many persons, family members provide comfort. The family also needs support and understanding from the health team.

CHAPTER 53 REVIEW QUESTIONS
Circle the BEST answer.
1. For a person who has AD, what would be the best way to accomplish morning care?
   a. Rotate nursing assistants to increase the person's socialization
   b. Follow the same routine every morning; assign same staff member
   c. Check the person every morning and adapt care as needed
   d. Complete care, whenever the person seems willing to participate
2. Which clothing item would be the best choice for a confused person?
   a. Wrap-around skirt that ties on the side
   b. Jeans that button in front
   c. Pullover sweatshirt
   d. Shoes with Velcro fasteners
3. When a person with AD wanders, the major risk is
   a. Potential for life-threatening accidents
   b. Disruption of routine activities of daily living
   c. Liability for the staff and facility
   d. Insufficient rest and sleep
4. You are tidying the room of a person who has AD, which item on the bedside table should be removed and given to the nurse?
   a. Plastic bottle of water
   b. Cigarette lighter
   c. Picture of deceased spouse
   d. Alarm clock
Answers to these questions are on p. 538.

CHAPTER 55 SEXUALITY
Sex and Sexuality
- **Sex** is the physical interactions between people involving the body and reproductive organs.
- **Sexuality** is the physical, emotional, social, cultural, and spiritual factors that affect a person's feelings, attitudes, and behaviors about one's gender identity and sexual behavior.
- Sexuality involves the personality and the body—how a person behaves, thinks, dresses, and responds to others.

Injury, Illness, and Surgery
- Injury, illness, and surgery can affect sexual function and ability. Chronic illnesses, such as heart disease, stroke, diabetes, and chronic obstructive pulmonary disease affect sexual function. Some drugs affect sexual desire or performance.

Sexuality and Older Persons
- Love, affection, and intimacy are needed throughout life. Older persons love, fall in love, and have intimate relationships and activities.
- Reproductive organs change with aging. Frequency of sex decreases for many older persons.
- Sexual partners are lost through death, divorce, and relationship break-ups. Or a partner needs hospital or nursing center care.

Meeting Sexual Needs
- The nursing team promotes the meeting of sexual needs.
- Review Box 55-1(p 811), Promoting Sexuality, in the Textbook.

Inappropriate Sexually Behavior

- Some persons flirt, make sexual advances or comments that are directed towards the health team members. Some expose themselves, masturbate, or touch the staff. This can anger and embarrass the staff member. These reactions are normal.
- Touch may have a sexual purpose. You must be professional about the matter.
  o Ask the person not to touch you. State the places where you were touched.
  o Tell the person that you will not do what he or she wants.
  o Tell the person what behaviors make you uncomfortable. Politely ask the person not to act that way.
  o Allow privacy if the person is becoming aroused.
  o Discuss the matter with the nurse. The nurse can help you understand the behavior.
  o Follow the care plan. Measures to deal with sexually aggressive behaviors are based on the cause of the behavior.

Protecting the Person

- The person must be protected from unwanted sexual comments and advances. This is sexual abuse (see Chapter 5 in the Textbook). Tell the nurse right away.
- No one should be allowed to sexually abuse another person. This includes staff members, patients, residents, family members or other visitors, and volunteers.

CHAPTER 55 REVIEW QUESTIONS

Circle the BEST answer.

1. There is a confused resident in a long-term care center who frequently masturbates in public and in his own room. Which care action is the nurse most likely to ask you to perform?
   a. Tell the person to stop masturbating whenever you notice the behavior
   b. Perform perineal hygiene and frequently check for wet or soiled underwear
   c. Interrupt the behavior and distract him with another activity
   d. Take him to a private room and watch him until he finishes
2. Which care measure promotes sexuality?
   a. Assisting the person to go to the bathroom
   b. Allowing brief public masturbation
   c. Encouraging the person to flirt with you
   d. Allowing the person to select their clothes

Answers to these questions are on p. 538.

CHAPTER 58 EMERGENCY CARE

Emergency Care

- Rules for emergency care include:
  o Call for help
  o Wait for help if the scene is not safe enough to approach
  o Know your limits. Do not do more than you are able.
  o Stay calm.
  o Know where to find emergency supplies.
  o Follow Standard Precautions and the Bloodborne Pathogen Standard to the extent possible.
  o Check for life-threatening problems. Check for breathing, a pulse, and bleeding.
  o Keep the person lying down or as you found him or her.
  o Move the person only if the setting is unsafe.
  o Perform necessary emergency measures.
  o Do not remove clothes unless necessary.
  o Keep the person warm. Cover the person with a blanket, coat, or sweater.
  o Re-assure the person. Explain what is happening and that help was called.
  o Do not give the person food or fluids.
  o Keep on-lookers away. They invade privacy.
- Review Box 58-1(p 847), Emergency Care Rules, in the Textbook for more information.

CPR

- Cardiopulmonary resuscitation (CPR) supports breathing and circulation. It provides blood and oxygen to the heart, brain, and other organs until advanced emergency care is given. See Figure 58-9(p 851), in the Textbook for additional information.
- CPR involves:
  o *Chest compressions*—person must be on a hard, flat surface. Compressions are given at a rate of 100-120/min
  o *Opening the airway and giving breaths*—airway is opened using the head tilt-chin lift method. For an adult, 2 breaths are delivered after 30 compressions.
  o *Defibrillation*—ventricular fibrillation (VF, V-fib) is an abnormal heart rhythm. Rather than beating in a regular rhythm, the heart shakes and quivers. The heart, brain, and other organs do not receive blood and oxygen. A *defibrillator* is used to deliver a shock to the heart and reestablish a regular rhythm. Defibrillation as soon as possible after the onset of VF (V-fib) increases the person's chance of survival.
  o *Child and Infant CPR*—CPR for children and infants is different from adults and varies by age range. Review Table 58-1(p 855), CPR-Differences by Age Group

Respiratory Arrest

- Breathing stops but the heart action continues for several minutes; if breathing is not restored cardiac arrest occurs.
- Open the airway
- Give 1 breath every 5 to 6 seconds for adults.
- Give 1 breath every 3 to 5 seconds for infants and children.

Heart Attack

- Heart attack (myocardial infarction) occurs when part of the heart muscle dies from the sudden blockage of blood flow in a coronary artery. If you suspect a heart attack, activate EMS
- Signs and symptoms include:
  o Chest pain (not relieved by rest)
  o Pain or discomfort in 1 or both arms, the back, neck, jaw, or stomach

o Shortness of breath
o Perspiration and cold, clammy skin
o Feeling light-headed
o Nausea and vomiting

Hemorrhage

- Hemorrhage is the excessive loss of blood in a short time. It can be internal or external. Follow the Emergency Care Rules in Box 58-1(p 847), in the Textbook; this includes activating the Emergency Medical Services (EMS) system;
- Internal bleeding can cause pain, shock, vomiting of blood, coughing up blood, cold and moist skin, and loss of consciousness. Keep the person warm, flat, and quiet until help arrives. Do not give fluids.
- To control external bleeding:
  o Do not remove any objects that have pierced or stabbed the person.
  o Place a sterile dressing directly over the wound. Or use any clean material.
  o Apply firm pressure directly over the bleeding site. Do not release pressure or remove the dressing.

Fainting

- **Fainting** is the sudden loss of consciousness from an inadequate blood supply to the brain.
- Warning signals are dizziness and perspiration, pale skin and weak pulse. Have the person sit or lie down before fainting occurs.

Shock

- **Shock** results when tissues and organs do not get enough blood. Blood loss, poisoning, heart attack (myocardial infarction), burns, and severe infection are causes. Allergic reactions can cause anaphylaxis. Anaphylactic shock is an emergency.

Stroke

- **Stroke** occurs when the brain is suddenly deprived of its blood supply.
- Major signs include:
  o Sudden numbness or weakness of the face, arm, or leg, especially on 1 side of the body
  o Sudden confusion or trouble speaking or understanding speech
  o Sudden trouble seeing in 1 or both eyes
  o Sudden trouble walking, dizziness, or loss of balance or coordination
  o Sudden, severe headache with no known cause
- If stroke is suspected, immediately activate the EMS system. The most effective stroke treatments must be given within 3 hours of symptom onset.

Seizures

- You cannot stop a seizure. However, you can protect the person from injury.
  o Lower the person to the floor.
  o Turn the person onto his or her side. Make sure the head is turned to the side. Do not put any object

or your fingers between the person's teeth. Follow the Emergency Care Rules in Box 58-1(p 847), in the Textbook. Know when to call EMS for seizures. Review Box 58-3(p 859), Seizures -Activating EMS

Concussion

- Head injuries can be minor or serious and life-threatening. Symptoms include difficulty thinking and concentrating, headaches, fuzzy or blurred vision, nausea and vomiting, feelings of tiredness or low energy, irritability and sadness, mood swings, and more or less sleep than usual. Some of the danger signs that signal the need for emergency care include: headache that gets worse or does not go away, weakness, numbness, or decreased coordination, nausea or vomiting more than once, slurred speech, and confusion.

Cold and Heat Related Illness

- **Hypothermia** is an abnormally low body temperature. Prolonged exposure to cold temperatures is the most common cause. Other causes include being cold and wet or being under cold water for too long.
- **Frostbite** is an injury to the body caused by freezing of the skin and underlying tissues. The nose, ears, cheeks, chin, fingers, and toes are the most common sites for frostbite. Damage can be permanent. Severe cases may require amputation
- **Heat related illness** is caused by staying out in the heat too long. Exercising and working outside during hot, humid weather are other causes. Persons at risk for heat related illness include infants, young children, and older persons. Other risk factors include obesity, fever, dehydration, heart disease, mental health disorders, poor circulation, prescription drug use, and alcohol use. Review Table 58-2(p 861), Heat Related Illness in the Textbook.
- **Burns** typically occur in the home. Infants, children, and older persons are at risk.
- First aid measures include:
  o Remove the person from the fire or burn source but do not touch the person if he or she is in contact with an electrical source.
  o Stop the burning process.
  o Apply cold or cool water for 10 to 15 minutes.
  o Remove hot clothing and jewelry that is not sticking to the skin.
  o Cover burns with sterile, dry dressings. Or use a sheet or any other clean cloth.
  o Keep blisters intact. Do not break blisters.
  o Elevate the burned area above heart level if possible.

CHAPTER 58 REVIEW QUESTIONS

Circle the BEST answer.

1. A resident in a long-term care center shows signs and symptoms of sudden cardiac arrest. Who determines when to activate the EMS system?
   a. The doctor on call
   b. The charge nurse

    c. The facility administrator

    d. The staff member who witnessed the symptoms

2. If you find a person lying on the floor, you should

    a. Keep the person lying down

    b. Help the person back to the bed

    c. Elevate the person's head

    d. Obtain a wheelchair

3. When preparing to give chest compressions, locate the hands

    a. On the sternum between the nipples

    b. On the upper half of the sternum

    c. On the left side of the sternum

    d. Slightly below the end of the sternum

4. If a person tells you she feels faint

    a. Hold her up to prevent injury from falling

    b. Let her walk around to increase circulation

    c. Have her sit or lie down before fainting occurs

    d. Fan her and have her drink cool fluids

5. Which observation indicates that rescue breathing is being performed correctly?

    a. The chest muscles expand and contract

    b. Air is heard passing in and out of the mouth

    c. The chest rises with each breath

    d. The abdomen inflates with each breath

Answers to these questions are on p. 538.

CHAPTER 59 END-OF-LIFE CARE

Attitudes About Death

- Attitudes about death often change as a person grows older and with changing circumstances.

Culture and Spiritual Needs

- Practices and attitudes about death differ among cultures.
- Many religions practice rites and rituals during the dying process and at the time of death.

Age

- For children, their understanding and interpretation of death is based on their developmental age.
- Adults fear pain and suffering, dying alone, and the invasion of privacy. They also fear loneliness and separation from loved ones. Adults often resent death because it affects plans, hopes, dreams, and ambitions.
- Older persons usually have fewer fears than younger adults. Some welcome death as freedom from pain, suffering, and disability. Like younger adults, they often fear dying alone.

The Stages of Dying

- Dr. Kübler-Ross described 5 stages of dying. They are:
  - *Stage 1: Denial.* The person refuses to believe he or she is going to die.
  - *Stage 2: Anger.* There is anger and rage, often at family, friends, and the health team.
  - *Stage 3: Bargaining.* Often the person bargains with God or a higher power for more time.
  - *Stage 4: Depression.* The person is sad and mourns things that were lost.
  - *Stage 5: Acceptance.* The person is calm and at peace. The person accepts death.

- Dying persons do not always pass through all 5 stages. A person may never get beyond a certain stage. Some move back and forth between stages.

Comfort Needs

- Comfort is a basic part of end-of-life care. It involves physical, mental and emotional, and spiritual needs. Comfort goals are to:
  - Prevent or relieve suffering to the extent possible.
  - Respect and follow end-of-life wishes.
- Dying persons may want to talk about their fears, worries, and anxieties. You need to listen and use touch.
  - *Listening.* Let the person express feelings and emotions in his or her own way. Do not worry about saying the wrong thing or finding the right words. You do not need to say anything.
  - *Touch.* Touch shows caring and concern. Sometimes the person does not want to talk but needs you nearby. Silence, along with touch, is a meaningful way to communicate.
- Some people may want to see a spiritual leader. Or they may want to take part in religious practices.

Physical Needs

- As the person weakens, basic needs are met. The person may depend on others for basic needs and activities of daily living (ADL). Every effort is made to promote physical and psychological comfort. The person is allowed to die in peace and with dignity.

Pain

- Some dying persons do not have pain. Others may have severe pain. Always report signs and symptoms of pain at once. Pain management is important. The nurse can give pain-relief drugs. Preventing and controlling pain is easier than relieving pain.

Breathing Problems

- Shortness of breath and difficulty breathing (dyspnea) are common end-of-life problems. The semi-Fowler's position and oxygen are helpful.
- Noisy breathing (death rattle) is common as death nears. This is due to mucus collecting in the airway. The side-lying position, suctioning by the nurse, and drugs to reduce the amount of mucus may help.

Vision, Hearing, and Speech

- Vision blurs and gradually fails. Explain what you are doing to the person or in the room. Provide good eye care.
- Hearing is one of the last functions lost. Always assume that the person can hear.
- Speech becomes difficult. Anticipate the person's needs. Do not ask questions that need long answers.

Mouth, Nose, and Skin
- Frequent oral hygiene is given as death nears.
- Crusting and irritation of the nostrils can occur. Carefully clean the nose.
- Skin care, bathing, and preventing pressure injuries are necessary. Change linens and gowns whenever needed.

Nutrition
- Nausea, vomiting, and loss of appetite are common at the end of life. Drugs for nausea and vomiting are given.
- Some persons are too tired or too weak to eat. You may need to feed them.
- As death nears, loss of appetite is common. The person may choose not to eat or drink. Do not force the person to eat or drink. Report refusal to eat or drink to the nurse.

Elimination
- Urinary and fecal incontinence may occur. Give perineal care as needed.

The Person's Room
- The person's room should be comfortable and pleasant. It should be well lit and well ventilated. Remove unnecessary equipment.
- Mementos, pictures, cards, flowers, and religious items provide comfort. The person and family arrange the room as they wish.

The Family
- This is a hard time for family. The family goes through stages like the dying person. Be available, courteous, and considerate.
- The person and family need time together. However, you cannot neglect care because the family is present. Most agencies let family members help give care.

Legal Issues
- *Advance directives*. Advance directives give persons rights to accept or refuse treatment. The advance directive is a document stating a person's wishes about health care when that person cannot make his or her own decisions.
- *Living wills*. A living will is a document about measures that support or maintain life when death is likely. A living will may instruct doctors not to start measures that prolong dying or to remove measures that prolong dying.
- *Durable power of attorney for health care*. This gives the power to make health care decisions to another person. When a person cannot make health care decisions, the person with durable power of attorney can do so.
- *"Do Not Resuscitate" (DNR) order*. This means the person will not be resuscitated. The person is allowed to die with peace and dignity. The orders are written after consulting with the person and family.

- You may not agree with care and resuscitation decisions. However, you must follow the person's or family's wishes and the doctor's orders. These may be against your personal, religious, and cultural values. If so, discuss the matter with the nurse. An assignment change may be needed.

Signs of Death
- There are signs that death is near.
  - Movement, muscle tone, and sensation are lost.
  - Abdominal distention, fecal incontinence, nausea, and vomiting are common.
  - Body temperature changes. The person feels cool, looks pale, and perspires heavily.
  - The pulse is fast or slow, weak, and irregular. Blood pressure starts to fall.
  - Slow or rapid and shallow respirations are observed. Mucus collects in the airway. You may hear the death rattle.
  - Pain decreases as the person loses consciousness. Some people are conscious until the moment of death.
- The signs of death include no pulse, no respirations, and no blood pressure. The pupils are dilated and fixed.

Care of the Body After Death
- Post-mortem care is done to maintain a good appearance of the body.
- Moving the body when giving post-mortem care can cause remaining air in the lungs, stomach, and intestines to be expelled. When air is expelled, sounds are produced.
- When giving post-mortem care, follow Standard Precautions and the Bloodborne Pathogen Standard.

CHAPTER 59 REVIEW QUESTIONS
Circle the BEST answer.
1. A person who is dying is having trouble speaking. Which action will you use?
   a. Smile frequently, but do not talk
   b. Speak slowly and clearly
   c. Ask the family to anticipate needs
   d. Ask a few yes or no questions
2. Persons in the denial stage of dying
   a. Are angry
   b. Bargain with God
   c. Refuse to believe that they are dying
   d. Are calm and at peace
3. When caring for a person who is dying and has advanced Alzheimer disease, what is the focus of care measures?
   a. The person's senses
   b. The person's routine
   c. The person's long-term memories
   d. The person's family

4. While caring for a dying person, you hear the *death rattle*. Which action would you take?
   a. Obtain the bag-valve mask with oxygen
   b. Turn the person to a side-lying position
   c. Take the person's hand: death is near
   d. Elevate the head of the bed
5. You are assisting with post-mortem care, you close the person's mouth, but it won't stay closed. What would you do?
   a. Place the neck in hyperextension
   b. Use a small strip of tape across the lips
   c. Place a rolled towel under the chin
   d. Roll an ace wrap around the chin and head
6. A document that states a person's wishes about health care when that person cannot make his or her own decisions is
   a. A living will
   b. An advance directive
   c. A durable power of attorney for health care
   d. A "Do Not Resuscitate" order

Answers to these questions are on p. 538.

Practice Examination 1

This test contains 79 questions. For each question, circle the BEST answer.

1. A nurse asks you to give a person his drug when he is done in the bathroom. What is the best response?
   A. "I will give the drug for you, but I don't know what to do if something goes wrong, or if he refuses it."
   B. "I will ask the other nursing assistant to give the drug. She has more experience and she knows what to do."
   C. "I am sorry but I cannot give that drug. I will let you know when he is out of the bathroom."
   D. "I refuse to give that drug. It's not part of my job responsibilities and we could both get fired."

2. Which person is demonstrating ethical behavior?
   A. Nurse remarks, "That IV was so hard to start; that patient had tattoos all over her arms."
   B. Nursing assistant says, "I prefer to take of people who have religious and moral values."
   C. Nurse states, "That man is refusing all life-saving treatments; I just can't stand it."
   D. Nursing assistant says, "I saw that nurse hit a patient; I have to report what I saw."

3. You smell alcohol on the breath of a co-worker. You
   A. Ignore the situation
   B. Tell the co-worker to get counseling
   C. Give the co-worker a breath mint
   D. Tell the nurse at once

4. A person's call light goes unanswered. He gets out of bed and falls. His leg is broken. This is
   A. Negligence
   B. Emotional abuse
   C. Physical abuse
   D. Malpractice

5. Your mom asks you about a person on your unit. How should you respond?
   A. "She is walking better now that she is receiving physical therapy."
   B. "It's a violation of privacy and confidentiality to talk about persons."
   C. "Don't tell anyone I told you but she is getting worse."
   D. "She has been very sad recently and needs visitors."

6. You are going off duty. The nursing assistant coming on duty is standing beside you. A call light goes on. Your response is
   A. "I'm ready to go. I will let you answer that light."
   B. "I've been here all day so I am not answering that light."
   C. "Everyone usually answers the lights when they come on duty."
   D. "I will answer the light; you can get organized for the shift."

7. Which nursing assistant has correctly used the computer to record patient information?
   A. Nursing Assistant A saves data and logs off after charting
   B. Nursing Assistant B gives care after lunch, but charts 0800
   C. Nursing Assistant C gets permission to use the nurse's password
   D. Nursing Assistant D does the recording for a co-worker to help out

8. You are answering the phone in the nurses' station. You
   A. Wait to answer the phone, until you can give your full attention to the caller
   B. Give a courteous greeting, identify the unit and give your name and title
   C. Ask the caller to call back, because the nurse is not available
   D. Give confidential information about a resident to a close family friend

9. A person who was admitted to the nursing center yesterday does not feel safe. What is the best action?
   A. Tell him that nothing in the routine care is harmful
   B. Reassure the person that he will soon feel at home
   C. Show the person around the nursing center
   D. Quickly care for the person so the nurse can talk to him

10. A person is angry and is shouting at you. You should
    A. Inform the person that shouting is unacceptable
    B. Stay calm and try to understand the person
    C. Remove the person away from others
    D. Call the family and explain the situation

11. Which nursing assistant is using a good communication technique?
    A. Nursing Assistant A says, "Oral hygiene prevents halitosis."
    B. Nursing Assistant B softly mumbles, "Good morning, sir."
    C. Nursing Assistant C says, "Do you want to bath, eat, rest, or talk?"
    D. Nursing Assistant D clearly says, "Please straighten your arm."

12. Which person has a condition that would prompt you to check with the nurse and the care plan before using a gait belt?
    A. Person has weakness in his right arm
    B. Person has urinary incontinence
    C. Person had recent abdominal surgery
    D. Person had a stroke several years ago

13. When you are listening to a person, you
    A. Say, "I only have a few minutes, what do you need?"
    B. Stand in the doorway and nod your head
    C. Say, "mmm" while you are performing tasks
    D. Face the person and make eye contact

14. Which nursing assistant displays the best interaction with the comatose person?
    A. Nursing Assistant A makes jokes that she thinks the person would like
    B. Nursing Assistant B skillfully cares for the person without talking
    C. Nursing Assistant C assumes that the person can hear and explains actions
    D. Nursing Assistant D talks to another nursing assistant while giving care.

15. You need to give care to an elderly woman when a visitor is present. You
    A. Politely show the visitor where to wait until the care is complete
    B. Do care in the presence of the visitor because she is a woman
    C. Tell the visitor that she needs the nurse's permission to stay
    D. Tell the visitor that you are not allowed to do the care if she stays

16. A person tells you he wants to talk with a minister. You
    A. Ask him to share concerns and listen carefully
    B. Tell him that you will notify the nurse right away
    C. Ask what he needs to discuss with the minister
    D. Tell him the minister only comes on Sunday

17. When you care for a person who has a restraint, you
    A. Observe the person every 15 minutes or as often as directed by the nurse
    B. Release the restraints and reposition the person every 4-6 hours
    C. Check to see if the restrained person is okay at the end of your shift
    D. Apply the restraint and cover the person with a warm blanket

18. You are caring for an elderly person who has night-time urination. Which care measure will you use?
    A. Put an extra diaper on the person.
    B. Wake the person during the night to void
    C. Withhold fluids throughout the day
    D. Give fluids before 1700 hours.

19. A person you are caring for touches your buttocks several times. You
    A. Joke around and then tell him to stop
    B. Ask the person not to touch you again
    C. Tell the nurse that you would like to be reassigned
    D. Ask the person if he thinks touching is appropriate

20. What do you do when you are pushing a person in a wheelchair up a ramp.
    A. Pull the chair backward
    B. Ask the person to help by using his feet
    C. Push the chair forward
    D. Ask the person to push on the wheel rims

21. You cannot read the person's name on the identification (ID) bracelet. You
    A. Tell the nurse so a new bracelet can be made
    B. Ignore the bracelet, because you know the person
    C. Ask another nursing assistant to identify the person
    D. Ask the family to verify the person's identity

22. The universal sign of choking is
    A. Holding the breath
    B. Clutching at the throat
    C. Waving the hands
    D. Coughing up mucus

23. A person is on a diabetic diet. You
    A. Serve meals early, so he or she has plenty of time to eat
    B. Give the person snacks whenever he or she is hungry
    C. Make the person finish any food that is left on the tray
    D. Tell the nurse about changes in the person's eating habits

24. With mild airway obstruction
    A. The person is usually unconscious
    B. The person cannot speak
    C. Finger sweep should be attempted
    D. Forceful coughing should be encouraged

25. To relieve severe airway obstruction in a conscious adult, you do
    A. Abdominal thrusts
    B. Back thrusts
    C. Chest compressions
    D. A finger sweep

26. Faulty electrical equipment
    A. Is used if it is functional
    B. Is reported to the nurse
    C. Is replaced as soon as possible
    D. Is used only with alert persons

27. A warning label has been removed from a hazardous substance container. You
    A. May use the substance if you know what is in the container
    B. Open the container to determine the properties of the substance
    C. Take the container to the nurse and explain the problem
    D. Discard the container and contents immediately in the trash

28. A person's beliefs and values are different from your views. What should you do?
    A. Refuse to care for the person.
    B. Delegate care to another nursing assistant.
    C. Tell the nurse about your concerns.
    D. Tell the person how you feel.

29. You find a person smoking in the nursing center. You should
    A. Ignore the smoking if no one is using oxygen.
    B. Tell the person to leave the nursing center
    C. Call security to report the smoking violation
    D. Remind the person about designated smoking areas

30. During a fire, what is the first thing you would do?
    A. Rescue persons in immediate danger
    B. Sound the nearest fire alarm
    C. Close doors and windows to confine the fire
    D. Extinguish the fire

31. A person with Alzheimer's disease has increased restlessness and confusion as daylight ends. You should
    A. Try to reason with the person
    B. Ask the person to tell you what is bothering him or her
    C. Provide a calm, quiet setting late in the day
    D. Complete the person's treatments and activities late in the day

32. During which nursing task, would you increase vigilance to prevent suffocation?
    A. Helping an elderly person to the toilet
    B. Supervising a person during smoking
    C. Assisting an older person during meal time
    D. Helping a person with morning hygiene

33. When using a wheelchair, you should
    A. Lock both wheels before you transfer a person to and from the wheelchair
    B. Lock one wheel to prevent the person from moving the wheelchair
    C. Let the person move his feet along the floor while you are pushing the chair
    D. Ask the person to step over the footplates before pivoting to sit

34. An obese elderly man has fallen to the floor, but he appears uninjured and wants you to help him get up. What should you do first?
    A. Apply a gait belt and assist him to stand up slowly
    B. Tell him to lie still; the nurse is coming to check him
    C. Inform him that you will get assistance and the manual lift
    D. Have him sit up first to see how he feels; then help him to stand

35. A person is wearing a vest restraint, but someone has put the restraint on backwards. You report your observation to the nurse to prevent which serious complication?
    A. Contracture
    B. Strangulation
    C. Humiliation
    D. Incontinence

36. Before feeding a person, you
    A. Ask the nurse if the person has a healthcare-associated infection
    B. Wash your hands with alcohol-based hand sanitizer
    C. Wash your hands with soap and water
    D. Put on personal protective equipment (PPE)

37. When wearing gloves, you remember to
    A. Wear them until they become visibly soiled or contaminated
    B. Wear the same gloves if you remain in the same room
    C. Use sterile gloves to give care if the person has risk for infection
    D. Change gloves when they become contaminated with urine

38. When washing your hands, you
    A. Use hot water and a disinfectant to create a rich lather
    B. Dry your hands and then use that towel to turn off the faucet
    C. Shake the excessive water from your hands before drying.
    D. Keep your hands and forearms lower than your elbows

39. You need to move a box from the floor to the counter in the utility room. You
    A. Bend from your waist to pick up the box
    B. Hold the box away from your body as you pick it up
    C. Bend your knees and squat to lift the box
    D. Stand with your feet close together as you pick up the box

40. The nurse asks you to place a person in Fowler's position. You
    A. Put the bed flat
    B. Raise the head of the bed between 45 and 60 degrees
    C. Raise the head of the bed between 80 and 90 degrees
    D. Raise the head of the bed 15 degrees

41. You accidentally scratch a person. This is
    A. Neglect
    B. Negligence
    C. Malpractice
    D. Physical abuse

42. You positioned a person in a chair. For good body alignment, you
    A. Have the person's back and buttocks against the back of the chair
    B. Leave the person's feet unsupported for freedom of movement
    C. Have the backs of the person's knees touch the edge of the chair
    D. Have the person sit on the edge of the chair and hold arm rests

43. You need to transfer a person with a weak left leg from the bed to the wheelchair. You
    A. Get the person out of bed on the left side
    B. Get the person out of bed on the right side
    C. Get help and manually lift the person out of bed
    D. Ask the person which side he/she prefers to move first

44. A person tries to scratch and kick you. Which action would you use first?
    A. Protect yourself from harm
    B. Restrain the person
    C. Tell the nurse about the patient
    D. Ignore the behavior and continue care

45. Which circumstance is most likely to cause shearing?
    A. Person is logrolled so that soiled under-pad can be removed.
    B. Person slips down in bed when head of the bed is raised
    C. Person reports feeling dizzy when first sitting up to dangle
    D. Person is sleeping in a supine position with pillow under the head.

46. For comfort, most older persons prefer
    A. Rooms that are cool with circulating ceiling fans
    B. Restrooms that resemble a home bathroom
    C. Cheerful talking and laughing at the nurses' station
    D. Lighting that meets their needs

47. Call lights are
    A. Placed on the person's strong side
    B. Answered in a chronologic order
    C. Stored in a bedside drawer
    D. Placed near the dominant hand

48. A nurse asks you to inspect a person's closet. You
    A. Ask the nurse for permission to handle the person's property
    B. Inspect the closet when the person is in the dining room
    C. Ask the person if you can inspect his or her closet
    D. Tell the nurse that inspecting the closet is not an assistant task.

49. When changing bed linens, you
    A. Take the linen cart from room to room
    B. Shake the linens to remove dust and debris
    C. Take only needed linens into the person's room
    D. Put dirty or used linens on the floor

50. In which circumstance would you attempt to fight the fire by using a fire extinguisher?
    A. There is a fire in the resident's trash can
    B. A grease fire in the kitchen is spreading.
    C. Cigarette ash ignites the blankets and mattress
    D. A resident is trapped behind a wall of flames

51. When doing mouth care for an unconscious person, you
    A. Wipe the mouth and teeth with a damp cloth
    B. Give mouth care at least every 2 hours
    C. Place the person in a supine position
    D. Open the mouth with your fingers

52. A person is angry because he did not get to the activity room on time because one of your co-workers did not come to work. How should you respond to him?
    A. "It's not my fault. A co-worker called off today and we are short-staffed."
    B. "I'm sorry you were late for activities. I will try to plan better."
    C. "I am doing the best I can. We had some unexpected problems today."
    D. "I have been very busy and you know that I usually get you there on time."

53. You are asked to clean a person's dentures. You
    A. Use hot water and scrub away food particles and mucous
    B. Hold the dentures firmly and line the sink with a towel
    C. Wrap the dentures in tissues after cleaning
    D. Store the denture cup with the person's room number on it

54. When bathing a person, you notice a rash that was not there before. You
    A. Apply a thin layer of lotion to soothe the rash
    B. Ask if the water temperature is causing the rash
    C. Tell the nurse and record it in the medical record
    D. Ask the person if the rash itches or is contagious

55. When washing a person's eyes, you
    A. Use irrigating eye drops
    B. Clean the eye near you first
    C. Wipe from the inner to the outer aspect of the eye
    D. Wipe beneath the eye but avoid the upper lid

56. When giving a back massage, you
    A. Use cool lotion to soothe the skin
    B. Use light feathery strokes
    C. Gently massage red bony areas
    D. Look for bruises and breaks in the skin

57. You need to give perineal care to a female. You
    A. Separate the labia and clean downward from front to back
    B. Separate the labia and clean upward from back to front
    C. Wear gloves only if there is drainage or secretions
    D. Use plain tap water and gently rub the tissue with a soft cloth

58. When giving a person a tub bath or shower, you
    A. Stand beside the person until he/she is finished
    B. Turn the hot water on first, then the cold water
    C. Stay within hearing distance if the person can be left alone
    D. Direct the person to adjust the water temperature

59. A person is on an anticoagulant. You
    A. Use a safety razor
    B. Use an electric razor
    C. Use a straight razor
    D. Use a pair of scissors

60. A person with a weak left arm wants to take off a sweater. You
    A. Encourage the person to independently take off the sweater
    B. Help the person remove the sweater from his or her right arm first
    C. Help the person remove the sweater from his or her left arm first
    D. Suggest that the person keep the sweater on

61. Which nursing assistant is demonstrating a communication barrier?
    A. Nursing Assistant A calls all the residents "Sir" or "Mam".
    B. Nursing Assistant B says, "Don't worry, everything will be alright."
    C. Nursing Assistant C is quiet and patient when the person seems tearful.
    D. Nursing Assistant says, "Could you say that again, please?"

62. A person has an indwelling catheter. You
    A. Instruct the person on how to position the tubing
    B. Disconnect the catheter from the drainage tubing every 8 hours
    C. Secure the catheter to the lower leg
    D. Measure and record the amount of urine in the drainage bag

63. A person needs to eat a diet that contains carbohydrates. Carbohydrates
    A. Are needed for tissue repair and growth
    B. Provide energy and fiber for bowel elimination
    C. Add flavor to food and help the body use certain vitamins
    D. Are needed for nerve and muscle function

64. You are taking a rectal temperature with an electronic thermometer. You
    A. Insert the thermometer, provide privacy and return in 2 minutes
    B. Place the person in a prone position
    C. Insert the thermometer 1 inch into the rectum
    D. Insert the thermometer ½ inch into the rectum

65. A patient has a blood pressure (BP) of 86/58 mm Hg. You
    A. Report the BP to the nurse at once
    B. Record the BP and tell the nurse at the end of the shift
    C. Report the BP along with vital signs from other patients
    D. Retake the BP in 30 minutes and then tell the nurse

66. For which person would you take an oral temperature?
    A. An unconscious person
    B. A person receiving oxygen
    C. A child who breathes through the mouth
    D. A cooperative adult

67. When caring for a person who is blind or visually impaired, you
    A. Offer your arm and the person walks a half step behind you
    B. Do as much for the person as possible
    C. Talk very loudly to get his or her attention
    D. Touch the person before indicating your presence

68. You are caring for a person with dementia. You
    A. Select the person's clothes for the day
    B. Choose the activities the person attends
    C. Send personal items home or lock them up for safety
    D. Let the family make choices if the person cannot

69. For a person who needs amputee rehabilitation, which information would you need to get from the nurse and the care plan?
    A. Type of dietary restrictions
    B. Type of communication device
    C. Type of prosthetic device
    D. Type of incontinence training

70. While bathing a person, you
    A. Keep the windows open for good ventilation
    B. Wash the dirtiest areas first; then change gloves
    C. Encourage the person to help as much as possible
    D. Rub the skin dry with several dry paper towels

71. When a person is dying
    A. Assume that the person can hear you
    B. Assume that the person cannot swallow
    C. Assume that the person can see you
    D. Assume that repositioning causes discomfort

72. A person is on intake and output. You
    A. Measure only liquids such as water and juice
    B. Measure ice cream and gelatin as part of intake
    C. Measure intravenous (IV) fluids
    D. Measure tube feedings

73. A person has been on bed rest. You need to have the person walk. What will you do first?
    A. Help the person to get up and encourage walking.
    B. Have the person dangle before getting out of bed.
    C. Have the person sit in a chair for at least 10 minutes.
    D. Help the person to do range-of-motion exercises

74. Which aspect of your personal grooming and attire can help to prevent skin tears when working with elderly patients?
    A. Wearing soft clothing and long sleeves
    B. Keeping fingernails short and smooth
    C. Wearing arm and leg protectors
    D. Keeping skin well moisturized

75. Which circumstance is an example of maintaining a person's privacy?
    A. You give care information to staff who are directly involved in the care of the patient
    B. You discuss the person's treatment with another nursing assistant in the lunch room
    C. You open the person's mail because you know she won't remember to open it herself.
    D. You keep the door open while assisting a resident with toileting because of the odors

76. You have assisted a person to get on the bedpan and provided privacy. When should you check on the person?
    A. Every 5 minutes
    B. Every 10 minutes
    C. After 30 minutes
    D. Wait until you are called

77. If a person is on bed rest, he or she
    A. May be allowed to perform some activities of daily living (ADL)
    B. Can use the bedside commode for elimination needs
    C. Will remain in bed and needs help with all ADLs
    D. Can use the bathroom for elimination needs

78. When admitting a person, identify him or her by
    A. Asking the person his or her name
    B. Checking the admission form and the ID bracelet
    C. Calling the admitting office to identify the person
    D. Asking the nurse to identify the person

79. Which body system brings O_2 into the lungs and removes CO_2?
    A. Renal system
    B. Circulatory system
    C. Nervous system
    D. Respiratory system

This test contains 77 questions. For each question, circle the BEST answer.

1. You can refuse to do a delegated task when
   A. You are too busy with other tasks
   B. You are not familiar with the task
   C. The task is not in your job description
   D. It is the end of the shift and need to leave

2. Mr. Smith does not want life-saving measures. You
   A. Explain to Mr. Smith why he should have life-saving measures
   B. Respect his decision and support his right to self-determination
   C. Ask the family to speak with him and change his mind
   D. Tell the spiritual advisor about Mr. Smith's decision

3. You are walking by a resident's room. You hear a nurse shouting at a person. This is
   A. Battery
   B. Malpractice
   C. Verbal abuse
   D. Neglect

4. When caring for a patient who speaks a different language, you should
   A. Speak loudly and clearly to the patient
   B. Change patient assignments
   C. Use words the patient seems to understand
   D. Speak quickly and pantomime actions

5. During a home visit, you observe that the elderly person is living with a daughter who is a hoarder. What would you do?
   A. Help the daughter clear pathways to exit the house
   B. Check the environment for unsafe sources of heat
   C. Report situation to the nurse and follow nurse's instructions
   D. Suggest that the daughter take the elderly person to a safer place

6. To prevent equipment accidents, you should
   A. Use 2-pronged plugs on all electrical devices
   B. Follow the manufacturer's instructions
   C. Place a barrier around spills and wipe up later
   D. Use old equipment if new equipment is unfamiliar

7. Which action is part of the safety check that you would perform after visitors leave?
   A. Make sure that the call light is within reach
   B. Straighten the bed linens and empty the trash cans
   C. Show interest in how the visit went
   D. Check to see if visitors had any problems

8. You need to wash your hands
   A. After you document a procedure
   B. After you remove gloves
   C. After you talk with a person
   D. After you eat your lunch

9. You need to move a person weighing 250 pounds in bed. You
   A. Do the procedure alone and ask the person to help
   B. Keep the door open in case you need to call for help
   C. Roll the person back and forth while shifting weight
   D. Ask for assistance from at least 2 other staff members

10. When transferring a person from a bed to a wheelchair, which action would you use?
    A. Lock the wheels on the bed and wheelchair before transfer
    B. Pull on the front of the transfer belt as the person stands up
    C. Have the person put his or her arms around your neck
    D. Have the person sit and dangle while you go get the wheelchair

11. When making a bed, you
    A. Keep the bed in the low position
    B. Wear gloves when removing linens
    C. Raise the head of the bed
    D. Raise the foot of the bed

12. To give perineal care to a male, you
    A. Use a circular motion and work toward the meatus
    B. Use a circular motion and start at the meatus and work outward
    C. Clean the shaft first using long firm upward strokes
    D. Clean the scrotum first using a circular motion

13. A person with a weak left arm wants to put on his or her sweater. You
    A. Put the sweater on the right arm; then pull and stretch the left sleeve
    B. Help the person put the sweater on his or her right arm first
    C. Help the person put the sweater on his or her left arm first
    D. Grasp the sweater at the shoulders and pull downwards

14. A person has an indwelling catheter. You
    A. Place the drainage bag on the floor
    B. Hang the drainage bag on the bedside stand
    C. Hang the drainage bag on a bed rail
    D. Hang the drainage bag from the bed frame

15. A person needs to eat a diet that contains protein. Protein
    A. Is needed for tissue repair and growth
    B. Provides energy and fiber
    C. Adds flavor to food
    D. Is needed for nerve conduction

16. Older persons
    A. Have an increased sense of thirst
    B. Need less water than younger persons
    C. May not feel thirsty
    D. Usually ask for water if they need it

17. A person is NPO. You
    A. Post a sign in the bathroom
    B. Keep the water pitcher filled at the bedside
    C. Remove the water pitcher and glass from the room
    D. Provide oral hygiene once a day

18. A person drank 3 oz of milk at lunch. He or she drank
    A. 30 mL
    B. 60 mL
    C. 90 mL
    D. 120 mL

19. When feeding a person, you
    A. Offer fluids at the end of the meal
    B. Use a fork and a knife
    C. Sit silently while the person talks
    D. Allow time to chew and swallow

20. In planning care, which person is likely to require the most assistance with range of motion (ROM) exercises?
    A. Person is in a coma and needs passive ROM
    B. Person is self-care, but needs reminders to do active ROM
    C. Person has some weakness in the arm and needs active-assistive ROM
    D. Person needs active ROM for legs and active-assistive ROM for left arm

21. A person has a weak left leg. The person should
    A. Hold the cane in his or her left hand
    B. Hold the cane in his or her right hand
    C. Use two canes; one in each hand
    D. Use a walker

22. To promote comfort and relieve pain, you
    A. Help the person get out of bed, so you can change the linens
    B. Place pillows to support the body in good alignment
    C. Talk, make jokes and distract the person from the pain
    D. Wait 10 minutes after pain medication is given before giving care

23. A person is receiving oxygen through a nasal cannula. You
    A. Turn the oxygen higher when he or she is short of breath
    B. Fill the humidifier when it is not bubbling
    C. Check behind the ears and under the nose for signs of irritation
    D. Remove the cannula when the person goes to the dining room

24. A glass thermometer accidentally breaks. What would you do?
    A. Tell the nurse at once
    B. Get a broom and sweep it up
    C. Put the glass in the sharps container
    D. Call the infection control nurse

25. When taking a person's pulse, you
    A. Locate the brachial pulse
    B. Take the pulse for 30 seconds if it is irregular
    C. Tell the nurse if the pulse is less than 60
    D. Place your thumb on the pulse

26. You are counting respirations on a person. You
    A. Make friendly conversation with the person to show interest
    B. Count for 1 minute if an abnormal breathing pattern is noted
    C. Report a rate of 16 to the nurse at once
    D. Check breaths with a stethoscope if an abnormal pattern is noted,

27. You are taking blood pressures on people assigned to you. An older person has a blood pressure (BP) of 158/96 mm Hg. You
    A. Report the BP to the nurse at once
    B. Finish taking everyone's blood pressures
    C. Tell the person to relax and recheck the BP in 20 minutes
    D. Look at the record to see if the BP is normal for that person

28. When would you take a rectal temperature?
    A. The person has diarrhea.
    B. The person is confused.
    C. The person is unconscious.
    D. The person is agitated.

29. A person has been admitted to the nursing center recently. You
    A. Check belongings for dangerous items
    B. Defer all questions to the nurse
    C. Speak in a gentle, calm voice
    D. Leave the person alone, for privacy

30. When taking a person's height and weight, you
    A. Have the person completely undress
    B. Have the person void before being weighed
    C. Weigh the person after a bath or shower
    D. Balance the scale after every usage

31. A person is bedfast. To prevent pressure injuries, you
    A. Re-position the person at least every 3 hours
    B. Gently massage reddened areas and bony prominences
    C. Perform range-of-motion on the lower extremities every 2 hours
    D. Keep the skin free of moisture from urine, stools, or perspiration

32. A person has a hearing problem you
    A. Invite the person to large social gatherings
    B. Chat about your personal interests
    C. Face the person when speaking
    D. Speak very loudly and give details

33. When caring for a person who is blind or visually impaired, you
    A. Position equipment for the staff's convenience
    B. Keep the lights off; the person can't see
    C. Explain the location of food and beverages
    D. Re-arrange furniture to minimize clutter

34. You are caring for a person with dementia. You
    A. Read the person's mail for him
    B. Tell the family about the person's condition
    C. Protect the person's confidential information
    D. Expose the person's body to expedite care

35. When caring for a confused person, you
    A. Use terms of endearment to increase trust
    B. Explain your actions only if the person shows interest
    C. Give simple, clear directions and answers to questions
    D. Remove clocks and calendars to decrease distractions

36. A person with Alzheimer's disorder likes to wander. You
    A. Keep the person in his or her room
    B. Restrain the person in a chair
    C. Follow the person around the facility
    D. Allow wandering in a safe space

37. The goal of restorative nursing programs is to
    A. Return the person to independent life at home
    B. Promote independence in performing self-care measures
    C. Assist the physician to repair the person's disability
    D. Help the person admit to limitations and restrictions

38. When caring for a person with a disability, you
    A. Sympathize with limitations and show kindness by taking over care
    B. Tell the person that progress is faster, if he or she cooperates
    C. Remind about progress made in the rehabilitation program
    D. Support denial of the disability if it helps the person to cope

39. After a person dies, which action violates the person's rights?
    A. Draping and screening the body during post-mortem care
    B. Collecting, bagging and labeling personal possessions
    C. Discussing the family's reactions with other staff members
    D. Allowing the family to view the body in a private area

40. You enter a person's room and find a fire in the wastebasket. Your first action is to
    A. Remove the person from the room
    B. Close the door
    C. Call for help
    D. Activate the fire alarm

41. A person is left lying in urine and a pressure injury develops. This is
    A. Fraud
    B. Neglect
    C. Assault
    D. Battery

42. A nurse asks you to assess a small foot wound, clean it, and then place a topical medication and a sterile dressing on the wound. You
    A. Agree to do the task if the nurse will show you how to do it.
    B. Ask another nursing assistant to help you with the task
    C. Politely tell the nurse you can't do all the steps to complete the task
    D. Do the task, but afterwards, report the nurse to the director of nursing

43. You observe a person's urine is foul-smelling and dark amber. Your first action is to
    A. Measure the urine
    B. Ask the person about fluid intake
    C. Tell the nurse
    D. Record the observation

44. A daughter asks you to get some water for her mom. Your response is
    A. "I am not caring for your mom. I will get her nursing assistant for you."
    B. "I do not have time right now, but if you can wait 30 minutes, I'll get it."
    C. "She might be on a special diet or fluid restrictions that I don't know about."
    D. "I will be happy to do that; first let me make sure she is not on fluid restrictions."

45. Which restraint alternative would be a good choice for a person with dementia who has wandering behavior?
    A. Take vital signs and give reassurance every 15 minutes
    B. Lock the person in his bedroom and turn on the television
    C. Alert staff and others about person's wandering behavior
    D. Tell the person to use the call bell whenever he begins to wander

46. The nurse asks you to place a person in the supine position. You
    A. Elevate the head of the bed 45 degrees
    B. Elevate the foot of the bed 15 degrees
    C. Place the person on his or her back with the bed flat
    D. Place the person on his or her abdomen

47. The most important way to prevent or avoid spreading infection is to
    A. Wash your hands
    B. Cover your nose when coughing
    C. Use disposable gloves
    D. Wear a mask

48. You are eating lunch and a nursing assistant begins to gossip about another person. You
    A. Join the conversation and talk about the person
    B. Remove yourself from the group
    C. Try to say something nice about the person
    D. Change the subject or talk about someone else

49. When moving a person up in bed, you should
    A. Raise the head of the bed
    B. Ask the person to remain still
    C. Apply a transfer belt
    D. Ask a co-worker to help you

50. A person is on a sodium-controlled diet. This means
    A. Canned vegetables are omitted from the diet
    B. Salt may be added to food at the table
    C. Salt is less harmful when it is cooked with foods
    D. Small servings of ham, sausage, or bacon are served

51. Elastic stockings
    A. Are applied after breakfast and hygiene
    B. Should be wrinkle free
    C. Help to prevent pneumonia
    D. Are applied at bedtime

52. While walking, the person begins to fall. You
    A. Call for help and ask for a wheelchair
    B. Grab the gait belt; hold him up to prevent a fall
    C. Bring him close to your body; ease him to the floor
    D. Quickly move items that could cause injury

53. Before assisting a person to bathe, you should
    A. Help him/her to go to the toilet
    B. Partially undress the person
    C. Raise the head of the bed
    D. Instruct him/her to brush the teeth

54. When taking a rectal temperature with an electronic thermometer, you insert the thermometer
    A. ½ inch
    B. 1½ inches
    C. 2 inches
    D. 2½ inches

55. Touch
    A. Is a form of nonverbal communication
    B. Is a form of verbal communication
    C. Is a form of physical aggression
    D. Is a form of care that is used only for children

56. You may share information about a person's care and condition with
    A. Staff caring for the person
    B. Person's only daughter
    C. Person's closest friends
    D. Other nursing assistants

57. A person tells you he or she has pain upon urination. You
    A. Tell the nurse
    B. Ask the person to describe the pain
    C. Ask the person how often it happens
    D. Tell the doctor

58. A person's culture and religion are different from yours. You
    A. Ignore the person's customs if they are unsafe or illogical
    B. Ask the family if the customs can be waived to accommodate care
    C. Ask the person to explain beliefs, customs and practices to you
    D. Explain how beliefs and customs can interfere with good health practices

59. You need to wear gloves when you
    A. Do range-of-motion exercises
    B. Feed a person
    C. Give perineal care
    D. Walk a person

60. An older person is normally alert. Today he is confused. What should you do?
    A. Try to stimulate the person with activities
    B. Ignore the confusion; this condition is common
    C. Check to see if the person is confused later in the day.
    D. Report specific behavioral changes to the nurse

61. While helping a person to ambulate, he tells you he feels faint. What do you do first?
    A. Have the person sit down.
    B. Call for the nurse.
    C. Obtain a wheelchair.
    D. Ask the person to take a deep breath.

62. You are asked to encourage fluids for a person. You
    A. Increase the person's fluid intake
    B. Measure the person's fluid intake
    C. Withhold food and have the person drink fluids first
    D. Offer the person coffee, soda, beer, or whatever he/she wants

63. Which nursing assistant is failing to effectively communicate?
    A. Nursing Assistant A uses words the other person understands.
    B. Nursing Assistant B always talks about herself and her own issues.
    C. Nursing Assistant C lets others express their feelings and concerns.
    D. Nursing Assistant D listens while a person talks about an uncomfortable topic.

64. During bathing, a person may
    A. Decide what products to use
    B. Share the shower room with others
    C. Have students assisting without his or her permission
    D. Have to bathe when scheduled to do so

65. Which child needs to be brought to the attention of the supervising nurse, because he may not be meeting the milestones for his age group?
    A. 4- month old rolls from front to back and reaches for toys
    B. 9-month old is afraid of strangers and clings to familiar adults
    C. 18-month old stands up alone, but is not taking steps
    D. 3-year old plays with toys, levers and moving parts

66. Which nursing assistant needs a reminder about measuring blood pressure?
    A. Nursing Assistant A applies the cuff to a bare upper arm
    B. Nursing Assistant B encourages 20 minutes of rest before the procedure
    C. Nursing Assistant C locates the brachial artery
    D. Nursing Assistant D uses the arm with an IV infusion

67. You find clean linens on the floor in a person's room. You
    A. Use the linens to make the bed
    B. Return the linens to the linen cart
    C. Put the linens in the laundry
    D. Tell the nurse

68. When doing mouth care on an unconscious person, you
    A. Use a large amount of fluid to rinse secretions
    B. Position the person on his or her side
    C. Entertain the person by talking about current events
    D. Insert his or her dentures when done

69. When brushing or combing a person's hair, you
    A. Cut matted or tangled hair
    B. Encourage the person to do as much as possible
    C. Style the hair as you want
    D. Perform the task weekly

70. When providing nail and foot care, you
    A. Cut fingernails with scissors
    B. Trim toenails for all assigned persons
    C. Carefully clip ingrown toenails
    D. Check between the toes for cracks and sores

71. An indwelling catheter becomes disconnected from the drainage system. You
    A. Quickly reconnect the tubing to the catheter
    B. Tell the nurse at once
    C. Get a new drainage system
    D. Flush the catheter with antiseptic solution

72. Urinary drainage bags are
    A. Discarded at the end of each shift
    B. Emptied and measured at the end of each shift
    C. Cleaned and rinsed out at the end of each shift
    D. Washed and stored away at the end of each shift

73. A person needs a condom catheter applied. You remember to
    A. Use a soft rubber band to secure the catheter
    B. Use adhesive tape to secure the catheter
    C. Use elastic tape to secure the catheter
    D. Use catheter adhesive cream to secure the catheter

74. To increase comfort and to facilitate the urge to have a bowel movement, what would you do?
    A. Have the person use the commode for privacy
    B. Talk to and distract the visitors while the person is on the toilet
    C. Keep the door slightly ajar and partially draw the privacy curtain
    D. Leave the person alone if possible

75. You are transferring a person with a weak left side from the wheelchair to the bed. You
    A. Place the wheelchair on the left side of the bed, with person facing the foot of the bed
    B. Place the wheelchair on the right side of the bed with person facing the foot of the bed
    C. Place the wheelchair at the bottom of the bed with person facing the head of the bed
    D. Place the wheelchair at the top of the bed with person facing the foot of the bed

76. You are asked to position an elderly person for a rectal examination. Which position would you help the person to assume?
    A. Knee-chest position
    B. Lithotomy position
    C. Sim's position
    D. Horizontal recumbent position

77. The leading cause of death in the United States is
    A. Cardiovascular and respiratory system disorders
    B. Cancer and immune disorders
    C. Strokes and nervous system disorders
    D. Accidents and musculo-skeletal disorders

Skills Evaluation Review

Each state has its own policies and procedures for the skills test. The following information is an overview of what to expect.

- To pass the skills evaluation, you typically will need to perform 5 of all the skills available.
- To pass the skills evaluation, you must perform skills correctly. Some states require all 5 to be performed correctly; others require 4 of 5.
- Be prepared to perform at least one measurement skill, such as blood pressure, radial pulse, respirations, urine output or weight; performance includes recording and documentation.
- A nurse aide evaluator evaluates your performance of certain skills. Having someone watch as you work is not a new experience. Your instructor evaluated your performance during your training program. While you are working, your supervisor evaluates your skills.
- Mannequins and people are used as "patients" or "residents," depending on the skills you are performing. Speak to the person as you would a patient or resident.
- If you make a mistake, tell the evaluator what you did wrong. Then perform the skill correctly. Do not panic.
- Take whatever equipment you normally take to or use at work. Wear a watch with a second hand. You may need it to measure vital signs and check how much time you have left.

Before and During the Procedure

- Hand-washing is evaluated at the beginning of the skills test. You are expected to know when to wash your hands. Therefore you may not be told to do so. Follow the rules for hand hygiene during the test.
- Before entering a person's room, knock on the door. Greet the person by name and introduce yourself before beginning a procedure. Check the identification (ID) or the photo ID to make certain you are giving care to the right person.
- Explain what you are going to do before beginning the procedure and as needed throughout the procedure.
- Always follow the rules of medical asepsis. For example, remove gloves and dispose of them properly. Keep clean linens separated from used linens.
- Always protect the person's rights throughout the skills test.
- Communicate with the person as you give care. Focus on the person's needs and interests. Always treat the person with respect. Do not talk about yourself or your personal problems.
- Provide privacy. This involves pulling the privacy curtain around the bed, closing doors, and asking visitors to leave the room.

- Promote safety for the person. For example, lock the wheelchair when you transfer a person to and from it. Place the bed in the lowest horizontal position when the person must get out of bed or when you are done giving care.
- Make sure the call light is within the person's reach. Attaching it to the bed or bed rail does not mean the person can reach it.
- Use good body mechanics. Raise the bed and over-bed table to a good working height.
- Provide for comfort.
  - Make sure the person and linens are clean and dry. The person may have become incontinent during the procedure.
  - Change or straighten bed linens as needed.
  - Position the person for comfort and in good alignment.
  - Provide pillows as directed by the nurse and the care plan.
  - Raise the head of the bed as the person prefers and allowed by the nurse and the care plan.
  - Provide for warmth. The person may need an extra blanket, a lap blanket, a sweater, socks, and so on.
  - Adjust lighting to meet the person's needs.
  - Make sure eyeglasses, hearing aids, and other devices are in place as needed.
  - Ask the person if he or she is comfortable.
  - Ask the person if there is anything else you can do for him or her.
  - Make sure the person is covered for warmth and privacy.

Skills

Ask your instructor to tell you which of the following skills are tested in your state. Place a checkmark in the box in front of each tested skill so it will be easy for you to reference. The skills marked with an asterisk (*) are used with permission of National Council of State Boards of Nursing (NCSBN). These skills are offered as a study guide to you. The word "client" refers to the resident or person receiving care. You are responsible for following the most current standards, practices, and guidelines in your state.

The steps in boldface type are critical element steps. Critical element steps must be done correctly to pass the skill. If you miss a critical element step, you will not pass the skills evaluation. For example, you are to transfer a client from the bed to a wheelchair. You will fail if you do not lock the wheels on the wheelchair before transferring the person. An automatic failure is one that could potentially cause harm to a person. Your state may mark critical element steps in another way—underline or italics. If your state has one, review the candidate's handbook.

❏*Hand Hygiene (Hand-Washing) (Chapter 16)

1. Addresses client by name and introduces self to client by name
2. Turns on water at sink
3. Wets hands and wrists thoroughly
4. Applies soap to hands
5. **Lathers all surfaces of wrists, hands, and fingers, producing friction for at least 20 (twenty) seconds keeping hands lower than the elbows and the fingertips down**
6. Cleans fingernails by rubbing fingertips against palms of the opposite hand
7. **Rinses all surfaces of wrists, hands, and fingers, keeping hands lower than the elbows and the fingertips down**
8. Uses clean, dry paper towel/towels to dry all surfaces of fingers, hands, wrists, starting at the fingertips and then disposes of paper towel/towels into waste container
9. Uses clean, dry paper towel/towels to turn off faucet then disposes of paper towel/towels into waste container or uses knee/foot control to turn off faucet
10. Does not touch inside of sink at any time

❏*Applies One Knee-High Elastic Stocking (Chapter 39)

1. Explains procedure, speaking clearly, slowly, and directly, maintaining face-to-face contact whenever possible
2. Privacy is provided with a curtain, screen, or door
3. Client is in supine position (lying down in bed) while stocking is applied
4. Turns stocking inside-out, at least to heel
5. Places foot of stocking over toes, foot, and heel
6. Pulls top of stocking over foot, heel, and leg
7. Moves foot and leg gently and naturally, avoiding force and over-extension of limb and joints
8. **Finishes procedure with no twists or wrinkles and heel of stocking, if present, is over heel and opening in toe area (if present) is either under or over toe area; if using mannequin, candidate may state stocking needs to be wrinkle-free**
9. Signaling device is within reach and bed is in low position
10. After completing skill, washes hands

❏*Assists to Ambulate Using a Transfer Belt (Chapters 14 and 34)

1. Explains procedure, speaking clearly, slowly, and directly, maintaining face-to-face contact whenever possible
2. Privacy is provided with a curtain, screen, or door
3. **Before assisting to stand, client is wearing non-skid shoes/footwear**
4. Before assisting to stand, bed is at a safe level
5. Before assisting to stand, checks and/or locks bed wheels
6. **Before assisting to stand, client is assisted to sitting position with feet flat on the floor**
7. Before assisting to stand, applies transfer belt securely at the waist over clothing/gown
8. Before assisting to stand, provides instructions to enable client to assist in standing including prearranged signal to alert client to begin standing
9. Stands facing client positioning self to ensure safety of candidate and client during transfer. Counts to three (or says other prearranged signal) to alert client to begin standing
10. On signal, gradually assists client to stand by grasping transfer belt on both sides with an upward grasp (candidate's hands are in upward position), and maintaining stability of client's legs by standing knee to knee, or toe to toe with client
11. Walks slightly behind and to one side of client for a distance of ten (10) feet, while holding onto the belt
12. Assists client to bed and removes transfer belt
13. Signaling device is within reach and bed is in low position
14. After completing skill, washes hands

❏*Assists With Use of Bedpan (Chapter 27)

1. Explains procedure speaking clearly, slowly, and directly, maintaining face-to-face contact whenever possible
2. Privacy is provided with a curtain, screen, or door
3. Before placing bedpan, lowers head of bed
4. Puts on clean gloves before placing bedpan under client
5. Places bedpan correctly under client's buttocks
6. Removes and disposes of gloves (without contaminating self) into waste container and washes hands
7. After positioning client on bedpan and removing gloves, raises head of bed
8. Toilet tissue is within reach
9. Hand wipe is within reach and client is instructed to clean hands with hand wipe when finished
10. Signaling device within reach and client is asked to signal when finished
11. Puts on clean gloves before removing bedpan
12. Head of bed is lowered before bedpan is removed
13. Ensures client is covered except when placing and removing bedpan

*Reproduced and used with permission from the *Nurse Assistant Candidate Handbook* from National Council of State Boards of Nursing (NCSBN), Chicago, Ill, © 2019.

14. Empties and rinses bedpan and pours rinse into toilet

15. Places bedpan in designated dirty supply area

16. Removes and disposes of gloves (without contaminating self) into waste container and washes hands

17. Signaling device is within reach and bed is in low position

❏*Cleans Upper or Lower Denture (Chapter 23)

1. Puts on clean gloves before handling dentures

2. Bottom of sink is lined and/or sink is partially filled with water before denture is held over sink

3. Rinses denture in moderate temperature running water before brushing them

4. Applies denture toothpaste to toothbrush

5. Brushes all surfaces of denture

6. Rinses all surfaces of denture under moderate temperature running water

7. Rinses denture cup and lid

8. Places denture in denture cup with moderate temperature water solution and places lid on cup

9. Rinses toothbrush and places in designated toothbrush basin/container

10. Maintains clean technique with placement of toothbrush and denture

11. Sink liner is removed and disposed of appropriately and/or sink is drained

12. Removes and disposes of gloves (without contaminating self) into waste container and washes hands

❏*Counts and Records Radial Pulse (Chapter 33)**

1. Explains procedure, speaking clearly, slowly, and directly, maintaining face-to-face contact whenever possible

2. Places fingertips on thumb side of client's wrist to locate radial pulse

3. Counts beats for one full minute

4. Signaling device is within reach

5. Before recording, washes hands

6. **Records pulse rate within plus or minus 4 beats of evaluator's reading**

❏*Counts and Records Respirations (Chapter 33)†

1. Explains procedure (for testing purposes), speaking clearly, slowly, and directly, maintaining face-to-face contact whenever possible

2. Counts respirations for one full minute

3. Signaling device is within reach

4. Washes hands

5. **Records respiration rate within plus or minus 2 breaths of evaluator's reading**

❏*Dresses Client With Affected (Weak) Right Arm (Chapter 26)

1. Explains procedure, speaking clearly, slowly, and directly, maintaining face-to-face contact whenever possible

2. Privacy is provided with a curtain, screen, or door

3. Asks which shirt he/she would like to wear and dresses him/her in shirt of choice

4. Avoids overexposure of client by ensuring client's chest is covered.

5. Removes gown from the left (unaffected) side first, then removes gown from the right (affected/weak) side

6. Before dressing client, disposes of gown into soiled linen container

7. **Assists to put the right (affected/weak) arm through the right sleeve of the shirt before placing garment on left (unaffected) arm**

8. While putting on shirt, moves body gently and naturally, avoiding force and over-extension of limbs and joints

9. Finishes with clothing in place

10. Signaling device is within reach and bed is in low position

11. After completing skill, washes hands

❏*Feeds Client Who Cannot Feed Self (Chapter 30)

1. Explains procedure to client, speaking clearly, slowly, and directly, maintaining face-to-face contact whenever possible

2. Before feeding, candidate looks at name card on tray and asks client to state name

3. **Before feeding client, client is in an upright sitting position (75–90 degrees)**

4. Places tray where the food can be easily seen by client

5. Candidate cleans client's hands before beginning feeding

6. Candidate sits facing client during feeding

7. Tells client what foods and beverages are on tray

8. Asks client what he/she would like to eat first

**Count for 1 full minute.
†Count for 1 full minute. For testing purposes you may explain to the client that you will be counting the respirations.

9. Using spoon, offers client one bite of each type of food on tray, telling client the content of each spoonful

10. Offers beverage at least once during meal

11. Candidate asks client if they are ready for next bite of food or sip of beverage

12. At end of meal, candidate cleans client's mouth and hands

13. Removes food tray

14. Leaves client in upright sitting position (75-90 degrees) with signaling device within client's reach

15. After completing skill, washes hands

❏*Gives Modified Bed Bath (Face and One Arm, Hand, and Underarm) (Chapter 24)

1. Explains procedure, speaking clearly, slowly, and directly, maintaining face-to-face contact whenever possible

2. Privacy is provided with a curtain, screen, or door

3. Removes gown and places directly in soiled linen container while ensuring client's chest and lower body are covered

4. Before washing, checks water temperature for safety and comfort and asks client to verify comfort of water

5. Puts on clean gloves before washing client

6. **Beginning with eyes, washes eyes with wet washcloth (no soap), using a different area of the washcloth for each stroke, washing inner aspect to outer aspect, then proceeds to wash face**

7. Dries face with dry cloth towel/washcloth

8. Exposes one arm and places cloth towel underneath arm

9. Applies soap to wet washcloth

10. Washes fingers (including fingernails), hand, arm, and underarm keeping rest of body covered

11. Rinses and dries fingers, hand, arm, and underarm

12. Moves body gently and naturally, avoiding force and over-extension of limbs and joints

13. Puts clean gown on client

14. Empties, rinses, and dries basin

15. Places basin in designated dirty supply area

16. Disposes of linen into soiled linen container

17. Avoids contact between candidate clothing and used linens

18. Removes and disposes of gloves (without contaminating self) into waste container and washes hands

19. Signaling device is within reach and bed is in low position

Makes an Occupied Bed (Client Does Not Need Assistance to Turn) (Chapter 22)

1. Explains procedure, speaking clearly, slowly, and directly, maintaining face-to-face contact whenever possible

2. Privacy is provided with a curtain, screen, or door

3. Lowers head of bed before moving client

4. Client is covered while linens are changed

5. Loosens top linen from the end of the bed

6. Raises side rail on side to which client will move and client moves toward raised side rail

7. Loosens bottom used linen on working side and fanfolds bottom used linen toward center of bed

8. Fanfolds and places clean bottom linen or fitted bottom sheet on working side and tucks linen folds under client

9. Before going to other side, client rolls back onto clean bottom linen

10. Raises side rail then goes to other side of bed

11. Removes used bottom linen

12. Pulls and tucks in clean bottom linen, finishing with bottom sheet free of wrinkles

13. Client is covered with clean top sheet and bath blanket/used top sheet has been removed

14. Changes pillowcase

15. Linen is centered and tucked at foot of bed

16. Avoids contact between candidate's clothing and used linens

17. Disposes of used linens into soiled linen container and avoids putting linens on floor

18. Signaling device is within reach and bed is in low position

19. Washes hands

❏*Measures and Records Blood Pressure (Chapter 33)

1. Explains procedure, speaking clearly, slowly, and directly, maintaining face-to-face contact whenever possible

2. Before using stethoscope, wipes bell/diaphragm and earpieces of stethoscope with alcohol

3. Client's arm is positioned with palm up and upper arm is exposed

4. Feels for brachial artery on inner aspect of arm, at bend of elbow

5. Places blood pressure cuff snugly on client's upper arm with sensor/arrow over brachial artery site

6. Earpieces of stethoscope are in ears and bell/ diaphragm is over brachial artery site

---

*Reproduced and used with permission from the *Nurse Assistant Candidate Handbook* from National Council of State Boards of Nursing (NCSBN), Chicago, Ill, © 2019.

7. Candidate inflates cuff between 160 mm Hg to 180 mm Hg. If beat heard immediately upon cuff deflation, completely deflate cuff. Re-inflate cuff to no more than 200 mm Hg.

8. Deflates cuff slowly and notes the first sound (systolic reading), and last sound (diastolic reading) (If rounding needed, measurements are rounded UP to the nearest 2 mm of mercury)

9. Removes cuff

10. Signaling device is within reach

11. Before recording, washes hands

12. **After obtaining reading using BP cuff and stethoscope, records both systolic and diastolic pressures each within plus or minus 8 mm Hg of evaluator's reading**

❑ *Measures and Records Urinary Output (Chapter 31)*

1. Puts on clean gloves before handling bedpan

2. Pours the contents of the bedpan into measuring container without spilling or splashing urine outside of container

3. Rinses bedpan and pours rinse into toilet

4. Measures the amount of urine at eye level with container on flat surface (if between measurement lines, round up to nearest 25ml/cc)

5. After measuring urine, empties contents of measuring container into toilet

6. Rinses measuring container and pours rinse water into toilet

7. Before recording output, removes and disposes of gloves (without contaminating self) into waste container and washes hands

8. **Records contents of container within plus or minus 25 mL/cc of evaluator's reading**

❑ *Measures and Records Weight of Ambulatory Client (Chapter 36)*

1. Explains procedure, speaking clearly, slowly, and directly, maintaining face-to-face contact whenever possible

2. Client has non-skid shoes/footwear on before walking to scale

3. Before client steps on scale, candidate sets scale to zero

4. Ask client to step on center of scale and obtains client's weight

5. Asks client to step off scale

6. Before recording, washes hands

7. **Records weight based on indicator on scale. Weight is within plus or minus 2 lbs of evaluator's reading (If weight recorded in kg, weight is within plus or minus 0.9 kg of evaluator's reading)**

❑ *Positions on Side (Chapter 19)*

1. Explains procedure, speaking clearly, slowly, and directly, maintaining face-to-face contact whenever possible

2. Privacy is provided with a curtain, screen, or door

3. Before turning, lowers head of bed

4. Raises side rail on side to which body will be turned

5. Candidate assists client to slowly roll onto side toward raised side rail

6. Places or adjusts pillow under head for support

7. Candidate repositions arm and shoulder so that client is not lying on arm

8. Supports top arm with supportive device

9. Places supportive device behind client's back

10. Places supportive device between legs with top knee flexed; knee and ankle supported

11. Signaling device is within reach and bed is in low position

12. After completing skill, washes hands

❑ *Provides Catheter Care for Female (Chapter 28)*

1. Explains procedure, speaking clearly, slowly, and directly, maintaining face-to-face contact whenever possible

2. Privacy is provided with a curtain, screen, or door

3. Before washing checks water temperature for safety and comfort and asks client to verify comfort of water

4. Puts on clean gloves before washing

5. Places linen protector under perineal area including buttocks before washing

6. Exposes area surrounding catheter (only exposing client between hip and knee)

7. Applies soap to wet washcloth

8. **While holding catheter at meatus without tugging, cleans at least four inches of catheter from meatus, moving in only one direction , away from meatus, using a clean area of the cloth for each stroke**

9. **While holding catheter at meatus without tugging, using a clean washcloth, rinses at least four inches of catheter from meatus, moving only in one direction,**

away from meatus, using a clean area of the washcloth for each stroke

10. While holding catheter at meatus without tugging, dries at least four inches of catheter moving away from meatus using a dry cloth towel/washcloth

11. Empties, rinses, and dries basin

12. Places basin in designated dirty supply area

13. Disposes of used linen into soiled linen container and disposes of linen protector appropriately

14. Avoids contact between candidate clothing and used linen

15. Removes and disposes of gloves (without contaminating self) into waste container and washes hands

16. Signaling device is within reach and bed is in low position

Provides Fingernail Care on One Hand (Chapter 25)

1. Explains procedure, speaking clearly, slowly, and directly, maintaining face-to-face contact whenever possible

2. Before immersing fingernails, checks water temperature for safety and comfort and asks client to verify comfort of water

3. Basin is in a comfortable position for client

4. Puts on clean gloves before cleaning fingernails

5. Fingernails are immersed in basin of water

6. Cleans under each fingernail with orangewood stick

7. Wipes orangewood stick on towel after each nail

8. Dries fingernail area

9. Candidate feels each nail and files as needed

10. Disposes of orangewood stick and emery board into waste container (for testing purposes)

11. Empties, rinses, and dries basin

12. After rinsing basin, places basin in designated used supply area

13. Disposes of used linens into used linens container

14. Removes and disposes of gloves (without contaminating self) into waste container and washes hands

15. Signaling device is within reach

❏*Provides Foot Care on One Foot (Chapter 25)

1. Explains procedure, speaking clearly, slowly, and directly, maintaining face-to-face contact whenever possible

2. Privacy is provided with a curtain, screen, or door

3. Before washing, checks water temperature for safety and comfort and asks client to verify comfort of water

4. Basin is in a comfortable position for client and on protective barrier

5. Puts on clean gloves before washing foot

6. Client's bare foot is placed into the water

7. Applies soap to wet washcloth

8. Lifts foot from water and washes foot (including between the toes)

9. Foot is rinsed (including between the toes)

10. Dries foot (including between the toes) with dry cloth towel/washcloth

11. Applies lotion to top and bottom of foot, (excluding between the toes) removing excess with a towel/washcloth

12. Supports foot and ankle during procedure

13. Empties, rinses, and dries basin

14. Places basin in designated dirty supply area

15. Disposes of used linen into soiled linen container

16. Removes and disposes of gloves (without contaminating self) into waste container and washes hands

17. Signaling device is within reach

❏*Provides Mouth Care (Chapter 23)

1. Explains procedure, speaking clearly, slowly, and directly, maintaining face-to-face contact whenever possible

2. Privacy is provided with a curtain, screen, or door

3. Before providing mouth care, client is in upright sitting position (75–90 degrees)

4. Puts on clean gloves before cleaning mouth

5. Places cloth towel across chest before providing mouth care

6. Secures cup of water and moistens toothbrush

7. Before cleaning mouth applies toothpaste to moistened toothbrush

8. **Cleans mouth (including tongue and all surfaces of teeth) using gentle motions**

9. Maintains clean technique with placement of toothbrush

10. Candidate holds emesis basin to chin while client rinses mouth

11. Candidate wipes mouth and removes clothing protector

12. Disposes of used linen into soiled linen container

---

*Reproduced and used with permission from the *Nurse Assistant Candidate Handbook* from National Council of State Boards of Nursing (NCSBN), Chicago, Ill, © 2019.

13. Rinses toothbrush and empties, rinses, and dries basin

14. Removes and disposes of gloves (without contaminating self) into waste container and washes hands

15. Signaling device is within reach and bed is in low position

❏ *Provides Perineal Care (Peri-Care) for Female (Chapter 24)*

1. Explains procedure, speaking clearly, slowly, and directly, maintaining face-to-face contact whenever possible

2. Privacy is provided with a curtain, screen, or door

3. Before washing checks water temperature for safety and comfort and asks client to verify comfort of water

4. Puts on clean gloves before washing perineal area

5. Places pad/linen protector under perineal area, including buttocks, before washing

6. Exposes perineal area (only exposing between hips and knees)

7. Applies soap to wet washcloth

8. **Washes genital area, moving from front to back, while using a clean area of the washcloth for each stroke**

9. **Using clean washcloth, rinses soap from genital area, moving from front to back, while using a clean area of the washcloth for each stroke**

10. Dries genital area moving from front to back with dry cloth towel/washcloth

11. After washing genital area, turns to side, then washes rectal area moving from front to back using a clean area of washcloth for each stroke.

12. Using clean washcloth, rinses soap from rectal area, moving from front to back, while using a clean area of washcloth for each stroke

13. Dries rectal area moving from front to back with dry cloth towel/washcloth

14. Repositions client

15. Empties, rinses, and dries basin

16. Places basin in designated dirty supply area

17. Disposes of used linen into soiled linen container and disposes of linen protector appropriately

18. Avoids contact between candidate clothing and used linen

19. Removes and disposes of gloves (without contaminating self) into waste container and washes hands

20. Signaling device is within reach and bed is in low position

❏ *Transfers From Bed to Wheelchair Using Transfer Belt (Chapter 20)*

1. Explains procedure, speaking clearly, slowly, and directly, maintaining face-to-face contact whenever possible

2. Privacy is provided with a curtain, screen, or door

3. Before assisting to stand, wheelchair is positioned along side of bed, at head of bed, facing the foot, or foot of bed facing head

4. Before assisting to stand, footrests are folded up or removed

5. **Before assisting to stand, locks wheels on wheelchair**

6. Before assisting to stand, bed is at a safe level

7. Before assisting to stand, checks and/or locks bed wheels

8. **Before assisting to stand, client is assisted to a sitting position with feet flat on the floor**

9. Before assisting to stand, client is wearing shoes

10. Before assisting to stand, applies transfer belt securely at the waist over clothing/gown

11. Before assisting to stand, provides instructions to enable client to assist in transfer including prearranged signal to alert when to begin standing

12. Stands facing client, positioning self to ensure safety of candidate and client during transfer. Counts to three (or says other prearranged signal) to alert client to begin standing

13. On signal, gradually assists client to stand by grasping transfer belt on both sides with an upward grasp (candidates hands are in upward position) and maintaining stability of client's legs by standing knee to knee, or toe to toe with the client

14. Assists client to turn to stand in front of wheelchair with back of client's legs against wheelchair

15. Lowers client into wheelchair

16. Positions client with hips touching back of wheelchair and transfer belt is removed

17. Positions feet on footrests

18. Signaling device is within reach

19. After completing skill, washes hands

❏ *Performs Modified Passive Range-of-Motion (PROM) for One Knee and One Ankle (Chapter 34)*

1. Explains procedure, speaking clearly, slowly, and directly, maintaining face-to-face contact whenever possible

2. Privacy is provided with a curtain, screen, or door

---

*Reproduced and used with permission from the *Nurse Assistant Candidate Handbook* from National Council of State Boards of Nursing (NCSBN), Chicago, Ill, © 2019.

3. Ensures that client is supine in bed and instructs client to inform candidate if pain is experienced during exercise

4. **While supporting the leg at knee and ankle, bends the knee then returns leg to client's normal position (extension/flexion) (AT LEAST 3 TIMES unless pain is verbalized). Moves joints gently, slowly, and smoothly through the range of motion, discontinuing exercise if client verbalizes pain.**

5. **While supporting the foot and ankle close to the bed, pushes/pulls foot toward head (dorsiflexion), and pushes/pulls foot down, toes point down (plantar flexion) (AT LEAST 3 TIMES unless pain is verbalized). Moves joints gently, slowly, and smoothly through the range of motion, discontinuing exercise if client verbalizes pain.**

6. Signaling device is within reach and bed is in low position

7. After completing skill, washes hands

❑ *Performs Modified Passive Range-of-Motion (PROM) for One Shoulder (Chapter 34)*

1. Explains procedure, speaking clearly, slowly, and directly, maintaining face-to-face contact whenever possible

2. Privacy is provided with a curtain, screen, or door

3. Instructs client to inform candidate if pain is experienced during exercise

4. **While supporting arm at the elbow and at the wrist, raises client's straightened arm from side position upward toward head to ear level and returns arm down to side of body (flexion/extension) (AT LEAST 3 TIMES unless pain is verbalized). Moves joint gently, slowly, and smoothly through the range of motion, discontinuing exercise if client verbalizes pain.**

5. **While supporting arm at the elbow and at the wrist, moves client's straightened arm away from the side of body to shoulder level and returns to side of body (abduction/adduction) (AT LEAST 3 TIMES unless pain is verbalized). Moves joint gently, slowly, and smoothly through the range of motion, discontinuing exercise if client verbalizes pain.**

6. Signaling device is within reach and bed is in low position

7. After completing skill, washes hands

❑ *Performs Passive Range-of-Motion of Lower Extremity (Hip, Knee, Ankle) (Chapter 34)*

1. Washes hands before contact with client

2. Identifies self to client by name and addresses client by name

3. Explains procedure to client, speaking clearly, slowly, and directly, maintaining face-to-face contact whenever possible

4. Provides for client's privacy during procedure with curtain, screen, or door

5. Positions client supine and in good body alignment

6. Supports client's leg by placing one hand under knee and other hand under heel

7. Moves entire leg away from body (performs AT LEAST 3 TIMES unless pain occurs)

8. Moves entire leg toward body (performs AT LEAST 3 TIMES unless pain occurs)

9. Bends client's knee and hip toward client's trunk (performs AT LEAST 3 TIMES unless pain occurs)

10. Straightens knee and hip (performs AT LEAST 3 TIMES unless pain occurs)

11. Flexes and extends ankle through range-of-motion exercises (performs AT LEAST 3 TIMES unless pain occurs)

12. Rotates ankle through range-of-motion exercises (performs AT LEAST 3 TIMES unless pain occurs)

13. **While supporting limb, moves joints gently, slowly, and smoothly through range-of-motion to point of resistance, discontinuing exercise if pain occurs**

14. Provides for comfort

15. Before leaving client, places signaling device within client's reach

16. Washes hands

❑ *Performs Passive Range-of-Motion of Upper Extremity (Shoulder, Elbow, Wrist, Finger) (Chapter 34)*

1. Washes hands before contact with client

2. Identifies self to client by name and addresses client by name

3. Explains procedure to client, speaking clearly, slowly, and directly, maintaining face-to-face contact whenever possible

4. Provides for client's privacy during procedure with curtain, screen, or door

5. Supports client's extremity above and below joints while performing range-of-motion

6. Raises client's straightened arm toward ceiling and back toward head of bed and returns to flat position (flexion/extension) (performs AT LEAST 3 TIMES unless pain occurs)

7. Moves client's straightened arm away from client's side of body toward head of bed, and returns client's straightened arm to midline of client's body (abduction/adduction) (performs AT LEAST 3 TIMES unless pain occurs)

8. Moves client's shoulder through rotation range-of-motion exercises (performs AT LEAST 3 TIMES unless pain occurs)

*Reproduced and used with permission from the *Nurse Assistant Candidate Handbook* from National Council of State Boards of Nursing (NCSBN), Chicago, Ill, © 2019.

9. Flexes and extends elbow through range-of-motion exercises (performs AT LEAST 3 TIMES unless pain occurs)

10. Provides range-of-motion exercises to wrist (performs AT LEAST 3 TIMES unless pain occurs)

11. Moves finger and thumb joints through range-of-motion exercises (performs AT LEAST 3 TIMES unless pain occurs)

12. **While supporting body part, moves joint gently, slowly, and smoothly through range-of-motion to point of resistance, discontinuing exercise if pain occurs**

13. Before leaving client, places signaling device within client's reach

14. Washes hands

❏ *Makes an Unoccupied (Closed) Bed (Chapter 22)*

1. Washes hands

2. Collects clean linens

3. Places clean linens on a clean surface

4. Raises the bed for good body mechanics

5. Puts on gloves

6. Removes linens without contaminating uniform. Rolls each piece away from self

7. Discards linens into laundry bag

8. Moves the mattress to the head of the bed

9. Applies mattress pad

10. Applies bottom sheet, keeping it smooth and free of wrinkles

11. Places the top sheet and bedspread on the bed, keeping them smooth and free of wrinkles

12. Tucks in top linens at the foot of the bed. Makes mitered corners

13. Applies clean pillowcase with zippers and/or tags to inside of pillowcase

14. Lowers the bed to its lowest position. Locks the bed wheels

15. Washes hands

❏ ***Donning and Removing PPE (Gown and Gloves) (Chapter 17)*

1. Picks up gown and unfolds

2. Facing the back opening of gown, places arms through each sleeve

3. Fastens the neck opening

4. Secures gown at waist making sure that back of clothing is covered by gown (as much as possible)

5. Puts on gloves

6. Cuffs of gloves overlap cuffs of gown

7. **Before removing gown, with one gloved hand, grasps the other glove at the palm, removes glove**

8. **Slips fingers from ungloved hand underneath cuff of remaining glove at wrist, and removes glove turning it inside out as it is removed**

9. Disposes of gloves into designated waste container without contaminating self

10. After removing gloves, unfastens gown at neck and at waist

11. After removing gloves, removes gown without touching outside of gown

12. While removing gown, holds gown away from body, without touching the floor, turns gown inward and keeps it inside out

13. Disposes of gown in designated container without contaminating self

14. After completing skill, washes hands

❏ *Performs Abdominal Thrusts (Chapter 13)*

1. Asks client if he or she is choking

2. Stands behind the client

3. Wraps arms around client's waist

4. Makes a fist with one hand

5. Places thumb side of fist against the client's abdomen

6. Positions fist in middle above navel and well below sternum (breastbone)

7. Grasps your fist with your other hand

8. Presses fist and other hand into abdomen with a quick upward thrust

9. Repeats thrusts until object is expelled or client becomes unresponsive

❏ *Ambulation With Cane or Walker (Chapter 34)*

1. Explains procedure to client, speaking clearly, slowly, and directly, maintaining face-to-face contact whenever possible

2. **Locks bed wheels or wheelchair brakes**

3. Assists client to a sitting position

4. **Before ambulating, puts on and properly fastens slip-resistant footwear**

5. Applies transfer belt (if directed by nurse or care plan)

6. Positions cane or walker correctly. Cane is on the client's strong side

7. Assists client to stand, using correct body mechanics

8. Stabilizes cane or walker and ensures that client stabilizes cane or walker

*Reproduced and used with permission from the *Nurse Assistant Candidate Handbook* from National Council of State Boards of Nursing (NCSBN), Chicago, Ill, © 2019.

9. Stands behind and slightly to the side of client on the person's weak side; grasps transfer belt (if used).

10. Ambulates client at least 10 steps

11. Assists client to pivot and sit, using correct body mechanics

12. Before leaving client, remove transfer belt (if used); places signaling device within client's reach

13. Washes hands

❏Fluid Intake (Chapter 31)

1. Observes dinner tray

2. Determines, in milliliters (mL), the amount of fluid consumed from each container

3. Determines total fluid consumed in mL

4. Records total fluid consumed on intake and output (I&O) sheet

5. Calculated total is within required range of evaluator's reading

❏Brushes or Combs Client's Hair (Chapter 25)

1. Explains procedure to client, speaking clearly, slowly, and directly, maintaining face-to-face contact whenever possible

2. Collects brush or comb and bath towel

3. Places towel across client's back and shoulders or across the pillow

4. Asks client how he or she wants his or her hair styled

5. Combs/brushes hair gently and completely

6. Leaves hair neatly brushed, combed, and/or styled

7. Removes towel

8. Removes hair from comb or brush

9. Before leaving client, places signaling device within client's reach

10. Washes hands

❏Transfers a Client Using a Mechanical Lift (Chapter 20)

1. Assembles required equipment; performs safety check of slings, straps, hooks, and chains

2. Checks client's weight to ensure it does not exceed the lift's capacity

3. Asks a co-worker to help

4. Explains procedure to client, speaking clearly, slowly, and directly, maintaining face-to-face contact whenever possible

5. Provides for privacy during procedure with curtain, screen, or door

6. Locks the bed wheels

7. Raises the bed for proper body mechanics

8. Lowers the head of the bed to a level appropriate for the client

9. Stands on one side of the bed; co-worker stands on the other side

10. Lowers the bed rails if up

11. Centers the sling under the client following the manufacturer's instructions

12. Ensures that the sling is smooth

13. Positions the client in semi-Fowler's position

14. Positions a chair to lower the client into it

15. Lowers the bed to its lowest position

16. Raises the lift to position it over the client

17. Positions the lift over the client

18. Attaches the sling to the sling hooks and checks fasteners for security

19. Crosses the client's arms over the chest

20. Raises the lift high enough until the client and sling are free of the bed

21. Instructs co-worker to support the client's legs as candidate moves the lift and the client away from the bed

22. Positions the lift so the client's back is toward the chair

23. Slowly lowers the client into the chair

24. Places client in comfortable position, in correct body alignment

25. Lowers the sling hooks and unhooks the sling

26. Removes the sling from under the client unless otherwise indicated. Moves lift away from client

27. Puts footwear on the client

28. Covers the client's lap and legs with a lap blanket

29. Positions the chair as the client prefers

30. Places signaling device within client's reach

31. Washes hands

❏Provides Mouth Care for an Unconscious Client (Chapter 23)

1. Explains procedure to client, speaking clearly, slowly, and directly, maintaining face-to-face contact whenever possible

2. Provides for privacy during procedure with curtain, screen, or door

3. Washes hands

4. Positions client on side with head turned well to one side

5. Puts on gloves

6. Places the towel under the client's face

7. Places the kidney basin under the chin

8. Uses swabs or toothbrush and toothpaste or other cleaning solution

9. Uses a plastic tongue depressor (if needed) to hold the person's mouth open
10. Cleans inside of mouth including the gums, tongue, and teeth
11. Cleans and dries face
12. Removes the towel and kidney basin
13. Applies lubricant to the lips
14. Positions client for comfort and safety
15. Removes and discards the gloves
16. Places signaling device within the client's reach
17. Washes hands

❏ *Provides Drinking Water (Chapter 31)*

1. Washes hands
2. Assembles equipment—ice, scoop, pitcher, cup, straw
3. Explains procedure to client, speaking clearly, slowly, and directly, maintaining face-to-face contact whenever possible
4. Uses the scoop to fill the pitcher with ice; does not let the scoop touch the rim or inside of the pitcher
5. Places scoop in appropriate receptacle after each use
6. Adds water to pitcher
7. Places the pitcher, disposable cup, and straw (if used) on the over-bed table, within the person's reach
8. Before leaving, places signaling device within client's reach
9. Washes hands

❏ *Provides Perineal Care for Uncircumcised Male (Chapter 24)*

1. Explains procedure to client, speaking clearly, slowly, and directly, maintaining face-to-face contact whenever possible
2. Provides for privacy during procedure with curtain, screen, or door
3. Washes hands
4. Fills basin with comfortably warm water
5. Puts on gloves
6. Elevates bed to working height
7. Places waterproof pad under buttocks
8. Gently grasps penis
9. Retracts the foreskin
10. Using a circular motion, cleans the tip by starting at the meatus of the urethra and working outward
11. Rinses the area with another washcloth
12. Returns the foreskin to its natural position
13. Cleans the shaft of the penis with firm, downward strokes and rinses the area
14. Cleans the scrotum

15. Pats dry the penis and the scrotum
16. Cleans the rectal area
17. Removes the waterproof pad
18. Lowers the bed
19. Removes and discards the gloves
20. Washes hands
21. Before leaving, places signaling device within client's reach

❏ *Empties and Records Content of Urinary Drainage Bag (Chapter 28)*

1. Explains procedure to client, speaking clearly, slowly, and directly, maintaining face-to-face contact whenever possible
2. Washes hands
3. Puts on gloves
4. Places a paper towel on the floor
5. Places the graduate on the paper towel
6. Places the graduate under the collection bag
7. Ensures that the bag is below the bladder and the drainage tube is not kinked
8. Opens the clamp on the drain
9. Lets all urine drain into the graduate—does not let the drain touch the graduate
10. Closes clamp and positions drain in holder
11. Measures urine
12. Removes and discards the paper towel
13. Empties the contents of the graduate into the toilet and flushes
14. Rinses and dries the graduate with clean, dry paper towels
15. Returns the graduate to its proper place
16. Removes the gloves
17. Washes hands
18. Records the time and amount on the intake and output (I&O) record
19. Provides for client comfort
20. Places the signaling device within reach of client

❏ *Applies a Vest Restraint (Chapter 15)*

1. Obtains the correct type and size of restraint
2. Checks straps for tears or frays
3. Washes hands
4. Explains procedure to client, speaking clearly, slowly, and directly, maintaining face-to-face contact whenever possible
5. Provides for privacy during procedure with curtain, screen, or door
6. Makes sure the client is comfortable and in good alignment

7. Assists the person to a sitting position; as far back in wheelchair as possible with buttocks against chair back.

8. Applies the restraint following the manufacturer's instructions—the "V" part of the vest crosses in front

9. Makes sure the vest is free of wrinkles in the front and back

10. Brings the straps through the slots if vest criss-crosses.

11. Makes sure the client is comfortable and in good alignment

12. Secures the straps to the chair or to the movable part of the bed frame

13. Uses buckle or a quick release tie

14. Makes sure the vest is snug—slide an open hand between the restraint and the client

15. Places the signaling device within the client's reach

16. Washes hands

❏ *Performs a Back Rub (Massage) (Chapter 35)*

1. Washes hands

2. Explains procedure to client, speaking clearly, slowly, and directly, maintaining face-to-face contact whenever possible

3. Provides for privacy during procedure with curtain, screen, or door

4. Raises the bed for good body mechanics

5. Lowers the bed rail near the candidate, if up

6. Positions the person in the prone or side-lying position

7. Exposes the back, shoulders, upper arms, and buttocks

8. Warms the lotion

9. Rubs entire back in upward, outward motion for approximately 2 to 3 minutes; does not massage reddened bony areas

10. Straightens and secures clothing or sleepwear

11. Returns client to comfortable and safe position

12. Places the signaling device within reach

13. Lowers the bed to its lowest position

14. Washes hands

❏ *Positions a Foley (indwelling) Catheter (Chapter 28)*

1. Explains procedure to client, speaking clearly, slowly, and directly, maintaining face-to-face contact whenever possible

2. Washes hands

3. Puts on gloves

4. Secures catheter and drainage tubing according to facility procedure

5. Places tubing over leg

6. Positions drainage tubing so urine flows freely into drainage bag and has no kinks

7. Attaches bag to bed frame, below level of bladder

8. Washes hands

❏ *Applies a Cold Pack or Warm Compress (Chapter 42)*

1. Washes hands

2. Collects needed equipment

3. Explains procedure to client, speaking clearly, slowly, and directly, maintaining face-to-face contact whenever possible

4. Provides for privacy during procedure with curtain, screen, or door

5. Positions the client for the procedure

6. Covers cold pack or warm compress with towel or other protective cover

7. Properly places cold pack or warm compress on site

8. Checks the client for complications every 5 minutes

9. Checks the cold pack or warm compress every 5 minutes

10. Removes the application at the specified time—usually after 15 to 20 minutes

11. Provides for comfort

12. Places the signaling device within reach

13. Washes hands

❏ *Positions for an Enema (Chapter 29)*

1. Washes hands

2. Explains procedure to client, speaking clearly, slowly, and directly, maintaining face-to-face contact whenever possible

3. Provides for privacy

4. Positions the client in Sims' position or in a left side-lying position

5. Covers client with a bath blanket

6. Provides for comfort

7. Places the signaling device within reach

8. Washes hands

❏ *Positions Client for Meals (Chapter 30)*

1. Washes hands

2. Explains procedure to client, speaking clearly, slowly, and directly, maintaining face-to-face contact whenever possible

3. If the person will eat in bed:
   a. Raises the head of the bed to a comfortable position—usually Fowler's or high-Fowler's position is preferred

b. Removes items from the over-bed table and cleans the over-bed table

c. Adjusts the over-bed table in front of the person

d. Places the client in proper body alignment

4. If the person will sit in a chair:

a. Positions the person in a chair or wheelchair

b. Provides support for the client's feet

c. Removes items from the over-bed table and cleans the table

d. Adjusts the over-bed table in front of the person

e. Places the client in proper body alignment

5. Places the signaling device within reach

6. Washes hands

❏ *Takes and Records Axillary Temperature, Pulse, and Respirations (Chapter 33)*

1. Washes hands before contact with client

2. Identifies self to client by name and addresses client by name

3. Explains procedure to client, speaking clearly, slowly, and directly, maintaining face-to-face contact whenever possible

4. Provides for client's privacy during procedure with curtain, screen, or door

5. Turns on digital oral thermometer

6. Dries axilla and places thermometer in the center of the axilla

7. Holds thermometer in place for appropriate length of time

8. Removes and reads thermometer

9. Records temperature on pad of paper

10. **Report abnormal temperature at once**

11. Discards sheath from thermometer

12. Places fingertips on thumb side of client's wrist to locate radial pulse

13. Counts beats for 1 full minute

14. Records pulse rate on pad of paper

15. **Report abnormal pulse at once**

16. Counts respirations for 1 full minute

17. Records respirations on pad of paper

18. **Report abnormal respirations at once**

19. Before leaving client, places signaling device within client's reach

20. Washes hands

❏ *Transfers Client From Wheelchair to Bed (Chapter 20)*

1. Washes hands before contact with client

2. Identifies self to client by name and addresses client by name

3. Explains procedure to client, speaking clearly, slowly, and directly, maintaining face-to-face contact whenever possible

4. Provides for client's privacy during procedure with curtain, screen, or door

5. Positions wheelchair close to bed with arm of wheelchair almost touching bed

6. Before transferring client, ensures client is wearing non-skid footwear

7. Before transferring client, folds up footplates

8. Before transferring client, places bed at safe and appropriate level for client

9. **Before transferring client, locks wheels on wheelchair and locks bed brakes**

10. a. *With transfer (gait) belt:* Stands in front of client, positioning self to ensure safety of candidate and client during transfer (for example, knees bent, feet apart, back straight), places belt around client's waist, and grasps belt. Tightens belt so that fingers of candidate's hand can be slipped between transfer/gait belt and client

b. *Without transfer belt:* Stands in front of client, positioning self to ensure safety of candidate and client during transfer (for example, knees bent, feet apart, back straight, arms around client's torso under arms)

11. Provides instructions to enable client to assist in transfer, including prearranged signal to alert client to begin standing

12. Braces client's lower extremities to prevent slipping

13. Counts to three (or says other prearranged signal) to alert client to begin transfer

14. On signal, gradually assists client to stand

15. Assists client to pivot and sit on bed in manner that ensures safety

16. Removes transfer belt, if used

17. Assists client to remove non-skid footwear

18. Assists client to move to center of bed

19. Provides for comfort and good body alignment

20. Before leaving client, places signaling device within client's reach

21. Washes hands

❏ *Applies an Incontinence Brief (Chapter 27)*

1. Washes hands before contact with client

2. Identifies self to client by name and addresses client by name

3. Explains procedure to client, speaking clearly, slowly, and directly, maintaining face-to-face contact whenever possible

4. Chooses correct brief and size per facility instructions

5. Provides privacy for the resident

6. Elevates bed to comfortable working height

7. Puts on gloves

8. Places waterproof under-pad under client, asking client to raise buttocks or turning the client to the side

9. Loosens tabs on each side of the product

10. Turns the client away from you

11. Removes the product from front to back, observes for urine amount (small, moderate, large) color, or blood; rolls the product up and places the product into trash bag

12. Opens the new brief, folding it in half, length-wise along the center, and inserts it between the client's legs from front to back; unfolds and spreads the back panel

13. Turns the client onto his or her back, with the product under buttocks with top of absorbent pad aligned just above the buttocks crease

14. Grasps and stretches the leg portion of front panel to extend elastic for groin placement

15. Rolls ruffles away from groin

16. Snuggly places bottom tabs angled toward abdomen on both sides

17. Places top tabs on each side angled toward bottom tabs

18. Removes gloves

19. Washes hands

20. Covers client appropriately and provides for comfort

21. Places signaling device within reach

After the Procedure

After you demonstrate a skill, complete a safety check of the room.

- The person is wearing eyeglasses, hearing aids, and other devices as needed.
- The call light is plugged in and within reach.
- Bed rails are up or down according to the care plan.
- The bed is in the lowest horizontal position.
- The bed position is locked if needed.
- Manual bed cranks are in the down position.
- Bed wheels are locked.
- Assistive devices are within reach. Walker, cane, and wheelchair are examples.
- The over-bed table, filled water pitcher and cup, tissues, phone, TV controls, and other needed items are within reach.
- Unneeded equipment is unplugged or turned off.
- Harmful substances are stored properly. Lotion, mouthwash, shampoo, after-shave, and other personal care products are examples.

After the Test

- Celebrate—you have completed the competency evaluation! The length of time for you to get your test results varies with each state. In the meantime, try to relax. Continue your daily routine and be the best nursing assistant you can be.

Answers to Review Questions in Textbook Chapters Review

Chapter 1
1. a
2. b
3. c

Chapter 2
1. d
2. a
3. b
4. d

Chapter 3
1. d
2. a
3. b
4. a

Chapter 4
1. b
2. a
3. d

Chapter 5
1. c
2. a
3. b
4. a
5. a
6. a
7. a
8. b

Chapter 6
1. b
2. c
3. a
4. d
5. a
6. b

Chapter 7
1. b
2. d
3. d
4. d

5. b
6. a
7. a
8. c
9. c
10. d
11. c
12. c
13. b
14. b

Chapter 8
1. a
2. d
3. c
4. c
5. a

Chapter 9
1. b
2. c
3. b

Chapter 11
1. d
2. b
3. b

Chapter 12
1. a
2. d
3. a
4. c
5. d
6. c

Chapter 13
1. b
2. d
3. c
4. b
5. c
6. c
7. b
8. a

9. a
10. b

Chapter 14
1. b
2. b
3. c
4. a
5. a
6. d

Chapter 15
1. d
2. c
3. b
4. a
5. b
6. c

Chapter 16
1. b
2. b
3. a
4. b
5. c

Chapter 17
1. c
2. d
3. a
4. c
5. b

Chapter 18
1. c
2. b
3. a
4. d

Chapter 19
1. d
2. a
3. b

Chapter 20
1. d
2. c
3. d

Chapter 21
1. c
2. b
3. a
4. a
5. d
6. c
7. d

Chapter 22
1. b
2. d
3. a
4. b
5. c

Chapter 23
1. b
2. a
3. b
4. a

Chapter 24
1. a
2. b
3. d
4. d
5. b
6. c

Chapter 25
1. d
2. c
3. d
4. b
5. d
6. d
7. a

8. b
9. a
10. b

Chapter 26
1. d
2. a
3. c
4. d
5. c

Chapter 27
1. d
2. a
3. c
4. a
5. c

Chapter 28
1. d
2. a
3. d
4. a

Chapter 29
1. b
2. d
3. b
4. a

Chapter 30
1. a
2. d
3. a
4. d
5. b

Chapter 31
1. b
2. a
3. c
4. c
5. b

Chapter 33
1. c
2. a
3. b
4. b

Chapter 34
1. c
2. a
3. c
4. a

Chapter 35
1. a
2. c
3. d
4. a
5. c

Chapter 36
1. c
2. a
3. a
4. b

Chapter 38
1. b
2. c
3. d
4. b

Chapter 39
1. b
2. d
3. d

Chapter 40
1. a
2. b
3. a

Chapter 41
1. b
2. c
3. b
4. c

Chapter 42
1. c
2. a

Chapter 43
1. b
2. b
3. a
4. b
5. a

Chapter 45
1. a
2. c

3. d
4. c
5. b

Chapter 46
1. d
2. c
3. b
4. c

Chapter 47
1. d
2. a
3. a
4. c

Chapter 48
1. b
2. a
3. c
4. b
5. d

Chapter 49
1. d
2. a
3. a
4. c

Chapter 50
1. c
2. c
3. a
4. b
5. d

Chapter 51
1. d
2. b
3. c

Chapter 52
1. a
2. b
3. b
4. d
5. b
6. c

Chapter 53
1. b
2. d
3. a
4. b

Chapter 55
1. b
2. d

Chapter 58
1. b
2. a
3. a
4. c
5. c

Chapter 59
1. d
2. c
3. a
4. b
5. c
6. b

1. **C** You never give drugs. You may politely refuse to do a task that you have not been trained to do. However, you need to tell the nurse. Do not ignore a request to do something. Page 26, Chapter 3.

2. **D** An ethical person does not judge others or cause harm to another person; harm must be immediately reported. Ethical behavior involves not being prejudiced or biased. Ethical behavior also involves not avoiding persons whose standards and values are different from your own. Page 40, Chapter 5.

3. **D** An ethical person is knowledgeable of what is right conduct and wrong conduct. Health care workers do not drink alcohol before coming to work and do not drink alcohol while working. Page 40, Chapter 5.

4. **A** Negligence is an unintentional wrong and a failure to act in a reasonable and prudent manner, that results in harm Page 42, Chapter 5.

5. **B** The person's information is confidential. Information about the patient or resident is shared only among health team members involved in his or her care. Page 40, Chapter 5.

6. **D** End-of-shift is a time for good teamwork. Continue to do your job. Your attitude is important. Page 98, Chapter 8.

7. **A** If data is not saved if can be lost. Logging off prevents someone else from using the computer under your password. The time should accurately reflect when the care was given. Using someone else's password or charting for a co-worker are incorrect actions. Page 99, Chapter 8.

8. **B** Give a courteous greeting and identify location and self. Answer calls promptly ideally on the first ring. Take a message if someone is not available to come to the phone, Confidential information about a resident or employee is not given to any caller. Page 102, Chapter 8.

9. **C** Showing the person the nursing center is the best action. Health care agencies are strange places with strange routines and equipment. People feel safer if they know what to expect. Reassuring and making vague statements or deferring to the nurse do not immediately reduce the person's anxiety. Page 71, Chapter 7.

10. **B** When a person is angry or hostile, stay calm and professional. The person is usually not angry with you. He or she may be angry at another person or situation. Page 83, Chapter 7.

11. **D** Use words that are familiar to the person. Speak clearly, slowly, and distinctly. Also, ask 1 question at a time and wait for an answer. Page 75, Chapter 7.

12. **C** Conditions that involve the chest or abdomen should be discussed with the nurse before using the gait belt. Weakness of the arm, urinary problems and history of stroke are not contraindications for use of a gait belt; however always check with the nurse if you are unsure. Pages 198, Chapter 14.

13. **D** Listening requires that you care and have interest in the other person. Have good eye contact with the person. Focus on what the person is saying. Page 78, Chapter 7.

14. **C** Assume that a comatose person hears and understands you. Talk to the person and tell him or her what you are going to do. Page 81, Chapter 7.

15. **A** Protect a person's right to privacy when giving care. Politely ask visitors to leave the room. Do not expose the person's body in front of them. Show visitors where to wait. Page 81, Chapter 7.

16. **B** If a person wants to talk with a minister or spiritual leader, tell the nurse. It is not your responsibility to act as a spiritual counselor. Page 81, Chapter 7.

17. **A** Observe the person with a restraint at least every 15 minutes (or as often as directed by the nurse or care plan). Remove the restraint and re-position the person every 2 hours. Checking the person at the end of your shift is not incorrect, but checks should be performed every 15 minutes throughout the shift. Restraints and the restrained body part should be in plain view. Page 208, Chapter 15.

18. **D** For night-time urination, most fluids are given before 1700. Diapering, withholding fluid and waking the person at night are incorrect measures. Consult the nurse if you are unsure. Page 149, Chapter 12.

19. **B** Act in a professional manner. Joking around may encourage the behavior. Refusing the assignment is not the best choice for the person and it is likely that the behavior will continue with another caregiver. Person may not be able to explain the behavior. Page 811, Chapter 55.

20. **C** Push the chair forward when transporting the person. Do not pull the chair backward unless going through a doorway. If the person tries to help, hands or feet could be injured. Page 289, Chapter 20.

21. **A** Tell the nurse at once. It is important to do the correct procedure on the right person. You must be able to read the person's name on the ID bracelet or use the photo ID to identify the person. Page 160, Chapter 13.

22. **B** Clutching at the throat is the "universal sign of choking." Page 170, Chapter 13.

23. **D** When a person is on a diabetic diet, tell the nurse about changes in the person's eating habits. The person's meals and snacks need to be served on time. If the person is snacking between meals, you should tell the nurse. You cannot make the person eat, but you should report amounts consumed. Page 466, Chapter 30.

24. **D** With mild airway obstruction, the person is conscious and can speak. Often forceful coughing can remove the object. Page 168, Chapter 13.

25. **A** Abdominal thrusts are used to relieve severe airway obstruction. Page 170, Chapter 13.

26. **B** Do not use faulty electrical equipment in nursing centers. Take the item to the nurse. Page 174, Chapter 13.

27. **C** If a warning label is removed or damaged, do not use the substance. Take the container to the nurse and explain the problem. Page 176, Chapter 13.

28. **C** An ethical person realizes that other people's values and standards may differ from one's own. Sharing concerns with the nurse is a good first step; the nurse can assist you with values clarification. Page 40, Chapter 5.

29. **D** Politely remind the person to smoke in designated smoking areas. Page 161, Chapter 13.

30. **A** During a fire, remember the word *RACE* (rescue, alarm, confine, extinguish). Page 180, Chapter 13.

31. **C** If a person with Alzheimer's disease has sundowning (increased restlessness and confusion as daylight ends), provide a calm, quiet setting late in the day. Do not try to reason with the person or ask the person to explain. Reason and communication are impaired and these attempts may increase agitation. Complete treatments and activities early in the day. Pages 788, Chapter 53.

32. **C** Meal time provides opportunities for choking. Remember to cut food into small pieces and make sure the person can chew and swallow the food served. Report loose teeth or dentures to the nurse. Page 169, Chapter 13.

33. **A** Lock both wheels before you transfer a person to and from the wheelchair. Locking wheels can be considered a form of restraint; follow agency's policy. The person's feet are on the footplates before moving the chair. The footplates should be raised before transfer. Page 289, Chapter 20.

34. **B** The nurse needs to check him for injuries before he gets up; then the nurse will determine which method should be used to move the person. Page 200, Chapter 14.

35. **B** Death from strangulation is the most serious risk factor if the vest restraint has been put on backwards. The other complications can be associated with restraint use, but are less directly related to the improper application of a vest restraint. Page 209, Chapter 15.

36. **C** Wash your hands with soap and water before eating or helping others to eat. Page 227, Chapter 16.

37. **D** Gloves need to be changed when they become contaminated (contamination is not always visible) with blood, body fluids, secretions, and excretions. Page 233, Chapter 16.

38. **D** When washing your hands, keep your hands and forearms lower than your elbows. Use warm water (not hot) and a mild soap (not a disinfectant) to protect the integrity of your skin. Use a clean dry paper towel to turn off the faucet. Do not shake or wave your hands during the procedure. Page 227, Chapter 16.

39. **C** Bend your knees and squat to lift a heavy object. Hold items close to your body when lifting a heavy object. For a wider base of support and more balance, stand with your feet apart. Do not bend from your waist when lifting objects. Pages 256, Chapter 18.

40. **B** The head of the bed is raised between 45 and 60 degrees for Fowler's position. Page 262, Chapter 18.

41. **B** Negligence—an unintentional wrong in which a person did not act in a reasonable and careful manner and causes harm to a person or the person's property. Page 42, Chapter 5.

42. **A** Have the person's back and buttocks against the back of the chair. Feet are flat on the floor or on the wheelchair footplates. The backs of the person's knees and calves are slightly away from the edge of the seat. Page 264, Chapter 18.

43. **B** Help the person out of bed on his or her strong side. In transferring, the strong side moves first. It pulls the weaker side along. Page 297, Chapter 20.

44. **A** When a person tries to bite, scratch, pinch, or kick you, you need to protect the person, others, and yourself from harm. Telling the nurse is the next action; the nurse may consult the health care provider if restraints are needed. The nurse may recommend ignoring the behavior, but this would be used in conjunction with other behavioral management techniques. Page 82, Chapter 7.

45. **B** When the head of the bed is raised, skin on the buttocks stays in place and internal structures move forward as the person slides down in bed. This creates a shearing force. Page 269, Chapter 19.

46. **D** For comfort, adjust lighting to meet the person's changing needs. Nursing centers maintain a temperature range of 71°F to 81°F. Home bathroom do not always have the safety features or assistive devices that older people need. Many older persons are sensitive to noise. Page 311, Chapter 21.

47. **A** Call lights are placed on the person's strong side and kept within the person's reach. The person's dominant side is usually stronger, but disease or injury can result in weakness. All call lights are answered promptly, but calls from the bathroom should be answered first if several lights are activated at the same time. Page 319, Chapter 21.

48. **C** You must have the person's permission to open or search closets or drawers. Page 320, Chapter 21.

49. **C** When handling linens, do not take unneeded linens to a person's room. Once in the room, extra linens are considered contaminated. The linen cart is kept in a

central location so that all staff have access to it. To prevent the spread of microbes, never shake linens. Never put clean or used linens on the floor. Page 324, Chapter 22.

50. **A** Hand-held fire extinguishers are used to fight small fires that have not spread. For personal safety and the safety of others, notify the fire department for large or spreading fires. Page 180, Chapter 13.

51. **B** Mouth care is given at least every 2 hours for an unconscious person. Wiping the teeth is insufficient. To prevent aspiration, you position the person on his/her side with the head turned well to the side. Use a plastic tongue depressor to keep the person's mouth open. Wear gloves. Page 344, Chapter 23.

52. **B** A good attitude is needed at work. Be pleasant and respectful. Avoid making excuses or being defensive. Page 62, Chapter 6.

53. **B** During cleaning, firmly hold dentures over a sink half-filled with water and lined with a towel. This prevents them from falling onto a hard surface and breaking. Clean and store dentures in cool water. Hot water causes dentures to lose their shape. To prevent losing dentures, label the denture cup with the person's name. Page 346, Chapter 23.

54. **C** Report and record the location and description of the rash. Page 356, Chapter 24.

55. **C** Gently wipe the eye from the inner aspect to the outer aspect of the eye. Clean the far eye first. The eye lids (upper and lower are cleansed with a clean damp washcloth). Page 358, Chapter 24.

56. **D** When giving a back massage, wear gloves if the person's skin has open areas. Warm the lotion before applying it to the person. Use firm strokes. Do not massage reddened bony areas. This can lead to more tissue damage. Page 553, Chapter 35.

57. **A** Separate the labia and clean downward from front to back. Wear gloves and use soap. Pages 368, Chapter 24.

58. **C** Stay within hearing distance if the person can be left alone. Standing close to the person is sometimes necessary to maintain safety, but privacy is respected whenever possible. Cold water is turned on first, then hot water. Some people are able to adjust the water temperature, but it is safer if you turn on the cold water first and then assist by adjusting the hot water Page 362, Chapter 24.

59. **B** Electric razors are used when a person is on an anticoagulant. An anticoagulant prevents or slows down blood clotting. Bleeding occurs easily. A nick or cut from a safety razor can cause bleeding. Page 383, Chapter 25.

60. **B** Remove clothing from the strong (unaffected) side first. Page 391, Chapter 26.

61. **B** Pat answers ("Don't worry) are barriers to communication. Using "Sir" or "Mam" can be used as a sign of respect, but many people prefer

to be addressed by name. Remaining silent when a person is upset and asking for clarification are good communication techniques. Page 80, Chapter 7.

62. **D** Measure and record the amount of urine in the drainage bag. The catheter is secured to the person's thigh or abdomen. Do not disconnect the catheter from the drainage tubing. The nurse may teach the person about positioning the tubing. Page 422, Chapter 28.

63. **B** Carbohydrates provide energy and fiber for bowel elimination. Page 462, Chapter 30.

64. **D** When taking a rectal temperature with an electronic thermometer, the thermometer is inserted ½ inch into the rectum. A glass thermometer is inserted 1 inch. Privacy is provide by drawing the curtain, but you must hold the thermometer in place. Sims position is preferred. Page 508, Chapter 33.

65. **A** It is your responsibility to immediately report any systolic pressure below 90 mm Hg and any diastolic pressure below 60 mm Hg. Page 523, Chapter 33.

66. **D** Oral temperatures are not taken on unconscious persons, persons receiving oxygen, or persons who breathe through their mouth. Page 505, Chapter 33.

67. **A** To assist with walking, offer the person your arm and have the person walk a half step behind you. When caring for a person who is blind or visually impaired, let the person do as much for himself or herself as possible. Use a normal voice tone. Do not shout at the person. Identify yourself when you enter the room. Do not touch the person until you have indicated your presence. Pages 699, Chapter 46.

68. **D** The family makes choices if the person cannot. The person with confusion and dementia has the right to personal choice. He or she also has the right to keep and use personal items. Page 796, Chapter 53.

69. **C** Persons requiring amputation rehabilitation will often (not always) need to learn how to use and adapt to a prosthetic (artificial) arm or leg. Special diets are used for many conditions, for example, those who have trouble swallowing may require a dysphagia diet. Communication devices, such as picture boards, are used to assist persons with speech disorders. Bowel and bladder programs are used for persons with various urinary disorders or spinal cord injuries. Pages 684, Chapter 45.

70. **C** Encourage the person to help as much as possible. Doors and windows are closed to reduce drafts. You wash from the cleanest areas to the dirtiest areas. Pat the skin dry with a soft towel to avoid irritating or breaking the skin. Page 354, Chapter 24.

71. **A** When a person is dying, always assume that the person can hear you. Re-position the person every 2 hours to promote comfort. Ability to swallow and see will vary. Skin care, personal hygiene, back massages, oral hygiene, and good body alignment promote comfort. Pages 868, Chapter 59.

72. **B** Foods that melt at room temperature (ice cream, sherbet, custard, pudding, gelatin, and Popsicles) are measured and recorded as intake. The nurse measures and records IV fluids and tube feedings. Page 465, Chapter 30.

73. **B** After bedrest, activity increases slowly and in steps. First the person dangles. Sitting in a chair follows. Next the person walks in the room and then in the hallway. Page 281, Chapter 19.

74. **B** For your personal grooming and attire, keeping your nails trimmed and smooth decreases the chances of tearing a person's fragile skin. The other options would be helpful and appropriate for the person's grooming and attire. Page 618, Chapter 40.

75. **A** Treat the resident with respect and ensure privacy. The resident has a right not to have his or her private affairs exposed or made public without giving consent. Only staff involved in the resident's care should see, handle, or examine his or her body. Page 14, Chapter 2.

76. **B** Check on the person every 5 minutes. Page 404 Chapter 27

77. **A** When a person is on bed rest, he or she is allowed to do some ADLs, such as self-feeding, oral hygiene, bathing, shaving, and hair care. For strict or complete bed rest, everything is done for the person who must remain in bed. For bed rest with commode privileges, the commode is at the bedside. For bed rest with bathroom privileges, the bathroom is used for elimination. Page 532 Chapter 34

78. **B** Identification is always done by using two identifiers. Upon admission, use the admission form and the ID bracelet. Asking the person to state his or her name is polite and correct, but some people are not able. If name is correctly stated a second identifier is still needed. Calling the admission office is incorrect. The nurse should be consulted if two identifiers are not available. Page 563 Chapter 36

79. **D** The respiratory system brings oxygen (O_2) into the lungs and removes carbon dioxide (CO_2). The renal system removes waste products; and maintains water, electrolyte, and acid base balance. The circulatory system pumps blood to the body. The nervous system controls, directs, and coordinates body functions. Page 743 Chapter 49

1. **C** You may politely refuse to do a task that is not in your job description. If you are not familiar with the task you should ask for instruction and supervision. Pages 33, Chapter 4.

2. **B** You may not agree with advance directives or resuscitation decisions. However, you must respect the person's wishes. In addition, it is not the nursing assistant's responsibility to have this discussion with the person, his family or others. Page 40, Chapter 5, and Page 872, Chapter 59.

3. **C** Verbal abuse is using oral or written words or statements that speak badly of, sneer at, criticize, or condemn a person. Page 47, Chapter 5.

4. **C** Speak in a normal tone. Use words the person seems to understand and speak slowly and distinctly. Asking for translation help is reasonable, changing assignments is not always possible and could be viewed as unethical. Page 80, Chapter 7.

5. **C** Report the situation to the nurse and follow the nurse's instructions. It is the nurse's responsibility to assess for dangers and talk to the daughter about solutions. Page 179, Chapter 13.

6. **B** Follow the manufacturer's instructions for equipment. Use 3-pronged plugs on all electrical devices. Wipe up spills right away. Ask for training if you are unfamiliar with something. Page 174, Chapter 13.

7. **A** After the visitors leave, the purpose of the safety check is too ensure that nothing was moved, removed or left behind. Unintentional alterations to the person's environment could cause harm. Pages 194, Chapter 14.

8. **B** Perform hand hygiene after removing gloves. Page 227, Chapter 16.

9. **D** Sometimes multiple people or a mechanical lift are needed for moving and turning persons in bed. If the person weighs more than 200 pounds, at least 3 staff members help with the move. Page 270, Chapter 19.

10. **A** The wheels of the bed and wheelchair should be locked before attempting the transfer. When using a transfer belt, grasp the belt from underneath and pull upward as the person stands up. A person must not put his or her arms around your neck. He or she can pull you forward or cause you to lose your balance. Equipment should be obtained before starting a procedure. Person may become dizzy while dangling and should not be left alone, Page 291, Chapter 20.

11. **B** Wear gloves when removing linens. Linens may contain blood, body fluids, secretions, or excretions. Raise the bed for good body mechanics. Put the bed flat, then place the clean linens. Page 325, Chapter 22.

12. **B** Use a circular motion, start at the meatus, and work outward. The shaft is cleaned after the tip of the penis using long firm downward strokes. The scrotum is cleaned with a clean washcloth. Page 370, Chapter 24.

13. **C** Put clothing on the weak (affected) side first. Page 391, Chapter 26.

14. **D** The drainage bag hangs from the bed frame. It must not touch the floor. The bag is always kept lower than the person's bladder. The drainage bag does not hang on the bed rail. Page 422, Chapter 28.

15. **A** Protein is needed for tissue repair and growth. Page 462, Chapter 30.

16. **C** Older persons may not feel thirsty (decreased sense of thirst). Offer water often. Page 481, Chapter 31.

17. **C** The water pitcher and glass are removed from the room. NPO means that the person should not take food or fluids by mouth. An NPO sign is posted above the bed. Oral hygiene is performed frequently. Page 482, Chapter 31.

18. **C** 1 oz equals 30 mL. 3 oz equals 90 mL. Page 482, Chapter 31.

19. **D** Allow time to chew and swallow. Fluids are offered during the meal. A teaspoon, rather than a fork and knife are used for feeding. Engage in normal conversation during the meal. Page 474, Chapter 30.

20. **A** A person in a coma, cannot move, turn, or transfer and needs frequent passive ROM. All motions must be done for the person. In active ROM, the person does the exercise by him or herself. In active-assisted the person does the exercise, but requires help. Page 535, Chapter 34.

21. **B** A cane is held on the strong side of the body. If the left leg is weak, the cane is held in the right hand. Pages 540, Chapter 34.

22. **B** Position the person in good alignment. Getting out of bed is generally encouraged, but for some people movement can disrupt comfort and increase pain. Consult the nurse when in doubt. Talk softly and gently; jokes could irritate or offend someone who is uncomfortable. Thirty minutes is usually the amount of time required for most oral pain medications to have effect. Page 552, Chapter 35.

23. **C** Check behind the ears and under the nose for signs of irritation. Notify the nurse if the person is short of breath, needs the oxygen removed (for any reason) or if the oxygen system is not working properly. Page 668, Chapter 43.

24. **A** Tell the nurse at once. Glass thermometers may contain mercury, which is a hazardous substance. Follow special procedures for handling hazardous materials. Page 506, Chapter 33.

25. **C** Record and report at once a pulse rate less than 60 or more than 100 beats per minute. The radial pulse is used for routine vital signs. If the pulse is

irregular, count it for 1 minute. Do not use your thumb to take a pulse. Page 529, Chapter 33.

26. **B** Count the respirations for 1 minute if an abnormal breathing pattern is noted. People change their breathing patterns if they are conversing. The healthy adult has 12 to 20 respirations per minute. Listening for breath sounds with a stethoscope is the nurse's responsibility. Page 521, Chapter 33.

27. **A** Report at once any systolic pressure above 120 mm Hg and any diastolic pressure above 80 mm Hg. Record the BP. Page 523, Chapter 33.

28. **C** Rectal temperatures are not taken if a person has diarrhea, is confused, or is agitated. Page 505, Chapter 33.

29. **C** Use tone of voice to convey dignity and self-esteem. Answer any questions that relate to your scope of practice. If you are not able to answer the question, tell the person that you will get the nurse. It is the nurse's responsibility to check for dangerous items. Before leaving the person, make sure that he/she is safe and comfortable. Page 16, Chapter 2.

30. **B** Have the person void before being weighed. A full bladder adds weight. Person should be clothed for privacy and dignity. Weigh the person at the same time of day, usually before breakfast. Balance the scale before weighing the person. Page 564, Chapter 36.

31. **D** Keep the skin free of moisture from urine, stools, or perspiration. Re-position the person at least every 2 hours. Do not massage reddened areas or bony prominences. Range of motion to the lower extremities is important, but this does not address pressure in other areas (e.g., back of head, sacrum, shoulders). Page 636, Chapter 41.

32. **C** Face the person when speaking. Large social gatherings create background noise that can be difficult for people with hearing problems. Chatting about your personal interests is generally not appropriate. Speak in a normal voice tone and do not include excessive details. Speak clearly, distinctly, and slowly. Page 699, Chapter 46.

33. **C** Explain the location of food and beverages. Furniture and equipment should be positioned according to the person's preferences, rather than the staff's convenience. Provide lighting as the person prefers. Do not re-arrange furniture and equipment. Pages 698, Chapter 46.

34. **C** The person with confusion and dementia has the right to privacy and confidentiality. Information about the person's care and condition is shared only with those involved in providing the care. Protect the person from exposure. Page 796, Chapter 53.

35. **C** Use simple, clear language. Explain what you are going to do and why. Call the person by name every time you are in contact with him or her. Terms of endearment (honey, sweetie) can be demeaning for some people. Keep calendars and clocks in the person's room. Page 783, Chapter 53.

36. **D** Wandering in a safe place allows exercise, which can reduce wandering. Do not keep the person in his or her room. Involve the person in activities. Following the person is impractical; all staff members should be alert for the person's whereabouts. Page 787, Chapter 53.

37. **B** Restorative nursing programs promote self-care measures. They help maintain the person's highest level of function; this could be at home or in a nursing care facility. Repair of the disability is not a realistic goal; however the person can regain health, strength, and independence. The focus is on abilities and progress, not restrictions or limitations. Page 680, Chapter 45.

38. **C** Remind the person of his or her progress in the rehabilitation program. Focus on the person's abilities and strengths. Progress may be slow, regardless of motivation or hard work. Denial is a coping mechanism but helping the person to deny the disability is not part of the nursing assistants' role. Page 684, Chapter 45.

39. **C** The final moments of death are kept confidential. So are family reactions. Draping the body, treating personal possessions with respect and allowing the family to have privacy for viewing are part of the dying person's rights. Page 872, Chapter 59.

40. **A** Remember the word *RACE*. Your first action is to Rescue the person in immediate danger. Then sound the Alarm, Confine the fire, and Extinguish the fire. Page 180, Chapter 13.

41. **B** Neglect is defined as failure to provide a person with the goods or services needed to avoid physical harm or mental anguish. Page 39, Chapter 5.

42. **C** Nursing assistants cannot perform assessment or give medications. Some facilities and state practice acts will allow nursing assistants to perform some wound care, if properly trained. Do not perform tasks that are not in your job description. Page 26, Chapter 3.

43. **C** Ask the nurse to observe urine that looks or smells abnormal. Then record your observation. Page 422, Chapter 28.

44. **D** A good attitude is needed at work. People rely on you to give good care. You are expected to be pleasant and respectful. Always be willing to help others. Page 62, Chapter 6.

45. **C** Staff, other departments, and others (visitors, volunteers, etc.) should be alerted to watch out for people who wander. Doors that open to the outside may also have alarms. Taking frequent vital signs is not necessary; locking the person in the room would be a violation of rights and a person with dementia who wanders is unlikely to be able to use the call bell for monitoring purposes. Pages 205, Chapter 15.

46. **C** The supine position is the back-lying position. For good alignment, the bed is flat and the head and shoulders are supported on a pillow. Place arms and hands at the sides. Page 263, Chapter 18.

47. **A** Hand-washing is the most important way to prevent or avoid spreading infection. Page 226, Chapter 16.

48. **B** To gossip means to spread rumors or talk about the private matters of others. Gossiping is unprofessional and hurtful. If others are gossiping, you need to remove yourself from the group. Do not make or repeat any comment that can hurt another person. Pages 62, Chapter 6.

49. **D** Ask a co-worker to help you. The head of the bed is lowered. The person flexes both knees. Assistive devices may be used, but a transfer belt is not the right device for this task. Pages 272, Chapter 19.

50. **A** On a sodium-controlled diet, high-sodium foods such as ham and canned vegetables are omitted. Salt is not added to food at the table. The amount of salt used in cooking is limited. Pages 467, Chapter 30.

51. **B** Elastic stockings should not have wrinkles or creases after being applied. Wrinkles and creases can cause skin breakdown. Apply stockings before the person gets out of bed. Apply the correct size. Purpose is to decrease risk for thrombus and embolus. Page 610, Chapter 39.

52. **C** When a person begins to fall, pull him/her close to your body and ease to the floor. Also protect the person's head. Page 200, Chapter 14.

53. **A** Before bathing, allow the person to use the bathroom, bedpan, or urinal. Page 356, Chapter 24.

54. **A** Insert an electronic thermometer ½ inch into the rectum. Page 508, Chapter 33.

55. **A** Touch is a form of nonverbal communication. It conveys comfort and caring. Touch means different things to different people. Some people do not like to be touched. Ask for permission; this decreases the threat of aggression. Touch can be used with all age groups. Page 77, Chapter 7.

56. **A** A person's information is confidential. The information is shared only among health team members involved in the person's care. Pages 62, Chapter 6.

57. **A** Report to the nurses and record complaints of urgency, burning, dysuria, or other urinary problems. Page 404, Chapter 27.

58. **C** Respect a person's culture and religion. Learn about his or her beliefs and practices. This helps you understand the person and give better care. If you feel the customs are unsafe, should be waived or discussed with the person, you should notify the nurse. Page 72, Chapter 7.

59. **C** Wear gloves when giving perineal care. Gloves are needed whenever contact with blood, body fluids, secretions, excretions, mucous membranes, and non-intact skin is likely. Pages 230, Chapter 16.

60. **D** Report any changes from normal or changes in the person's condition to the nurse at once. Then record your observations. Page 97, Chapter 8.

61. **A** If a person is standing (or walking), have him or her sit before fainting occurs. Page 858, Chapter 58.

62. **A** The person drinks an increased amount of fluid. You would measure the fluids, but this action does not encourage fluids. Withholding food is punitive and violates the rights of the person. Consult the nurse and the care plan before offering fluids, such as beer, coffee or soda. These fluids might be harmful to some people because of medical conditions or medications. Page 482, Chapter 31.

63. **B** Communication fails when you talk too much and fail to listen. Page 80, Chapter 7.

64. **A** During bathing, a person has the right to privacy and the right to personal choice. Page 353, Chapter 24.

65. **C** At 18-months children can usually stand, walk alone, walk up steps and may run. At 12 months, children are walking by holding on to furniture and will attempt several without holding on. Page 136, Chapter 11.

66. **D** Blood pressure is not taken on an arm with an IV infusion. When taking a blood pressure, apply the cuff to the bare upper arm. Ten to 20 minutes of rest prior to the procedure is correct technique. The diaphragm of the stethoscope is placed over the brachial artery. Page 525, Chapter 33.

67. **C** Never put clean or used linens on the floor. The floor is dirty. You cannot use the linens. Page 324, Chapter 22.

68. **B** To prevent aspiration, position the unconscious person on his/her side when you do mouth care. Use a small amount of fluid to clean the mouth. Tell the person what you are doing. Dentures are not worn when the person is unconscious. Page 345, Chapter 23.

69. **B** Encourage people to do their own hair care. Do not cut matted or tangled hair. The person chooses his or her hairstyle. Brushing and combing are done with morning care and whenever needed. Page 377, Chapter 25.

70. **D** Check between the toes for cracks and sores. If left untreated, a serious infection could occur. Fingernails are cut with nail clippers, not scissors. You do not trim or cut toenails if a person has diabetes or poor circulation or if he/she takes anticoagulant medications or has thickened nails, ingrown toenails or nail fungus. Page 386, Chapter 25.

71. **B** If an indwelling catheter becomes disconnected from the drainage system, you tell the nurse at once. Page 426, Chapter 28.

72. **B** Urinary drainage bags are emptied, and the contents measured at the end of each shift. Drainage bags must not touch the floor. The bag is always kept lower than the person's bladder. Drainage bags are discarded, but not at the end of each shift. They are never stored. Cleaning and rinsing leg bags may be done (in the home setting), but the larger drainage bags are usually discarded and replaced. Page 422, Chapter 28.

73. **C** Use elastic tape to secure a condom catheter. Elastic tape expands when the penis changes size. Adhesive tape and rubber bands do not. There is no adhesive cream that is used to secure catheters. Page 432, Chapter 28.

74. **D** For comfort during bowel elimination, leave the person alone if possible. Provide for privacy. Maintaining privacy is a little more difficult to ensure if the person is using the commode. Page 440, Chapter 29.

75. **A** Help the person from the wheelchair to the bed on his or her strong side. In transferring, the strong side moves first. It pulls the weaker side along. Placing the wheelchair at the head or bottom of the bed, increases the transfer distance from wheelchair to bed. Page 295, Chapter 20.

76. **C** The Sim's or side-lying position is the choice for elderly patients if the examiner needs to do a rectal examination. For adults or children, the knee-chest (genupectoral) position, would be the first choice if they are able to assume that position. Page 576 Chapter 37

77. **A** Respiratory and cardiac disorders are among the leading causes of death in the United States. Page 736, Chapter 49

Notes

Notes

Notes

Notes